DuVries'
SURGERY OF THE FOOT

EDITOR
ROGER A. MANN, M.D.

Associate Clinical Professor, Department of
Orthopaedic Surgery, University of California School of Medicine;
Director, Gait Analysis Laboratory, Shriner's Hospital
for Crippled Children, San Francisco;
Chief, Foot Surgery, Children's Hospital of the
East Bay and Samuel Merritt Hospital;
Consultant, Foot Surgery, Oak Knoll Naval Hospital,
Oakland, California

FOURTH EDITION
with **936** illustrations

The C. V. Mosby Company

Saint Louis   1978

FOURTH EDITION

Copyright © 1978 by The C. V. Mosby Company

All rights reserved. No part of this book may be reproduced
in any manner without written permission of the publisher.

Previous editions copyrighted 1959, 1965, 1973

Printed in the United States of America

The C. V. Mosby Company
11830 Westline Industrial Drive, St. Louis, Missouri 63141

Library of Congress Cataloging in Publication Data

DuVries, Henri L
   DuVries' Surgery of the foot.

   Bibliography: p.
   Includes index.
   1. Foot—Surgery.   I. Mann, Roger A., 1936-
II. Title.   III. Title: Surgery of the foot.
[DNLM: 1. Foot—Surgery. WE880 D987s]
RD563.D94   1978   617'.585   78-10829
ISBN 0-8016-2333-2

TS/CB/B 9 8 7 6 5 4 3 2 1

Contributors

Donald E. Baxter, M.D.

Assistant Clinical Professor of Orthopaedic Surgery and Chief, Foot Surgery Clinic, University of Texas at Houston; Assistant Surgeon, Shriner's Hospital for Crippled Children; Consultant in Foot Surgery, Veterans Administration Hospital; Assistant Clinical Professor of Orthopedic Surgery, Baylor College of Medicine, Houston, Texas

Michael W. Chapman, M.D.

Associate Professor of Orthopaedic Surgery, University of California School of Medicine, San Francisco, California

Igor Z. Drobocky, M.D.

Staff Diagnostic Radiologist, Doctors' Hospital, San Leandro, and Laurel Grove Hospital in Castro Valley; Consultant Radiologist, U.S. Navy, Oakland Naval Hospital, Oakland, California

Henri L. DuVries, M.D., D.P.M.

Assistant Clinical Professor of Orthopaedic Surgery (retired), University of California School of Medicine; Clinical Professor of Surgery, California College of Podiatric Medicine, San Francisco; Member, Senior Surgical Staff, Samuel Merritt Hospital, Oakland, California

Earl N. Feiwell, M.D.

Chief Orthopaedic Surgeon, Myelodysplasia Team, Rancho Los Amigos Hospital, Downey; Instructor of Orthopaedic Surgery, University of Southern California School of Medicine, Los Angeles, California

Douglas E. Garland, M.D.

Chief, Problem Fracture Service, Rancho Los Amigos Hospital, Downey, California

James M. Glick, M.D.

Assistant Clinical Professor of Orthopaedic Surgery, University of California School of Medicine; Associate Professor of Physical Education and Team Physician, San Francisco State University; Team Physician, City College of San Francisco, San Francisco, California

M. Mark Hoffer, M.D.

Chief of Children's Orthopaedic Service, Rancho Los Amigos Hospital, Downey, California

John D. Hsu, M.D., C.M.

Assistant Professor, Department of Surgery (Orthopaedics), University of Southern California School of Medicine; Director, M.D.A.A. Clinic, Orthopaedic Hospital, Los Angeles; Attending Orthopaedic Surgeon and Chief, Muscle Disease Clinics, Rancho Los Amigos Hospital, Downey, California

Walter W. Huurman, M.D.

Assistant Professor, Department of Orthopaedic Surgery and Rehabilitation; Assistant Professor, Department of Pediatrics, and Head, Division of Pediatric Orthopaedics, The University of Nebraska Medical Center, Omaha, Nebraska

Verne T. Inman, M.D., Ph.D.

Professor of Orthopaedic Surgery and Director, Biomechanics Laboratory (Emeritus), University of California School of Medicine, San Francisco, California

James O. Johnston, M.D.

Chief of Orthopaedics, Kaiser Hospital, Oakland; Associate Clinical Professor of Orthopaedics, University of California School of Medicine, San Francisco, California

Roger A. Mann, M.D.

Associate Clinical Professor, Department of Orthopaedic Surgery, University of California School of Medicine; Director, Gait Analysis Laboratory, Shriner's Hospital for Crippled Children, San Francisco; Chief, Foot Surgery, Children's Hospital of the East Bay and Samuel Merritt Hospital; Consultant, Foot Surgery, Oak Knoll Naval Hospital, Oakland, California

Stanford F. Pollock, M.D.

Assistant Clinical Professor of Orthopaedic Surgery, University of California School of Medicine; Research Associate, Veterans Administration Hospital, San Francisco; Active Staff, Mills Memorial Hospital, San Mateo, California

Jerral S. Seibert, M.D.

Associate Clinical Professor of Dermatology, University of California School of Medicine, San Francisco; Chief Physician of Dermatology, Samuel Merritt Hospital; Chief, Dermatology Service, Providence Hospital, Oakland, California

F. William Wagner, Jr., M.D.

Associate Clinical Professor, Orthopaedic Surgery, University of Southern California School of Medicine, Los Angeles; Co-Director, Orthopaedic Diabetic Service, Rancho Los Amigos Hospital, Downey, California

Robert L. Waters, M.D.

Chief, Surgical Services, and Chief, Stroke Service, Rancho Los Amigos Hospital, Downey, California

To

my parents

for the opportunities presented to me

To

my wife and family

for their patience and understanding

PREFATORY NOTE TO FOURTH EDITION

I am deeply indebted to my associate, Dr. Roger A. Mann, for his diligent editing and his original contributions to this edition and to the second and third editions. I am also extremely grateful to my many other colleagues who submitted new chapters.

It has been very gratifying to observe the tremendous interest and progress the healing arts have made in recent years in both the care and the knowledge of the diseases and deformities of the human foot—disorders that, although they have comprised a most common human ailment, have been practically ignored in the past. This marked advancement is evidenced within the fields of orthopaedic surgery and podiatry.

Henri L. DuVries, M.D., D.P.M.
Oakland, California

Foreword

In an energy era it has been easy to overlook basic forms and sources of locomotion, yet their contribution is constantly being reasserted. Our foot, to a degree, has somewhat similarly suffered. We require reexamination of anatomical and physiological fundamentals to interpret reactions to new stresses. We have not ever been standing on the same type of terrain over the centuries as we are now, moss to resilient cork, natural to artificial turf; the present gamut brings to mind examples which are likely to proliferate profoundly.

Structural interplay has emerged as the dominant influence in evaluating regional disorders in the body. The role of the foot in increased speed of ambulation, running, now must be assimilated for accurate identification of limb impairment in the huge field of athletic disorders. The greatly increased intrusion of artificial elements, now of established acceptance, to provide artificial joints is a modern miracle we need to grow with.

Such principles have been interpreted, and solutions presented, in this text as an up-to-date aid in treating the increasingly broad field of foot disorders. The book represents a distillation of new clinical syndromes, experience, conservative and practical aids, and appropriate surgical solutions, which combination should facilitate immensely its use by physician, surgeon, and all paramedical personnel.

James E. Bateman, M.D., F.R.C.S.(C)

Surgeon-in-Chief,
Orthopaedic and Arthritic Hospital,
Toronto, Ontario

Preface

It has been twenty years since the first edition of DuVries' *Surgery of the Foot* appeared. At the time of the first writing, Dr. Henri DuVries had thirty years' experience in the treatment of foot problems. I am glad to say that he is still going strong twenty years later. I was greatly honored to be asked to edit the fourth edition of this book, which from its inception has been one of the mainstays of knowledge regarding the function, diagnosis, and treatment of conditions of the foot and ankle.

My interest in the foot began in my second year of medical school, and after listening to the stimulating biomechanics lectures of Verne T. Inman, editor of the third edition, I became interested in the lower extremity, especially the foot. My first year of orthopaedic residency was spent with Verne Inman in the Biomechanics Laboratory at the University of California Medical Center in San Francisco, studying human gait and particularly the intrinsic muscles of the foot.

In my second year of residency, I met Henri DuVries, who as consultant to the Foot Clinic taught me how to evaluate and treat problems of the foot. After my orthopaedic residency I spent a year of fellowship with Dr. DuVries furthering my knowledge about the clinical aspects of the foot. It was during this year of fellowship that I realized that, although Dr. DuVries did not possess the biomechanical background of Dr. Inman nor Dr. Inman the clinical background of Dr.

DuVries, I had been placed in the unique position of bringing together the basic principles advocated by these two brilliant men. Working together with these men in the past fifteen years has given me the basic biomechanical and clinical knowledge I needed to approach and treat patients with foot problems. It is with this background that I approached the task as editor of the fourth edition.

The first edition of *Surgery of the Foot* was the labor of Henri DuVries, who presented to the medical world his vast clinical experience in foot problems. In the second edition he included other contributors to help expand specific sections of the book. The third edition, edited by Dr. Inman, changed the basic format of the book to include the ankle joint and expanded the number of contributors to specific sections.

As editor of the fourth edition, I have obtained contributors who have shown a specific interest in the topic they present. Thus the discussions on children's feet, neuromuscular diseases, the diabetic foot, dermatology, pathology, and radiology have been extensively rewritten. In the sections previously written by Dr. DuVries, I have attempted to reorganize the material to specifically indicate the etiology, pathophysiology, and various methods of treatment. I have also pointed out the surgical techniques that Dr. DuVries and I consider to be the procedures of choice for specific foot problems.

Needless to say, even after four editions, I still feel that further changes will become necessary as medicine continues to progress but the principles presented throughout this book are basic in their approach and will not change significantly over the years.

Roger A. Mann

Contents

PART THREE

Treatment

PART ONE

Basic considerations

1

BIOMECHANICS OF THE FOOT AND ANKLE

Verne T. Inman and Roger A. Mann

The initial chapters of this text on surgery will be concerned not with anatomy, as is customary, but with a discussion of the biomechanics of the foot and ankle. The specific relationships will be emphasized and some methods for functional evaluation of the foot will be presented. These alterations were initiated for several reasons.

First, it has been assumed that the orthopaedic surgeon possesses an accurate knowledge of the anatomic aspects of the foot and ankle. If this knowledge is lacking, textbooks of anatomy are available that depict in detail the precise anatomic structures comprising this part of the human body. It seems redundant to devote space here to what can only be a superficial review of the anatomy of the foot and ankle.

Second, it seems mandatory that any textbook on surgery of the foot should begin with a discussion of the biomechanics of the foot and ankle as an integral part of the locomotor system. The human foot is an intricate mechanism that functions interdependently with other components of the locomotor system. No text is readily available to the surgeon that clearly enunciates the functional interrelationships of the various parts of the foot. Interference with the functioning of a single part may be reflected in altered functions of the remaining parts. Yet the surgeon is constantly

called upon to change the anatomic and structural components of the foot. When so doing, he should be fully aware of the possible consequences of his actions.

Third, wide variations are known to occur in the component parts of the foot and ankle, and these variations are reflected in the degree of contribution of each part to the behavior of the entire foot. Depending on the contributions of an individual component, the loss or functional modification of that component by surgical intervention may result in either minimal or major alterations in the functional behavior of adjacent components. An understanding of basic interrelationships may assist the surgeon in explaining to himself why the same procedure performed on the foot of one person produced a satisfactory result while in another person the result was unsatisfactory.

Fourth, by being alert to the mechanical behavior of the foot, the physician may find that some foot disabilities caused by malfunction of a component part can be successfully treated by nonsurgical procedures rather than attacked surgically as has been customary. Furthermore, some operative procedures that fail to achieve completely the desired result can be further improved by minor alterations in the behavior of adjacent components through shoe modification or the use of inserts. An understanding of the biomechanics of the foot and ankle should, therefore, be an essential aid in surgical decision making and contribute to the success of postoperative treatment.

LOCOMOTOR SYSTEM

The human foot is too often viewed as a semirigid base whose principal function is to provide a stable support for the superincumbent body. In reality the foot is poorly designed for this purpose. Standing for prolonged periods of time can result in a feeling of fatigue or can produce actual discomfort in the feet. One always prefers to sit rather than stand. Furthermore, it is far less tiring to walk, run, jump, or dance on normally functioning feet—either barefooted or in comfortable shoes—than it is to stand. The foot, therefore, appears to have evolved as a dynamic mechanism functioning as an integral part of the locomotor system and should be studied as such rather than as a static structure designed exclusively for support.

Since human locomotion involves all major segments of the body, obviously certain suprapedal movements demand specific functions from the foot and alterations in these movements from above may be reflected below by changes in the behavior of the foot. Likewise, the manner in which the foot functions may be reflected in patterns of movement in the other segments of the body. Therefore the basic functional interrelationships between the foot and the remainder of the locomotor apparatus must be clearly understood.

To begin a review of the locomotor system, one must recognize that ambulating man is both a physical machine and a biologic organism. The former makes him subject to the physical laws of motion, the latter to the laws of muscular action. All characteristics of muscular behavior are exploited in locomotion; for example, when called upon to perform such external work as initiating or accelerating angular motion around joints, muscles rarely contract at lengths below their resting lengths (Bresler and Berry, 1951; Ryker, 1952; Close and Inman, 1953). When motion in the skel-

etal segments is decelerated or when external forces work upon the body, activated muscles become efficient. Activated muscles, in fact, are approximately six times as efficient when resisting elongation as when shortening to perform external work (Abbott et al., 1952; Asmussen, 1953; Banister and Brown, 1968). In addition, noncontractile elements in muscles and specific connective tissue structures assist muscular action. Thus human locomotion is a blending of physical and biologic forces which compromise to achieve maximal efficiency at minimal cost.

Man uses a unique and characteristic orthograde bipedal mode of locomotion. This method of locomotion imposes gross similarities in the manner in which all of us walk. However, each of us exhibits minor individual differences that permit us to recognize a friend or acquaintance even when he is viewed from a distance. The causes of these individual characteristics of locomotion are many. Each of us differs somewhat in the length and distribution of mass of the various segments of the body—segments that must be moved by muscles of varying fiber lengths. Furthermore, individual differences occur in the position of axes of movement of the joints, with concomitant variations in effective lever arms. Such factors as these and many more combine to establish in each of us a final idiosyncratic manner of locomotion.

A smoothly performing locomotor system results from the harmonious integration of many components. This final integration does not require that the specific contribution of a single isolated component be identical in every individual, nor must it even be identical within the same individual. The contribution of a single component varies under different circumstances. Type of shoe, amount of fatigue, weight of load carried, and other such variables can cause diminished functioning of some components with compensatory increased functioning of others. An enormous number of variations in the behavior of individual components is possible; however, the diversely functioning components, when integrated, are found to be complementary and will produce smooth bodily progression.

Average values of single anthropometric observations are, in themselves, of little value. The surgeon should be alert to the anthropometric variations that occur within the population, but it is more important for him to understand the functional interrelationships among the various components. This is particularly true in the case of the foot, where anatomic variations are extensive. If average values are the only bases of comparison, it becomes difficult to explain why some feet function adequately and asymptomatically, although their measurements deviate from the average, while others function symptomatically, even though their measurements approximate the average. It appears reasonable therefore to use average values only to provide a mathematical reference for demonstrating the extent of possible deviations from these averages. Therefore emphasis will be placed upon functional interrelationships and not upon descriptive anatomy.

Human locomotion is a learned process; it does not develop as the result of an inborn reflex. This statement is supported by Popova (1935), who studied the changing gait in growing children. The first few steps of an infant holding onto his mother's hand exemplify the learning process necessary to achieve orthograde progression. Scott (1969) of the Canadian National Institute for the Blind noted that congenitally blind children never attempt to stand and walk spontaneously but must be carefully taught. The result of this learning process is the integration of the neuromusculoskeletal mechanisms, with their gross similarities and individual variations, into an adequately functioning system of locomotion. Once a person has learned to walk and has attained maximal growth, a built-in regulatory mechanism is a part of his physiologic makeup and works whether the person is an amputee learning to use a new prosthesis, a long distance runner, or a woman wearing high heels.

Ralston (1958) has noted that nature's sole aim with all of us seems to be to achieve a system which will take us from one spot to another with the least expenditure of energy.

KINEMATICS OF HUMAN LOCOMOTION

Walking is more than merely placing one foot before the other. During walking all major segments of the body are in motion and displacements of the body occur that can be accurately described.

Vertical displacements of the body

The rhythmic upward and downward displacement of the body during walking is familiar to everyone and is particularly noticeable when someone is out of step in a parade. These displacements in the vertical plane are obviously a necessary concomitant of bipedal locomotion. When the legs are separated, as during the period of transmission of the body weight from one leg to the other (double weight bearing), the distance between the trunk and the floor must be less than when it passes over a relatively extended leg as it does during midstance. Since the nature of bipedal locomotion demands such vertical oscillations of the body, they should occur in a smooth manner for the conservation of energies. Fig. 1-1 shows that the center of gravity of the body does displace in a smooth sinusoidal path; the amplitude of displacement is approximately 4 to 5 cm (Ryker, 1952; Saunders et al., 1953).

Although movements of the pelvis and hip modify the amplitude of the sinusoidal pathway, the knee, ankle, and foot are particularly involved in converting what would be a series of intersecting arcs into a smooth, sinusoidal curve (Saunders et al., 1953). This conversion requires both simultaneous and precise sequential motions in the knee, ankle, and foot.

The center of gravity of the body reaches its maximal elevation immediately after passage over the weight-bearing leg; it then begins to fall. This fall must be stopped at the termination of the swing phase of the other leg as the heel strikes the ground. If one were forced to walk stiff-kneed and without the foot and ankle, the downward deceleration of the center of gravity at this point would be instantaneous. The body would be subject to a severe jar and the locomotor system would

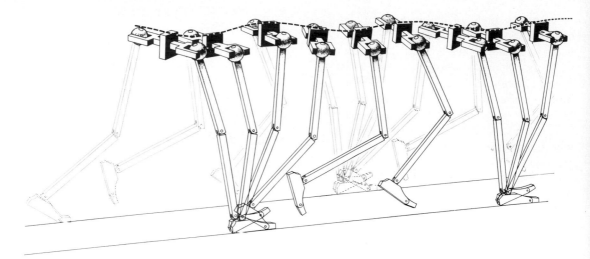

Fig. 1-1. Displacement of the center of gravity of the body in a smooth sinusoidal path. (From Saunders, J. B. C. M., Inman, V. T., and Eberhart, H. D.: J. Bone Joint Surg. **35A**:552, 1953.)

lose kinetic energy. Actually the falling center of gravity of the body is smoothly decelerated, because relative shortening of the leg occurs at the time of impact against a gradually increasing resistance. The knee flexes against a graded contraction of the quadriceps muscle; the ankle plantar flexes against the resisting anterior tibial muscles. After foot-flat position is reached, further shortening is achieved by pronation of the foot to a degree permitted by the ligamentous structures within.

Although the occurrence of this pronatory movement is more important in regard to other functions of the foot, it must be mentioned here since it constitutes an additional factor to that of knee flexion and ankle plantar flexion needed to smoothly decelerate and finally to stop the downward path of the body.

After decelerating to zero, the center of gravity must now evenly accelerate upward to propel it over the opposite leg. The kinetics of this phenomenon are complex, but the kinematics are simple. The leg is relatively elongated by transitory extension of the knee; further plantar flexion of the ankle elevates the heel, and supination of the foot occurs. Elevation of the heel is the major component contributing to upward acceleration of the center of gravity at this time.

Horizontal displacements of the body

In addition to vertical displacements of the body, a series of axial rotatory movements occur which can be measured in a horizontal plane. Rotations of the pelvis and the shoulder girdle are familiar to any observant person. Similar horizontal rotations occur in the femoral and tibial segments of the extremities. The tibias rotate about their long axes—internally during swing phase and into the first part of stance phase and externally during the latter part of stance. This motion continues until the toes leave the ground; the degree of these rotations is subject to marked individual variations. Levens et al. (1948), in a study of a series of twelve male subjects, recorded the minimal amount of horizontal rotation of the tibia in space at 13° and the maximal at 25° with an average of 19°. A great portion of this rotation occurs when the foot is firmly placed on the floor; the shoe normally does not slip but remains fixed. The rotations, however, generate a torque of 7 to 8 newton-meters, which is one of considerable magnitude (Cunningham, 1950).

In order for these movements to occur, a mechanism must exist in the foot which will permit the rotations but will offer resistance to them of a magnitude such that they will be transmitted through the foot to the floor and

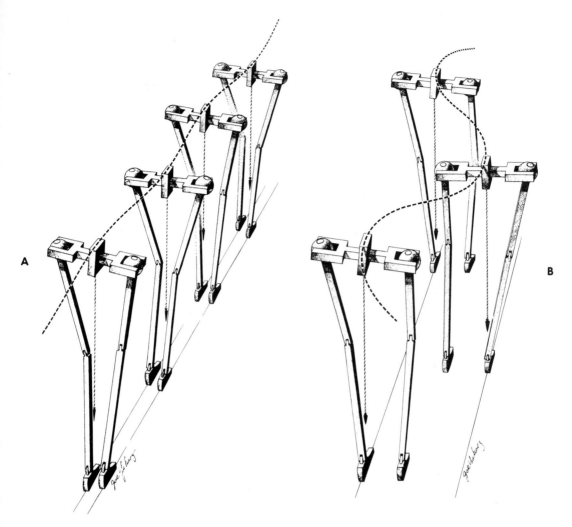

Fig. 1-2. A, Slight lateral displacement of the body occurring during walking with the feet close together. **B,** Increased lateral displacement of the body occurring during walking with the feet wide apart. (From Saunders, J. B. C. M., Inman, V. T., and Eberhart, H. D.: J. Bone Joint Surg. **35A:**552, 1953.)

will be recorded on the force plate as torques. The ankle and subtalar joints are such mechanisms and will be described.

Lateral displacements of the body

When a person is walking, his body does not remain precisely in the plane of progression but oscillates slightly from side to side to keep the center of gravity approximately over the weight-bearing foot. Everyone has experienced this lateral shift of the body with each step but may not have consciously appreciated its cause. Everyone has at some time walked side by side with a companion. If one gets out of step with the other, their bodies are likely to bump.

The body is shifted slightly over the weight-bearing leg with each step; therefore, a total lateral displacement of the body occurs from side to side of approximately 4 to 5 cm with each complete stride. This lateral displacement can be increased by walking with the feet more widely separated and decreased by keeping the feet close to the plane of progression (Fig. 1-2). Normally the presence of the tibiofemoral angle (slight genu valgum) permits the tibia to remain essentially vertical and the feet close together while the femurs diverge to articulate with the pelvis. Again the lateral displacement of the body is through a smooth sinusoidal pathway.

KINETICS OF HUMAN LOCOMOTION

The only forces that can produce motion in the human body are obviously those created by gravity, by muscular activity, and in a few instances by the elasticity of specific connective tissue structures. A force plate is used to record accurately the gravitational effects upon the whole body while walking (Cunningham, 1950). The principle of the force plate can be demonstrated by the bathroom scale. When one stands on the scale quietly and then flexes and extends the knees to raise and lower the body, the indicator on the dial moves abruptly as vertical floor reaction is being registered.

The force plate records instantaneously the forces imposed by the body upon the foot, which are transmitted through the interface between the sole of the shoe and the walking surface. These measurements include vertical floor reactions, fore-and-aft shears, medial-lateral shears, and horizontal torques. During the stance phase of walking, the floor reactions in all four categories are continuously changing. The changes indicate that the foot is being subjected to varying forces imposed upon it by movements of the superincumbent body.

Although floor reactions are important in demonstrating the totality of the forces transmitted through the foot, they give little information concerning the movements in the several articulations of the foot and ankle or about the activity of the muscles controlling these movements. Continuous goniometric recordings and electromyographic studies are required to indicate joint motion and phasic activity of the intrinsic and extrinsic muscles.

From the moment of heel strike to the instant of toe-off, floor reactions, joint motions, and muscular activity are changing constantly. Thus one cannot summarize this information for the entire period of stance and hope to even approximate what in reality is occurring in the foot and ankle. If, however, the stance phase is roughly divided into three intervals, a reasonably accurate summary of all factors can be presented. The division consists of the first interval, extending from heel strike to foot flat; the second interval, occurring at the period of foot flat with the body passing over the foot; and the third interval, extending from the moment of heel rise to toe-off. The second interval is approximately twice as long as either the first or the third interval.

Many of the activities that occur during stance phase have been studied. Levens et al. (1948) recorded the rotation of the tibia during locomotion; Cunningham (1950) recorded shifts in body weight reflected in floor reaction; Ryker (1952) and Wright et al. (1964) recorded ankle rotation; Mann and Inman (1964) reported on the phasic activity of muscles; and Wright et al. (1964) reported studies of the action of the subtalar and ankle joint complex which account for the amount of pronation or supination of the foot.

Walking cycle

The walking cycle consists of the stance phase of one foot, including the double–weight-bearing period, and the swing phase of the same leg. The weight-bearing period, or stance phase, comprises (within a 5% variation) 65% of the entire cycle. If we look at the walking cycle in greater detail, we see that the events during the stance phase include a period of double-limb support (from 0% to 12% of the cycle), a period of single-limb support (from 12% to 50%), and a second period of double-limb support (from 50% to 65% of the cycle), following which the swing phase begins.

First interval. The first interval occurs during approximately the first 15% of the walking cycle. The center of gravity of the body must be decelerated and then immediately accelerated to carry it over the extended leg. The heel's impact and shift of the center of gravity account for a vertical floor reaction that exceeds the body weight by 25% (Fig. 1-3, A). Characteristically the first interval begins with plantar flexion of the ankle and

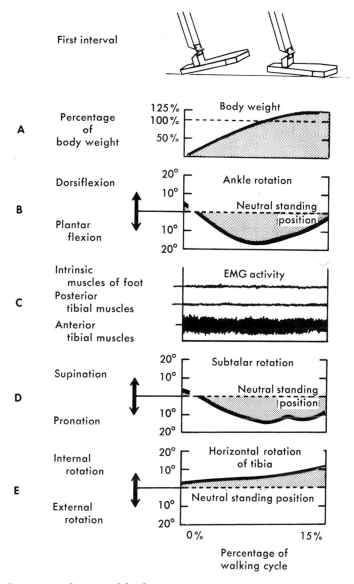

First interval

Percentage
A   of
body weight

125%
100%
50%

Body weight

Dorsiflexion

20°
10°

Ankle rotation

B

Neutral standing
position

Plantar
flexion

10°
20°

Intrinsic
    muscles of foot

EMG activity

Posterior
C   tibial muscles

Anterior
    tibial muscles

Supination

20°
10°

Subtalar rotation

D

Neutral standing
position

Pronation

10°
20°

Internal
    rotation

20°
10°

Horizontal rotation
of tibia

E

External
    rotation

10°
20°

Neutral standing position

0%   15%

Percentage of
walking cycle

Fig. 1-3. Composite of events of the first interval of walking or the period that extends from heel strike to foot flat.

continues toward dorsiflexion (Fig. 1-3, *B*).

During the first interval the anterior tibial and the extensor muscles of the toes are functioning to prevent foot slap (Fig. 1-3, *C*). The triceps surae, the peroneals, and the tibialis posterior are all electrically quiet, as are the intrinsic muscles in the sole of the foot and the long flexors of the toes. These is no muscular response in those muscles that are usually

considered important in supporting the longitudinal arch of the foot.

At this time the foot is being loaded with the weight of the body, and pronation of the foot occurs (Fig. 1-3, *D*). Careful inspection of the feet of individuals during walking will reveal this momentary pronation of the foot as it receives the impact of the body weight. Interestingly, this pronation of the foot is recorded as motion originating in the subtalar joint. The amount of pronation appears to depend entirely upon the joints of the foot—upon their capsular and extra-articular ligaments.

Because of the specific linkage of the leg to the foot through the subtalar articulation, pronation of the foot and internal rotation of the leg, as indicated by the direction of the curve in Fig. 1-3, *E*, must occur simultaneously.

Second interval. The second interval extends throughout 15% to 45% of the walking cycle. The center of gravity of the body passes over the weight-bearing leg at 30% of the walking cycle, after which it commences to fall.

Force-plate recordings show that the foot is now supporting less than the actual body weight. In normal walking the least load on the foot may be only 50% to 60% of the actual body weight (Fig. 1-4, *A*). The second interval is characterized by dorsiflexion, reaching a peak at 40% of the walking cycle, and then plantar flexion begins. Heel rise, however,

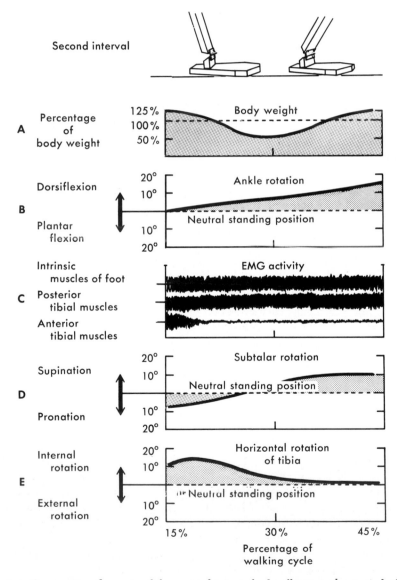

Fig. 1-4. Composite of events of the second interval of walking or the period of foot flat.

precedes the plantar flexion and begins at 35% of the cycle (Fig. 1-4, *B*).

During the second interval important functional changes occur in both the foot and the leg which are the result of muscular action. The triceps surae, the peroneals, the tibialis posterior, the long flexors of the toes, and all the intrinsic muscles in the sole of the foot spring into action (Fig. 1-4, *C*). The activity in the intrinsic muscles of the normal foot begins at 30% of the cycle. In an individual with a flat foot, activity begins at 15% of the cycle. The combined action of these muscles causes the heel to invert; supination of the foot, recorded as motion in the subtalar joint, begins (Fig. 1-4, *D*). Besides the action of these muscles on the foot per se, the posterior calf muscles during this interval also function to control the forward motion of the tibia upon the foot that is fixed to the floor. Restraint of the tibia brings about the knee extension during stance and permits the body to take a longer stride.

Since the forefoot is fixed to the floor, inversion of the heel must be accompanied by external rotation of the leg. The direction of the curve in Fig. 1-4, *E*, indicates the beginning of this rotation. The mechanical linkage provided by the subtalar joint makes this rotation effect inevitable. Fortunately these skeletal movements, produced by muscular effort, occur while the foot is subjected to a load that is less than the total body weight. Furthermore, inversion of the heel with the forefoot fixed is the very process which transforms a flexible midfoot into a rigid structure.

The rearrangements of the skeletal components of the foot necessary in preparation for heel rise and lift-off can be demonstrated by simple manipulation of the normal foot (Fig. 1-5). If they did not occur when they do, abnormal stresses would be placed on the ligamentous structures of the foot which could result in pain and disability.

Third interval. The third interval comprises the last of the stance phase, or the period that extends from 45% to 65% of the walking cycle.

Force-plate recordings show an increase in

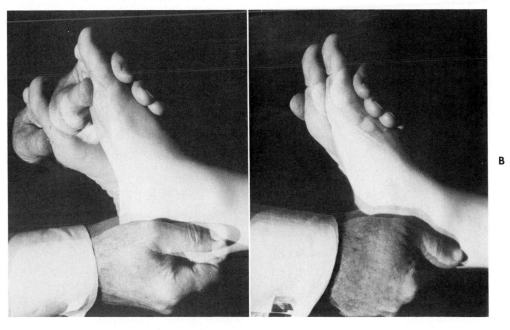

A   B

Fig. 1-5. Rearrangement of skeletal components of the foot. **A**, Supination of the forefoot and eversion of the heel permitting maximal motion in all components of the foot. **B**, Pronation of the forefoot and inversion of the heel resulting in locking of all components of the foot and producing a rigid structure.

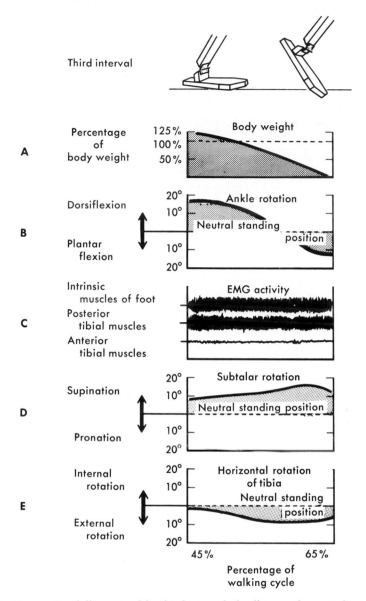

Fig. 1-6. Composite of all events of the third interval of walking or the period extending from foot flat to toe-off.

the percentage of body weight due to the falling of the center of gravity at the beginning of this interval; the load on the foot again exceeds the body weight by approximately 25%. However, the vertical floor reaction promptly falls to zero during this interval, since the body weight is being transferred to the other foot (Fig. 1-6, A). Plantar flexion of the foot occurs during this interval (Fig. 1-6,

B). It is caused primarily by the contraction of the triceps surae and leads to relative elongation of the extremity.

During the third phase the long flexors of the toes assist the triceps surae. The peroneals and the tibialis posterior assist in plantar flexion but also stabilize the leg upon the foot. Additionally, the tibialis posterior functions to aid the intrinsic muscles in the sole of the foot,

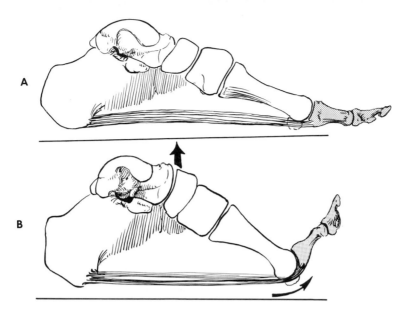

Fig. 1-7. Diagrammatic representation of "windlass action." **A,** Foot flat. **B,** Increased tension of the plantar aponeurosis caused by dorsiflexion of the toes with resultant elevation of the longitudinal arch.

which cannot by themselves invert the heel and raise the longitudinal arch (Fig. 1-6, *C*). The inability of the intrinsic muscles to raise the arch is strikingly apparent in individuals who have lost the function of the tibialis posterior through rupture or paralysis.

During the third interval the foot progressively supinates (Fig. 1-6, *D*) and the leg continues to rotate externally (Fig. 1-6, *E*).

Another mechanism that aids the intrinsic muscles in the inversion of the heel and the raising of the longitudinal arch has been emphasized by Hicks (1954). Since the plantar aponeurosis is attached distally to the base of the proximal phalanges, extension of the metatarsophalangeal joints causes relative shortening of the plantar aponeurosis, which exerts tension upon the calcaneus, thus passively inverting the heel and raising the longitudinal arch. Hicks named this mechanism "windlass action" (Fig. 1-7).

AXES OF ROTATION
Ankle joint

It is easy to visualize that the direction of the ankle axis in the transverse plane of the leg will dictate the vertical plane in which the foot will flex and extend. In the clinical literature this plane of ankle motion in relation to the sagittal plane of the leg is referred to by orthopaedists as the degree of tibial torsion and by podiatrists as malleolar torsion. Whereas it is common knowledge that the ankle axis is directed laterally and posteriorly as projected on the transverse plane of the leg, it is not widely appreciated that the ankle axis is also directed laterally and downward as seen in the coronal plane. Isman and Inman (1969), in anthropometric studies, found that in the coronal plane the functional axis of the ankle may deviate 68° to 88° from the vertical axis of the leg (Fig. 1-8). Since the axis of the ankle passes just distal to the tip of each malleolus, the examiner should be able to obtain a reasonably accurate estimate of the position of the axis by placing the ends of his index fingers at the most distal bony tips of the malleoli (Fig. 1-9).

A horizontal axis that remains normal to the vertical axis of the leg can affect only the amount of toeing out or toeing in of the foot; no rotatory influence can be imposed in a transverse plane on either the foot or the leg during flexion and extension of the ankle.

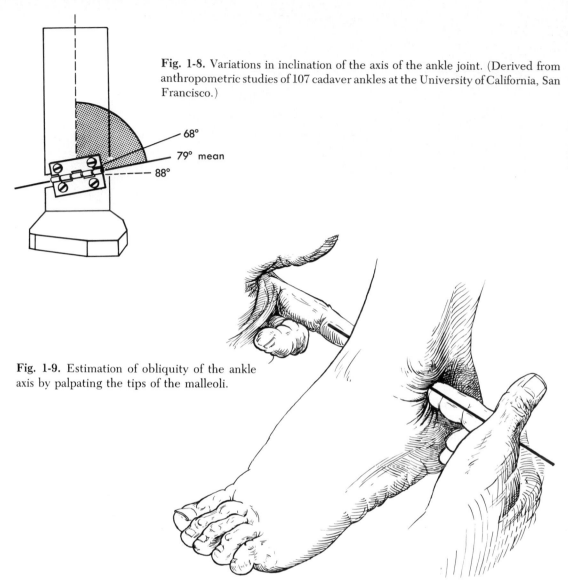

Fig. 1-8. Variations in inclination of the axis of the ankle joint. (Derived from anthropometric studies of 107 cadaver ankles at the University of California, San Francisco.)

68°

79° mean

88°

Fig. 1-9. Estimation of obliquity of the ankle axis by palpating the tips of the malleoli.

However, since the ankle joint axis is an obliquely oriented axis, it allows horizontal rotations to occur in the foot or the leg with movements of the ankle.

These rotations are clearly depicted in Figs. 1-10 and 1-11. With the foot free and the leg fixed, the oblique ankle joint axis causes the foot to deviate outward on dorsiflexion and inward on plantar flexion. The projection of the foot onto the transverse plane, as shown by the shadows in the sketches, reveals the extent of this external and internal rotation of the foot (Fig. 1-10). The amount of this rotation will vary with the obliquity of the ankle axis and the amount of dorsiflexion and plantar flexion.

With the foot fixed on the ground during midstance, the body passing over the foot produces dorsiflexion of the foot relative to the leg (Fig. 1-11). The oblique ankle axis then imposes an internal rotation on the leg (Levens et al., 1948). Again, the degree of internal rotation of the leg on the foot will depend upon the amount of dorsiflexion and the obliquity of the ankle axis. As the heel rises in preparation for lift-off, the ankle is plantar flexed. This in turn reverses the horizontal rotation, causing the leg to rotate externally.

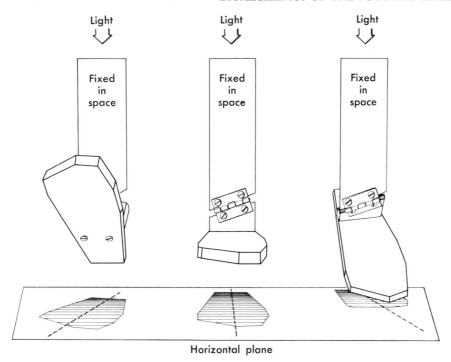

Fig. 1-10. Effect of obliquely placed ankle axis upon rotation of the foot in the horizontal plane during plantar flexion and dorsiflexion, with the foot free. The displacement is reflected in the shadows of the foot.

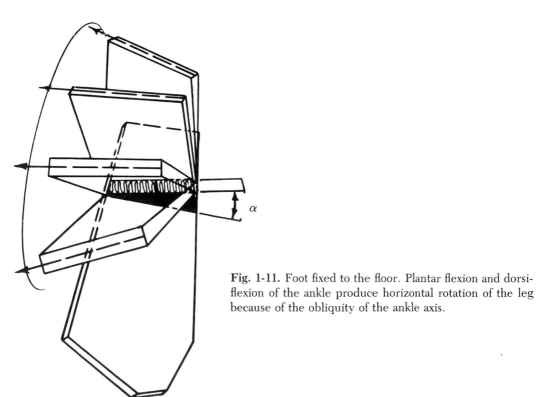

Fig. 1-11. Foot fixed to the floor. Plantar flexion and dorsiflexion of the ankle produce horizontal rotation of the leg because of the obliquity of the ankle axis.

When the horizontal rotations of the leg are studied independently, the foregoing sequence of events can be seen to be precisely what occurs in human locomotion. The lower part of the leg rotates internally during the first third and externally during the last two thirds of stance. The average amount of this rotation is 19°, within a range of from 13° to 25° (Levens et al., 1948). The recording of torques imposed on a force plate substantiates these rotations. Magnitudes vary from individual to individual but range from 7 to 8 newton-meters (Cunningham, 1950).

In summary, the oblique ankle axis produces the following series of events: from the instant of heel contact to the time the foot is flat, plantar flexion occurs and the foot appears to toe in. The more oblique the axis, the more apparent will be the toeing in. During midstance, the foot is fixed on the ground; relative dorsiflexion, with resulting internal rotation of the leg, occurs as the leg passes over the foot. As the heel rises, plantar flexion takes place and causes external rotation of the leg.

Rotations of the leg and movements of the foot caused by an oblique ankle axis, when observed independently, are seen to be qualitatively and temporarily in agreement. However, when the magnitudes of the various displacements are studied, irreconcilable disparities are evident. In normal locomotion ankle motion ranges from 20° to 36°, with an average of 24° (Berry, 1952; Ryker, 1952). The obliquity of the ankle axis ranges from 68° to 88°, with an average of 78° from the vertical (Isman and Inman, 1969). Even in the most oblique axis and movement of the ankle through the maximal range of 36°, only 11° of rotation of the leg around a vertical axis will occur. This is less than the average amount of horizontal rotation of the leg as measured independently in normal walking. The average obliquity of the ankle, together with the average amount of dorsiflexion and plantar flexion, would yield values for the horizontal rotation of the leg that were much smaller than the degree of horizontal rotation of the leg that actually occurs while the foot remains stationary on the floor and is carrying the superincumbent body weight.

Subtalar joint

It is necessary to examine other articulations in the foot which could, in cooperation with the ankle, allow the leg to undergo the additional amount of internal and external rotation. The mechanism that appears to be admirably designed for this very function is the subtalar joint.

The subtalar joint is a single-axis joint which acts like a mitered hinge connecting the talus and the calcaneus. The direction of its axis is backward, downward, and lateral (Manter, 1941; Close and Inman, 1953). Individual variations are extensive and imply variations in the behavior of this joint during locomotion. Furthermore, the subtalar joint appears to be a determinative joint of the foot influencing the performance of the more distal articulations and modifying the forces imposed upon the skeletal and soft tissues. Therefore we must understand the anatomic and functional aspects of this joint.

Based upon the anatomic fact that the subtalar joint moves around a single inclined axis and functions essentially like a hinge connecting the talus and the calcaneus, the functional relationships that result from such a mechanical arrangement are easily illustrated. Fig. 1-12, *A*, shows two boards joined by a hinge. If the axis of the hinge is at 45°, a simple torque converter has been created. Rotation of the vertical member causes equal rotation of the horizontal member. Changing the angle of the hinge will alter this one-to-one relationship. A more horizontally placed hinge will cause a greater rotation of the horizontal member for each degree of rotation of the vertical member; the reverse holds true if the hinge is placed more vertically. In Fig. 1-12, *B*, to prevent the entire horizontal segment from participating in the rotatory displacement, the horizontal member has been divided into a short proximal and a long distal segment with a pivot in between. Thus the distal segment remains stationary while only the short segment adjacent to the hinge rotates.

To approach more closely the true anatomic situation of the human foot, in Fig. 1-13, *A* and *B*, the distal portion of the horizontal member has been replaced by two structures.

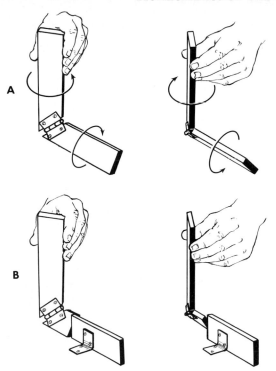

Fig. 1-12. Simple mechanism demonstrating functional relationships. **A,** Action of a mitered hinge. **B,** Addition of a pivot between two segments of the mechanism.

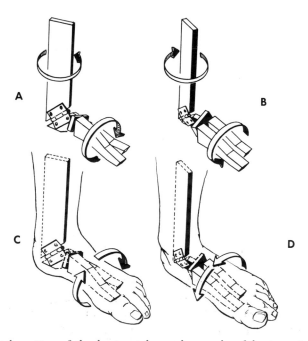

Fig. 1-13. Distal portion of the horizontal member replaced by two structures. **A** and **B,** Mechanical analog of the principal components of the foot. **C** and **D,** Mechanical components inserted into the foot and leg.

The medial represents the three medial rays of the foot that articulate through the cuneiforms to the talus; the lateral represents the two lateral rays which articulate through the cuboid to the calcaneus. In Fig. 1-13, C and D, the entire mechanism has been placed into the leg and foot to demonstrate the mechanical linkages resulting in specific movements in the leg and the foot. External rotation of the leg causes inversion of the heel, elevation of the medial side of the foot, and depression of the lateral side. Internal rotation of the leg produces the opposite effect on the foot.

Interestingly, in persons with flat feet the axis of the subtalar joint is more horizontal than in persons with "normal" feet; therefore the same amount of rotation of the leg imposes a greater supinatory and pronatory effect upon the foot. This may partially explain why some individuals with asymptomatic and flexible pes planus break down their shoes and frequently prefer to go without shoes, which they find restrictive. Furthermore, people with asymptomatic flat feet usually show a greater range of subtalar motion than do persons with "normal" feet. The reverse holds true for people with pes cavus; in them, one is often surprised at the generalized rigidity of the foot and the limited motion in the subtalar joint. According to Wright et al. (1964) the range of motion in the subtalar joint during walking is approximately 6° for a normal foot and 12° for a flat foot.

Transverse tarsal articulation

The calcaneocuboid and the talonavicular articulations together are often considered to make up the transverse tarsal articulation. Each possesses some independent motion and has been subjected to intensive study (Elftman, 1960). However, from a functional standpoint they perform together. In most textbooks of anatomy, movement is described as if the foot did not bear the weight of the body. The following statement is illustrative: Movement in the transverse tarsal articulation "consists of a sort of rotation by means of which the foot may be slightly flexed or extended, the sole being at the same time carried medially (inverted) or laterally (everted)."*

Actually, the importance of the transverse tarsal articulation lies not in its axes of motion while non–weight bearing but in how it behaves during the stance phase of motion when the foot is required to support the body weight. Some specific changes occur in the amount of motion sustained by the transverse tarsal articulation with the forefoot fixed and the heel everted or inverted. Everting the heel produces relative pronation of the foot; varying amounts of flexion and extension in the sagittal plane, adduction and abduction in the transverse plane, and rotation between the forefoot and the heel now occur. The examiner gets the impression that the midfoot has become "unlocked" and that maximal motion is possible in the transverse tarsal articulation. However, if the forefoot is held firmly in one hand, something happens in the transverse tarsal articulation to make it appear "locked." The previously elicited motions all become suppressed and the midfoot becomes rigid (Fig. 1-5).

The mechanisms that might produce this dramatic change from flexibility to rigidity in the midfoot have not been adequately studied. Elftman (1960) has described one such mechanism, but others may exist which are as yet unidentified. In any case, inversion of the heel in the normal foot promptly occurs as weight is transferred from heel to forefoot when a person rises on his toes. As previously mentioned, such inversion of the heel causes the midfoot to convert from a mobile structure to a rigid lever. The reorientation of the skeletal components is obviously the result of activity in the intrinsic and extrinsic muscles of the foot. Obviously also it is the result of activity in the intrinsic and extrinsic muscles of the foot, the ligamentous structures, and the rotation imparted to the foot by the leg.

Metatarsophalangeal break

After wearing a new pair of shoes for a while, one notices the appearance of an oblique crease in the area overlying the meta-

*Goss, C. M., editor: Gray's anatomy, ed. 28, Philadelphia, 1970, Lea & Febiger, p. 368.

tarsophalangeal articulation (Fig. 1-14). Its obliquity is due, of course, to the unequal forward extension of the metatarsals. The head of the second metatarsal is the most distal head; that of the fifth metatarsal is the most proximal. Although the first metatarsal is usually shorter than the second (because the first metatarsal head is slightly elevated and is supported by the two sesamoids), it often

functionally approximates the length of the second.

When the heel is elevated during standing or at the time of lift-off, the weight of the body is normally shared by all the metatarsal heads. To achieve this fair division of the body weight among the metatarsals, the foot must supinate slightly and deviate laterally. The oblique crease in the shoe gives evidence that these

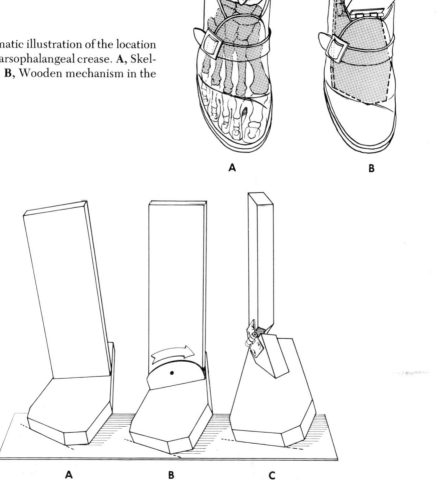

Fig. 1-14. Diagrammatic illustration of the location of the oblique metatarsophalangeal crease. **A,** Skeletal foot in the shoe. **B,** Wooden mechanism in the shoe.

Fig. 1-15. Supination and lateral deviation of the foot during raising of the heel caused by an oblique metatarsophalangeal break. **A,** Wooden mechanism without articulation. If no articulation were present, the leg would also deviate laterally. **B,** Wooden mechanism with articulation. The leg remains vertical; hence some type of articulation must exist between the foot and the leg. **C,** Articulation similar to that of the subtalar joint. Fortunately, in addition to its other complex functions, the subtalar joint also functions to permit the leg to remain vertical.

motions occur with every step. It has been demonstrated that the angle between the metatarsophalangeal break and the long axis of the foot may vary from 50° to 70° (Isman and Inman, 1969). Obviously, the more oblique the metatarsophalangeal break the more the foot must supinate and deviate laterally.

If the leg and foot acted as a single rigid member without ankle, subtalar, or transverse tarsal articulations, the metatarsophalangeal break would cause lateral inclination and external rotation of the leg (Fig. 1-15, A). However, to permit the leg to remain in a vertical plane during walking, an articulation must be provided between leg and foot (Fig. 1-15, B). Such an articulation is supplied by the subtalar joint (Fig. 1-15, C). Because of its anatomic arrangement, it is ideally suited to permit the foot to respond to the supinatory forces exerted by the oblique metatarsophalangeal break and still allow the leg to remain in a vertical plane.

All the essential mechanisms discussed in this chapter are pictorially summarized in Fig. 1-16. The two lower photographs were taken with the subject standing on a barograph; they reveal the distribution of pressure between the foot and the weight-bearing surface. (A barograph records reflected light through a transparent plastic platform; the intensity of the light is roughly proportionate to the pressure the foot imposes on the plate.)

In Fig. 1-16, A, the subject was asked to stand with muscles relaxed. Note that the leg is moderately rotated internally and the heel is slightly everted (in valgus position). The body weight is placed upon the heel, the outer side of the foot, and the metatarsal heads.

In Fig. 1-16, B, the subject was asked to rise on his toes. Note that the leg is now externally rotated, the heel is inverted (in varus position), and the longitudinal arch is elevated. The weight is concentrated upon the metatar-

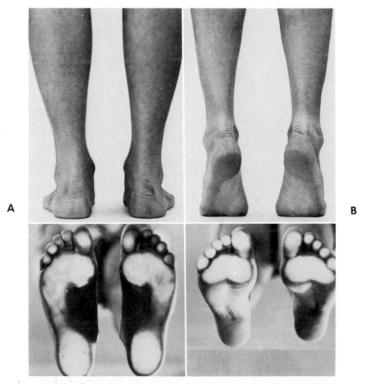

Fig. 1-16. Feet and legs of a person standing on a barograph. **A,** Weight bearing with muscles relaxed. **B,** Rising on the toes.

sal heads and is equally shared by the metatarsal heads and the toes.

Even though such movements cannot be illustrated pictorially, it is easy to imagine the contraction of the intrinsic and extrinsic muscles that is necessary to stabilize the foot and ankle as the subject transfers the body weight to the forefoot and raises the heel. It should also be recalled that dorsiflexion of the toes tightens the plantar aponeurosis and assists in the inversion of the heel. The supinatory twist activates the "locking" mechanism in the foot, thus converting a flexible foot (Fig. 1-16, *A*) into a rigid lever (Fig. 1-16, *B*), an action that is necessary at lift-off.

REFERENCES

Abbott, B. C., Bigland, B., and Ritchie, J. M.: The physiological cost of negative work, J. Physiol. (Lond.) **117**:380, 1952.

Asmussen, E.: Positive and negative muscular work, Acta Physiol. Scand. **28**:364, 1953.

Banister, E. W., and Brown, S. R.: The relative energy requirements of physical activity. In Falls, H. B., editor: Exercise physiology, New York, 1968, Academic Press, Inc.

Berry, F. R., Jr.: Angle variation patterns of normal hip, knee and ankle in different operations, Univ. Calif. Prosthet. Devices Res. Rep., Ser. 11, issue 21, February 1952.

Bresler, B., and Berry, F. R.: Energy and power in the leg during normal level walking, Univ. Calif. Prosthet. Devices Res. Rep., Ser. 11, issue 15, May 1951.

Close, J. R., and Inman, V. T.: The action of the ankle joint, Univ. Calif. Prosthet. Devices Res. Rep., Ser. 11, issue 22, April 1952.

Close, J. R., and Inman, V. T.: The action of the subtalar joint, Univ. Calif. Prosthet. Devices Res. Rep. Ser. 11, issue 24, May 1953.

Cunningham, D. M.: Components of floor reactions during walking, Univ. Calif. Prosthet. Devices Res. Rep. Ser. 11, issue 14, November 1950.

Elftman, H.: The transverse tarsal joint and its control, Clin. Orthop. **16**:41, 1960.

Hicks, J. H.: The mechanics of the foot. II. The plantar aponeurosis and the arch. J. Anat. **88**:25, 1954.

Isman, R. E., and Inman, V. T.: Anthropometric studies of the human foot and ankle, Bull. Prosthet. Res. **10-11**:97, 1969.

Levens, A. S., Inman, V. T., and Blosser, J. A.: Transverse rotation of the segments of the lower extremity in locomotion, J. Bone Joint Surg. **30A**:859, 1948.

Mann, R., and Inman, V. T.: Phasic activity of intrinsic muscles of the foot, J. Bone Joint Surg. **46A**:469, 1964.

Manter, J. T.: Movements of the subtalar and transverse tarsal joints, Anat. Rec. **80**:397, 1941.

Popova, T.: Quoted in Issledovaniia po biodinamike lokomotsii. Chapter 3, Vol. 1. Biodinamika khod'by normal'nogo vzroslogo muzhchiny (edited by N. A. Bernstein), Moscow, 1935, Idat. Vsesoiuz. Instit. Eksper. Med.

Ralston, H. J.: Energy-speed relation and optimal speed during level walking, Int. Z. Angew. Physiol. **17**:277, 1958.

Ryker, N. J., Jr.: Glass walkway studies of normal subjects during normal walking, Univ. Calif. Prosthet. Device. Res. Rep. Ser. 11, issue 20, January 1952.

Saunders, J. B. C. M., Inman, V. T., and Eberhart, H. D.: The major determinants in normal and pathological gait, J. Bone Joint Surg. **35A**:543, 1953.

Scott, E.: Personal communication.

Wright, D. G., Desai, M. E., and Henderson, B. S.: Action of the subtalar and ankle-joint complex during the stance phase of walking, J. Bone Joint Surg. **46A**:361, 1964.

2

PRINCIPLES OF EXAMINATION OF THE FOOT AND ANKLE

Verne T. Inman and Roger A. Mann

Fortunately the foot, ankle, and leg are parts of the body that are readily accessible to adequate physical examination. Usually a specific diagnosis can be reached by obtaining a careful history, by conducting a proper physical examination, and by using the indicated ancillary laboratory procedures. The techniques of examination available to the practitioner in his attempt to gather information concerning the foot and to make proper diagnoses vary with the age of the patient. In examining the preambulatory infant the practitioner must rely upon inspection, palpation, and manipulation. In examining the toddler, inspection, palpation, and manipulation may be supplemented with observations on the emerging patterns of locomotion. However, one should be aware that this period is a time of experimentation for the child, whose behavioral patterns are constantly changing. Since they may be based upon transitory findings, definitive surgical procedures at this stage of a child's development should be undertaken with caution. Only in the older child and in the adult can all the anatomic features and the functional behavior of the various components be realistically evaluated.

NEONATE AND PREAMBULATORY INFANT—CONGENITAL ABNORMALITIES

Gross abnormalities of the lower limbs of children are easily recognized at birth or shortly thereafter. These congenital abnormalities present themselves in many different forms. During the past decade several attempts have been made to name and classify congenital limb defects based upon the site and extent of the skeletal abnormality. Universal acceptance and use of such a system of classification with its standardized nomenclature would do much to improve communication and expedite the development of therapeutic principles. Currently the various types of limb deficiencies are reasonably well classified under the general heading of dysmelia, with the subdivisions of ectromelia, phocomelia, and amelia. Other abnormalities of the lower limb are still classified under specific descriptive names.

In a book of this nature, it is impossible to be encyclopedic. Therefore we are providing the reader with an extensive bibliography at the end of the present chapter as a vehicle for obtaining information of a more detailed nature than is here offered or for acquiring knowledge about deformities that occur infrequently. The following list attempts to be all-inclusive but should serve only as a reminder to the examiner. If more extensive discussions are available in chapters that follow, the chapter containing such discussion is indicated; if the subject is covered minimally or not at all, the reader is referred to the bibliography.

Dysmelia. Under this heading are found all limb deficiencies, including congenital absence of skeletal parts and aplasia. See Bibliography and Chapter 4.

Dimelia. For supernumerary bones and skeletal elements see Chapter 4.

Anterior or posterior bowing of tibia. See Bibliography.

Length of leg discrepancies. See Bibliography.

Hemihypertrophy and local gigantism. See Bibliography and Chapter 4.

Calcaneovalgus foot. See Bibliography and Chapter 4.

Clubfoot. See Chapter 4.

Congenital metatarsus varus. See Chapter 5.

Congenital hammertoes. See Chapter 4.

Flatfoot. See Chapters 4 and 8.

The appearance of low arches in neonates and infants is primarily caused by the presence of fat deposits in the soles of the feet. However, it is mandatory during an examination to manipulate the feet gently in order to check the motion of the major articulations. There are two general categories of flatfoot—mobile and spastic—and the examiner should discern which type of flatfoot he is observing.

Mobile flatfoot. Mobile flatfoot is a condition in which there is a wide range of motion in the hindfoot and midfoot. The important factor to determine is whether there is a short tendo Achillis that may impose abnormal forces on the foot when the child begins to walk.

Rigid flatfoot. In the presence of rigid flatfoot, passive inversion of the heel and pronation of the forefoot will not produce elevation of the longitudinal arch, which is the case in the normal foot. Rigid flatfoot occurs in two conditions that should be recognized early: tarsal coalition and congenital vertical talus (Chapter 4).

THE TODDLER

As the child begins to walk, it becomes possible to examine the behavior of all segments of the lower extremity and to observe the effects of weight bearing upon them.

The degree of toeing in or toeing out should be observed. The position of the foot during stance is determined by (1) the degree of anteversion or retroversion of the neck of the femur (see Bibliography), (2) tibial or malleolar torsion (see Bibliography), (3) the mobility of the major joints, and (4) the musculature.

The degree of anteversion or retroversion of the neck of the femur should be checked. This position can be clinically determined by noting the amount of passive internal and external rotation that is possible in the extended leg. Also, as the child walks, the position and degree of horizontal motion of the patellas should be observed. To facilitate observation of the patella as the child walks, it is helpful to place a dot on the middle of each patella. As the child walks toward the examiner, the rotation of these dots to the plane of progression and to one another can be readily observed.

Tibial or malleolar torsion is still a controversial subject among clinicians; the measurements reported by many investigators vary widely. However, it is clear that when the child sits on the edge of the examining table with the knees flexed and the patellas and feet facing forward the plane of the long axes of the feet should not deviate markedly from the sagittal plane.

The degree of pronation of the foot while the child walks or stands barefoot is readily observed by the examiner. By encouraging the child to rise on tippy-toes or to walk on tiptoe and then on heels, the examiner is quickly able to determine the mobility of the major joints and the adequacy of the musculature.

A rough check of the musculature can often

be made by tickling the feet and observing the various displacements of the feet and toes. Possible shortening of the tendo achillis should be investigated.

OLDER CHILD AND ADULT

To prevent overlooking pertinent findings, every examiner should follow a rigorous routine. The particular routine adopted will vary depending upon personal preference and arrangement of office facilities. However, it appears appropriate to emphasize that no matter what procedure he adopts, the examiner must consider the foot and ankle from three different points of view.

First, the foot and ankle should be seen as parts of the entire body. Since their examination may reveal the presence of systemic disease, evidence of circulatory, metabolic, and cutaneous abnormalities should be sought.

Second, the foot and ankle should be considered as important constituents of the locomotor system. They play reciprocal roles with the suprapedal segments, and abnormal function of any part of the locomotor apparatus is reflected in adaptive changes in the remaining parts. Therefore it is essential for the examiner to observe the patient walking over an appreciable distance in order to do the following:

1. Detect obvious abnormalities of locomotion (For example, unequal step length or limp must be investigated.)
2. Perceive asymmetric behavior of the two sides of the body (For example, asymmetric arm swing denotes unequal horizontal rotation of the components of the torso.)
3. Observe the position of the patellas, which are indicators of the degree of horizontal rotation of the leg in the horizontal plane
4. Observe the degree of toeing in or out (Toeing in or out that is relatively constant during the walk cycle indicates the degree of malleolar torsion; toeing in or out occurring only during the interval between heel strike and foot flat indi-

cates the degree of obliquity of the ankle axis.)
5. Observe the amount of pronation of the foot during the first half of stance-phase walking
6. Note the amount of heel inversion and supination of the foot during lift-off, together with presence or absence of rotatory slippage of the forefoot on the floor (These motions indicate the amount of movement in the subtalar joint at that moment.)
7. Observe the position of the foot in relation to the floor at the time of heel strike (Normally the heel strikes the ground first, after which rapid plantar flexion occurs. If this sequence does not occur, further investigation is indicated. The time of heel rise should also be carefully noted, occuring normally at 34% of the walking cycle just after the swinging leg has passed the stance foot. Early heel rise may be indicative of tightness of the gastrocsoleus muscle complex. A delay in heeel rise can indicate weakness in the same muscle group.)

It must be stressed that one sees only what one is looking for. If the implications of the preceding statements are not readily apparent, it is suggested that the reader review Chapter 1 at this time.

Third, the human foot and ankle should be viewed as relatively recent evolutionary acquisitions; thus they are subject to considerable individual anatomic and functional variation. It is regretable that in most of the anatomic and orthopaedic literature, only average values for the positions of axes of the major articulations and for ranges of motion about these axes are given (see Chapter 1). It so happens that an average individual is difficult to find, particularly among patients seeking help in the practitioner's office. The examiner should be aware of these variations and should also be cognizant of their functional implications. Only with such knowledge and insight will he be able to determine the proper therapeutic procedure to use and to evaluate realistically his success or failure with that procedure.

Sequence of examination

When examining the foot and ankle, the examiner should follow as closely as possible the procedural sequence taught in courses in introductory physical diagnosis. After taking an adequate history, the examiner first *inspects*, then *palpates*, and finally (in an orthopaedic examination) *manipulates*. This sequence must be modified and repeated several times as the patient performs tasks with and without shoes, while walking, standing, and sitting on the edge of the examining table.

The following outline for the examination of the foot and ankle has proved adequate in our experience; to increase its value, annotations have been inserted to elucidate the significance of some findings and to explain the use of special diagnostic procedures. Even if one does not wish to adopt the routine as presented here, it may prove useful as a checklist.

The patient generally presents himself dressed in customary street clothes. It is usually convenient at that time for the examiner to observe the patient walking at various speeds, with shoes on, hands empty, and arms hanging freely at the sides. The following observations should be made:

Type of limp, if present. A pathologic condition of the lower extremity may produce a limp that is characteristic of the particular disorder. A patient with a painful hip, for example, will throw himself over the painful side during walking.

Symmetry of arm swing. As a rule, the shoulders rotate 180° out of phase with the pelvis; this is a passive response to pelvic rotation. If there are no abnormalities in the spine or upper extremities, rotation of the shoulders is reflected in equal and symmetric arm swing. If the arm swing is asymmetric, horizontal rotation of the pelvis is also asymmetric. Since such asymmetric pelvic rotation may be the result of abnormality in any of the components of the lower extremity, it is mandatory that the practitioner take extra care in examining not only the foot and ankle, but the knees and hips as well.

Degree of toe-in or toe-out. At toe-off the leg has achieved its maximal external rotation and the foot toes out slightly. During swing phase the entire leg and foot rotate internally The average amount of rotation is about 15° but varies greatly among individuals. It may be almost imperceptible (3°) or considerable (30°) (Levens et al., 1948). At the time of heel strike the long axis of the foot has approached, to a varying degree, the plane of progression. The degree of parallelism between the long axis of the foot and the plane of progression at this point is subject to considerable individual variation. However, the transition from heel strike to foot flat, which occurs rapidly, should be carefully observed. Some individuals will show an increase in toe-in during the very short period of plantar flexion of the ankle, indicating a greater degree of obliquity of the ankle axis (see Chapter 1).

Amount of pronation of foot during early stance phase. Normally the foot will pronate as it is loaded with the body weight during the first half of stance phase. The amount of pronation is subject to extreme individual variation. The important factor, however, is whether the foot remains pronated during the period of heel rise and lift-off. In the normally functioning foot, as the heel rises, an almost instantaneous inversion of the heel occurs. If the heel fails to invert at this time, the examiner should check the strength of the intrinsic and extrinsic muscles of the foot, as well as the ranges of motion in the articulations of the hindfoot and midfoot.

Nature of heel strike and heel rise. The foot should contact the ground heel first, after which it rapidly plantar flexes so it is flat on the ground by 7% of the walking cycle. In pathologic conditions the patient may contact the ground with the foot flat or possibly on his toes. The time when the heel begins to rise off the ground is at approximately 35% of the walking cycle, i.e., when the swinging leg is passing by the stance leg. If heel rise occurs too early in the walking cycle, tightness in the gastrocsoleus musculature is most likely the cause. If the heel-rise time is delayed significantly, this can be due to weakness of the calf musculature.

Rotatory slippage of shoe on floor at lift-off. Except on slippery surfaces, the shoe does not visibly rotate externally or slip on the floor at the time of lift-off. Failure of the ankle and subtalar joints to permit adequate external rotation of the leg during this phase of walking may result in direct transmission of the rotatory forces to the interface between the sole of the shoe and the walking surface, with resultant rotatory slippage of the shoe on the floor. Upon noting slippage, the examiner should look for possible muscular imbalance and should check the obliquity of the ankle axis and the range of motion in the subtalar joint.

Type of shoe and height of heel. Since the type of shoe worn and its heel height affect the way a person walks, they must be noted. When wearing high heels, for example, women show less ankle-joint motion than when wearing flat heels, and in tennis shoes, show little difference from men in gait.

While the patient is disrobing, it is convenient for the examiner to inspect the shoes and note the following:

1. The path of wear from heel to toe
2. Presence of supportive devices or corrections in the shoes (Arch supports, Thomas heels, sole wedges, or metal tabs indicate previous difficulties.)
3. Obliquity of the angle of the crease in the toe of the shoe (The angle varies from person to person; the greater the obliquity of the crease in the shoe to its long axis, the greater the amount of subtalar motion that is required to distribute the body weight evenly over the metatarsal heads.)
4. The impression the forefoot has made on the insole of the shoe, which often gives important information about the patient's symptoms
5. Presence or absence of circular wear on the sole of the shoe (Such wear indicates rotatory slippage of the foot on the floor during lift-off from suppressed subtalar motion.)
6. The location of the wear pattern on the bottom of the shoe to ascertain whether it is too big or too small (The shape of the shoe, i. e., narrow pointed shoe or broad toe box, as well as the overall shape of the foot when the patient is weight bearing should be carefully observed.)

The patient, now barefoot, is requested to walk. The same sequence of observation is repeated. Any gross abnormalities that were obscured by stockings and shoes can now be seen.

For the convenience of the examiner who is seated, the patient is next requested to stand upon a raised platform or lift, distributing his weight equally on the two feet. The examiner makes a preliminary evaluation of the patient's posture and a cursory inspection of the lower extremities from both front and back, taking note of the following.

Presence of pelvic tilt. To estimate pelvic tilt from the front, the examiner places his index fingers on either the anterior superior iliac spines or the iliac crests; from the back, he observes the gluteal creases. An anatomic or functional shortening of one leg can readily be seen if the shortening is greater than one-quarter inch. Inspection of the popliteal creases will reveal whether major shortening is in the thigh or in the leg.

Gross abnormalities of components of lower extremity. These abnormalities include differences in circumferences of the thigh and calves, excessive deviations in skeletal alignment, and the degree of pes planus or pes cavus.

There appear to be at least two general categories of pes planus. In one category the longitudinal arch is depressed, without the complicating factors of everted heel, abducted forefoot, or longitudinal rotation of the metatarsals and phalanges (Fig. 2-1). This type of flatfoot is seen typically in individuals with a plantar-flexed talus (Fig. 2-2). In the other category the foot appears to have fallen inward like the tilting of a half-hemisphere; the heel is everted, the outer border of the foot shows angulation at the midfoot, and the forefoot is abducted. There may also be varying degrees of rotation of the metatarsals and phalanges around their long axes (Fig. 2-3). In the first category the tendo Achillis remains relatively straight; in the second the tendo

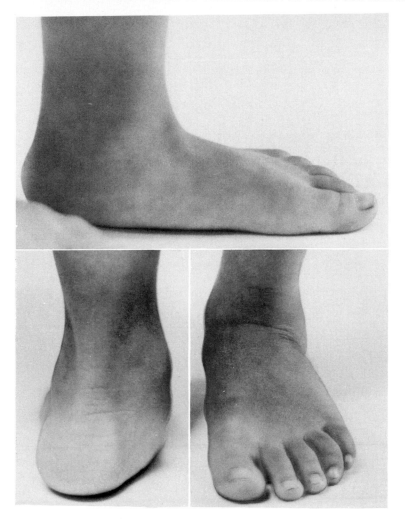

Fig. 2-1. One type of pes planus. Note the depression of the longitudinal arch, without everted heel, abducted forefoot, or longitudinal rotation of the metatarsals and phalanges.

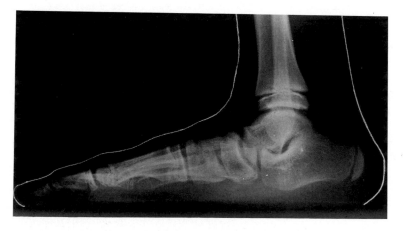

Fig. 2-2. Weight-bearing radiograph of the foot of a black youth. Note the flatfoot and the plantar-flexed talus.

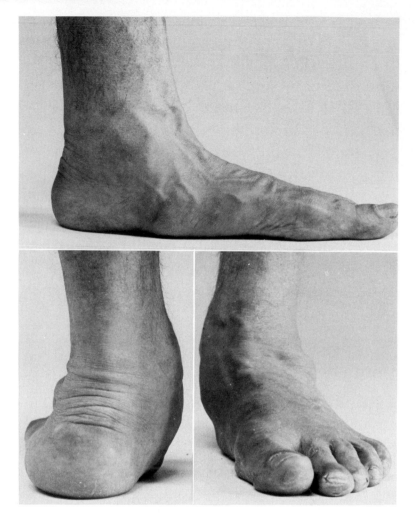

Fig. 2-3. Another type of pes planus. The foot appears to have fallen inward like a half-hemisphere.

Achillis deviates laterally when the patient bears weight upon the relaxed foot. The pathologic implications of these two types of flatfoot are different.

Movements occurring when patient rises on toes. When the patient is asked to rise onto his toes, if the foot is functioning normally, the heel will promptly invert, the longitudinal arch will rise, and the leg will rotate externally. Failure of these movements to occur may indicate a weak foot or a specific pathologic process.

Since inversion of the heel is achieved through proper performance of the subtalar and transverse tarsal articulations, failure to invert the heel should immediately focus the examiner's attention upon possible malfunction of these structures. Conditions that may limit activity in these joints are muscular weakness, rupture or weakness of the tibialis posterior, arthritic changes in the subtalar joint, and such skeletal abnormalities as vertical talus and tarsal coalition.

Windlass action. Normally dorsiflexion of the toes increases the tension of the plantar aponeurosis, which causes the longitudinal arch to rise (Fig. 2-4, A and B). Failure of the longitudinal arch to rise suggests the presence

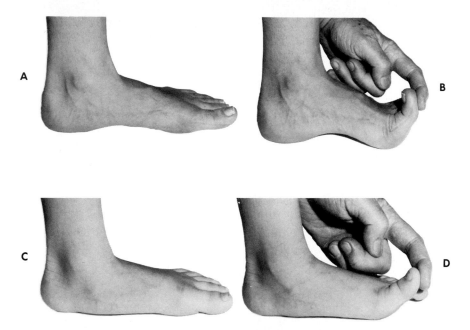

Fig. 2-4. A, "Normal" weight-bearing foot. **B,** Dorsiflexion of the great toe causes elevation of the arch because of the windlass action of the aponeurosis. **C,** Flat weight-bearing foot. **D,** Dorsiflexion of the great toe does not cause the arch to rise.

of prolonged pes planus with attendent abnormal stretching and elongation of the plantar aponeurosis (Fig. 2-4, *C* and *D*).

Stability of subtalar joint. The weight-bearing line of the body normally falls medial to the axis of the subtalar joint; therefore, when the patient stands on one foot with muscles relaxed, the foot pronates. Because of the linkage between the foot and the leg provided by the subtalar articulation, when the examiner rotates the leg externally the heel will invert and the weight-bearing line will move laterally. This position creates a metastable state, which in the normal foot extends over a moderate range of longitudinal rotation of the leg (10° to 15°). When the examiner exerts minimal external rotatory force upon the leg with his hand, the patient's full body weight can be transmitted through the hindfoot to the floor. However, in some patients this metastable state cannot be achieved even if the examiner applies maximal external rotatory force to the leg. In others the metastable state is so tenuous that if the examiner exerts a few degrees of internal

or external rotatory force upon the leg the foot will promptly pronate or supinate.

The patient is next instructed to sit on the examining table with legs and feet hanging over the side. A more detailed examination is now possible.

Surface of foot, ankle, and leg. Any vascular abnormalities such as varicosities, areas of telangiectasia, and edema should be noted. The dorsalis pedis and posterior tibial pulses should be palpated. The speed of capillary filling after compression of the nail bed should be checked. The skin over joints is normally cooler than the skin over muscular areas of the extremity; inflammatory processes in or around deep structures cause increased temperature of the overlying skin. The examiner, by gently passing his hand over the extremity, can frequently localize "hot spots" that, when located, should alert him to investigate the underlying components. The distribution of hair on the foot should be carefully noted. The skin on the plantar aspect of the foot and about the toes is carefully inspected for callus formation, which often indicates abnormal pressure upon the foot.

Skeletal structures (general appraisal).
Gross skeletal deformities are readily discernible and can hardly be overlooked even by the most inexperienced examiner. Difficulties in making a diagnosis are more likely to arise in patients whose feet, on casual inspection, appear to be relatively normal.

Ranges of motion

After a sequential examination has been described in some detail, it is appropriate to discuss techniques of eliciting other pertinent information.

The passive ranges of motion of all the major articulations of the foot should be rapidly checked for limitation of motion, painful movement, and crepitus. These symptoms may occur separately or in any combination.

The ankle joint should be moved through its full range of motion. Although the ankle is essentially a single-axis joint, its axis is skewed to both the transverse and the coronal planes of the body passing downward and backward from the medial to the lateral side. A reasonably accurate estimate of the location of the ankle axis can be obtained by placing the tips of the index fingers just below the most distal projections of the two malleoli (Fig. 2-5). Depending upon the degree of obliquity of the axis, dorsiflexion and plantar flexion produce medial and lateral deviation of the foot. If the examiner has noted previously that the patient tended to toe in during the interval between heel strike and foot flat, an oblique axis of the ankle as projected on the coronal plane of the body is to be expected. Since an oblique axis of the ankle will assist in absorbing the horizontal rotation of the leg, its range of motion is related to the range of motion in the subtalar joint. Thus range of subtalar motion should also be estimated.

The amount of motion in the subtalar joint varies; however, Isman and Inman (1969) found that in a series of feet in cadaver specimens a minimum of 20° and a maximum of 60° of motion were present. The simplest method of determining the degree of subtalar motion

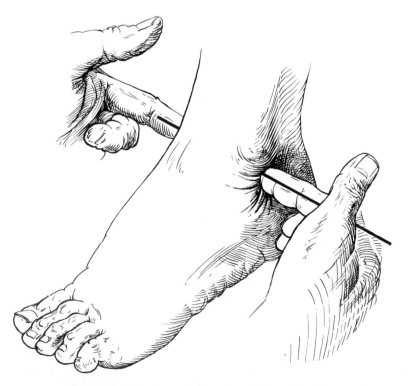

Fig. 2-5. Estimating the location of the ankle axis.

is to apply rotatory force on the calcaneus while permitting the rest of the foot to move passively. When rotatory force is applied to the forefoot, abnormally large displacements may be obtained through movements of the articulations in the midfoot that are additive to subtalar motion. By far the most accurate method of determining the degree of subtalar motion is to place the patient prone and flex his knee to approximately 135°. The axis of the subtalar joint now lies close to the horizontal plane. The examiner then passively inverts and everts the heel while measuring the extent of motion by attaching a gravity goniometer or level to the calcaneus with a metal spring clip (Fig. 2-6). Lack of subtalar motion should alert the examiner to the possibility of an arthritic process in the subtalar joint, of peroneal spastic flatfoot, or of an anatomic abnormality such as tarsal coalition.

Normally there is no lateral play of the talus in the mortise even when the foot is in full plantar flexion. Any lateral displacement that can be imposed on the talus in its mortise by the examiner is indicative of abnormal widening of the mortise. Frequently the talus can be displaced forward and backward a millimeter or so in the mortise, but this is a normal finding.

Occasionally a degree of lateral talar tilt can be demonstrated in the normal ankle joint in the following manner: The examiner places the ankle in full plantar flexion, thus displacing the trochlea anteriorly. He forcibly inverts the foot while placing his thumb just in front of the lateral malleolus and pressing against the anterior portion of the trochlea. He can then feel a slight medial rocking of the talus. Excessive talar tilt should alert the examiner to suspect injury to the lateral ligaments. The range of motion of the transverse tarsal, metatarsophalangeal, and interphalangeal joints should be observed for pain, joint stiffness, and deformities.

Ligamentous and muscular structures

The attachments of the collateral ligaments of the ankle should be palpated for tenderness. The deltoid, anterior talofibular, and calcaneofibular ligaments are readily palpable. The posterior talofibular ligament is too deeply situated to be felt.

Injuries to the distal fibular syndesmosis are too frequently overlooked by orthopaedists, even though patients with such injuries may suffer pain when walking, jumping, and running. The construction of this articulation is such that the fibula is nestled into a groove on the lateral side of the tibia (Fig. 2-7). The anterior lip of the tibial groove is prominent

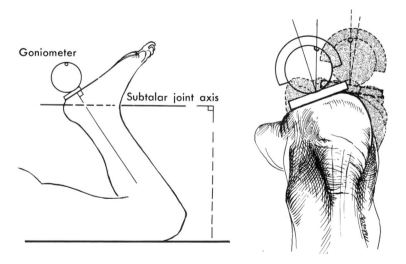

Fig. 2-6. Spherical goniometer attached to the calcaneus to measure the degree of subtalar motion.

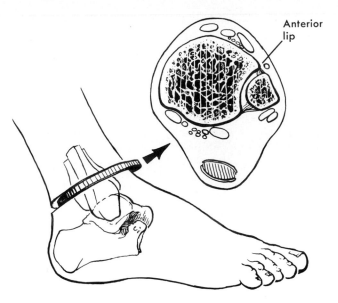

Fig. 2-7. Cross section of the leg just proximal to the ankle joint showing the fibula nestled in its groove in the tibia. Note the prominent anterior lip. (Adapted from Eycleshymer, A. C., and Schoemaker, D. M.: A cross-section anatomy, New York, 1970, Appleton-Century-Crofts.)

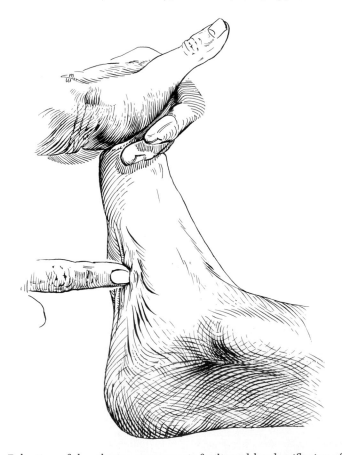

Fig. 2-8. Palpation of the plantar aponeurosis facilitated by dorsiflexion of the toes.

whereas the posterior lip is less pronounced. When attempting to displace the fibula anteriorly in an uninjured ankle, the examiner cannot elicit movement; but he frequently can feel movement, even in a normal ankle, when he attempts to displace the fibula posteriorly. In patients who have sustained injuries to the ligamentous structures supporting the syndesmosis, rarely can he initiate an increase in anterior displacement of the fibula; only occasionally does the attempt produce an increase in pain. He usually can, however, initiate an increase in posterior displacement and is likely to elicit the particular pain of which the patient complains. In all patients who complain of vague ankle pain when they walk, run, or jump, the stability of the fibular syndesmosis should be investigated.

The ability of the heel to invert adequately determines the effectiveness of the foot to fulfill its role as a rigid lever at the time of push-off. If inversion of the heel is insufficient to achieve skeletal stability, abnormal stresses may be placed upon the ligamentous and muscular components of the foot. Such stresses may produce areas of tenderness, which should be sought by applying deep pressure on the plantar aponeurosis, calcaneal tuberosity, and plantar calcaneonavicular ligament.

Plantar aponeurosis. This area should be palpated along its entire surface. Dorsiflexion of the toes will make the fascia more prominent and will facilitate palpation (Fig. 2-8).

Calcaneal tuberosity. The plantar aponeurosis is attached proximally to the calcaneal tuberosity. Tenderness here is indicative of abnormal tension in the aponeurosis. The presence of calcaneal spur is confirmatory evidence of this condition.

Plantar calcaneonavicular (spring) ligament. The examiner can most effectively test for tenderness by applying pressure to the area immediately below the head of the talus, with the foot completely relaxed.

Calcaneocuboid, talonavicular, and cuneonavicular articulations

Abnormal stresses are often imposed upon the capsular structures of the joints of the midfoot; hence these articulations should all be palpated for areas of tenderness and should be stressed for pain.

Of course, no examination is complete without a rough check of the strengths of the various major muscle groups controlling the movements of the foot and ankle. When checking the strength of the muscle groups, the examiner should palpate the tendons while they contract. Abnormal shortening of the triceps surae should always be investigated. In patients with pes planus, the examiner frequently finds that a shortened triceps surae will prevent sufficient dorsiflexion of the foot to allow the heel, if held in inversion, to contact the floor. Until the tendon is surgically lengthened or the triceps surae is stretched by assiduous exercise, wedged heels, heel cups, inserts, and arch supports will probably be ineffective. To check the degree of shortening, the examiner should initiate forceful dorsiflexion of the foot with the heel in a fully inverted position. He may determine whether the shortening is in the soleus, the gastrocnemius, or both, by checking the amount of dorsiflexion with the knee extended and with the knee flexed. In the latter position the gastrocnemius is relaxed.

Metatarsalgia

Pain in the region of the metatarsophalangeal articulation is a frequent complaint. When it occurs in the first metatarsophalangeal joint, it is usually caused by (1) lateral angulation of the first phalanx (hallux valgus) with or without medial exostosis and overlying bunion, (2) injury or degenerative changes with resultant arthritis (hallux rigidus), or (3) arthritic changes in the sesamoid articulation. The latter changes are frequently overlooked, particularly when hallux valgus is present, in which case the sesamoids may be displaced laterally. Fractures of the sesamoids are infrequent and must be distinguished from bipartite sesamoids. When the patient reacts with pain to pressure or attempted displacement of the sesamoids, an abnormality should be suspected.

The second metatarsal is mortised between the three cuneiform bones, making it relatively immobile in relation to the midfoot. It is usually the longest of the metatarsals. Unless the foot is free to deviate laterally, the second metatarsal takes an undue share of the body weight at lift-off—weight that otherwise would be distributed among the other metatarsals. Frequently the concentration of forces on the second metatarsal head is revealed by the presence of plantar callosities.

Many types of metatarsalgia are commonly seen in women who wear heels that are too high to permit adequate lateral deviation of the foot. Other causes of the concentration of body weight upon the second metatarsal with resultant pain in that area of the foot are (1) absolute weakness of the intrinsic muscles of the foot, with functional inability to depress adequately the more movable metatarsals, and (2) insufficient supination of the forefoot at lift-off because of functional abnormality of the midfoot and hindfoot.

Palpation of each metatarsophalangeal joint and the adjacent web spaces to localize the involved areas is essential. The toes should be carefully examined and the range of motion of the joints recorded with the ankle joint in both equinus and full dorsiflexion as well as with the patient standing. Contractures of the flexor tendons can be identified in this manner. Abnormal callus formation about the toes can likewise lead the examiner to the source of the patient's problem (e.g., clawing of the toes when standing).

Peripheral nerves

When the patient complains of a burning type of pain, often accompanied by a feeling of numbness, a careful sensory examination should be conducted. Such complaints frequently indicate peripheral nerve disorders and may be early symptoms of a generalized neuritis or neuropathy. The examiner should check not only for deficits in cutaneous sensation, but also for diminished positional and vibratory sensation.

Two areas exist in the foot where peripheral nerves may be locally entrapped and irritated: (1) where the posterior nerve passes posteriorly to the medial malleolus (tarsal tunnel syndrome) and (2) where the digital nerves (particularly the second and third) pass between the metatarsal heads (Morton's neuralgia). Patients with tarsal tunnel syndrome experience pain when pressure is applied over the posterior tibial nerve and behind the medial malleolus. They may demonstrate a positive Tinel sign to percussion of this area. Patients with Morton's neuralgia experience characteristic pain when pressure is applied to the interspaces on the plantar aspect of the foot between the metatarsal heads. At times the thickened nerve can be rolled under the examiner's fingers, reproducing the patient's pain symptoms. Evidence of delayed conduction time confirms the presence of peripheral nerve abnormality in cases of the tarsal tunnel syndrome.

REFERENCES

Isman, R. E., and Inman, V. T.: Anthropometric studies of the human foot and ankle, Bull. Prosthet. Res. **10** 11:97, 1969.

Levens, A. S., Inman, V. T., and Blosser, J. A.: Transverse rotation of the segments of the lower extremity in locomotion, J. Bone Joint Surg. **30A:** 859, 1948.

BIBLIOGRAPHY
Classifications and general discussion

Burtch, R. L.: Nomenclature for congenital skeletal limb deficiencies: a revision of the Frantz and O'Rahilly classification, Artif. Limbs **10:**24, 1966.

Frantz, C. H., and O'Rahilly, R.: Congenital skeletal limb deficiences, J. Bone Joint Surg. **43A:**1202, 1961.

Henkel, L., and Willert, H. G.: Dysmelia: a classification and a pattern of malformation in a group of congenital defects of the limbs, J. Bone Joint Surg. **51B:**399, 1969.

O'Rahilly, R.: Morphological patterns in limb deficiencies and duplications, Am. J. Anat. **89:**135, 1951.

Wiedemann, H. R.: Derzeitiges Wissen über Exogenese von Missbildungen im Sinne von Embryopathien beim Menschen, Med. Welt. **24:**1343, 1962.

Congenital absence of fibula and tibia

Aitken, G. T.: Amputation as a treatment for certain low extremity congenital anomalies, J. Bone Joint. Surg. **41A:**1267, 1959.

Coventry, M. B., and Johnson, E. W.: Congenital absence of the fibula, J. Bone Joint Surg. **34A:**941, 1952.

Dankmeijer, J.: Congenital absence of the tibia, Anat. Rec. **62:**179, 1935.

Dennison, W. M.: Delayed ossification of the tibia in apparent congenital absence, Br. J. Surg. **28:**101, 1940.

Duraiswami, P. K.: Experimental causation of congenital skeletal defects and its significance in orthopaedic surgery, J. Bone Joint Surg. **34B**:646, 1952.

Evans, E. L., and Smith, N. R.: Congenital absence of tibia, Arch. Dis. Child. **1**:194, 1926.

Farmer, A. W., and Laurin, C. A.: Congenital absence of the fibula, J. Bone Joint Surg. **42A**:1, 1960.

Frantz, C. H., and O'Rahilly, R.: Congenital skeletal limb deficiencies, J. Bone Joint Surg. **43A**:1202, 1961.

Caenslen. F. J.: Congenital defects of tibia and fibula, Am. J. Orthop. Surg. **12**:453, 1914.

Gray, J. E.: Congenital absence of the tibia, Anat. Rec. **101**:265, 1948.

Harmon, P. H., and Fahey, J. J.: The syndrome of congenital absence of the fibula: report of three cases with special reference to pathogenesis and treatment, Surg. Gynecol. Obstet. **64**:876, 1937.

Harris, R. I.: The history and development of Syme's amputation, Artif. Limbs **6**:4, 1961.

Hootnick, D., Boyd, N. A., Fixsen, J. A., and Loyd-Roberts, D. C.: The natural history and management of congenital short tibia with dysplasia or absence of the fibula, J. Bone Joint Surg. **59B**:267, 1977.

Kruger, L. M., and Talbott, R. D.: Amputation and prosthesis as definitive treatment in congenital absence of the fibula, J. Bone Joint Surg. **43A**:625, 1961.

Nutt, J. J., and Smith, E. E.: Total congenital absence of the tibia, Am. J. Roentgenol. Radium Ther. **46**:841, 1941.

Ollerenshaw, R.: Congenital defects of the long bones of the lower limbs: a contribution to the study of their causes, effects, and treatment, J. Bone Joint Surg. **7**:528, 1925.

Putti, V.: The treatment of congenital absence of the tibia or fibula, Int. Abstr. Surg. **50**:42, 1930.

Thompson, T. C., Straub, L. R., and Arnold, W. D.: Congenital absence of the fibula, J. Bone Joint Surg. **39A**:1229, 1957.

Westin, G. W., Sakai, D. N., and Wood, W. L.: Congenital longitudinal deficiency of the fibula, J. Bone Joint Surg. **58A**:492, 1967.

Wood, W. L., Zlotsky, N., and Westin, G.W.: Congenital absence of the fibula: treatment by Syme amputation—indications and technique, J. Bone Joint Surg. **47A**:1159, 1965.

Congenital bowing and pseudarthrosis of tibia

Aegerter, E. E.: The possible relationship of neurofibromatosis, congenital pseudarthrosis, and fibrous dysplasia, J. Bone Joint Surg. **32A**:618, 1950.

Aegerter, E. E., and Kirkpatrick, J. A., Jr.: Orthopedic diseases, ed. 2, Philadelphia, 1963, W. B. Saunders Co.

Badgley, C. E.: Primary and secondary congenital deformities. In American Academy of Orthopaedic Surgeons, Instructional Course Lectures, vol. 10, Ann Arbor, 1953, J. W. Edwards.

Badgley, C. E., O'Connor, S. J., and Kudner, D. F.: Congenital kyphosocoliotic tibia, J. Bone Joint Surg. **34A**:349-371, 1952.

Barber, C. G.: Congenital bowing and pseudarthrosis of the lower leg: Manifestations of von Recklinghausen's neurofibromatosis, Surg. Gynecol. Obstet. **69**:618, 1939.

Birkett, A. N.: Note on pseudarthrosis of the tibia in childhood, J. Bone Joint Surg. **33B**:47, 1941.

Boyd, H. B., and Fox, K. W.: Congenital pseudarthrosis: follow-up study after massive bone grafting, J. Bone Joint Surg. **30A**:274, 1948.

Crenshaw, A. H., editor: Campbell's operative orthopaedics, vol. 2, ed. 5, St. Louis, 1971, The C. V. Mosby Co.

Charnley, J.: Congenital pseudarthrosis of the tibia treated by the intramedullary nail, J. Bone Joint Surg. **38A**:283, 1956.

Compere, E. L.: Localized osteitis fibrosa in the newborn and congenital pseudarthrosis, J. Bone Joint Surg. **18**:513, 1936.

Duraiswami, P. K.: Experimental causation of congenital skeletal defects and its significance in orthopaedic surgery, J. Bone Joint Surg. **34B**:646, 1952.

Eyre-Brook, A. L., Baily, R. A. J., and Price, D. H. G.: Infantile pseudarthrosis of the tibia: three cases treated successfully by delayed autogenous by-pass graft, with some comments on the causative lesion, J. Bone Joint Surg. **51A**:604, 1969.

Freund, E.: Congenital defects of femur, fibula, and tibia, Arch. Surg. **33**:349-376, 1936.

Green, W. T., and Rudo, N.: Pseudarthrosis and neurofibromatosis, Arch. Surg. **46**:639, 1943.

Hallock, H.: The use of multiple small bone transplants in the treatment of pseudarthrosis of the tibia of congenital orgin or following osteotomy for the correction of congenital deformity, J. Bone Joint Surg. **20**:648, 1938.

Henderson, M. S.: Congenital pseudarthrosis of the tibia, J. Bone Joint Surg. **10**:483, 1928.

Heyman, C. H., and Herndon, C. H.: Congenital posterior angulation of the tibia, J. Bone Joint Surg. **31A**:571, 1949.

Heyman, C. H., Herndon, C. H., and Kingsbury, G. H.: Congenital posterior angulation of the tibia with talipes calcaneus, J. Bone Joint Surg. **41A**:476, 1959.

Jaffe, H. L.: Tumors and tumorous conditions of the bones and joints, Philadelphia, 1958, Lea & Febiger.

Kite, J. H.: Congenital pseudarthrosis of tibia and fibula: report of fifteen cases, South, Med. J. **34**:1021, 1941.

Kite, J. H.: Congenital deformities of lower extremity. In Bancroft, F. W., and Marble, H. C., editors: Surgical treatment of the motor-skeletal system, ed. 2, vol. 1, Philadelphia, 1951. J. B. Lippincott Co.

Krida, A.: Congenital posterior angulation of the tibia: a clinical entity unrelated to congenital pseudarthrosis, Am. J. Surg. **82**:98, 1951.

Madsen, E. T.: Congenital angulation and fractures of extremities, Acta Orthop. Scand. **25**:242, 1956.

McElvenny, R. T.: Congenital pseudo-arthrosis of the tibia, Q. Bull. Northwest. Univ. Med. Sch. **23**:413, 1949.

McFarland, B.: Birth fracture of the tibia, Br. J. Surg. **27**:706, 1940.

McFarland, B.: Pseudarthrosis of the tibia in childhood, J. Bone Joint Surg. **33B**:36, 1951.

Middleton, D. S.: Studies on prenatal lesions of striated muscle as a cause of congenital deformity, Edinburgh Med. J. **41**:401, 1934.

Milgram, J. E.: Impaling (telescoping) operation for pseudarthrosis of long bones in childhood, Bull. Hosp. Joint Dis. **17**:152, 1956.

Moore, B. H.: Some orthopaedic relationships of neurofibromatosis, J. Bone Joint Surg. **29**:199, 1941.

Moore, J. R.: Delayed autogenous bone graft in the treatment of congenital pseudarthrosis, J. Bone Joint Surg. **31A**:23, 1949.

Moore, J. R.: Congenital pseudarthrosis of the tibia. In American Academy of Orthopaedic Surgeons, Instructional Course Lectures, vol. 14, Ann Arbor, 1957, J. W. Edwards.

Nicoll, E. A.: Infantile pseudarthrosis of the tibia, J. Bone Joint Surg. **51B**:589, 1969.

Purvis, G. D., and Holder, J. E.: Dual bone graft for congenital pseudarthrosis of the tibia: variations of technic, South. Med. J. **53**:926, 1960.

Sofield, H. A., and Millar, E. A.: Fragmentation, realignment and intramedullary rod fixation of deformities of the long bones in children. A ten-year appraisal, J. Bone Joint Surg. **41A**:1371, 1959.

Williams, E. R.: Two congenital deformities of the tibia. Congenital angulation and congenital pseudarthrosis, Br. J. Radiol. **16**:371, 1943.

Wilson, P. D.: A simple method of two-stage transplantation of the fibula for use in cases of complicated and congenital pseudarthrosis of the tibia, J. Bone Joint Surg. **23**:639, 1941.

Congenital vertical talus

Axer, A.: Into-talus transposition of tendons for correction of paralytic valgus foot after poliomyelitis in children, J. Bone Joint Surg. **42A**:1119, 1960.

Clark, M. S., Dambrosia, R. D., and Ferguson, A. B., Jr.: Congenital vertical talus, J. Bone Joint Surg. **59A**:861, 1977.

Dickson, J. W.: Congenital vertical talus, J. Bone Joint Surg. **44B**:229, 1962.

Eyre-Brook, A. L.: Congenital vertical talus, J. Bone Joint Surg. **49B**:618, 1967.

Grice, D. S.: The role of subtalar fusion in the treatment of valgus deformities of the feet. In American Academy of Orthopaedic Surgeons, Instructional Course Lectures, vol. 16, St. Louis, 1959. The C. V. Mosby Co.

Hark, F. W.: Rocker-foot due to congenital subluxation of the talus, J. Bone Joint Surg. **32A**:344, 1950.

Harrold, A. J.: Congenital vertical talus in infancy, J. Bone Joint Surg. **49B**:634, 1967.

Herndon, C. H., and Heyman, C. H.: Problems in the recognition and treatment of congenital convex pes valgus, J. Bone Joint Surg. **45A**:413, 1963.

Heyman, C. H.: The diagnosis and treatment of congenital convex pes valgus or vertical talus. In American Academy of Orthopaedic Surgeons, Instructional Course Lectures, vol. 16, St. Louis, 1959, The C. V. Mosby Co.

Hughes, J. R.: On congenital vertical talus, J. Bone Joint Surg. **39B**:580, 1957.

Lamy, L., and Weissman, L.: Congenital convex pes valgus, J. Bone Joint Surg. **21**:79, 1939.

Lloyd-Roberts, G. C., and Spence, A. J.: Congenital vertical talus, J. Bone Joint Surg. **40B**:33, 1958.

Mead, N. C., and Nast, G.: Vertical talus (congenital talonavicular dislocation), Clin. Orthop. **21**:198, 1961.

Osmond-Clarke, H.: Congenital vertical talus, J. Bone Joint Surg. **38B**:334, 1956.

Outland, T., and Sherk, H. H.: Congenital vertical talus, Clin. Orthop. **16**:214, 1960.

Silk, F. F., and Wainwright, D.: The recognition and treatment of congenital flat foot in infancy, J. Bone Joint Surg. **49B**:628, 1967.

Steindler, A.: Orthopedic operations, Springfield, Ill. 1940, Charles C Thomas, Publisher.

Stone, K. H.: Congenital vertical talus: a new operation, Proc. R. Soc. Med. **56**:12, 1963.

Thompson, J. E. M.: Treatment of congenital flatfoot, J. Bone Joint Surg. **28**:787, 1946.

Townes, P. L., DeHart, G. K., Hecht, F., and Manning, J. A.: Trisomy 13-15 in a male infant, J. Pediatr. **60**:528, 1962.

Uchida, I. A., Lewis, A. J., Bowman, J. M., and Wang, H. C.: A case of double trisomy: trisomy no. 18 and triplo-X, J. Pediatr. **60**:498, 1962.

Wainwright, D.: The recognition and cure of congenital flat foot, Proc. R. Soc. Med. **57**:357, 1964.

White, J. W.: Congenital flatfoot: a new surgical approach, J. Bone Joint Surg. **22**:547, 1940.

Whitman, A.: Astragalectomy and backward displacement of the foot: an investigation of its practical results, J. Bone Joint Surg. **4**:266, 1922.

Hemihypertrophy and gigantism

Barsky, A. J.: Macrodactyly, J. Bone Joint Surg. **49A**:1255, 1967.

Ben-Bassat, M., Casper, J., Kaplan, I., and Laron, Z.: Congenital macrodactyly, J. Bone Joint Surg. **44B**:359, 1966.

Bryan, R. S., Lipscomb, P. R., and Chatterton, C. C.: Orthopedic aspects of congenital hypertrophy, Am. J. Surg. **96**:654, 1958.

Charters, A. D.: Local gigantism, J. Bone Joint Surg. **39B**:542, 1957.

Dennyson, W. D., Bear, J. N., and Bhoola, K. D.: Macrodactyly in the foot, J. Bone Joint Surg. **59B**:355, 1977.

Goidanich, I. F.,, and Campanacci, M: Vascular hamartomata and infantile angioectatic osteohyperplasia of the extremities: a study of ninety four cases, J. Bone Joint Surg. **44A**:815, 1962.

Hutchison, W. J., and Burdeaux, B. D., Jr.: The influence of stasis on bone growth, Surg. Gynecol. Obstet. **99**:413, 1954.

Peabody, C. W.: Hemihypertrophy and hemiotrometry: congenital total unilateral somatic asymetry, J. Bone Joint Surg. **18**:466, 1936.

Pease, C. N.: Local stimulation of growth of long bones, J. Bone Joint Surg. **34A**:1, 1952.

Peremans, G.: An unusual case of congenital asymmetry of the pelvis and of the lower extremities, J. Bone Joint Surg. **5**:331, 1923.

Sabanas, A. O., and Chatterton, C. C.: Crossed congenital hemihypertrophy, J. Bone Joint Surg. **37A**:871, 1955.

Strobino, L. J., French. G. O., and Colonna, P. C.: The effect of increasing tensions on the growth of epiphyseal bone, Surg. Gynecol. Obstet. **95**:694, 1952.

Thomas, H. B.: Partial gigantism: overgrowth and asymmetry of bones and skeletal muscle, Am. J. Surg. **32**:108, 1936.

Thorne, F. L., Posch, J. L., and Mladick, R. A.: Megalodactyly, Plast. Reconstr. Surg. **41**:232, 1968.

Trueta, J.: The influence of the blood supply in controlling bone growth, Bull. Hosp. Joint Dis. **14**:147, 1953.

Ward, J., and Lerner, H. L.: A review of the subject of congenital hemihypertrophy and a complete case report, J. Pediatr. **31**:403, 1947.

Inequality of length of leg

Abbott, L. C.: The operative lengthening of the tibia and fibula, J. Bone Joint Surg. **9**:128, 1927.

Aitken, A. P.: Overgrowth of the femoral shaft following fracture in children, Am. J. Surg. **49**:147, 1940.

Anderson, M. S., Green, W. T., and Messner, M. B.: Growth and predictions of growth in the lower extremities, J. Bone Joint Surg. **45A**:1, 1963.

Arkin, A. M., and Katz, J. F.: The effects of pressure on epiphyseal growth, J. Bone Joint Surg. **38A**:1057, 1956.

Barfod, B., and Christensen, J.: Fractures of the femoral shaft in children with special reference to subsequent overgrowth, Acta Chir. Scand. **116**:235, 1959.

Barr, J.: Growth and inequality of leg length in poliomyelitis, N. Engl. J. Med. **238**:737, 1948.

Barr, J. S., Lingley, J. R., and Gall, E. A.: The effect of roentgen irradiation on epiphyseal growth. I. Experimental studies upon the albino rat, Am. J. Roentgenol. Radium Ther. **49**:104, 1943.

Barr, J. S., Stinchfield, A. J., and Reidy, J. A.: Sympathetic ganglionectomy and limb length in poliomyelitis, J. Bone Joint Surg. **32A**:793, 1950.

Bell, J. S., and Thompson, W. A. L.: Modified spot scanography, Am. J. Roentgenol. Radium Ther. **63**:915, 1950.

Bisgard, J. D.: Longitudinal bone growth: the influence of sympathetic deinnervation, Ann. Surg. **97**:374, 1933.

Bisgard, J. D., and Bisgard, M. E.: Longitudinal growth of long bones, Arch. Surg. **31**:568, 1935.

Blount, W. P.: Unequal leg length in children, Surg. Clin. North Am. **38**:1107, 1958.

Blount, W. P.: Unequal leg length. In American Academy of Orthopaedic Surgeons, Instructional Course Lectures, vol. 17, St. Louis, 1960, The C. V. Mosby Co.

Blount, W. P., and Clarke, G. R.: control of bone growth by epiphyseal stapling: a preliminary report, J. Bone Joint Surg. **31A**:464, 1949.

Blount, W. P., and Zeier, F.: Control of bone length, J.A.M.A. **148**:451, 1952.

Bohlman, H. R.: Experiments with foreign materials in the region of the epiphyseal cartilage plate of growing bones to increase their longitudinal growth, J. Bone Joint Surg. **11**:365, 1929.

Bost, F. C., and Larsen, L. J.: Experiences with lengthening of the femur over an intramedullary rod, J. Bone Joint Surg. **38A**:567, 1956.

Brockway, A., Craig, W. A., and Cockrell, B. R., Jr.: End-result of sixty-two stapling operations, J. Bone Joint Surg. **36A**:1063, 1954.

Brodin, H.: Longitudinal bone growth, the nutrition of the epiphyseal cartilages and the local blood supply, Acta Orthop. Scand. (supp.) **20**:1, 1955.

Brookes, M.: Femoral growth after occlusion of the principal nutrient canal in day-old rabbits, J. Bone Joint Surg. **39B**:563, 1957.

Cameron, B. M.: A technique for femoral-shaft shortening: a preliminary report, J. Bone Joint Surg. **39A**:1309, 1957.

Carpenter, E. B., and Dalton, J. B.: A critical evaluation of a method of epiphyseal stimulation, J. Bone Joint Surg. **38A**:1089, 1956.

Coleman, S. S., and Noonan, T. D.: Anderson's method of tibial-lengthening by percutaneous osteotomy and gradual distraction. Experience with thirty-one cases, J. Bone Joint Surg. **49A**:263, 1967.

Compere, E. L., and Adams, C. O.: Studies of longitudinal growth of long bones. I. The influence of trauma to the diaphysis, J. Bone Joint Surg. **19**:922, 1937.

Dalton, J. B., Jr., and Carpenter, E. B.: Clinical experiences with epiphyseal stapling, South. Med. J. **47**:544, 1954.

David, V. C.: Shortening and compensatory overgrowth following fractures of the femur in children, Arch. Surg. **9**:438, 1924.

Doyle, J. R., and Smart, B. W.: Stimulation of bone growth by short-wave diathermy, J. Bone **45A**:15, 1963.

Duthie, R. B.: The significance of growth in orthopaedic surgery, Clin. Orthop. **14**:7, 1959.

Ferguson, A. B.: Surgical stimulation of bone growth by a new procedure: preliminary report, J.A.M.A. **100**:26, 1933.

Ferguson, A. B.: Growth as a factor in relation to deformity and disease. In American Academy of Orthopaedic Surgeons, Instructional Course Lectures, vol. 9, Ann Arbor, 1952, J. W. Edwards.

Ford, L. T., and Key, J. A.: A study of experimental trauma to the distal femoral epiphysis in rabbits, J. Bone Joint Surg. 38A:84, 1956.

Gardner, E.: The development and growth of bones and joints. In American Academy of Orthopeadic Surgeons, Instructional Course Lectures, vol. 13, Ann Arbor, 1956, J. W. Edwards.

Gatewood and Mullen, B. P.: Experimental observations on the growth of long bones, Arch. Surg. 15:215, 1927.

Geiser, M., and Trueta, J.: Muscle action, bone rarefaction and bone formation: an experimental study, J. Bone Joint Surg. 40B:282, 1958.

Gelbke, H.: The influence of pressure and tension on growing bones in experiments with animals, J. Bone Joint Surg. 33A:947, 1951.

Gill, G. G., and Abbott, L. C.: Practical method of predicting the growth of the femur and tibia in the child, Arch. Surg. 45:286, 1942.

Goetz, R. H., Du Toit, J. G., and Swart, B. H.: Vascular changes in poliomyelitis and the effect of sympathectomy on bone growth, Acta Med. Scand. (supp.) 306:56, 1955.

Goff, C. W.: Growth determinations, In American Academy of Orthopaedic Surgeons, Instructional Course Lectures, vol. 8, Ann Arbor, 1951, J. W. Edwards.

Goff, C. W.: Surgical care of unequal extremities: Measuring and predicting growth. In American Academy of Orthopaedic Surgeons, Instructional Course Lectures, vol. 16, St. Louis, 1959, The C. V. Mosby Co.

Goff, C. W.: Surgical treatment of unequal extremities, Springfield, 1960, Charles C Thomas, Publisher.

Green, W. T.: Discussion following prediction of unequal growth of the lower extremities in anterior poliomyelitis, J. Bone Joint Surg. 31A:485, 1949.

Green, W. T., and Anderson, M.: Experiences with epiphyseal arrest in correcting discrepancies in length of the lower extremities in infantile paralysis, J. Bone Joint Surg. 29:659, 1947.

Green, W. T., and Anderson, M.: Discrepancy in length of the lower extremities. In American Academy of Orthopaedic Surgeons, Instructional Course Lectures, vol. 8, Ann Arbor, 1951, J. W. Edwards.

Green, W. T., and Anderson, M.: The problem of unequal leg length, Pediatr. Clin. North Am. 2:1137, 1955.

Green, W. T., and Anderson, M.: Epiphyseal arrest for the correction of discrepancies in length of the lower extremities, J. Bone Joint Surg. 39A:853, 1957.

Green, W. T., and Anderson, M.: Skeletal age and control of bone growth. In American Academy of Orthopaedic Surgeons, Instructional Course Lectures, vol. 17, St. Louis, 1960, The C. V. Mosby Co.

Green, W. T., Wyatt, G. M., and Anderson, M. S.: Orthoroentgenography as a method of measuring the bones of the lower extremities, J. Bone Joint Surg. 28:60, 1946.

Gruelich, W. W., and Pyle, S. I.: Radiographic atlas of skeletal development of the hand and wrist, Stanford, Calif., 1950, Stanford University Press.

Greville, N. R., and Ivins, J. C: Fractures of the femur in children. An analysis of their effect on the subsequent length of both bones of the lower limb, Am. J. Surg. 93:376, 1957.

Greville, N. R., and Janes, J. M.: An experimental study of overgrowth after fractures, Surg. Gynecol. Obstet. 105:711, 1957.

Gross, R. H.: An evaluation of tibial lengthening procedures, J. Bone Joint Surg. 53A:693, 1971.

Gullickson, G., Jr., Olson, M., and Koettke, F. J,.: The effect of paralysis of one lower extremity on bone growth, Arch. Phys. Med. Rehabil. 31:392, 1950.

Haas, S. L.: The relation of the blood supply to the longitudinal growth of bone, Am. J. Orthop. Surg. 15:157, 1917.

Haas, S. L.: Interstital growth in growing long bones, Arch. Surg. 12:887, 1926.

Haas, S. L.: Retardation of bone growth by a wire loop, J. Bone Joint Surg. 27:25, 1945.

Haas, S. L.: Femoral shortening in subtrochanteric region combined with angulation at site of resection, Am. J. Surg. 80:461, 1950.

Haas, S. L.: Restriction of bone growth by pins through the epiphyseal cartilaginous plate, J. Bone Joint Surg. 32A:338, 1950.

Haas, S. L.: Stimulation of bone growth, Am. J. Surg. 95:125, 1958.

Harris, H. A.: The growth of the long bones in childhood. (With special reference to certain bony striations of the metaphysis and to the role of vitamins.) Arch. Intern. Med. 38:785, 1926.

Harris, H. A.: Lines of arrested growth in the long bones in childhood: the correlation of histological and radiographic appearances in clinical and experimental conditions, Br. J. Radiol. 4:561, 1931.

Harris, H. A.: Bone growth in health and disease, London, 1933, Oxford University Press.

Harris, R. I., and McDonald, J. L.: The effect of lumbar sympathectomy upon the growth of legs paralyzed by anterior poliomyelitis, J. Bone Joint Surg. 18:35, 1936.

Hayes, J. T., and Brody, G. L.: Cystic lymphangiectasis of bone, J. Bone Joint Surg. 43A:107, 1961.

Herndon, C. H., and Spencer, G. E.: An experimental attempt to stimulate linear growth of long bones in rabbits, J. Bone Joint Surg. 35A:758, 1953.

Hiertonn, T.: Arteriovenous anastomoses and acceleration of bone growth, Acta Orthop. Scand. 26:322, 1956.

Hutchinson, W. J., and Burdeaux, B. D.: The influence of stasis on bone growth, Surg. Gynecol. Obstet. 99:413, 1954.

James, C. C. M., and Lassman, L. P.: Spinal dysraphism: the diagnosis and treatment of progressive lesions in spina bifida occulta, J. Bone Joint Surg. **44B**:828, 1962.

Janes, J. M., and Musgrove, J. E.: Effect of arteriovenous fistula on growth of bone: an experimental study, Surg. Clin. North Am. 30:1191, 1950.

Kruger, L. M., and Talbott, R. D.: Amputation and prosthesis as definitive treatment in congenital absence of the fibula, J. Bone Joint Surg. **43A**:625, 1961.

Maresh, M. M.: Linear growth of long bones of extremities from infancy through adolescence, Am. J. Dis. Child. **89**:725, 1955.

Marino-Zuco, C: Treatment of length discrepancy of the lower limbs, J. Bone Joint Surg. **38B**:934, 1956.

Moore, B. H.: A critical appraisal of the leg lengthening operation, Am. J. Surg. **52**:415, 1941.

Morgan, J. D., and Somerville, E. W.: Normal and abnormal growth at the upper end of the femur, J. Bone Joint Surg. **42B**:264, 1960.

Neer, C. S., II, and Cadman, E. F.: Treatment of fractures of the femoral shaft in children, J.A.M.A. **163**:634, 1957.

Park, E. A., and Richter, C. P.: Transverse lines in bone: mechanism of their development, Johns Hopkins Med. J. **93**:234, 1953.

Pearse, H. E., and Morton, J. J.,: The stimulation of bone growth by venous stasis, J. Bone Joint Surg. **12**:97, 1930.

Pease, C. N.: Local stimulation of growth of long bones: a preliminary report, J. Bone Joint Surg. **34A**:1, 1952.

Phemister, D. B.: Operative arrestment of longitudinal growth of bones in the treatment of deformities, J. Bone Joint Surg. **15**:1, 1933.

Ratliff, A. H. C.: The short leg in poliomyelitis, J. Bone Joint Surg. **41B**:56, 1959.

Reidy, J. A.: Lingley, J. R., Gall, E. A., and Barr, J. S.: The effect of roentgen irradiation on epiphyseal growth. II. Experimental studies upon the dog, J. Bone Joint Surg. **29**:853, 1947.

Rezaian, S. M.: Tibial lengthening using a new extension device. Report of thirty-two cases, J. Bone Joint Surg. **58A**:239, 1976.

Richards, V., and Stofer, R.: The stimulation of bone growth by internal heating, Surgery **46**:84, 1959.

Ring, P. A.: Shortening and paralysis in poliomyelitis, Lancet, **2**:980, 1957.

Ring, P. A.: Experimental bone lengthening by epiphyseal distraction, Br. J. Surg. **46**:169, 1958.

Ring, P. A.: Congenital short femur: simple femoral hypoplasia, J. Bone Joint Surg. **41B**:73, 1959.

Ring, P. A.: The influence of the nervous system upon the growth of bones, J. Bone Joint Surg. **43B**:121, 1961.

Ring, P. A., and Less, J.: The effect of heat upon the growth of bone, J. Pathol. **75**:405, 1958.

Schneider, M.: Experimental epiphyseal arrest by intra-osseous injection of papain, J. Bone Joint Surg. **45A**:25, 1963.

Siffert, R.: The effect of staples and longitudinal wires on epiphyseal growth, J. Bone Joint Surg. **38A**:1077, 1956.

Siffert, R. S.: The effect of juxta-epiphyseal pyogenic infection on epiphyseal growth, Clin. Orthop. **10**:131, 1957.

Sofield, H. A., Blair, S. J., and Millar, E. A.: Leg-lengthening, J. Bone Joint Surg. **40A**:311, 1958.

Sofield, H. A., and Millar, E. A.: Fragmentation, realignment and intramedullary rod fixation of deformities of the long bones in children, J. Bone Joint Surg. **41A**:1371, 1959.

Stewart, S. F.: Effect of sympathectomy on the leg length in cortical rigidity, J. Bone Joint Surg. **19**:222, 1937.

Stinchfield, A. J., Reidy, J. A., and Barr, J. S.: Prediction of unequal growth of the lower extremities in anterior poliomyelitis, J. Bone Joint Surg. **31A**:478, 1949.

Straub, L. R., Thompson, T. C., and Wilson, P. D.: The results of epiphyseodesis and femoral shortening in relation to equilization of limb length, J. Bone Joint Surg. **27**:255, 1945.

Strobino, L. J., Colonna, P. C., Brodey, R. D., and Leinbach, T.: The effect of compression on the growth of epiphyseal bone, Surg. Gynecol. Obstet. **103**:85, 1956.

Strobino, L. J., French, G. O., and Colonna, P. C.: The effect of epiphyseal bone, Surg. Gynecol. Obstet. **95**:694, 1952.

Thompson, T. C., Straub, L. R., and Arnold, W. D.: Congenital absence of the fibula, J. Bone Joint Surg. **39A**:1229, 1957.

Thompson, T. C., Straub, L. R., and Campbell, R. D.: An evaluation of femoral shortening with intramedullary nailing, J. Bone Joint Surg. **36A**:43, 1954.

Truesdell, E. D.: Inequality of the lower extremities following fracture of the shaft of the femur in children, Ann. Surg. **74**:498, 1921.

Trueta, J.: Stimulation of bone growth by redistribution of the intra-osseous circulation, J. Bone Joint Surg. **33B**:476, 1951.

Trueta, J.: The influence of the blood supply in controlling bone growth, Bull. Hosp. Joint Dis. **14**:147, 1953.

Trueta, J., and Amato, V. P.: The vascular contribution to osteogenesis, J. Bone Joint Surg. **42B**:571, 1960.

Tupman, G. S.: Treatment of inequality of the lower limbs, J. Bone Joint Surg. **42B**:489, 1960.

Tupman, G. S.: A study of bone growth in normal children and its relationship to skeletal maturation, J. Bone Joint Surg. **44B**:42, 1962.

White, J. W.: A simplified method for tibial lengthening, J. Bone Joint Surg. **12**:90, 1930.

White, J. W.: Femoral shortening for equalization of leg length, J. Bone Joint Surg. **17**:597, 1935.

White, J. W.: A practical graphic method of recording leg length discrepancies, South. Med. J. **33**:946, 1940.

White, J. W.: Leg-length discrepancies. In American Academy of Orthopaedic Surgeons, Instructional Course Lectures, vol. 6, Ann Arbor, 1949, J. W. Edwards.

White, J. W.: A method of subtrochanteric limb shortening, J. Bone Joint Surg. **31A**:86, 1949.

White, J. W., and Stubbins, S. G.: Growth arrest for equalizing leg lengths, J.A.M.A. **126**:1146, 1944.

White, J. W., and Warner, W. P.: Experiences with metaphyseal arrests, South. Med. J. **31**:41, 1938.

Wilson, C. L., and Percy, E. C.: Experimental studies on epiphyseal stimulation, J. Bone Joint Surg. **38A**:1096, 1956.

Wise, C. S., Castlemann, B., and Watkins, A. L.: Effect of diathermy (short wave and microwave) on bone growth in the albino rat, J. Bone Joint Surg. **31A**:487, 1949.

Wu, Y. K., and Miltner, L. J.: A procedure for stimulation of longitudinal growth of bone, J. Bone Joint Surg. **19**:909, 1937.

Tarsal coalitions

Anderson, R. J.: The presence of an astralagoscaphoid bone in man, J. Anat. **14**:452, 1880.

Austin, F. H.: Symphalangism and related fusions of tarsal bones, Radiology **56**:882, 1951.

Badgley, C. E.: Coalition of the calcaneus and the navicular, Arch. Surg. **15**:75, 1927.

Bersani, F. A., and Samilson, R. L.: Massive familial tarsal synotosis, J. Bone Joint Surg. **39A**:1187, 1957.

Boyd, H. B.: Congenital talonavicular synostosis, J. Bone Joint Surg. **26**:682, 1944.

Bullitt, J. B.: Variations of the bones of the foot: fusion of the talus and navicular, bilateral and congenital, Am. J. Roentgenol. Radium Ther. **20**:548, 1928.

Conway, J. J., and Cowell, H. R.: Tarsal coalition: clinical significance and roentgenographic demonstration, Radiology **92**:799, 1969.

Cowell, H. R.: Talo-calcaneal coalition and new causes of peroneal spastic flat foot, Clin. Orthop. **85**:16, 1972.

Harris, B. J.: Anomalous structures in the developing human foot (abstr.), Anat. Rec. **121**:399, 1955.

Harris, R. I.: Rigid valgus foot due to talonaccaneal bridge, J. Bone Joint Surg. **37A**:169, 1955.

Harris, R. I.: Peroneal spastic flatfoot. In American Academy of Orthopaedic Surgeons, Instructional Course Lectures, vol. 15, Ann Arbor, 1958, J. W. Edwards.

Harris, R. I.: Follow-up notes on articles previously published in this journal, J. Bone Joint Surg. **47A**:1657, 1965.

Harris, R. I., and Beath, T.: Etiology of peroneal spastic flat foot, J. Bone Joint Surg. **30B**:624, 1948.

Harris, R. I., and Beath, T.: John Hunter's specimen of talocalcaneal bridge, J. Bone Joint Surg. **32B**:203, 1950.

Hodgson, F. G.: Talonavicular synostosis, South. Med. J. **39**:940, 1946.

Holl, M: Beiträge zur chirurgischen Osteologie des Fusses, Arch. Klin. Chir. **25**:211, 1880.

Illievitz, A. B.: Congenital malformations of the feet: Report of a case of congenital fusion of the scaphoid with the astragalus, and complete absence of one toe, Am. J. Surg. **4**:550, 1928.

Jack, E. A.: Bone anomalies of the tarsus on relation to "peroneal spastic flat foot," J. Bone Joint Surg. **36B**:530, 1954.

Kendrick, J. I.: Treatment of calcanconavicular bar, J.A.M.A. **172**:1242, 1960.

Lapidus, P. W.: Congenital fusion of the bones of the foot: with a report of a case of congenital astragaloscaphoid fusion, J. Bone Joint Surg. **14**:888, 1932.

Lapidus, P. W.: Bilateral congenital talonavicular fusion: report of a case, J. Bone Joint Surg. **20**:775, 1938.

Lapidus, P. W.: Spastic flat-foot, J. Bone Joint Surg. **28**:126, 1946.

Mahaffey, H. W.: Bilateral congenital calcaneocuboid synostosis: a case report, J. Bone Joint Surg. **27**:164, 1945.

Nievergelt, K.: Positiver Vaterschaftsnachweis auf Grund erblicher Missbildungen der Extremitäten, Arch. Julius Klaus-Stiftg. Vererbungsforschg. **19**:157, 1944.

O'Donoghue, D. H., and Sell, L. S.: Congenital talonavicular synostosis: a case report of a rare anomaly, J. Bone Joint Surg. **25**:925, 1943.

Outland, T., and Murphy, I. D.: Relation of tarsal anomalies to spastic and rigid flatfeet, Clin. Orthop. **1**:217, 1953.

Outland, T., and Murphy, I. D.: The pathomechanics of peroneal spastic flat foot, Clin. Orthop. **16**:64, 1960.

Pearlman, H. S., Edkin, R. E., and Warren, R. F.: Familial tarsal and carpal synostosis with radialhead subluxation (Nievergelt's syndrome), J. Bone Joint Surg. **46A**:585, 1964.

Pfitzner, W.: Ein Beitrag zur Kenntniss der sekundären Geschlectsunterschiede beim Menschen, Morphol. Arb. **7**:473, 1897.

Schreiber, R. R.: Talonavicular synostosis, J. Bone Joint Surg,. **45A**:170, 1963.

Seddon, H. J.: Calcaneo-scaphoid coalition, Proc. R. Soc. Med. **26**:419, 1933.

Shands, A. R., Jr., and Wentz, I. J.: Congenital anomalies, accessory bones and osteochondritis in the feet of 850 children, Surg. Clin. North Am. **33**:1643, 1953.

Simmons, E. H.: Tibialis spastic varus foot with tarsal coalition, J. Bone Joint Surg. **47B**:533, 1965.

Slomann: On coalition calcaneo-navicularis, J. Orthop. Surg. **3**:586, 1921.

Vaughan, W. H., and Segal, G.: Tarsal coalition, with special reference to roentgenographic interpretation, Radiology **60**:855, 1953.

Wagoner, G. W.: A case of bilateral congenital fusion of the calcanei and cuboids, J. Bone Joint Surg. **10**:220, 1928.

Waugh, W.: Partial cubo-navicular coalition as a cause of peroneal spastic flat foot, J. Bone Joint Surg. **39B**:520, 1957.

Webster, F. S., and Romerts, W. M.: Tarsal anomalies and peroneal spastic flatfoot, J.A.M.A. **146**:1099, 1951.

Weitzner, I.: Congenital talonavicular synostosis associated with its hereditary multiple ankylosing arthropathies, Am. J. Roentgenol. Radium Ther. **51**:185, 1946.

Wray, J. B., and Herndon, C. N.: Hereditary transmission of congenital coalition of the calcaneus to the navicular, J. Bone Joint Surg. **45A**:365, 1963.

Torsional deformities of lower extremities

Appleton, A. B.: Postural deformities and bone growth, Lancet **1**:451, 1934.

Arkin, A. M., and Katz, J. F.: Effects of pressure on epiphyseal growth, J. Bone Joint Surg. **38A**:1056, 1956.

Backman, S.: The proximal end of the femur: investigations with special reference to the etiology of femoral neck fractures, Acta Radiol. (supp.) **146**:1, 1957.

Badgley, C. E.: Correlation of clinical and anatomical facts leading to a conception of the etiology of congenital hip dysplasias, J. Bone Joint Surg. **25**:503, 1943.

Badgley, C. E.: Etiology of congenital dislocation of the hip, J. Bone Joint Surg. **31A**:341, 1949.

Baker, L. D., and Hill, L. M.: Foot alignment in the cerebral palsy patient, J. Bone Joint Surg. **46A**:1, 1964.

Bergmann, G. A.: Die Bedeutung der Innendrehung der Unterschenkel für die Entwicklung des Senk-Knickfusses mit der Angabe einer Messmethode von Messergebnissen, Acta Orthop. **96**:177, 1962

Billing, L.: Roentgen examination of the proximal femur end in children and adolescents, Acta Radiol. (supp.) **110**:1, 1954.

Blount, W. P.: Bow leg, Wis. Med. J. **40**:484, 1941.

Blumel, J., Eggers, G. W. N., and Evans, E. B.: Eight cases of hereditary bilateral medial tibial torsion in four generations, J. Bone Joint Surg. **39A**:1198, 1957.

Böhm, M.: The embryologic orgin of club-foot, J. Bone Joint Surg. **11**:229, 1929.

Böhm, M.: Infantile deformities of the knee and hip, J. Bone Joint Surg. **15**:574, 1933.

Browne, D.: Congenital deformities of mechanical orgin, Proc. R. Soc. Med. **29**:1409, 1936.

Chapple, C. C., and Davidson, D. T.: A study of the relationship between fetal position and certain congenital deformities, J. Pediatr. **18**:483, 1941.

Crane, L.: Femoral torsion and its relation to toeing-in and toeing-out, J. Bone Joint Surg. **41A**:421, 1959.

Doyle, M. R.: Sleeping habits of infants, Phys. Ther. Rev. **25**:74, 1945.

Dunlap, K., Shands, A. R., Hollister, L.C., Gahl, J. S., and Streit, H. A.: A new method for determination of torsion of the femur, J. Bone Joint Surg. **35A**:289, 1953.

Dunn, D. M.: Anteversion of the neck of the femur, J. Bone Joint Surg. **34B**:181, 1952.

Durham, H. A.: Anteversion of the femoral neck to the normal femur and its relation to congenital dislocation of the hip, J.A.M.A. **65**:223, 1915.

Elftman, H.: Torsion of the lower extremity, Am. J. Phys. Anthropol. **3**:255, 1945.

Fitzhugh, M. L.: Faulty alignment of the feet and legs in infancy and childhood, Phys. Ther. Rev. **21**:239, 1941.

Garden, R. S.: The structure and function of the proximal end of the femur, J. Bone Joint Surg. **43B**:576, 1961.

Geist, E. S.: An operation for the after treatment of some cases of congenital club-foot, J. Bone Joint Surg. **6**:50, 1924.

Howorth, M. B.: A textbook of orthopedics, Philadelphia, 1952, W. B. Saunders Co.

Hutter, C. G., and Scott, W.: Tibial torsion, J. Bone Joint Surg. **31A**:511, 1949.

Irwin, C. E.: The iliotibial band: its role in producing deformity in poliomyelitis, J. Bone Joint Surg. **31A**:141, 1949.

Kaplin, E. B.: The iliotibial tract: clinical and morphological significance, J. Bone Joint Surg. **40A**:817, 1958.

Khermosh, O., Lior, G., and Weissman, S. L.: Tibial torsion in children, Clin. Orthop. **79**:25, 1971.

Kingsley, P. C., and Olmstead, K. L.: A study to determine the angle of anteversion of the neck and of the femur, J. Bone Joint Surg. **30A**:745, 1948.

Kite, J. H.: Torsion of the lower extremities in small children, J. Bone Joint Surg. **36A**:511, 1954.

Kite, J. H.: Torsion of the legs in small children, Med. Assoc. Georgia **43**:1035, 1954.

Kite, J. H.: Torsional deformities of the lower extremities, West Va. Med. J. **57**:92, 1961.

Knight, R. A.: Developmental deformities of the lower extremities, J. Bone Joint Surg. **36A**:521, 1954.

Lanz-Wachsmuth: Praktische Anatomie, Berlin, 1938, Springer-Verlag.

LeDamany, P.: La torsion du tibia, normale, pathologique, expérimentale, J. Anat. Physiol. **45**:598, 1909.

Lowman, C. L.: Rotation deformities, Boston Med. Surg. J. **21**:581, 1919.

Lowman, C. L.: The sitting position in relation to pelvic stress, Phys. Ther. Rev. **21**:30, 1941.

MacKenzie, I. G., Seddon, H. J., and Trevor, D.: Congenital dislocation of the hip, J. Bone Joint Surg. **42B**:689, 1960.

Majestro, T. C., and Frost, H. M.: Spastic internal femoral torsion, Clin. Orthop. **79**:44, 1971.

Milch, H.: Subtrochanteric osteotomy, Clin. Orthop. **22**:145, 1962.

Morgan, J. D., and Somerville, E. W.,: Normal and abnormal growth at the upper end of the femur, J. Bone Joint Surg. **42B**:264, 1960.

Nachlas, I. W.: Medial torsion of the leg, Arch. Surg. **28**:909, 1934.

Nachlas, I. W.: Common defects of the lower extremity in infants, South. Med. J. **41**:302, 1948.

O'Donoghue, D. H.: Controlled rotation osteotomy of the tibia, South. Med. J. **33**:1145, 1940.

Rabinowitz, M. S.: Congenital curvature of the tibia, Bull. Hosp. Joint Dis. **12**:63, 1951.

Rosen, H., and Sandick, H.: The measurement of tibiofibular torsion, J. Bone Joint Surg. **37A**:847, 1955.

Sell, L. S.: Tibial torsion accompanying congenital clubfoot, J. Bone Joint Surg. 23:561, 1941.

Statham, L., and Murray, M. P.: Early walking patterns
of normal children, Clin. Orthop. 79:8, 1971.

Sterling, R. I.: "Derotation" of the tibia, Br. Med. J.
1:581, 1936.

Sutherland, D. H., Schottstaedt, E. R., Larsen, L. S.,
Ashley, R. K., Callander, J. N., and James, P. M.:
Clinical and electromyographic study of seven spastic
children with internal rotation gait, J. Bone Joint Surg.
51A:1070, 1969.

Swanson, A. B., Green, P. W., and Allis, H. D.: Rotational deformities of the lower extremity in children
and their clinical significance, Clin. Orthop. 27:157,
1963.

Thelander, H. E., and Fitzhugh, M. L.: Posture habits in
infancy affecting foot and leg alignments, J. Pediatr.
21:306, 1942.

Yount, C. C.: The role of tensor fasciae femoris in certain
deformities of the lower extremities, J. Bone Joint
Surg. 8:171, 1926.

3

RADIOGRAPHIC EXAMINATION OF THE NORMAL FOOT

Igor Z. Drobocky

In this day of tomography, xeroradiography, magnification and fine-detail radiography, and computed tomography, the standard radiographic film examination of the foot still offers the best overall detail for the rapid analysis of foot morphology. The standard radiographic projections of the foot are the best means by which the numerous variations of normal can be examined fully. Special projections, together with the standard projections are usually all that is necessary for full evaluation of the precise interrelationships of the individual digits and other small bones of the foot.

STANDARD RADIOGRAPHIC PROJECTIONS

Standard radiographic projections of the foot can be either weight-bearing or passive views. If the biomechanics of the foot are to be evaluated, the weight-bearing views in anteroposterior (dorsoplantar) and lateral projections (Figs. 3-1 and 3-2) are chosen. For completeness the recumbent oblique projections can be added. For an analysis of function, standing lateral views centered at the first metatarsophalangeal joint and standing AP views of the talotarsal joints with various degrees of flexion of the foot are used. If only the structural anatomy of the foot is to be evaluated, the recumbent or non-weight-

supporting views are sufficient, easier, and quicker to perform—i.e., the standard AP lateral and oblique views (Figs. 3-3 to 3-6).

SPECIAL RADIOGRAPHIC PROJECTIONS

It may be necessary to evaluate certain areas of interest in the foot. For these, special projections are used. The most common regions of interest are the *individual digits*. To visualize the digits adequately, the examiner must direct his attention to the variable length and direction of the digits. The position of the AP projection is standard, but the lateral projection must be adapted to the requirements of the patient; usually modified oblique projections are necessary. The *middle* and *distal phalanges* can sometimes best be demonstrated with placement of a dental film between the individual digits, extending to the midproximal phalanx; and with flexion of the adjacent toes, the particular area can be seen (Fig. 3-7).

Regardless of the area of interest to be examined, at least two projections at right angles to each other must be obtained.

1. Attention to the *great toe* is given by dorsoplantar (AP) and lateral projections. The AP view is standard, but the lateral projection is usually a modification of the true lateral. To obtain the most satisfactory projection of the

Text continued on p. 50.

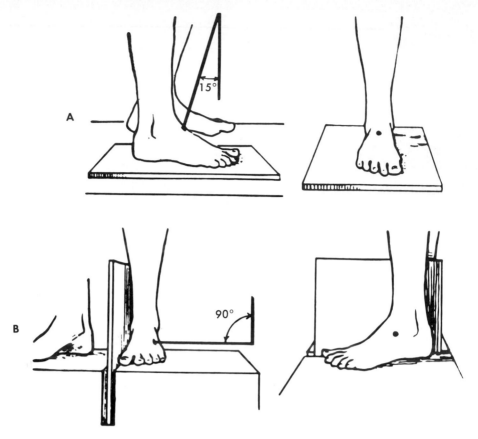

Fig. 3-1. Standard positioning for projections of the foot in weight bearing. **A,** Weight-bearing anteroposterior view. **B,** Weight-bearing lateral view. (From Meschan, I.: Semin. Roentgenol. **5:**327, 1970. By permission of Grune & Stratton, Inc.)

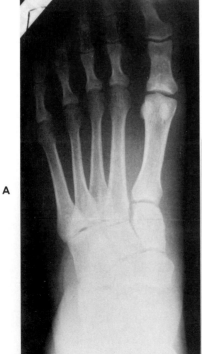

Fig. 3-2. Standard projections of the foot in weight bearing. **A,** Weight-bearing anteroposterior view. **B,** Weight-bearing lateral view.

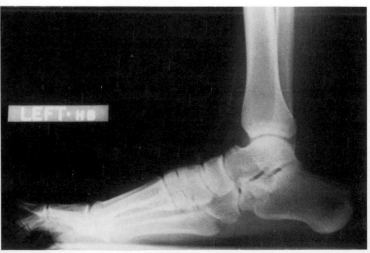

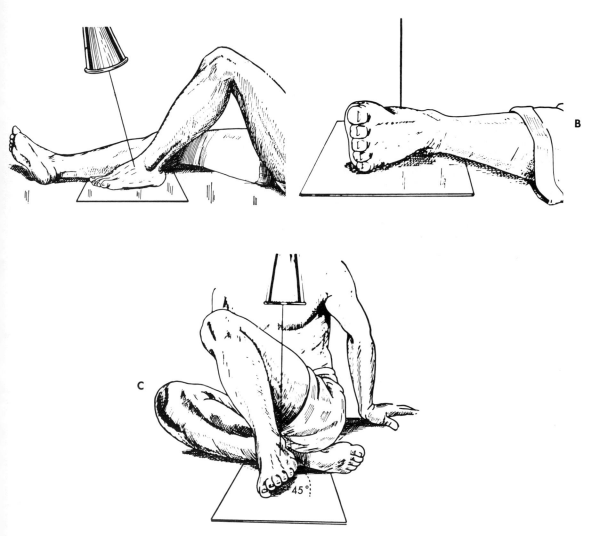

Fig. 3-3. Standard positioning for projections of the foot in recumbency. **A,** Anteroposterior view. **B,** Lateral view. **C,** Oblique view. (From Meschan, I.: An atlas of anatomy basic to radiology, vol. 1, Philadelphia, 1975, W. B. Saunders Co.)

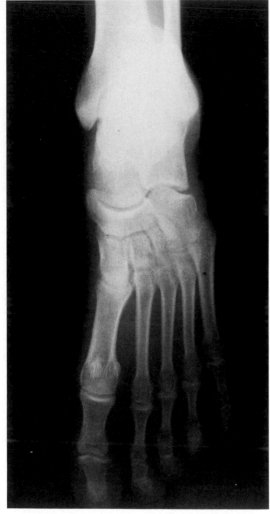

A

Fig. 3-4. A, Standard anteroposterior view of the foot. **B,** Line drawing for anatomic points of interest.

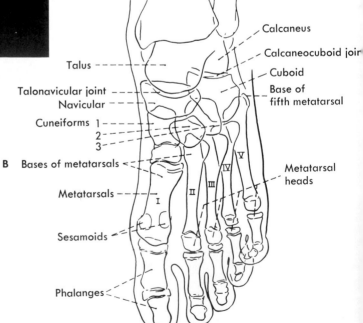

Talus

Talonavicular joint

Navicular

Cuneiforms 1

2

3

B Bases of metatarsals

Metatarsals

Sesamoids

Phalanges

Calcaneus

Calcaneocuboid joint

Cuboid

Base of
fifth metatarsal

Metatarsal
heads

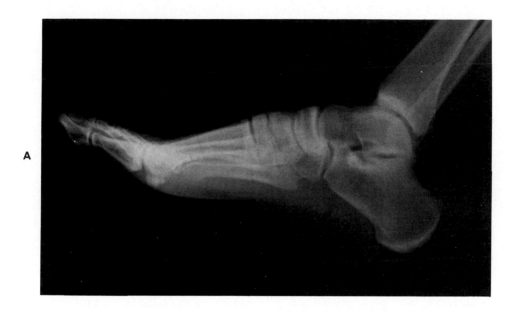

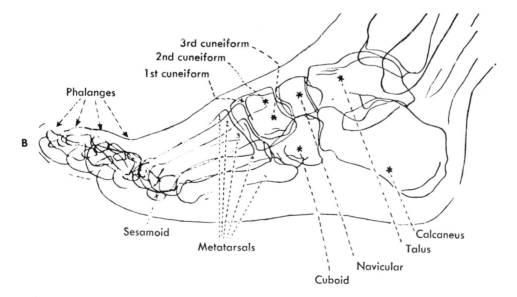

Fig. 3-5. A, Standard lateral view of the foot. **B,** Line drawing for anatomic points of interest.

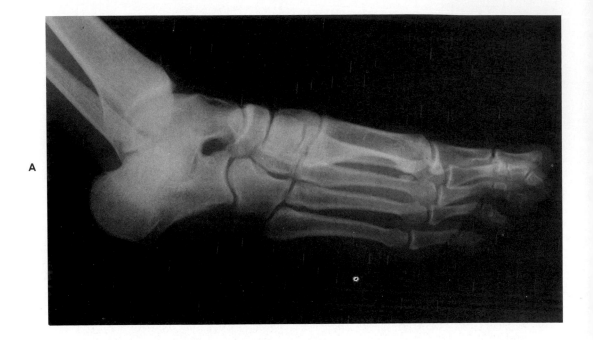

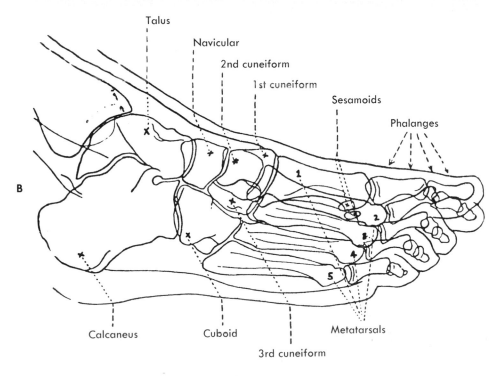

Fig. 3-6. A, Standard oblique view of the foot. **B,** Line drawing for anatomic points of interest.

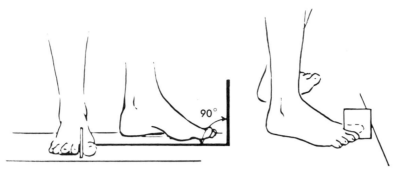

Fig. 3-7. Special projection for individual digits of the foot. Here for the great toe. (From Meschan, I.: Semin. Roentgenol. **5:**327, 1970. By permission of Grune & Stratton, Inc.)

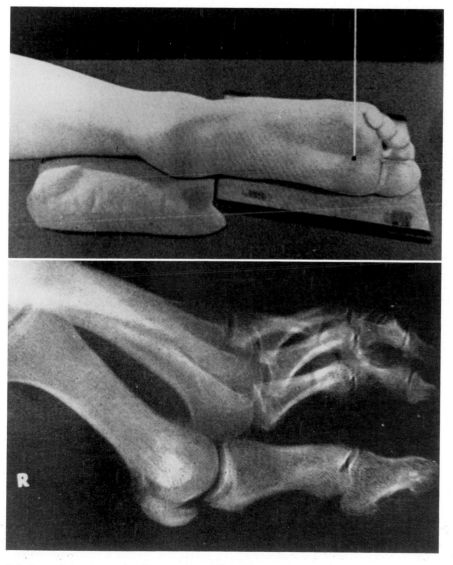

Fig. 3-8. Special projection for the great toe in lateral projection. The entire toe from the base to the distal aspect. (From Clarke, K. C.: Positioning in radiography, ed. 9, London, 1973, Ilford, Ltd.)

great toe, from the base of the metatarsal bone to the distal aspect, the technician should place the foot with the great toe and medial aspect of the leg in contact with the table and the heel raised on a sandbag so the film will be in contact with the foot. In this position the plantar aspect of the foot is obliquely forward relative to the film (Fig. 3-8) and an unobscured lateral of the great toe is obtained. The AP view of the great toe is the basic dorsiplantar projection.

2. Special projections of the *first metatarsophalangeal sesamoid bones* are sometimes necessary. These are gained usually well enough in the standard AP and lateral views; but an axial projection of this area is sometimes diagnostic (Fig. 3-9).

3. To examine the *os calcis* adequately, the physician must employ AP, lateral, oblique, and axial projections. The AP, lateral, and oblique projections are standard but the axial views may be a number of variations. The axial projection generally employed is centered on the plantar aspect between both heels with the tube angled 40° from the vertical and the patient supine with ankles flexed and film placed under the heels (Fig. 3-10). A variation of this is to place the patient prone, ankle extended, with the tube angled 60° from the vertical and the film placed perpendicular to the table against the plantar aspect of the foot. These same projections can be used with the patient laterally positioned when necessary to maintain the position without discomfort. When this is done, attention must be given to maintaining the limbs in horizontal alignment by the use of pads and by making the exposure with the tube in a horizontal projection.

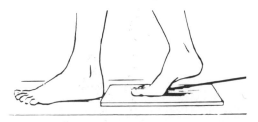

Fig. 3-9. Special axial projection for the ball of the foot and the sesamoids. (From Meschan, I.: Semin. Roentgenol. **5:**327, 1970. By permission of Grune & Stratton, Inc.)

Another method of obtaining the axial projection of the calcaneus is to place the patient in the erect position, provided the patient's state allows such positioning. The patient then stands on the film and the tube is angled 30° from the vertical toward the heels.

4. The *talocalcaneal joints* present special problems in positioning, and a number of variations are necessary to demonstrate the three articular surfaces on the superior aspect of the calcaneus. An oblique projection is required for the posterior talocalcaneal articulation, and in conjunction the middle subtalar articulation with the sustentaculum tali can be shown. An oblique medial projection with varying tube angulation toward the head is used at 40°, 30°, 20°, and 10° (Fig. 3-11). Generally the 40° angulation demonstrates the anterior portion of the posterior talocalcaneal joint; the 30° to 20° angulation demonstrates the articulation between the talus and the sustentaculum tali; the 10° angulation demonstrates the posterior portion of the posterior talocalcaneal articulation. An oblique lateral projection can be used to show the sulcus calcanei. To obtain this view, flexion is maintained at the ankle joint and the limb is rotated laterally until the foot is again at an angle of 45° to the table. It is difficult for the patient to maintain the position for this view, and immobilization is required (Fig. 3-12).

In certain cases even *greater detail of the talocalcaneal joint* is necessary as when evaluating the need for arthrodesis and follow-up postarthrodesis surgery. For such a survey, various oblique lateral views are necessary. From the standard lateral position the limb is rotated toward the film holder at an angle of approximately 40°. In this position the patella is against the table. The center point for the view is the ankle joint with the tube angled 20° caudally (Fig. 3-13). Using this position as the starting point, the examiner then performs a complete survey with a 45° oblique medial and a 10° cephalic tilt view or a 45° oblique lateral and a 15° to 18° cephalic tilt. Finally, he obtains a standard oblique foot view concentrating over the ankle.

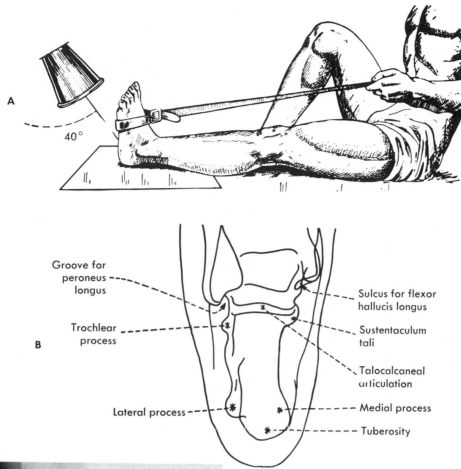

B

Groove for
peroneus
longus

Trochlear
process

Lateral process

Sulcus for flexor
hallucis longus

Sustentaculum
tali

Talocalcaneal
articulation

Medial process

Tuberosity

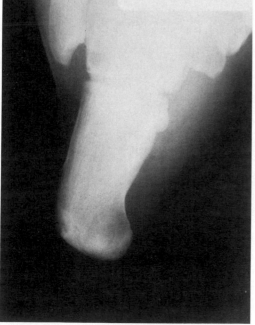

C

Fig. 3-10. Special axial projection for the calcaneus. **A,** Positioning for calcaneus view. **B,** Line drawing for anatomic points of interest. **C,** Axial projection of calcaneus. (From Meschan, I.: An atlas of anatomy basic to radiology, vol. 1, Philadelphia, 1975, W. B. Saunders Co.)

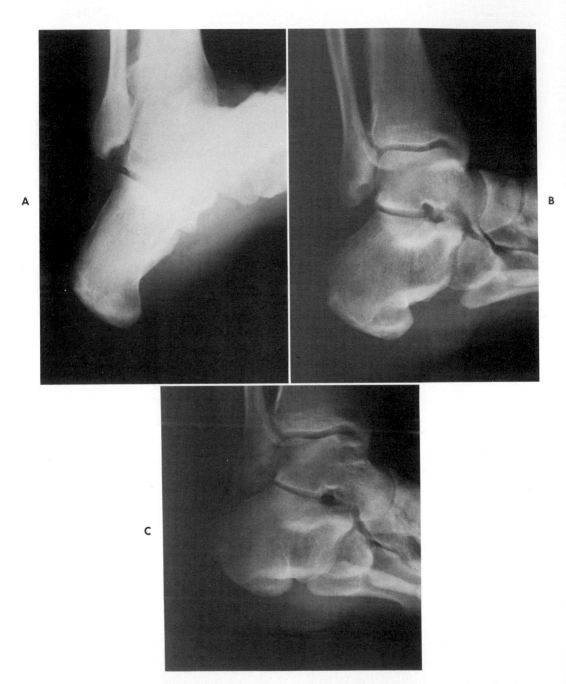

Fig. 3-11. Special projections of the talocalcaneal joints. **A,** 40°; **B,** 20°; **C,** 10°. **D,** Line drawing of anatomic points of interest.

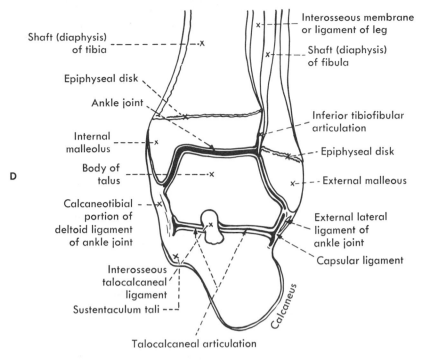

Shaft (diaphysis) of tibia ------- x

Interosseous membrane or ligament of leg

Shaft (diaphysis) of fibula

Epiphyseal disk

Ankle joint

Internal malleolus

Body of talus

Calcaneotibial portion of deltoid ligament of ankle joint

Interosseous talocalcaneal ligament

Sustentaculum tali ---

D

Inferior tibiofibular articulation

Epiphyseal disk

External malleous

External lateral ligament of ankle joint

Capsular ligament

Calcaneus

Talocalcaneal articulation

Fig. 3-11, cont'd. For legend see opposite page.

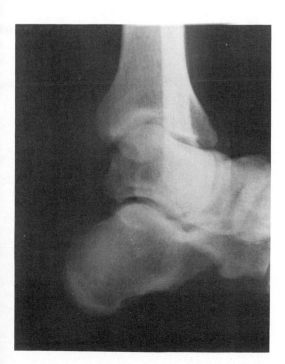

Fig. 3-12. Special projection of the talocalcaneal joint, oblique lateral view, to disclose any dorso-plantar compression and demonstrate the sulcus calcanei.

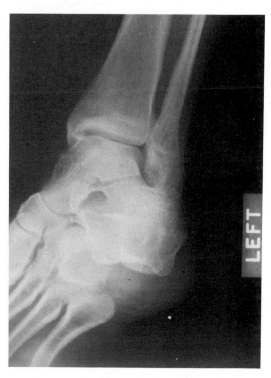

Fig. 3-13. Special projection of the talocalcaneal joint, oblique lateral view with 20° caudal tilt, for arthrodesis evaluation.

SPECIAL TECHNIQUES FOR CHILDREN

Infants and children present problems in examination of the foot, and immobilization becomes critical to obtaining adequate views. Immobilization is achieved with the tape band over the dorsum of the foot and pressure applied to the dorsum and the plantar aspect. Even though the child is lying down, a standing view relationship can be obtained for the dorsal view. This same relationship can be obtained for the lateral view by placing a flat wooden block against the plantar aspect of the foot in the immobilized lateral projection. Each lateral projection is taken separately (Fig. 3-14). It has been noted that simultaneous lateral projections of the feet with the lower extremities in the frogleg position produce distortion and should be avoided.

For the majority of congenital foot deformities in children, the dorsal, plantar, and lateral views of the feet will suffice to demonstrate the abnormality. For congenital clubfoot studies the Kite positions, similar to that illustrated in Fig. 3-14, are sufficient. In general, no attempt should be made to alter the abnormal relationship of the osseous structures when the foot is being placed on the cassette. If stress views are necessary, these can be obtained as a separate series after the baseline views are obtained. In the dorsoplantar projections the central ray is directed vertically to the tarsus, and in the lateral projections the vertical ray is directed vertically to the midtarsal area. These views then demonstrate an anterior talar subluxation and the degree of plantar equinus flexion.

NORMAL AXIAL AND ANGULAR MEASUREMENTS OF THE FOOT

In references to the arches of the feet, the longitudinal and transverse arches have been used in orthopaedic and radiologic literature. Though these are good for "eyeballing the x-ray," a more specific approach should be used in defining alteration of the anatomy of the foot.

The *calcaneal pitch* (Fig. 3-15) is the true measurement of the longitudinal arch of the foot. It is an index of the height of the foot and component structures. By convention it is considered low between 10° and 20°, medium between 20° and 30°, and high if greater than 30°.

Another indicator of the relationship of the os calcis to the surrounding framework is the *Böhlers critical angle*—for defining the integrity of the plantar arch–os calcis–talus relationships (Fig. 3-16). The Böhlers angle for the normal calcaneus is formed between a line tangent to the upper contour of the tuberosity of the calcaneus and a line uniting the highest point of the anterior process with the highest point of the posterior articular surface. This angle normally averages 30° to 35°. Less than

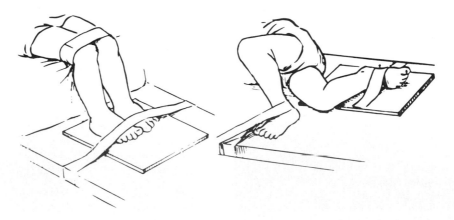

Fig. 3-14. Special technique for anteroposterior and lateral views of the feet in children. (From Meschan, I.: Semin. Roentgenol. **5:**327, 1970. By permission of Grune & Stratton, Inc.)

28° is definitely abnormal and represents poor position.

The *diagonal axis of the talus* (Fig. 3-17) also complements the examination of the talo-calcaneal relationship. Normally it is horizontal or nearly so.

The *midtarsal joint line* is a quick reference line for evaluating the talus–os calcis relationship. It is an unbroken line along the anterior margin of the talus and os calcis in the lateral view (Fig. 3-18). The normal relationship is such that the distal margin of the head of the talus is continuous with the anterior joint surface of the os calcis.

Important anatomic landmarks which are useful in evaluating the structural integrity of the foot include the *sinus tarsi*, the *sustentaculum tali* and *lateral tuberosity* of the os calcis, and the *groove on the cuboid* produced by the *peroneus longus* (Fig. 3-19, *A*).

1. The sinus tarsi is evident as an oval area of decreased density above the sustentaculum tali. This is the transition point between the neck of the talus and the

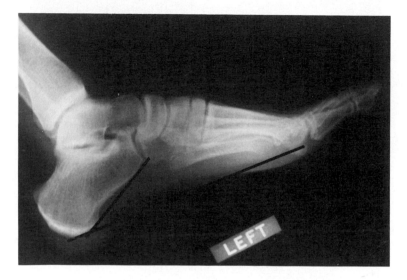

Fig. 3-15. Calcaneal pitch as an index of the height of the foot framework.

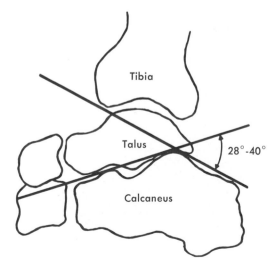

Fig. 3-16. Böhlers critical angle.

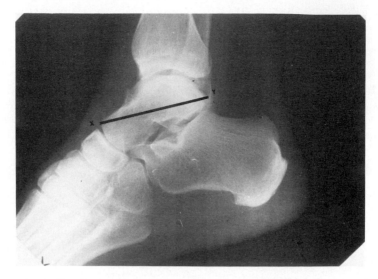

Fig. 3-17. The diagonal axis of the talus is normally horizontal or nearly so.

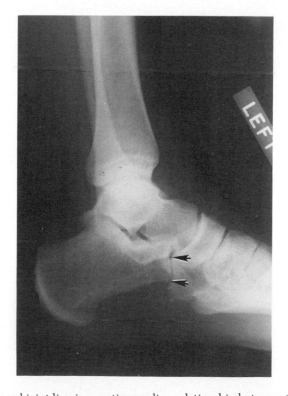

Fig. 3-18. The midtarsal joint line is a continuous line relationship between the os calcis and the cuboid.

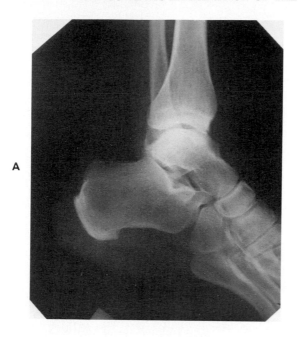

A

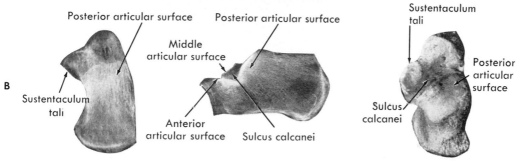

B

Fig. 3-19. Anatomic landmarks in evaluating the structural integrity of the foot. **A,** Lateral projection. **B,** Anatomic specimen. (From Clarke, K. C.: Positioning in radiography, ed. 9, London, 1973, Ilford, Ltd.)

body along the inferior surface. Visualization of the complete sinus tarsi as an unbroken oval indicates a proper framework to the subtalar joint.

2. The sustentaculum tali and the lateral tuberosity of the os calcis should be well seen on the lateral view (Fig. 3-19, *B*) in a normal foot. Inability to see these on a standard lateral projection in proper position may indicate an abnormal eversion of the os calcis.

3. The integrity of the arch of the tarsal bones can be further evaluated by noting the groove on the cuboid produced by the peroneus longus and seen on the standard lateral projection. Its full visualization and normal position also confirm the normal interrelationships of the tarsal bones.

PART TWO

Injuries, diseases, and deformities

4

CONGENITAL FOOT DEFORMITIES

Walter W. Huurman

Congenital deformities, those present at or before birth, may result from inherited (genetic) or extrinsic (environmental) influences. In order to understand the pathophysiology of congenital foot disorders, one must have a working knowledge of prenatal growth and foot development. Only with this as a background can one competently approach treatment of these disorders.

Embryology. The skeletal elements of the foot are blastemal by the fifth gestational week; all are present and begin to chondrify between 5 and 6½ weeks. The cartilage anlage of each individual bone begins to ossify at a particular time in development; the pattern of ossification is quite regular. The metatarsals and distal phalanges demonstrate a periosteal collar of bone at 9 weeks; the calcaneus demonstrates a lateral perichondral area of ossification at 13 weeks; and the talus shows an enchondral center after 8 months. The tarsonavicular does not ossify until the third to fourth postnatal year.

Joints are formed with the appearance of homogeneous interzones—intermediate cell masses—beginning at 6 weeks. The interzones then become fissured (9½ weeks), followed by synovial tissue invasion after 11 weeks.

Differentiation of tendons begins as early as the sixth week, and by the eighth week most ligaments of the foot and ankle are differentiated as cellular condensations (Blechschmidt, 1961).

Hence we see that differentiation of the blastema into elements arranged like those of the adult occurs between 5 and 7 weeks after conception. These elements of the limbs appear generally in a proximal-distal sequence, and the specific time of differentiation has been determined with reasonable accuracy (Gardner et al., 1959). Knowing the time of blastemal insult in the case of a specific skeletal abnormality may guide one to search for less obvious congenital malformations in organs differentiating at precisely the same time (Fuller and Duthie, 1974).

Growth and development. Maturation begins during the fetal period and continues postnatally through adolescence. Extrinsic and intrinsic influences which are separate from the genetic code can affect growth and development of the foot at any time during these years. Because of the unique properties of the growing foot, maturation can adversely affect the developing limb by furthering a pathologic condition. Conversely, the same function of growth can be turned to advantage by the knowledgeable clinician to lessen or eliminate the functional effects of an abnormal condition. In turn, the physician must not forget the potential for reappearance of the

Table 1. Foot deformities associated with other primary problems*

Planovalgus

Achondrogenesis (type 1)
Chromosome 18 trisomy
Chromosome 13 trisomy
Dysplasia epiphysealis hemimelica
Larsen syndrome
Marfan syndrome
Mucopolysaccharidosis IV
Multiple exostoses
Popliteal pterygium syndrome
Ehlers-Danlos syndrome
Bird-headed dwarfism
Chromosome 5P syndrome
Diaphyseal dysplasia

Metatarsus adductus

Acrocephalosyndactyly
Smith-Lemli-Opitz syndrome
Carpenter syndrome
Cerebrohepatorenal syndrome
Clasped thumbs

Equinovarus

Arthrogryposis multiplex congenita
Bird-headed dwarfism
Chromosome 18Q syndrome
Chromosome 13 trisomy
Craniocarpotarsal dystrophy
Diastrophic dwarfism
Ehlers-Danlos syndrome
Larsen syndrome
Oculoauriculovertebral dysplasia
Radioulnar synostosis
Situs inversus viscerum
Stippled epiphyses

Varus

Carpenter syndrome (acrocephalopoly-
    syndactyly, type II)
Hypochondroplasia
Laryngeal web or atresia

Calcaneus

Chromosome 18 trisomy
Chromosome 13 trisomy

Cavus

Mucopolysaccharidosis
Homocystinuria
Carpal tarsal osteolysis and
    chronic progressive glomerulopathy
Phytamic acid storage disease
Urticaria, deafness, and amyloidosis

Polydactyly

Chondroectodermal dysplasia
Chromosome 13 trisomy
Cleft lip without cleft palate
Cleft tongue
Cyclopia
Focal dermal hypoplasia
Orofaciodigital syndrome II
Polysyndactyly
Retinal dysplasia
Stippled epiphyses

Syndactyly

Acrocephalosyndactyly
Aglossia-adactyly
Ankyloblepharon
Chromosome 18P syndrome
Oligophrenia
Familial static ophthalmoplegia
Focal dermal hypoplasia
Holoprosencephalus
Hypertelorism
Laryngeal web or atresia
Lissencephaly
Meckel syndrome
Monosomy G syndrome, type II
Oculomandibulofacial syndrome
Orocraniodigital syndrome
Orofaciodigital syndrome, I and II
Popliteal web syndrome
Retinal dysplasia
Silver syndrome
Smith-Lemli-Opitz syndrome
Stippled epiphyses

*From Zimbler, S., Craig, C., Oh, W. H., and Iacono, V.: Exhibit presented at the annual meeting of the American Academy of Orthopaedic Surgeons, Las Vegas, 1977.

deformity or development of a compensating iatrogenic deformity after treatment, due to the inevitable effect of growth and development.

Genetics in the foot. Congenital anomalies of the foot may be seen as part of a genetic disorder following the Mendelian rules of inheritance. As such, the foot abnormality frequently appears in association with other obvious anomalies or, on occasion, may be the only phenotypic indication of a generalized syndrome. Heritable abnormalities follow either the dominant or the recessive mode of transmission and may be due to influence of an autosome or of the sex chromosome. Furthermore, expressivity may be variable (different effect of the same gene in different individuals) and penetrance may be incomplete (normal-appearing individual with an abnormal gene).

In 1976 Zimbler and Craig presented a large series of birth defect syndromes with identification of the disorder via the abnormalities of the foot. Missing from this list were foot disorders unassociated with other defects. McKusick (1975) lists several isolated anomalies (relative length of the first and second metatarsals, rotational deformity of the fifth toe, number of phalanges contained in the fifth toe) which demonstrate a dominant mode of inheritance.

Review of Zimbler and Craig's (1976) description enables classification of most disorders according to the mode of inheritance (Table 1). Some (Silver syndrome) have yet to show a clear genetic code but quite possibly will be classified in the future (Blechschmidt, 1961). For problems more specifically dealt with in the text, genetics are discussed under the individual disorder.

TALIPES DEFORMITIES

Talipes, derived from the Latin *talus* (ankle bone) and *pes* (foot), is a term properly describing any congenital foot deformity. Congenital hindfoot deformities are correctly designated talipes, followed by a descriptive term for the morbid anatomy. A plantar-flexed hindfoot therefore is talipes equinus; if dorsiflexed, talipes calcaneus; if inverted,

talipes varus; and when everted, talipes valgus.

Currently the simple contraction *talipes* is used in reference to the classic clubfoot deformity. Clinically the true clubfoot presents with a triad of (1) midfoot and forefoot adductus, (2) hindfoot varus, and (3) heel equinus. Anatomically, then, talipes equinovarus is the appropriate descriptive term and usage of simple "talipes" should probably be avoided.

Clubfoot (talipes equinovarus)

A relatively common malformation, and certainly the continuing subject of heated discussion among experts, clubfoot remains an unsolved and enigmatic congenital foot deformity. Orthopaedic literature abounds with articles on the topic and methods of treatment which are nearly as numerous as the number of authors. Despite this vast experience, the etiology remains obscure and the single best form of treatment is elusive.*

Incidence. The commonly accepted incidence in the general population is approximately 1 per 1,000 births. Wynne-Davies (1964) notes the incidence to be 1.24 per 1,000; when broken down by sex, the male incidence is 1.62 per 1,000 births and the female 0.8 per 1,000. This represents a distinct 2.17 to 1 predominance of male over female. There are strong hereditary factors active; and if one child in a family has the deformity, the incidence among siblings rises to 2.9 per 100 or 1 in every 35 births. If the index patient is female, the incidence among male siblings rises to 1 in 16; however, if the index patient is male, there appears to be no significant increase in the 1 per 35 sibling incidence. Although there may be a genetic factor involved, the specific Mendelian characteristics with regard to sex linkage, dominance or recessiveness, etc. have not been worked out; but penetrance does appear to be variable.

---

*As Lloyd-Roberts (1964) has knowingly stated: "This is an undeniably disheartening state of affairs which is in no way redeemed by the knowledge that little or no improvement has occurred since Brockman's review was published 35 years ago."

Pathologic anatomy. Despite the fact that since ancient times clubfoot has been recognized as a handicapping deformity, relatively few anatomic studies have been published. Careful review of most writings reveals that dissections were usually performed on a fetus or infant who also had other significant congenital malformations.

The anatomic findings in the deformed foot of a stillborn anencephalic, myelodysplastic, or fetus with other congenital malformations potentially affecting foot development should not be used as the anatomic basis for discussion of idiopathic clubfoot. Prior to the excellent studies of Irani and Sherman in 1963, no satisfactory series of dissections on the isolated idiopathic deformity have been reported. Although Settle (1963) confirmed the findings of Irani and Sherman later the same year, fourteen of his sixteen specimens had other significant deformities. Waisbrod, in 1973, contributed the study of eight additional idiopathic clubfeet occurring without any other significant congenital anomaly. At the present time these studies provide the basis for our knowledge of the pathologic anatomy.

The reason for the rather sparse information seems clear: isolated clubfoot deformity is not a cause of fetal or infant mortality and, hence, specimens are not readily available for study. Nonetheless, those idiopathic clubfeet studied have had rather constant findings. The primary deformity seems to be in the neck and head of the talus: the neck foreshortened to absent, medially deviated, and the articular surface of the head inclined plantarward. Other bony and soft tissue abnormalities which may be present seem to be adaptive to this primary talar deformity.

The normal talar neck has an angle of incidence with its body of 150° to 155° (Paturet, 1951; Gardner, 1956). Irani and Sherman (1963) found in their dissected specimens an angle varying between 115° and 135°. Other than adaptive changes resulting from this primary deformity, the muscles, tendons, and neurovascular and other osseous structures of the foot and leg seemed to be basically normal.

Because of plantarward declination of the talar neck, a portion of the body of the talus lies anterior in the ankle mortise. This pulls the hindfoot into equinus and causes developmental contracture of both ankle and subtalar joint capsules as well as atrophy and contracture of the triceps surae (Wiley, 1959). Adaptive changes are present in the osseous structure of the talus itself. The articulations of the subtalar joint are mildly deformed, the medially and plantar-deviated head of the talus articulating with the anteromedial portion of the calcaneus. Settle (1963) found the subtalar joints to be slanted somewhat medially with a single large articular facet. The effect of this was to push the calcaneus into varus, widening the sinus tarsi and bringing the tendo Achillis insertion medial to the midline axis. Medial displacement of the tendo Achillis causes its line of pull to promote further hindfoot varus (Fried, 1959) (Fig. 4-1).

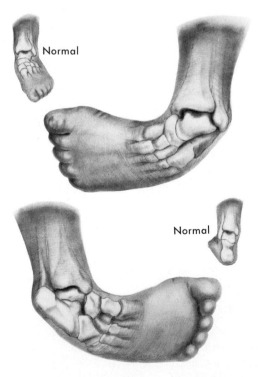

Fig. 4-1. Pathologic anatomy of clubfoot. The medially and plantar-deviated talar neck is the primary deformity; medial deviation of the navicular and hindfoot varus and equinus are adaptive. (From Settle, G. W.: Surg. **45A:**1341, 1963.)

The midfoot, likewise, adapts to changes in the head and neck of the talus. The navicular is smaller than normal and medially dislocated (Brockman, 1930; Ponseti and Smoley, 1963). This medial dislocation, however, is apparent only insofar as the navicular articulates properly with the talar head, covering its articular surface (Settle, 1963; Waisbrod, 1973). True, the navicular is deviated medially relative to the longitudinal axis of the talar body; but this is because the anterior talus is inclined medially and plantarward. On occasion, depending upon the angle of incidence of the talar neck, the navicular may be so far swung around that its medial margin articulates with the medial malleolus. The remainder of the midfoot seems to follow the talar neck; the cuboid is actually displaced slightly beneath the third cuneiform and rotated toward the medial side of its normal articulation with the calcaneus. The forefoot follows the varus and adducted contour of the midfoot, completing the clinical equinovarus appearance.

If the talar deformity is severe, all adaptive changes are accentuated. The medial border of the calcaneus may be concave, the lateral column of the foot elongated, and the medial column foreshortened. With the foot swung around into equinovarus, ligamentous and capsular structures on the posterior and medial side eventually become foreshortened, thickened, and quite rigid. This includes capsules of the ankle, subtalar, talonavicular, and naviculocuneiform joints. Furthermore, the deltoid and talocalcaneal interosseous ligaments similarly become contracted. The tendinous structures (tibialis posterior, tibialis anterior, tendo Achillis), if allowed to come into opposition with deformed osseous structures, may adhere to them. This apparent abnormality of tendon insertion is adaptive and secondary to the distorted hindfoot and midfoot. When dissected, the normal insertion of these tendinous structures is always present.

While treating the idiopathic clubfoot, the physician must constantly keep in mind the pathologic anatomy and dynamics of the growing foot. Successful treatment relies primarily on the ability of growing osseous structures to adapt and alter their shape in response to the influence of extrinsic force.

Etiology. Because the literature contains no report of an idiopathic clubfoot dissection in a fetus under 7 weeks of gestation, it has not been established whether the deformity is blastemal in origin or arises during the embryonic period. However, the presence of significantly fewer vessels in the talar neck of a fetal clubfoot, with marked disorganization of these vessels, seems to indicate that the deformity is probably blastemal in origin (Waisbrod, 1973).

Bohm (1929) described four stages of normal fetal foot positioning, proceeding from a stance of equinovarus immediately after the embryonic period and progressing through gradual supination, ankle dorsiflexion, and finally, by the fourth month, pronation. A partial arrest of development during the blastemal or early embryonic stage may well be the insult causing the deformity recognized at birth.

Radiographic evaluation. Because the osseous structures of the infant foot are small, it is nearly impossible to ascertain their true anatomic relationship by simple clinical examination. Indeed, the rather abundant heel fat pad can easily hide a great deal of hindfoot equinus. Likewise, the absence of soft tissue definition can make even a moderate amount of hindfoot varus clinically difficult to appreciate. For this reason, radiographic evaluation performed initially and intermittently during the course of treatment is necessary to adequately assess correction.

Standard radiographic views should be obtained in AP and lateral projections. The AP view is obtained with the plantar surface flat on the film cassette in a pseudostanding position. The ankle should be slightly plantar flexed and the x-ray tube caudally directed 30°. This positioning will permit visualization of the hindfoot and allow accurate measurement of the talocalcaneal (Kite's) angle (Kite, 1930) (Fig. 4-2). The lateral view should likewise be obtained in a pseudostanding position with the ankle as near neutral as possible. If the film cassette is aligned parallel with the lateral border of the foot, an oblique view of

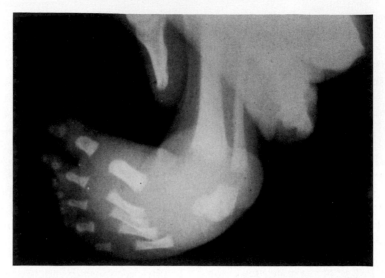

Fig. 4-2. AP view of a clubfoot in a neonate. Note the reduction in Kite's angle; the talus is nearly parallel with the calcaneus. Neither of the hindfoot structures aligns with the forefoot.

the hindfoot will result and the talus will spuriously appear to be flat topped and the fibula displaced posteriorly (Swann et al., 1969). An accurate lateral is obtained when the hindfoot is parallel with the cassette, and in the true projection the talus is recognized as having a normal dorsally convex articular surface.

In the AP view the longitudinal axis of the normal talus aligns well with a similar axis of the first metatarsal and the longitudinal axis of the calcaneus with the fifth metatarsal. These two axes converge posteriorly, forming Kite's angle (normally 20° to 40°). With hindfoot varus the calcaneus is rotated beneath the talus, plantar flexed, and, if the deformity is severe, medially bowed. This causes a decrease of Kite's angle, occasionally to 0°. With correction of hindfoot varus, the abnormal talocalcaneal relationship reverses and the calcaneus rotates laterally and everts. Without a normal talocalcaneal angle in the AP projection, the hindfoot varus has not been fully corrected.

In the lateral view the talocalcaneal angle is derived from a line drawn through the longitudinal axis of the talus at the midpoint of the talus and a second converging line drawn along the plantar surface of the calcaneus. This angle is not static and in the normal foot will decrease with plantar flexion and increase

with dorsiflexion. In the normal standing lateral projection the talocalcaneal angle measures between 35° and 50° (Heywood, 1964). A distinct overlap of the anterosuperior margin of the calcaneus on the anteroinferior margin of the talus is normally present. With clubfoot deformity and hindfoot varus, the normal lateral talocalcaneal angle is reduced and parallelism exists between the two structures. Furthermore, relatively little change in the angle occurs with dorsiflexion and plantar flexion (Fig. 4-3).

Careful evaluation of the calcaneotibial relationship will demonstrate hindfoot equinus uncorrected with forced dorsiflexion. The ossific nucleus of the talus is displaced anteriorly because of the equinus deformity and, when severe, the posterior calcaneus nearly approximates the posterior malleolus.

Forefoot deformity is seen in both anteroposterior and lateral projections. On the AP projection both adduction and inversion with shortening of the medial column and lengthening of the lateral column are present. Viewed laterally, the plantar soft tissue structures may be foreshortened and cause forefoot equinus.

Until all of the radiographic alterations have returned to normal, one cannot be satisfied that the clubfoot deformity has been cor-

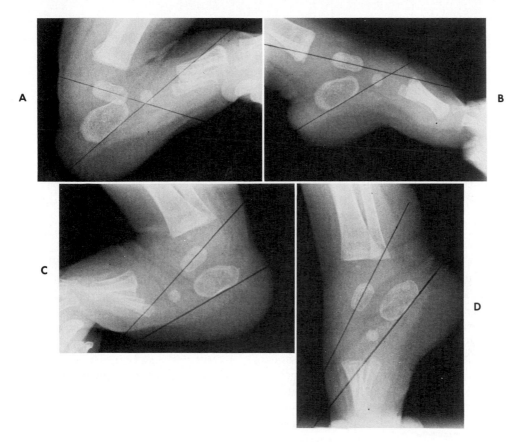

Fig. 4-3. Clubfoot in a 3-month-old child. **A** and **B,** Stress dorsiflexion–plantar flexion views of the normal foot. On stress dorsiflexion the lateral talocalcaneal angle measures 45°; on stress plantar flexion, 58°. Note the overlap of the anteroinferior talus and anterosuperior calcaneus on dorsiflexion. **C** and **D,** Stress dorsiflexion–plantar flexion lateral views of the opposite clubfoot. Despite stress, the talocalcaneal angle is reduced and remains unchanged at 17°. On dorsiflexion the calcaneus remains in equinus and the talus does not overlap the anterior process of the os calcis.

rected. Active treatment should continue until talocalcaneal parallelism is reversed in both AP and lateral views and until the stress plantar flexion–dorsiflexion radiographs demonstrate unlocking of the subtalar articulation with adequate dorsiflexion of the hindfoot. The standing lateral radiograph should present a normal plantigrade appearance with no hindfoot equinus, cavus deformity, or break of the midfoot.

Treatment. As each color has many shades and hues, so are there many degrees of clubfoot deformity. Treatment necessary to bring the foot to a plantigrade longitudinally aligned posture depends on the degree of deformity present. Each foot must be carefully examined, both clinically and radiographically, and the treatment program must be designed to meet the demands of the deformity present.

Waisbrod (1973), in studying his eight specimens, found the response to manual manipulation dependent upon the degree of deformity present in the talar neck. In his series he was able to passively correct three feet and found, on dissection, the talar neck in each of these to have an angle in excess of 150° with the body. It is quite likely that the apparent clubfoot which responds rapidly and readily to manipulation and casting has, in fact, little deformity in the talar neck; the initial clinical presentation may be more a postural problem. This is not to ignore these feet or to downgrade the importance of early active treatment, for the postural deformity, if persistent, can result in secondary structural change. A rather large number of clubfeet belong in the postural deformity category; and if they are treated early (from day of birth), secondary resistant changes do not have an opportunity to develop. The longer one waits before initiating treatment, the more significant and resistant are the secondary structural changes. Active treatment should begin as soon after birth as possible.

If plantar and medial inclination of the foreshortened distal talus exists to any degree, the osseous structures must be placed in an aligned position and held there during the formative years of growth and development for the foot to anatomically permit normal ambulation and normal footwear. To align the foot with the extremity may require dividing secondarily shortened and thickened capsules and ligaments as well as lengthening secondarily abbreviated muscle-tendon units (Lowe and Hannon, 1973). One must always remember that the talar neck deformity persists but may be altered over a period of time by utilization of Wolff's law. Holding the foot in a corrected position during growth and development will create adaptive changes in the distal talus (Denham, 1967), reverting it to near normal. However, it will continue to have a short neck with a somewhat flattened head, the navicular and talar body may continue to be smaller than normal, and, indeed, the entire foot and calf will probably never match the opposite member in size. If, after alignment of the foot is obtained by either serial casting or soft tissue release, the foot is not held in the corrected position for a significant period of growth and development, the neck of the talus will continue to deviate medially and the navicular and calcaneus will gradually realign with the abnormal talar neck, the hindfoot will drift back into varus and equinus, and the forefoot into cavus and adduction.

It would therefore seem reasonable that, once alignment is obtained and reasonably stable, the foot should be held in position day and night for a moderate period of time and subsequently at night alone through at least the second period of accelerated growth and development (7 to 8 years of age). Anything less may lead to reappearance of the deformity.

Treatment at birth. The foot of a neonate with talipes equinovarus deformity is oftentimes no larger than the thumb of the treating physician. This small structure on careful examination is frequently quite supple.

Longitudinal traction applied at the distal first through third metatarsals with the heel plantar flexed will result in gradual formation of a dimple over the superolateral aspect of the midfoot and represents gradual lateral subluxation of the navicular on the medially deviated talar head as the medial column elongates with traction. The dimple or void develops at the lateral junction of the talar neck with the talar body (Fig. 4-4). Lateral subluxation of the midfoot produces normal forefoot alignment with the tibia and, if held in this position, will allow soft tissue structures of the medial column to elongate and stretch. With traction on the forefoot, the physician stretches the tightened deltoid and talocalcaneal interosseous ligaments by pushing the calcaneus into eversion with thumb and forefinger of the opposite hand. Forceful attempts at dorsiflexing the ankle against tightened posterior ligaments will result in a nutcracker effect (Keim and Ritchie, 1964; Dunn and Samuelson, 1974), with the contracted posterior structures acting like a hinge and the talar body within the mortise like the fulcrum. To prevent a longitudinal break and development of a rocker-bottom deformity, the physician should not attempt forceful ankle dorsiflexion.

After manipulation the foot can be held in its realigned position by application of a corrective cast or, as is my preference, adhesive strapping. The taping technique, a modification of the Jones method, is preferred because of the difficulty encountered in attempting to apply a corrective cast with

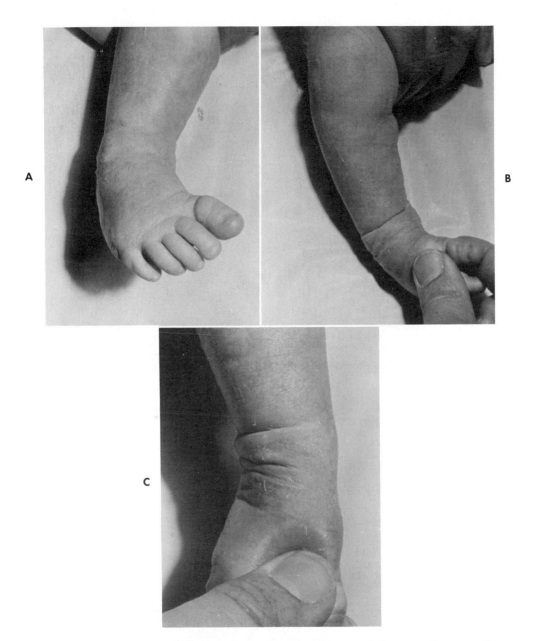

Fig. 4-4. Neonatal clubfoot deformity. **A,** Moderate equinovarus deformity. This responds to traction on the medial metatarsal heads, **B,** by developing a recess at the lateral border of the talar neck, **C,** as the navicular and forefoot are brought into alignment with the tibia. It represents lateral subluxation of the midfoot on the medially deviated head of the talus.

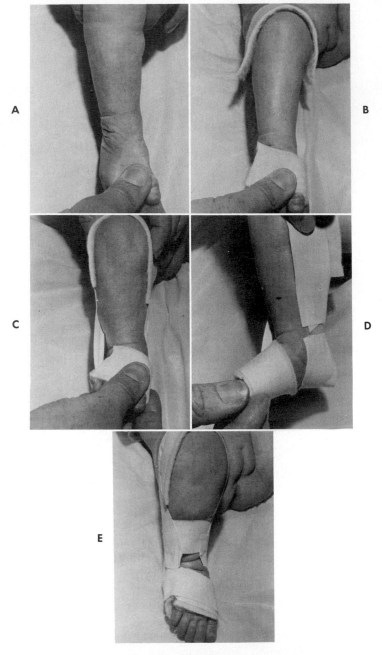

Fig. 4-5. Adhesive strapping of the neonatal clubfoot **A,** Gentle traction for several minutes applied to the medial metatarsal heads aligns the foot with the leg. Note the recess at the lateral margin of the talar neck. **B,** The areas to be covered by tape are painted with tincture of benzoin. A 1¼-inch-wide strip of orthopaedic felt covers the distal thigh, and a second strip surrounds the forefoot. **C,** A long strip of 1-inch adhesive tape encircles the foot and courses up the lateral leg, over the distal thigh (knee flexed), and three fourths of the way down the medial leg. **D,** A second long strip of tape beginning just at the medial malleolus runs under the calcaneus, up the lateral leg, over the distal thigh, and down the medial leg (overlying the initial tape). **E,** Two short anchoring strips encircle the distal leg and foot. The foot is held in a corrected position. Active and passive stretching exercises are still possible.

appropriately placed pressure points on the extremely small foot of a neonate. Furthermore, taping the newborn foot permits dynamic and passive stretching exercises during the entire time of treatment, thereby avoiding progressive joint stiffness and further muscle atrophy (Fig. 4-5).

Tape application

1. After manipulation and reduction of the clubfoot deformity and with traction applied to the distal first through third metatarsals by an assistant, apply tincture of benzoin to the foot, leg, and distal thigh in the areas to be covered by tape.

2. Place a piece of felt about 1¼ inches wide over the distal thigh with the knee flexed 90°, the free ends extending 1½ inches down the medial and lateral aspects of the leg.

3. Wrap a piece of felt of similar width about the forefoot, the free ends meeting on the lateral border of the foot.

4. At this point, or earlier, it is most helpful to follow Dr. Kite's suggestion: Give the baby a bottle in an attempt to promote muscle relaxation. Mother may play an active role in the treatment by assisting with this task.

5. Apply the first strip of tape, a long one, over the felt surrounding the forefoot. Begin at the lateral plantar margin, course medially over the dorsum of the foot, make the turn around the medial border, continue laterally on the plantar surface, and complete the circle about the foot. At all times be sure the assistant maintains the foot in a corrected position. Continue the strip up the lateral border of the leg (it tends to bowstring a bit at the ankle) over the felt draped on the distal thigh (the knee must be flexed 90°) and halfway down the medial side of the leg. This initial strip serves to align the forefoot, correcting the adductus and supination

6. Use the second long strip to correct heel varus and equinus. Begin just below the medial malleolus (do not overlap or connect with the end of the first strip), course beneath the heel medial to lateral, and push the calcaneus out of varus. Make sure this strip is no further distal than the cuboid. Continue up the lateral leg, overlying for the most part the first applied strip, over the distal thigh felt and

again down the medial leg. Final corrected position has now been accomplished.

7. The last two strips of tape, 4 to 6 inches in length, are used to anchor the longer pieces. With the first, circle the distal leg above the malleoli. This will tend to contain (but not eliminate) the bowstringing. Encircle the foot with the second, overlapping the felt and previously applied adductus correcting tape. If necessary, you can use a small strip to connect the skin of the distal thigh to the tape coursing over the knee to keep the latter from slipping off the thigh.

During the immediate postnatal period the strapping is changed daily. Nurses and the mother are encouraged to exercise and stretch the foot frequently during the day; and after leaving the hospital, the mother is instructed to perform stretching exercises with each diaper change. After discharge, usually on the third or fourth postdelivery day, the tape is changed in the physician's office at least twice weekly for the first 3 to 4 weeks. During this period of rapid growth and development, plantigrade alignment and progressive correction are encouraged by the corrective taping and stretching. If the plantar deviation of the talar neck is not too severe, the foot can be nearly or completely corrected by just the adhesive strapping for a period of 2 to 3 months. By 12 weeks of age, the foot is usually large enough to allow application of a corrective cast with discretely applied pressure points (Fig. 4-6). If radiographs demonstrate adequate dorsiflexion of the hindfoot with unlocking of the subtalar joint and a normal Kite's angle, the foot may be merely held in the corrected position by plaster until large enough to be fitted with a shoe.

Despite the fact that separate centers of ossification appear at radiographic examination to have normal relationships, you must remember that the unossified anterior talus is still directed medially and plantarward and, unless the foot is held in a corrected position, the forefoot will realign itself with the maldirected anterior talus. All three components of the deformity—hindfoot equinus, inversion, and forefoot adduction-suppination—will recur. For this reason, once radiographic evi-

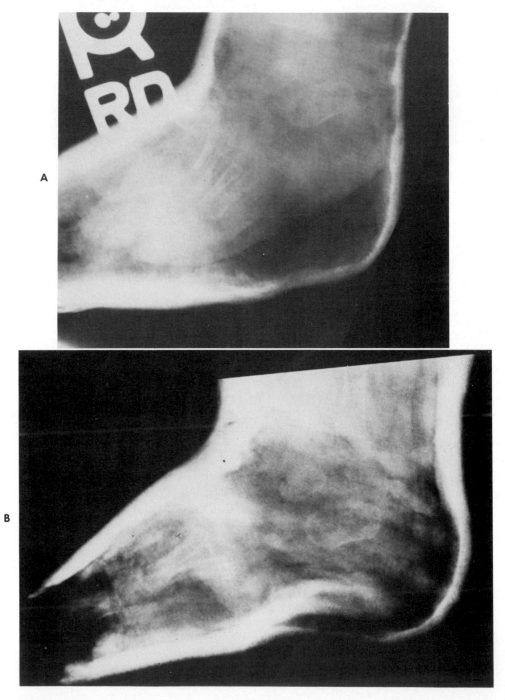

Fig. 4-6. A, Poorly molded cast. Externally it gives the impression of clubfoot correction; however, a radiograph demonstrates the loose fit and the persistent hindfoot equinus and varus. Note the absence of molding beneath the calcaneocuboid joint and behind the tendo Achillis. B, With better molding the foot is locked in position and will not slide up into the cast. The calcaneocuboid joint is further posterior than would be clinically suspected. An occasional radiographic check to verify placement of the mold is advisable.

dence of full correction has been obtained, the foot must be held in the corrected position with either plaster or a well-fitting brace. The device is worn day and night until walking age has been reached (10 to 12 months). As long as the radiograph continues to show adequate correction of the deformity, the child may then wear the brace at night only.

With single foot involvement a Phelps brace with a medial upright lateral valgus—inducing T-strap and 90° downstop is recommended. A plastic window at the counter of the shoe will allow the mother to visualize the heel of the child as it is placed in the shoe, assuring proper heel seating. A good practice is to obtain lateral radiographs in the brace to be sure the hindfoot has not persisted in equinus. If both feet are under treatment, bilateral Phelps braces are joined by a Denis-Browne bar bent into some valgus.

Surgical treatment. When treatment is begun at birth, the foot is usually supple enough to obtain at least some correction of the secondary deformity. Depending upon the severity of the primary talar deformity, a time usually arises at about 3 or 4 months of age when further correction is not possible by nonoperative means.

Surgery on an infant's foot is technically demanding because of the small structures being dealt with. Violation of any articular cartilage during an operative procedure can, and frequently does, result in permanent stiffness and deformity. Surgery should be delayed until it can safely be performed without damaging articular cartilage and until tendons, nerves, and vascular structures can be readily identified. Even at 3 to 4 months of age, the foot is often so small that the use of magnifying loupes during surgery is recommended.

The most frequent deformities remaining after conservative treatment are hindfoot varus and equinus. Taping, stretching, and casting usually correct the forefoot adduction-supination. Surgical release of posterior and posteromedial soft tissue structures will often allow completion of the correction (Fig. 4-7).

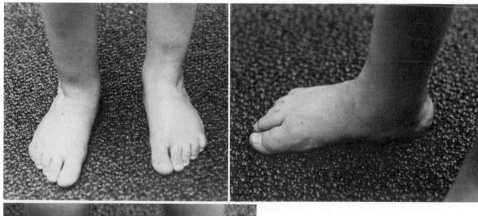

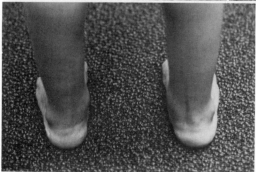

Fig. 4-7. Appearance of bilateral clubfeet at 3½ years of age treated by adhesive strapping until 3 months of age, corrective casts until 6 months, and then a posteromedial release; continued in casts until 11 months of age, and followed with night braces.

Although the tendo Achillis may appear to be the primary impediment to equinus correction, this is rarely the case. In a true clubfoot, the entire posterior capsule and posterior ligamentous structures are contracted and thickened (Smith, 1976). Therefore subcutaneous tenotomy of the tendo Achillis should rarely be performed without a formal division of the remaining resistent posterior soft tissues.

Posteromedial release

1. Make a longitudinal skin incision medial to the tendo Achillis, extending from the musculotendinous junction to the plantar margin of the calcaneus.

2. Longitudinally open the sheath and divide the tendo Achillis, bisecting it in the sagittal plane. Complete the tenotomy by freeing its lateral half proximally at the musculotendinous junction and its medial half distally at the insertion into the calcaneal tuberosity. When repaired, this will decrease the tendency for the triceps to invert the heel on plantar flexion.

3. Critical evaluation of dorsiflexion will usually demonstrate little correction of equinus after heel cord tenotomy. Identify the flexor hallucis longus deep to the tendo Achillis. Place the foot in plantar flexion and identify and medially retract the flexor digitorum longus, posterior tibial tendons, and neurovascular bundle, exposing the posterior surface of the tibia.

4. Make a longitudinal incision in the posterior retinaculum and dense ankle capsule; this allows identification of the joint without injury to the distal tibial epiphysis. With care and using small scissors, transversely divide the entire posterior capsule. Division should be carried laterally as far as the fibular malleolus. A rather dense structure, the calcaneofibular ligament, will be encountered coursing from the posterior aspect of the lateral malleolus to the calcaneus; this should be divided.

5. Continue the release medially and include the posterior fibers of the deltoid ligament; protect the neurovascular contents of the tarsal tunnel. Lloyd-Roberts (1964) extends the posteromedial release distally, stripping the abductor hallucis from its calcaneal origin.

6. Dorsiflex the foot to bring the articular surface of the talar dome into view. Divide the posterior inferior tibiofibular ligament.

7. Identify the subtalar joint in the same manner as done for the ankle: begin with a longitudinal incision and, after the joint space is visualized, divide its posterior capsule from the lateral malleolus to the midportion of the medial malleolus.

8. Intraoperative stress radiographs should demonstrate correction of both equinus and varus. If the posterior tibial tendon appears tight, lengthen it near its musculotendinous junction.

9. Reapproximate the tendo Achillis by placing two or three sutures in its raw surface. Hold the ankle at neutral; note that lengthening of ¾ to 1¼ inches has been accomplished.

10. Insert a smooth K-wire transversely through the posterior calcaneus, medial to lateral. Close the skin with subcuticular suture or Steri-Strips. Apply a long-leg cast with the pin incorporated; do not attempt maximum correction until the wound has healed.

11. Two weeks later, change the cast under anesthesia and, using the calcaneal pin, obtain maximum correction of hindfoot equinus and varus. Leave the second cast on for 6 weeks; remove the K-wire 8 weeks postoperatively.

When severe medial and plantar deviation of the talar neck exists, forefoot correction is occasionally not possible by conservative means. In such an instance an extended posterior and medial release according to the method of Turco (1971, 1975) is recommended, again with precision by an experienced surgeon using iris scissors and with the assistance of magnification if necessary to avoid damage to articular cartilage. For this reason the extended release should probably be delayed until at least 6 months of age, when the osseous structures have reached a size that makes identification of the small joints more certain. After the extended release, postoperative casting in a manner similar to the method just described is carried out and bracing instituted *as* the child nears walking age. If the child is older when the extended release procedure is first performed, postoperative casting should be continued for at least 4 to 6 months. Night bracing is recommended until the child has passed through the second growth spurt (usually age 7 to 8).

Uncorrected or residual clubfoot in older child. After the age of 2 years, clubfoot correction by soft tissue release alone becomes more difficult. By the time the child is 4, some form of bony reconstruction is usually necessary. The goal in these late cases is not to create a normal foot but rather to convert the existing deformity to one which is plantigrade and allows normal shoe wear.

Many procedures have been described, including metatarsal osteotomy, lateral wedge resection of the tarsus, excochleation of the cuboid (Johanning, 1958), fusion of the calcaneocuboid joint (the Dilwyn-Evans procedure) (Evans, 1961; Abrams, 1969), calcaneal osteotomy after the method of Dwyer (Dwyer, 1963; Fisher and Schaffer, 1970), and ultimately triple arthrodesis. Each of these procedures has its place in the armamentarium of reconstructive clubfoot surgery, and each case must be individually evaluated to select the appropriate form of treatment.

Metatarsus adductus and metatarsus varus

Much confusion surrounds the terminology of these deformities. Many authors use the words adductus and varus interchangeably; to additionally confuse the issue, metatarsus adductus varus has been further delineated as a separate entity (Lloyd-Roberts and Clark, 1973). As noted in earlier editions, the distinction may be academic and the difference merely a matter of degree.

If we assume the two entities metatarsus adductus and metatarsus varus are merely variations in degree of the same deformity, metatarsus varus is the more involved of the two (Kite, 1950). Metatarsus adductus varus is perhaps the severest grade of the deformity. The most important thing to recognize is that the hindfoot is in neither equinus nor varus (Peabody and Muro, 1933). In the mildest form of the problem, metatarsus adductus, little or no supination persists with weight bearing.* Today it appears at least ten times as frequently as clubfoot deformity (Wynne-Davies, 1964), is quite supple, and can be

---

*Just after the turn of the century, the problem was not widely recognized—only four cases noted among 5,000 patients in Hoffa's clinic (Helbing, 1905).

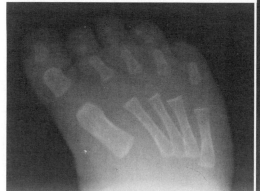
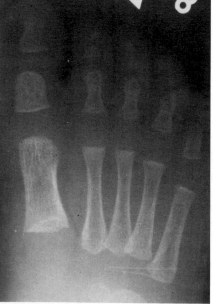

Fig. 4-8. Metatarsus adductus. **A,** At 3 months of age; convexity of the lateral border of the foot. The lateral three metatarsals have a slight medial bow, with the actual inturning (adductus) greatest in the first metatarsal and least in the fifth. **B,** Standing radiograph at age 18 months; treated with serial casting for 8 weeks beginning at 3 months of age.

corrected easily with passive stretching and corrective immobilization (Fig. 4-8).

As the degree of deformity progresses, metatarsus varus occurs and in this case the forefoot demonstrates supination as well as adduction with weight bearing. Metatarsus varus tends to be hereditary (Kite, 1967), is a more resistant problem, and more frequently requires surgical intervention.

Anatomy. In metatarsus adductus or varus the head of the talus is directed inward but not plantarward as in clubfoot deformity. No hindfoot equinus is present; but the hallmark of the problem, incurving of the lateral border of the foot, is noted. The metatarsal shafts are deviated medially, the deviation increasing from lateral to medial. Actual incurving of the lateral metatarsal diaphyses may occur as the child grows. The first metatarsal is straight, but at the metatarsal base the first cuneiform articulates with its mesial aspect. Generally the cuneiforms are rotated into varus—each, however, remaining lateral to the navicular. The heel is never in varus, either remaining neutral or deviating into valgus. With weight bearing the lateral border of the foot is in contact with the ground and the medial border is elevated.

In the absence of hindfoot varus or equinus, Kite (1967) termed the deformity one third of a clubfoot. The probable interrelationship of these deformities is noted in the common finding of talar neck medial deviation. Bleck's (1976) explanation and description of persistent medial deviation of the talar neck as a cause for childhood toe-in may point out the clinical presentation of the same deformity of an even lesser degree.

When forefoot and midfoot varus is very severe, combined with cavus and hindfoot valgus, McCormick and Blount (1949) termed this degree of deformity "skewfoot." Lloyd-Roberts and Clark (1973) have termed the deformity *metatarsus adductus varus* when fixed adduction and supination of the forefoot are accompanied by valgus deformity of the heel. It would appear that both McCormick and Blount (1949) and Lloyd-Roberts and Clark (1973) were using different terminology to describe the same problem.

Etiology. As yet no microscopic studies have been performed to investigate the possibility that a developmental defect in the fetal talar neck can, if mild, lead to metatarsus adductus or metatarsus varus.

Kite (1967) felt that muscle imbalance with overpull of the tibialis anterior and tibialis posterior may be the cause. Abnormal insertion of the tibialis anterior into the base of the first metatarsal, with slips of tendon extending to the neck of the first metatarsal and without insertional fibers into the first cuneiform, has also been implicated as a cause of forefoot imbalance leading to metatarsus adductus.

Treatment of metatarsus adductus. In general, milder cases of metatarsus adductus recognized in early infancy respond promptly to conservative management (Ponsetti and Becker, 1966). Often, the early deformity is merely dynamic due to overpull of the anterior tibial or posterior tibial tendon. If a dynamic deformity is allowed to persist, however, a more fixed adductus will develop (Reimann and Werner, 1975). Hence, early intervention is preferred, simplifying treatment.

The small foot of a neonate is quite supple, and because of its small size a well-molded cast with appropriately placed pressure points is difficult to apply. Passive stretching of the forefoot by the mother at each diaper change, combined with frequent stroking of the lateral border during the day, stimulating active forefoot eversion, may be enough to reverse the inturning. In North America, infants are placed prone to sleep. The resultant reflex posture of hip and knee flexion, combined with internal rotation of the foot, promotes structural change in metatarsus adductus. Since very young infants are not capable of rolling over, the inturned foot remains in this position so long as the baby is left prone. The adverse effect of such posturing can be reversed by poking two holes in the heel of soft infant shoes. When a shoelace, woven through the four holes, is tied together and the shoes placed upon the infant's feet, the baby will then lie with the feet externally rotated even when prone. This may reverse the tendency for progression of dynamic metatarsus adductus to a structural deformity.

If the child is over 3 months of age and the deformity persists, no matter to what degree, it is best to initiate cast treatment. The ideal goal in treating metatarsus deformity is to limit the treatment to nonsurgical means and complete treatment prior to walking age. Therefore, as soon as the foot is large enough and if any degree of deformity persists, one should proceed directly to serial casting (Reimann, 1975). In the absence of equinus, a below-knee well-molded cast is adequate. Since in the first few months of life the child is growing quite rapidly, osseous structures and articular surfaces remodel readily; hence permanent correction can be achieved. The cast should be changed weekly, with progressive correction obtained until the lateral border of the foot is either straight or slightly concave. It is probably best to continue casting until slight overcorrection is noted; a final holding cast should be applied for 2 weeks after overcorrection has been achieved. Despite the fact that the soft bones of the infant's foot should remodel, with correction permanent, it has been our practice to place the child in either straight-last shoes or sneakers with a straight lateral border. Reversing normal shoes, right for left, is inadvisable since this may tend to promote heel valgus. When the child reaches walking age, he should be able to proceed directly to normal footwear.

The approach toward the more resistant metatarsus varus deformity is essentially the same as that used for metatarsus adductus. More time may be required for correction and, unless full correction with slight overcorrection is achieved, recurrence is common. Again, aiming for completion of treatment prior to walking age is important. If the child is over 1 year of age, growth of the foot slows considerably and, hence, remodeling takes much longer. Cast treatment of a child over 1 year of age tends to be measured in months rather than weeks as in the infant. However, plaster treatment can be effective.

Application of cast. Following are the basic steps in applying a cast:

1. A knowledgeable assistant stands at the outer side of the leg, grasping the foot with index and long fingers between the heads of the first and second metatarsals. With the other hand the thigh is held, stabilizing the extremity with the knee flexed 90°.

2. Place a 3-inch length of 2-inch Stockinet on the upper calf to serve as a cuff for the proximal end of the cast.

3. Wrap the extremity from the tip of the toes to just below the knee with a single layer of Webril. Place extra padding under the heel, over the lateral border of the cuboid, and medial to the first metatarsal head.

4. With 2-inch wide extra–fast-setting plaster, wrap from medial to lateral across the plantar surface of the forefoot. The cast may be applied in one stage; incorporate a small splint covering the plantar surface of the foot and posterior calf as reinforcement. When the final 2 inches of bandage is reached, fashion a small tag to initiate removal if the mother is to soak the cast off just prior to recasting.

5. Apply molding pressures by stabilizing the hindfoot with the outer hand. The calcaneus is held in a neutral position, the heel cradled so the thenar eminence falls at the calcaneocuboid joint. There it will serve as a fulcrum over which the forefoot can be laterally displaced. The ankle should be maintained at neutral or in slight equinus, and the index finger of the outer hand creates an impression over the distal tendo Achillis. This prevents the foot from sliding and/or the child from kicking the cast off.

6. With the inner hand, apply forefoot abduction pressure pushing the head of the first metatarsal laterally. The pressure should never be applied distal to the first metatarsophalangeal joint (creating a hallux valgus). Also resist the tendency to force the forefoot into pronation.

7. After the cast has dried, the Stockinet may be turned down over the proximal margin and held in place with a single strip of plaster. The lateral margin of the cast at the small toe should be split and turned back to allow visualization of all lateral toes.

In the small infant we soak the cast off rather than remove it with a cast saw. The noise of the saw is frightening and causes the child to cry and the foot to go tense. A good cast can be applied only over a relaxed foot; the child should be given a bottle or pacifier during cast application.

Operative treatment. By the time the child reaches 2 years of age, growth has slowed considerably and cast treatment, although occasionally effective, must be unduly prolonged. In this age group, soft tissue procedures are effective for gaining permanent correction.

In some feet with metatarsus adductus deformity, the abductor hallucis tendon is the primary deforming force (Lichtblau, 1975). When attempts at passive correction of the adducted forefoot lead to bowstringing of the abductor hallucis, lengthening of this tendon can result in permanent correction (Fig. 4-9). The procedure is simple, carried out through a small longitudinal incision over the distal medial first metatarsal. The abductor tendon is identified and divided obliquely or in Z fashion. This allows the tendon to lengthen; reattachment is not necessary. The skin is then closed and a corrective cast is applied for 6 weeks. Overcorrection of forefoot adduction can result; but if the tendon is lengthened rather than excised, overcorrection is unlikely to occur (Fig. 4-10).

After 3 years of age, Heyman et al. (1958) recommend mobilization of the tarsometatarsal and intermetatarsal joint for correction of resistant forefoot adduction. Transfer of the anterior tibial tendon laterally into the cuboid has been recommended but runs a significant risk of creating a pes valgus deformity (Specht, 1973). Splitting the tibialis anterior longitudinally and moving the lateral portion

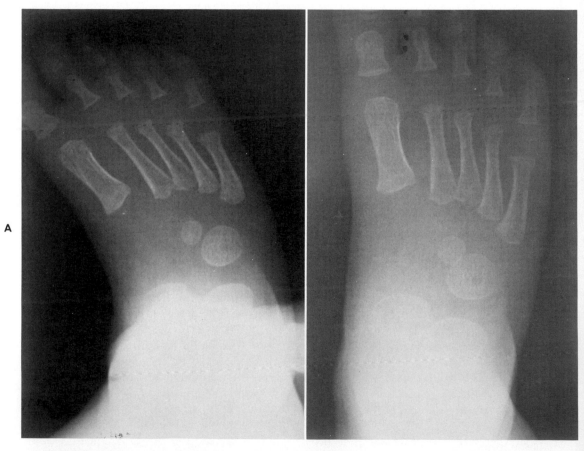

A

Fig. 4-9. A, Metatarsus adductus in a child 1 year 8 months old. **B,** At age 1 year 10 months, after lengthening of the abductor hallucis tendon.

of the tendon into the third cuneiform has been recommended as an alternative to avoid creation of the opposite deformity.

Split anterior tibial transfer

1. Make a longitudinal incision over the dorsal aspect of the first cuneiform at the insertion of the tibialis anterior tendon.

2. Make a second linear incision about 1½ inches long on the lateral side of the tibial crest at the junction of its middle and lower thirds.

3. Divide the lateral half of the tendon near its insertion and begin a longitudinal incision in the tendon which courses proximally, thereby creating a free lateral slip of tendon.

4. Insert a tendon passer into the sheath of the anterior tibialis at the proximal incision; guide it under the extensor retinaculum and pass it into the distal wound.

5. Attach a silk whip suture to the free lateral portion of the tendon, grasp it with the tendon passer, and withdraw the suture into the proximal wound. Traction on the suture will then draw the lateral half of the tibialis anterior into the proximal wound.

6. Make a short longitudinal incision over the third cuneiform. Insert the tendon passer into the third incision, guiding it under the transverse retinacular ligament and out the proximal wound.

7. Pull the tendon through the subcutaneous tunnel, under the transverse retinacular ligament, and into the incision over the third cuneiform.

8. Weave a stainless steel wire through the distal inch of the withdrawn tibialis anterior tendon after the method of Bunnell and insert a pullout wire through its most proximal loop.

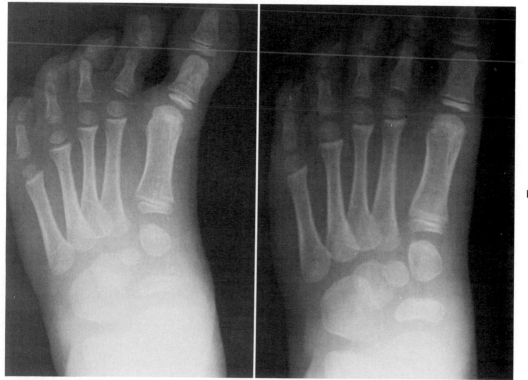

Fig. 4-10. A, Persistent metatarsus adductus in a 5-year-old boy who was casted for clubfoot from birth to 11 months of age. Note the continuing medial deviation of the talar head. **B,** Six months after lengthening of the abductor hallucis. Hallux valgus has not occurred.

9. Drill a hole through the tarsus at the third cuneiform and pass the wire through the bone and plantar skin using straight needles. Pass the pullout loop through skin on the dorsum of the foot.

10. Anchor the tendon in bone by passing the free ends of wire through a foam sponge and tying them over a button.

11. Close all incisions, making certain that the foot is held in dorsiflexion and mild eversion at all times by an assistant.

12. Apply a plaster cast from toes to knee. The cast and pullout wires can be removed after 8 weeks. Correction of forefoot varus should be permanent.

Mobilization of tarsometatarsal joints. Releasing soft tissues and aligning the forefoot to correct adductus are effective so long as sufficient growth remains to allow for remodeling of deformed articular surfaces (Kendrick et al., 1970) (Fig. 4-11). Capsulotomies and soft tissue release should therefore be limited to

the child under 7 years of age with persistent adduction deformity. Since treatment using this method relies on the remodeling potential of bone, the foot must be held in the corrected position until such remodeling can occur.

1. The approach can be made via a distally curved incision across the dorsum of the foot. Begin medially at the first tarsometatarsal joint, extending laterally to the base of the fifth metatarsal. Alternatively, two longitudinal incisions may avoid the occasional complication of skin slough and transection of longitudinal neurovascular structures. Visualization, however, is better with a transverse incision. Make longitudinal incisions between the first and second metatarsal and between the fourth and fifth. Capsulotomies proceed similarly by either approach.

2. Retract the skin flap to expose the deep fascia covering the tarsal articulation at the base of the first metatarsal. Identify the tib-

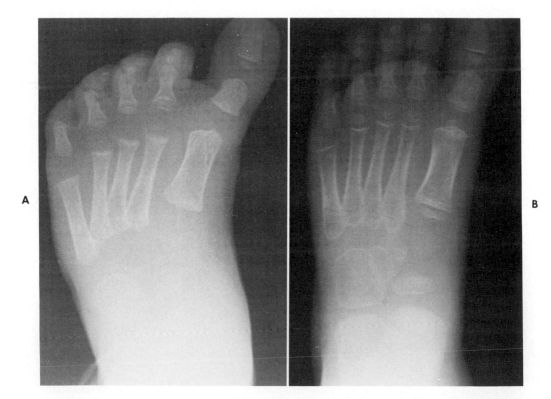

Fig. 4-11. A, Persistent metatarsus adductus at age 2 years 11 months. **B,** At 3 years 10 months, correction after tarsometatarsal and intermetatarsal capsulotomies. The second metatarsal was not osteotomized.

ialis anterior tendon and protect its insertion.

3. Make a longitudinal incision in the deep fascia overlying the interosseous space between the first and second metatarsals. Divide the interosseous ligaments, beginning distally and proceeding proximally. This permits accurate identification of the first metatarsocuneiform joint. Avoid damage to the physeal plate of the first metatarsal.

4. Incise the entire dorsal and medial capsule of the first tarsometatarsal joint; flex the metatarsal to expose and carefully divide the entire medial two thirds of the plantar capsule. Leave the lateralmost margin of the plantar capsule intact.

5. The second tarsometatarsal articulation is proximal to the others. Because of this variation osteotomy of the second metatarsal alone at the level of the other tarsometatarsal joints more readily permits adductus correction than capsulotomy; a transverse osteotomy done subperiosteally is sufficient. During exposure of the second metatarsal, carefully protect the extensor tendons and longitudinally running neurovascular structures.

6. Proceed laterally, completely dividing all ligaments and capsules at each tarsometatarsal articulation medially and dorsally; on the plantar aspect divide only the medial two thirds of each ligament and capsule.

7. After the intermetatarsal ligaments and tarsometatarsal capsules have been thoroughly divided, the forepart of the foot will swing laterally at the tarsometatarsal joints. Close the skin and apply a well-molded corrective cast to hold the forefoot in as much abduction as possible, however, avoid excessive forefoot pronation or hindfoot valgus.

8. Remove the cast under anesthesia after 2 weeks to examine the wound and gain further correction if necessary. A casting program should continue for an extended period of time to allow articular surface remodeling at the tarsometatarsal joints. Depending on the age of the child (longer in the older child), immobilization should continue for 3 to 5 months.

Treatment of resistant metatarsus varus in older children. Over the age of 8 years soft tissue release is insufficient to effect adequate correction of significant metatarsus varus (Kendrick et al., 1970; Lincoln et al., 1976). Correction of the deformity is assured only by osteotomizing and realigning the bony structures of the forefoot. If the primary deformity is metatarsus adductus with little forefoot supination, metatarsal osteotomies will correct the deformity.

Metatarsal osteotomy can be performed through the same approach used for capsulotomies of Heyman et al. (1958). Either a curving transverse or two longitudinal incisions may be utilized. Berman and Gartland (1971) have recommended using a hollow drill, making dome-shaped apex-proximal osteotomies in each of the metatarsals. Special care and occasionally even radiograph localization must be taken to avoid damaging the epiphyseal plate at the proximal end of the first metatarsal. Carrying out the osteotomy subperiosteally tends to promote union and avoid displacement of the fragments.

After osteotomies it is safest to hold the foot in a corrected position with longitudinal pins through the first and fifth metatarsals. A cast to maintain the foot in the corrected position is applied at surgery and is left intact until the pins are removed at 6 weeks. If union at this point is radiographically limited, further casting for an additional 3 to 4 weeks may be necessary. However, bony union is usually rapid; and recurrence after successful osteotomy is rare.

If significant forefoot supination or cavovarus is present, plantar release accompanied by abductor hallucis tenotomy may be combined with the metatarsal osteotomy or open wedge osteotomy of the tarsal bones to correct the deformity (Fowler et al., 1959; Lincoln et al., 1976). In older children, shortening the lateral column of the foot by excising a wedge of tarsus based laterally may likewise be indicated.

Talipes calcaneovalgus

Reported to be the most common congenital foot malformation (Wetzenstein, 1970), this deformity may exist to some degree in up to 50% of all births (Larsen et al., 1974). Its most striking feature is marked dorsiflexion of the foot, the dorsal aspect of the metatarsals approximating the anterior tibia. There is significant increase in hindfoot valgus with occasional contracture of dorsiflexion musculature. There seem to be abnormal mobility in pronation and frequently a significant decrease in active or passive plantar flexion.

Differential diagnosis is most important. The appearance of the foot with calcaneovalgus deformity can simulate that of congenital convex pes valgus. The basic anatomic difference between the two abnormalities is the position of the calcaneus: in congenital convex pes valgus the calcaneus is fixed in plantar flexion with contracture of the tendo Achillis and dislocation of the navicular onto the dorsal neck of the talus; in talipes calcaneovalgus the calcaneus is dorsiflexed, somewhat in valgus, and most important the relationships between all osseous structures are normal. There are no luxations and, therefore, no adaptive bony changes.

Active treatment of the deformity has generally been recommended; however, a follow-up of 110 calcaneovalgus feet by Larsen et al. (1974) indicated that no significant difference was later found between patients treated actively and those allowed to go untreated. The experience of these authors would indicate that even in the presence of dorsiflexor contracture, the ultimate result is excellent, with or without treatment.

The only residual seen after congenital talipes calcaneovalgus is persistent hindfoot valgus and slight depression of the medial arch. Neither of these problems is often symptomatic, and the occasional case may respond to orthotic support.

In our practicee the mother is taught to manipulate and massage the foot into plantar flexion. Since no abnormal bony relationship exists and secondary adaptive changes do not occur, maintenance of the corrected position in plaster is not necessary. If plantar flexion is limited to less than a neutral ankle position, we have sometimes undertaken a short period of adhesive strapping (taping into plantar flexion) to accelerate correction.

FLAT FEET

Two of the more common reasons a child is brought to a physician with lower extremity complaints are flat feet and intoeing. An analytic scientific approach to either of these problems paves the way to successful treatment.

Pes planus may be congenital in nature if the normal anatomy is distorted at birth. As in other congenital anomalies, degree of deformity varies from patient to patient. Treatment depends upon the degree of deformity and the resistance to passive correction. Pes planus may also exist in the absence of congenital bony anomalies and then is due to abnormality of soft tissue structures, loose ligaments, contracted tendo Achillis, etc. Indeed, in children the vast majority of flat feet are flexible, correct passively, and develop a longitudinal arch with non–weight bearing.

The common finding on examination of either flexible or rigid flatfoot is depression or loss of the longitudinal arch on weight bearing. The head of the talus or medial aspect of the navicular may be prominent at the normal midarch position. The forefoot is abducted, and the calcaneus may be in valgus (Fig. 4-12). Sometimes the normal longitudinal arch can be restored by external rotation of the tibia with the foot fixed in a weight-bearing position (Rose, 1962). Excessive internal tibial torsion, or genovalgum, and simple ligamentous laxity are the common causes when such a response is noted.

Weight-bearing radiographs should be obtained prior to initiation of treatment. The lateral view must include the entire foot and ankle; the AP view is taken with the x-ray tube angled 30° toward the heel to enable the talocalcaneal angle to be better visualized (Fig. 4-13).

Flexible pes planus

Although most flat feet are flexible and passively correct early in life, persistence of deformity can result in structural change as the foot grows and develops (Miller, 1977). The deformity disappears with non–weight bearing and frequently with exteranl rotation of the leg. Oftentimes the patient is capable of

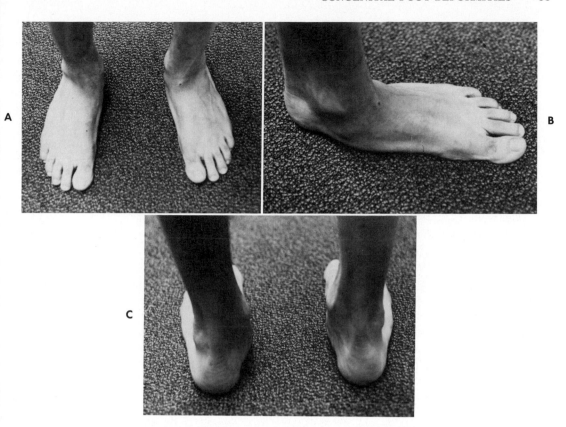

Fig. 4-12. A, Symptomatic flat feet in a 16-year-old boy. **B,** The medial arch is depressed, and the head of the talus is prominent on the plantar aspect of the arch. **C,** Slight hindfoot valgus when viewed from behind.

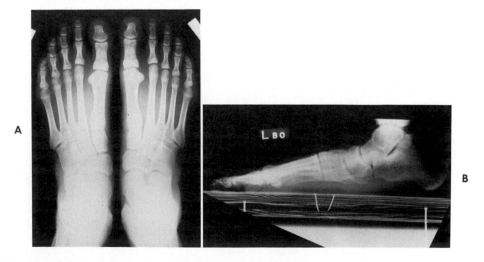

Fig. 4-13. Radiograph of the feet in Fig. 4-12. **A,** AP view. Note the medial deviation of the talar neck. The longitudinal axis of the talus falls medially, away from the axis of the first metatarsal. **B,** Lateral view. The talus is plantar flexed, and the navicular sags but is not dislocated on the talar neck.

actively correcting the deformity by contracting the tibialis anterior.

Heel alignment is normal with 0° to 5° of valgus and the forefoot straight (Bleck, 1971). In children up to 2 or 3 years of age, the normal arch is obscured by an overabundance of fat tissue on the plantar aspect of the heel. Hence one cannot use the clinical appearance of the toddler's foot to diagnose flat feet. Radiographs must be obtained.

Normal weight-bearing radiographs show divergence of the talus and calcaneus in the AP projection of approximately 20° (18° ± 5°). In the lateral view a line bisecting the body of the talus is inclined in plantar flexion approximately 25° from the horizontal; a line drawn along the inferior border of the calcaneus shows 15° of dorsiflexion (Bleck, 1977). With flexible flatfoot the talocalcaneal angle in the AP projection is increased due to divergence of talus and calcaneus, and on lateral views an interruption in the longitudinal arch is noted. Normally the line through the body and neck of the talus is parallel with the first metatarsal; with loss of the longitudinal arch, the talar neck is depressed to some degree and this line lies at an angle and inferior to the shaft of the

first metatarsal (Templeton, 1965) (Fig. 4-14). Sagging of the talonavicular and/or naviculo-cuneiform joints is often noted.

Treatment. Symptoms are rarely present during childhood. However, the stresses of weight bearing, shoe wear, and hard surfaces may result in fatigue-type discomfort during the teen-age years.

Few truly scientific reports documenting the lasting value of corrective devices are present in the literature. Bleck (1977) has shown that passive correction with an orthotic device in early childhood may result in permanent and significant restoration of the longitudinal arch.

As in other congenital abnormalities, growth and development can be effectively used to gain permanent correction so long as the orthotic device is worn faithfully and for a prolonged period of time. If the talar plantar flexion angle exceeds 45° the UCBL insert has achieved improvement in 74% of cases (Henderson and Campbell, 1967). For less severe deformity, with the talus plantar flexed 35° to 45°, the Helfet heel seat is reportedly effective in 85% of cases (Helfet, 1956). As might be expected, the longer the corrective device

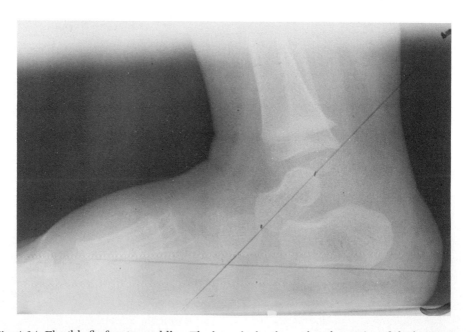

Fig. 4-14. Flexible flatfoot in a toddler. The lateral talocalcaneal angle is 50°, and the longitudinal axis of the talus falls at a significant angle below the axis of the first metatarsal. There is no fixed hindfoot (calcaneal) equinus.

is used the greater will be the improvement.

An occasional cause of flatfoot, one often overlooked when the patient presents for examination and treatment, is contracture of the tendo Achillis. If flatfoot is found in conjunction with a tight tendo Achillis, the heel cord stretching exercises or serial casting may restore the longitudinal arch (Harris and Beath, 1948; Helfet, 1956; Miller, 1977).

Unless osseous abnormalities are evident, flexible flatfoot in childhood rarely requires surgery. The operations of Miller (1927) and Hoke (1931) involve arthrodesis of midfoot joints and hence are inappropriate for the very young growing foot. Even in the adolescent we find that symptoms significant enough to require surgical intervention are extremely rare. In a five-year postoperative review of forty-six naviculocuneiform fusions performed for mobile flatfoot, Jack (1953) reported 82% good or excellent results among adolescents. Longer follow-up of the same group at sixteen years postoperative revealed deterioration to unsatisfactory in 50%, due primarily to stress-induced degenerative change in other joints (Semour, 1967). When the tendo Achillis is contracted and compression of the longitudinal arch in the young adolescent is symptomatic, the technique of Young (1939) remains the treatment of choice. Miller (1977) has recently reported excellent or good results using Chamber's (1946) procedure in 95% of eighty-one feet.

Accessory navicular (prehallux)

On occasion, a patient will present with flat feet and complain of tenderness over a palpable prominence at the medial aspect of the depressed longitudinal arch (Kidner, 1929). Radiographs demonstrating the presence of an accessory ossicle adjacent to the proximal medial aspect of the navicular confirm the diagnosis of prehallux. The navicular is described as cornuate when the ossicle has fused with the main body of the bone (Fig. 4-15). Because of this osseous overgrowth, a painful bursa aggravated by footwear frequently forms directly over the prominence.

Normally the tibialis posterior swings under the medial aspect of the navicular to insert into the plantar aspect of the first and second cuneiforms as well as the base of the second and fourth metatarsals. With either a cornuate or an accessory navicular, the major insertion of the tibialis posterior is often into the abnormal projection of bone (Zadek, 1948). Surgical treatment of the condition according to the method of Kidner (1929) relieves the local discomfort secondary to the bursa and elevates the longitudinal arch by realigning the tendon of the tibialis posterior. (See Chapter 5, p. 00.)

Rigid flat feet

The flatfoot whose abnormal appearance does not correct when non–weight bearing requires more attention and often a more aggressive approach.

Rigid flat feet tend to have a greater incidence of symptomatology and cause more disability. Physical examination reveals prom-

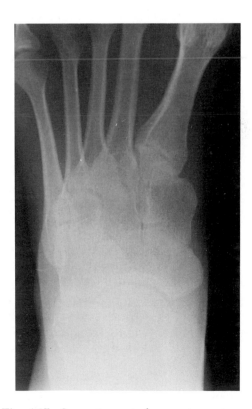

Fig. 4-15. Cornuate navicular causing pain and discomfort in a 15-year-old girl. After a Kidner procedure, symptoms resolved.

inence of the talar head or navicular along the medial border of the longitudinal arch as well as loss or limitation of subtalar motion', persistant equinus, and painful callosities signifying abnormal mechanics. Radiographs often demonstrate osseous abnormalities, and more frequently surgical intervention is required.

Several types of rigid flatfoot exist. These are grouped according to etiology in the discussions which follow.

Peroneal spastic flatfoot (tarsal coalition). Various abnormalities in the development of normal articulations between the tarsal bones have long been recognized. Union between the talus and navicular, the calcaneus and talus, the calcaneus and navicular, and the calcaneus and cuboid has been noted. This union can take the form of a fibrous connection (syndesmosis), a cartilaginous bond (synchondrosis), or a bony bridge (synostosis). These are grouped together into a common category termed tarsal coalition.

Slomann (1921) was the first to recognize the association of peroneal tendon spasm in a rigid flatfoot with coalition of the tarsal bones. In 1927, Badgley described the anatomy of a coalition of the navicular and calcaneus. He, too, observed that certain severe cases of rigid flatfoot seemed to be associated with a calcaneonavicular coalition.

Tarsal coalition is an autosomal dominant condition, the talocalcaneal type being most common (Wray and Herndon, 1963). There does not appear to be any association between fusion of the tarsal bones and fusion of the carpus. Leonard (1972) in a review of thirty-one patients with calcaneonavicular or talocalcaneal coalitions, found similar deformities in 50% of first-degree relatives.

Conway and Cowell (1969) postulated that the congenital deformity does not begin as a failure of segmentation but rather is seen in early childhood as a syndesmosis. Although the union remains fibrous, motion appears to be near normal and no symptoms are noted. Hence identification of the problem in infancy or early childhood is rare. As time passes, the syndesmosis becomes a cartilaginous bar and motion is progressively restricted. By the time early adolescence is reached, the carti-

laginous bar becomes ossified and significant restriction of hindfoot motion occurs.

This restriction places an abnormal stress upon the tarsus. Abnormal stress in the region results in pain and discomfort leading to protective spasm of the peroneal muscles. As motion is progressively restricted and the peroneal muscles become tightened, the midfoot is forced into more pronation and a rigid type of flatfoot develops. Symptoms often appear following a rather minor wrenching-type injury to the foot after the bridge has become cartilaginous or osseous. Actual fracture of the coalition has been noted, and healing of such a fracture can occur.

An individual complaining of discomfort and demonstrating a rigid-type flatfoot must be carefully examined, including appropriate radiographic views. Physical findings include significant loss of subtalar motion, which may be demonstrated with the foot at 90° to the leg and the hand of the examiner firmly grasping the calcaneus. In this position the talus is well locked in the ankle mortise and passive inversion and eversion of the calcaneus create motion only in the subtalar joint. In the presence of tarsal coalition, such motion is markedly reduced or absent. When the coalition has been present a long time, hindfoot valgus results in shortening of the peroneal muscle-tendon unit. Attempts at inverting the midfoot cause the peroneal tendon to stand out, as if in spasm. In an instance such as this, the peroneal spasm only is apparent. However, when ligamentous strain in the hindfoot has occurred due to loss of flexibility, the peroneal spasm can be real and painful (Harris, 1955).

Peroneal spasm may also be caused by degenerative arthritis or inflammatory processes within the midfoot or hindfoot. In such instances, unless marked gross deformity has occurred, subtalar motion is less limited (Outland and Murphy, 1960; Cowell, 1972).

Radiographic examination should be performed in the standing AP and lateral projections, and in addition an oblique view should be obtained at approximately 45° to delineate a calcaneonavicular coalition (Korvin, 1934) (Fig. 4-16, *A*). An axial view of the hindfoot

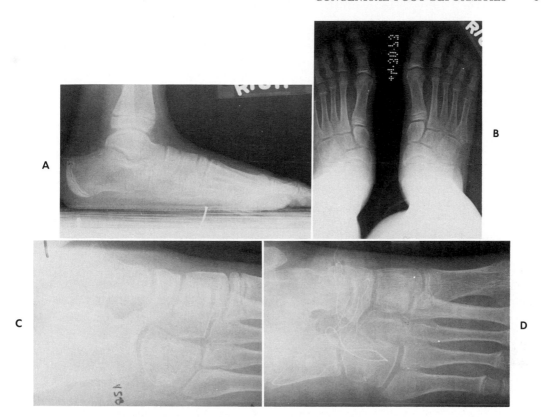

Fig. 4-16. Calcaneonavicular coalition. **A** to **C,** Not easily appreciated on the routine lateral or AP views. The oblique view, however, obtained at 45° clearly shows the bar. **D,** After resection of the bar and interposition of the extensor brevis orgin. The wire is a pull-out suture, tied over a button, holding the muscle in place immediately after the operation.

acquired at a 45° angle normally will demonstrate the joints of the posterior facet and sustentaculum tali, the middle facet. If a bony coalition is present, the facet joint is obliterated on this tangential view. Occasionally the x-ray beam does not pass directly through the joint when tilted 45°; if the joint on such a film appears abnormal, the lateral standing radiograph should be examined to determine the actual angle of the joint. If significantly different from 45°, a film with the tube tilted appropriately so the beam passes through the subtalar joint should be obtained.

Recently it has been pointed out that a syndesmosis or synchondrosis of the middle facet is present if the facet joint appears oblique rather than horizontal on the tangential view (Fig. 4-17). Only if the union is

osseous does complete obliteration of the joint occur and, if cartilaginous or fibrous, coalition may be difficult to appreciate. A radiographic finding of facet obliquity and/or irregularity, however, is strong evidence that a coalition is probably present (Jayakumar and Cowell, 1977).

The most difficult area to examine radiographically for a coalition is the anterior facet between the calcaneus and talus. Conway and Cowell (1975) recommend tomography in the lateral projection to demonstrate this joint.

In addition to the primary radiographic findings of coalition, secondary changes at radiography are also noted. Most significant of these is the "talar beak." Lipping of the superoanterior surface of the talar head at the talonavicular joint is secondary to abnormal

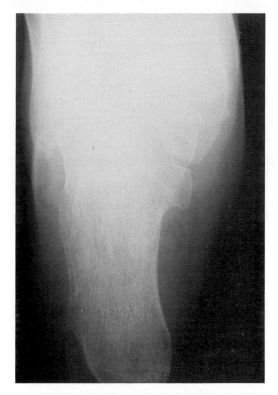

Fig. 4-17. Synchondrosis of the middle facet (talocalcaneal coalition). Note the obliquity of the joint. Resection is not usually successful; if the condition is symptomatic, resection and talocalcaneal fusion are necessary. Degenerative changes in the talonavicular joint may additionally necessitate fusion there.

motion of the tarsal complex. Talar beaking is not present early in life but, as time passes, develops as a remodeling process. Other secondary changes include narrowing of the talocalcaneal joint as seen on lateral views (Harris and Beath, 1948).

Treatment. As previously mentioned, symptomatology does not usually occur until early adolescence. Talonavicular coalition rarely is the cause of symptomatology and is usually an incidental radiographic finding.

When an individual first notices symptoms secondary to calcaneonavicular or talocalcaneal coalition, 6 weeks of immobilization in a short-leg walking cast often results in resolu-

tion of the discomfort. If not completely resolved or if shortly thereafter recurring, a second period in plaster may be necessary. Further treatment is dependent upon age of the patient and the presence or absence of degenerative changes in other joints.

If coalition has occurred between the calcaneus and navicular and the patient is less than 12 years of age, resection of the bar may be carried out. Structural changes are unlikely to have occurred yet in other joints, and normal pain-free motion may be surgically restored. Through a standard lateral approach to the sinus tarsi, a rectangular portion of the bar is removed with interposition of the extensor digitorum brevis (Cowell, 1975) (Fig. 4-16, *D*). If the patient is beyond early adolescent years or if the coalition is between the talus and calcaneus, successful resection is not routinely possible. In such instances arthrodesis of the talonavicular, calcaneocuboid, and subtalar joints is necessary. For middle facet coalition, Harris (1955) recommends a medial approach with resection of the bar followed by talonavicular and subtalar fusion. Arthrodesis of this type should be delayed until the individual is 11 or 12 years of age and the foot has obtained nearly full growth. Symptomatic talocalcaneal coalition of the anterior facet unresponsive to a period of cast immobilization should be treated similarly at an appropriate age with triple arthrodesis.

Congenital convex pes valgus (congenital vertical talus). Rigid flatfoot, other than that seen with peroneal spasm, is also noted with this deformity. The imprecise term congenital vertical talus should probably be abandoned since the talus is vertically inclined to a varying degree with any significant flatfoot, both flexible and rigid. Preferably the term congenital convex pes valgus is more appropriate and more descriptive.

The essential difference between the flexible flatfoot and congenital convex pes valgus is dorsal dislocation of the navicular onto the neck of the talus in the latter. In flexible flatfoot the navicular may sag plantarward but articulates more normally with the head of the talus. Other salient findings are additional hallmarks of congenital convex pes valgus:

fixed equinus deformity of the calcaneus, lateral rotation of the anterior calcaneus, dorsiflexion and supination of the forefoot, and a typical rocker-bottom appearance. The talar head is prominent on the medial plantar aspect of the midfoot.

Concerning differential diagnosis, other entities may present a similar superficial appearance. With congenital calcaneal valgus, hindfoot equinus is absent; this is therefore a different problem. Unlike flexible flatfoot and tarsal coalition, congenital convex pes valgus can usually be recognized at birth (Osmond-Clarke, 1966). If it remains untreated, initial problems concern footwear. Because of the shape of the foot, the gait is awkward and shoe wear, particularly along the medial border, excessive. As the child approaches adolescence, callosities form over the medial aspect of the tarsus, ligamentous structures are strained, and the foot becomes painful.

Herndon and Heyman (1963) believe the abnormality is caused by an insult during the first trimester of pregnancy and may well be related to clubfoot deformity. To date, however, no absolute proof exists that either congenital convex pes valgus or clubfoot is due to changes during the embryonic period. Congenital convex pes valgus is frequently seen in association with other neurologic abnormalities such as myelodysplasia, neurofibromatosis, or arthrogryposis. Because of the association of congenital convex pes valgus with congenital neurologic abnormalities, such problems should be carefully searched for when the deformity is encountered (Lamy and Weissman, 1939; Lloyd-Roberts and Spence, 1958; Drennan and Sharrard, 1971). As with clubfoot, very little specimen dissection has been reported.

Patterson et al. (1968) described the anatomic findings at dissection of a 6-week-old infant who died of congenital heart disease; the spinal cord of the specimen was not examined. Findings in their study indicated that not until the shortened extensor tendons—including the tibialis anterior, extensor hallucis longus, extensor digitorum longus, and peronei—were serially lengthened was re-duction of the talonavicular subluxation possible. Correction of hindfoot equinus was possible only after heel cord lengthening. Section of the talonavicular, subtalar, and posterior ankle capsules was carried out prior to tendon division but did not reduce the navicular on the talus. Moderate abnormalities in the talus and calcaneus were felt to be secondary changes and not the primary cause of the deformity. Therefore these authors contended that the primary abnormality was shortening of the muscle-tendon unit.

Drennan and Sharrard (1971) pointed out the marked association of congenital convex pes valgus with central nervous system abnormalities and presented their dissection of this deformity in a myelodysplastic child. They, too, felt the deformity was secondary to shortening or overpull of the dorsiflexors and evertors of the foot unopposed by a weakened invertor—the tibialis posterior.

Physical findings. The problem as it presents clinically is a rigid foot with the heel in equinus, a convex sole with the head of the talus prominent on the plantar medial aspect of the tarsus. The forefoot is dorsiflexed and everted; passive correction of the deformity is not possible.

Radiographic findings. AP radiographs of the foot in a standing position demonstrate increased divergence of the talus and calcaneus. On lateral views the calcaneus is noted to be in equinus, the talus vertical, and, if ossified, the navicular dislocated onto the dorsal neck of the talus. If plantar flexion, non–weight-bearing stress projections are obtained; unlike the flexible flatfoot, the abnormal relationship between talus and the forefoot persists (Fig. 4-18). Jayakumar and Ramsey (1977) point out the essential difference between x-ray findings of the oblique or plantar-flexed talus seen in association with a flexible flatfoot and the vertical talus of congenital convex pes valgus.

Treatment. Conservative treatment, although usually unsuccessful, should be initiated as soon as possible after the patient is first seen (Becker-Anderson and Reimann, 1974). Efforts should be made at stretching the contracted anterior structures by maxi-

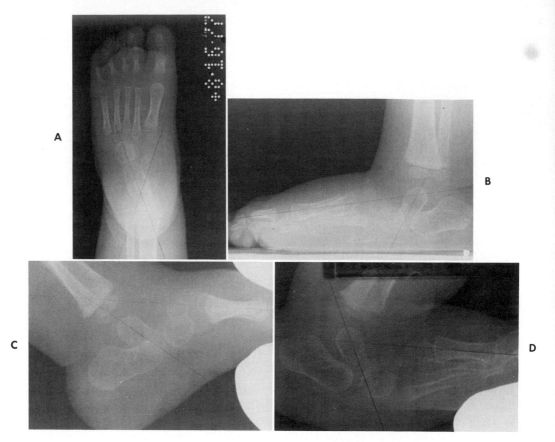

Fig. 4-18. Congenital convex pes valgus in an 18-month-old child. **A** and **B,** The talar axis falls at an angle medial and plantar to that of the first metatarsal. **C,** Plantar flexion stress fails to align the talus and first metatarsal. **D,** Dorsiflexion stress demonstrates persistence of hindfoot equinus. The unossified navicular is dislocated on the talar neck.

mally plantar flexing and inverting the forefoot, pressing the talar head dorsally, and attempting to push the navicular into a more normal relationship with the talus. Although it is not likely, serial casting after these maneuvers may result in correction of the deformity; more likely, casting will assist in making surgical correction more successful by stretching contracted dorsal soft tissue structures (Coleman et al., 1970).

Operative treatment as advocated by Lamy and Weissman (1939) combines partial or total talectomy with lengthening of peroneal and extensor tendons as necessary. Colton (1973) has recommended peritalar release with navicular excision as described by Stone. Most

authors agree that soft tissue procedures necessary to effect reduction include capsulotomies of the talonavicular, subtalar, and ankle joints and routine lengthening of the tendo Achillis (Hark, 1950; Coleman and Jarrett, 1966). Peroneal, anterior tibial, extensor digitorum communis, extensor hallucis longus, and posterior tibial tendons may be lengthened as necessary. In addition, Eyre-Brook (1950) excised a dorsally based wedge from the navicular and placed it beneath the neck of the talus for support. He also shortened the spring ligament. Because he believed the calcaneus was not in equinus, he did not recommend posterior release. Jayakumar and Ramsey (1977) have recommended transplantation of the anterior tibial tendon into the talar neck after reduction has been obtained, thus providing dynamic support to the reduction.

We would generally recommend soft tissue release of tightened talonavicular, subtalar, calcaneocuboid, and posterior ankle capsules through both medial and lateral incisions. The tendo Achillis should be lengthened and reduction of the deformity attempted by plantar flexing the forefoot; if tight, dorsal tendons should be lengthened as necessary. Reduction, once obtained, should be maintained by K-wire fixation through the first metatarsal and navicular and into the neck and body of the talus. Reduction of the deformity is possible only by acutely plantar flexing the forefoot, bringing the navicular into normal relationship with the talar head. If reduction following complete capsular and extensor tendon division is still impossible, navicular excision should be carried out. A second K-wire, transversely placed through the tuberosity of the calcaneus, is incorporated in plaster and serves as a lever to gradually bring the hindfoot out of equinus. Correction should be maintained in long-leg casts for 4 to 6 months; the K-wires may be removed at 3 months.

If the patient is adolescent or older, reduction of the deformity by soft tissue release and navicular excision is unlikely to be successful. By this time, foot strain and abnormal mechanics have altered other joints; and triple arthrodesis with resection of enough bone to create a plantigrade foot is the only solution. Heel cord lengthening and posterior capsulotomy may be required along with the triple arthrodesis to bring the calcaneus out of equinus.

ARTHROGRYPOSIS MULTIPLEX CONGENITA

In this congenital affection multiple rigid joint deformities are evident at birth (Mead et al., 1958). Severity of both deformity and rigidity may vary from patient to patient and joint to joint. More commonly involved regions of the skeleton include the fingers, wrists, elbows, and shoulders as well as hips, knees, and feet. Not infrequently the spine is involved with a congenital-type scoliosis. Normally the skin is smooth, muscle bulk is diminished, and fingers are rather long and slender (Sheldon, 1932). In even the mildest cases the presence of long tapered fingers may be a tip-off to the diagnosis of arthrogryposis.

Two types exist, a neuropathic form and a myopathic form (Adams et al., 1953). In many circles it is felt that the myopathic form is a type of muscular dystrophy and should be classified with the myodistrophias (Middleton, 1934; Banker et al., 1957). Etiology of arthrogryposis is generally unknown. Because many of the deformities appear to be teratologic in nature, the problem must arise sometime during the prenatal period (Drachman and Coulombre, 1962). Several causes have been proposed: intrauterine disturbances (decreased amniotic fluid, increased intrauterine pressure, mechanical compression of the fetus), inflammatory processes (rubella, viral infections, central nervous system infections) (Drachman and Banker, 1961), and environmental damage (teratogenic agents). Several attempts to work out the genetics have been made but published series tend to be too small for any definite conclusions to be reached. At the present time most authorities believe heredity does not play a significant role.

Microscopic studies of arthrogrypotic specimens have shown major abnormalities in both muscle and nerve tissue. Involved muscles tend to be small, pale, and pink; some muscles are simply not present. In other areas muscle fibers may be extensively replaced by fat and connective tissue. Nervous tissue involvement includes abnormalities of the spinal cord (i.e., a decrease or absence of anterior horn cells in the thoracic and lumbar regions). In addition, anterior roots have few fibers. Posterior roots and posterior horn cells appear to be normal (Adams et al., 1953; Drummond et al., 1974).

In arthrogryposis the foot tends to manifest the severest and most resistant of all deformities. Equinovarus is the commonest foot deformity, varying from quite mild to quite severe (Gibson and Urs, 1970). The most resistant and the most difficult to treat clubfeet are seen in arthrogryposis (Fig. 4-19). Although principles of management follow those for idiopathic clubfoot, conservative treatment often fails and the surgical approach must be extensive and radical.

As with the idiopathic clubfoot, treatment should begin as soon as possible after birth. Adhesive strapping in the nursery with frequent passive manipulation by nurses and mother should begin promptly. The deformity will generally not correct with longitudinal traction at the head of the first and second metatarsals, and its rigidity can be appreciated immediately.

After some foot growth and with the assumption that correction although slow is progressing, serial casting should begin as soon as the foot is large enough. Unlike other congenital problems, arthrogryposis does not tend to be progressive; but suspension of treatment commonly results in relapse to the initial deformity (Oh, 1976). Since the basic problem is abnormal or absent muscles and abnormal nerve structures, the goal of treatment in the arthrogryotic clubfoot differs from that in an idiopathic condition. In arthrogryposis the attempt is to change a stiffened, rigid, deformed foot to one which is stiff, rigid, and plantigrade (Lloyd-Roberts and Lettin, 1970). To date, no form of treatment has been successful in obtaining or restoring any significant degree of increased mobility.

If after a period of conservative treatment it becomes obvious that full correction has not been obtained (and this is usually the case), operative intervention should proceed directly. Correction of the hindfoot is of prime importance; and if the equinus and varus can be neutralized, any residual forefoot deformity is unlikely to interfere with function. If the deformity is mild or moderate, posterior release with capsulotomy of the ankle and subtalar joints with segmental excision (not lengthening) of the tendo Achillis and posterior tibial tendon, accompanied by division of the posterior talofibular and deltoid ligaments, may result in a plantigrade foot. Under such circumstances the foot should be maintained in plaster in the corrected position for 3 or 4 months postoperatively. It is then advisable to continue maintenance of correction in an appropriate day-night brace.

Often a moderate deformity will require a formal medial as well as posterior release. In

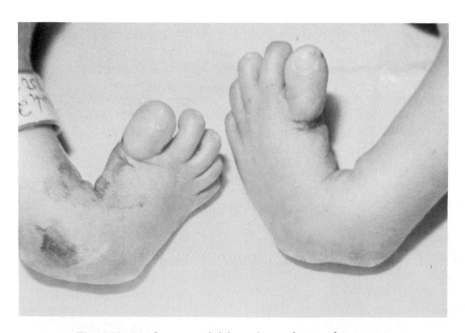

Fig. 4-19. Rigid, severe clubfeet of a newborn arthrogryptotic.

addition to those structures released via the posterior approach, the capsules of the talo-navicular, subtalar, and naviculocuneiform joints must be excised. Postoperative treatment is the same as for posterior release alone (Drummond et al., 1974). When the foot deformity is severe, soft tissue release can effect correction only by widely opening joints on the medial side of the foot. The situation has been likened to the opening of a suitcase; often there is insuffucient skin and subcutaneous tissue for adequate wound closure. With such severe deformity, after removal of cast immobilization, the suitcase simply closes again and the deformity recurs. In this instance correction of the deformity can be obtained only by shortening skeletal elements (Menelaus, 1971).

In a young child, arthrodesis of the growing foot is inappropriate. Excision of the talus is an effective method of gaining alignment and allows skin closure without tension. In an immature severely involved foot, talectomy results are best when carried out between ages 1 and 5 years; the procedure can result in a plantigrade functional foot.

Talectomy. A lateral curved incision following the line of the subtalar and talonavicular joints provides adequate exposure. Subcutaneous tissues should be protected and the incision carried directly to the capsules of these joints. The joints should be entered and the capsule excised; to prevent damage to the articular cartilage, an iris scissors should be used. As the dissection proceeds, the hindfoot can be manipulated into equinovarus, permitting division of the posterior and posteromedial ligaments. The entire talus must be excised; any remnants left behind can grow and produce a recurrent progressive deformity. After excision of the talus, a portion of the tendo Achillis should be excised. The calcaneus may then be placed in the ankle mortise; if it does not fit well, partial excision of the tip of the lateral malleolus and division of the anterior tibiofibular ligament may be necessary. The calcaneus is usually fairly stable within the ankle mortise, but a good practice is to hold the reduction with a K-wire or small Steinmann pin placed up through the

heel into the tibia. If excision of the talus is inadequate and the deformity is not fully corrected, the navicular may also be excised to provide further correction. One must avoid, however, excising any portion of the calcaneus because this will have an adverse effect on the size of the foot. Postoperatively the foot should be maintained in plaster for 6 weeks; the K-wire can be removed at 3 to 4 weeks.

Follow-up of talectomy for arthrogryposis has generally demonstrated good results, with a plantigrade functional foot, so long as the appropriate indications for surgery were present (Tompkins et al., 1956). The procedure is indicated for badly deformed rigid equinovarus feet when additional musculoskeletal abnormalities make prolonged standings and extended ambulation unlikely.

For the older child, triple arthrodesis is the procedure of choice. Adequate shortening of the skeletal elements to effect correction and closure of the skin without tension can be carried out during the procedure. If the triple arthrodesis does not effect complete correction, fusion of the ankle joint with appropriate resection of bone from the distal tibia may be necessary in the severely involved arthrogrypotic foot (Carmack and Hallock, 1947). Triple arthrodesis should probably not be performed when significant foot growth remains (i.e., below the age of 12 years).

Midtarsal wedge resection is effective in correcting cavus or forefoot equinus deformity. Supramalleolar osteotomy can be used to correct hindfoot equinus in the older child, although Drummond et al. (1974) believe this should be the last line of defense.

ABNORMALITIES OF THE TOES

Congenital abnormalities of the toes include polydactyly, syndactyly, macrodactyly, congenital hammertoe, and overlapping and underlapping toes. Congenital abnormalities of the great toe include hallux rigidus, hallux varus, and interphalangeal valgus. More than any other group of foot abnormalities, congenital toe deformities tend to be hereditary. Furthermore, some toe abnormalities are found in concert with generalized syndromes as noted in the compilation by Zimbler et al. (1977) (Table 1).

Abnormalities of the great toe

Congenital hallux varus. This is a rare deformity, differing from that seen as an adducted first toe accompanying metatarsus primus varus. There is no hereditary tendency for this deformity and it is often associated with supernumerary phalanges or metatarsals; on occasion, the first metatarsal is duplicated and fused.

Clinically the deformity presents as an adduction deviation of the great toe, occasionally as much as 90° to the long axis of the foot (Fig. 4-20). Most often the deformity occurs at the metatarsophalangeal joint; however, it is sometimes seen at the interphalangeal joint. McElvenny (1941) described hallux varus in association with (1) a short thick metatarsal, (2) accessory bones or toes, (3) varus deformity of one or more of the lateral four metatarsals,

and (4) a firm fibrous band along the medial aspect of the foot. This firm band, interpreted as being the abductor hallucis, has been implicated (Thompson, 1960) as a causative factor.

Surgery for the condition must be tailored to meet the needs of the individual deformity. In general, sufficient skin must be retained by fashioning appropriate flaps to provide cover for the inner border of the foot. Farmer (1958) described a skin-fat flap which he uses to lengthen the short medial side of the foot, adapting the technique to the demands of the deformity. To obtain reduction, all structures along the medial side, including the metatarsophalangeal joint capsule, must be transected. To obtain correction and prevent recurrence of the deformity, the abductor hallucis must be divided. If the deformity is limited to the distal phalanx or the interphalangeal joint, symptoms may develop in adolescence and require surgical intervention.

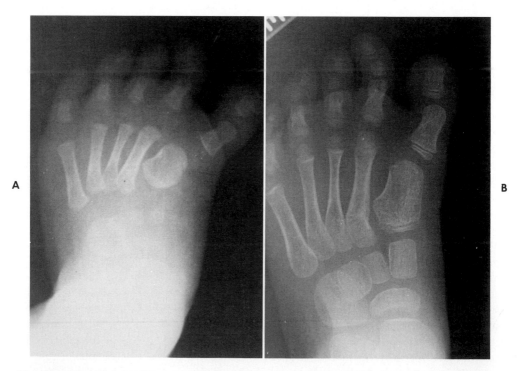

A

B

Fig. 4-20. Congenital hallux varus (atavistic first toe). **A,** At 10 months of age; shortening of the first metatarsal accompanied by medial subluxation of the metatarsophalangeal joint. **B,** At 3 years 7 months; early release of the abductor hallucis. This resulted in better cosmesis and alignment.

Angular deformity of the distal phalanx, either varus or valgus, can be corrected by appropriate osteotomy.

Congenital hallux rigidus. This deformity is extremely rare. Its presence has been ascribed to an abnormality of the first metatarsal: elevation, excessive length, or hypermobility. More commonly the deformity appears secondary to trauma, with involvement of the first metatarsophalangeal joint or development of osteochondritis dessicans of the first metatarsal head (Kessel and Bonney, 1958). Anomalies of the first metatarsal head which cause abnormal joint surfaces can have the same effect as trauma, leading to abnormal stress and degenerative joint disease. Treatment of symptomatic congenital hallux rigidus is the same as for the acquired type. Since symptoms are not usually present prior to adolescence, interference with future growth of the toe is not necessarily a consideration.

Abnormalities of the smaller toes

Polydactyly. Often inherited as an autosomal dominant (Kirtland and Russell, 1976), polydactyly is frequently part of a generalized syndrome and may be accompanied by supernumerary fingers. If the extra digit occurs on the tibial side of the foot, it is termed preaxial; on the fibular side, postaxial (Nathan and Keniston, 1975). The literature contains many references to polydactyly, but for the most part these references are made only in passing when describing the clinical characteristics of a generalized syndrome.

Recognition of the deformity in biblical times is found in Samuel 21:20: "And there was again war at Goth, where there was a man of great stature who had six fingers on each hand and six toes on each foot, 24 in number; and he also was descended from the giants." Frazier (1960) noted a twelvefold increase in polydactyly among the southern black population as compared with southern whites. He described an incidence of 3.6 per 1,000 live births among black children born in Baltimore.

Supernumerary toes are a clinical problem since they interfere with footwear. For this reason surgical excision is often indicated, but one must adhere to a few basic principles. Unlike the hand, the foot does not necessitate making a decision as to which is the most rudimentary of the digits and then excising that particular one. More appropriately, the contour of the entire foot should be considered and, for the most part, the peripheral extra digit excised (Tachdjian, 1972). This is irrespective of whether it appears to be the more major digit. On the medial side of the foot, the tibialmost toe is usually excised; and on the lateral side the fibularmost. If an abnormality of the metatarsals (bifurcation, duplication) is demonstrated radiographically, appropriate excision to obtain a normal contour of the entire foot must be considered (Fig. 4-21).

Surgical technique should be tailored to the individual case. In the usual circumstances disarticulation is carried out via a racquet-shaped incision with division and repair of ligaments and tendons as needed to prevent progressive deformity. Damage to remaining growth plates and articular cartilage must be avoided.

Muscle attachment is a more significant consideration with an accessory hallux than with other accessory toes. If the tibialmost hallux is excised, the abductor hallucis must be reinserted into the remaining proximal phalanx to avoid a hallux valgus deformity. Similarly, if the fibular hallux is grossly deformed and is to be excised, the adductor hallucis must be resutured into the proximal phalanx of the remaining hallux to avoid a hallux varus deformity secondary to overpull of the adductor hallucis.

Syndactyly. Like polydactyly, syndactyly is also seen in association with other congenital anomalies and syndromes. McKusick (1968) described five types of syndactyly, all transmitted as autosomal dominant traits. In the feet three types are seen:

Type I (zygodactyly). Partial or complete webbing of the second and third toes; hands also involved at times

Type II (synpolydactyly). Syndactyly of the lateral two toes and polydactyly of the fifth toe in the syndactyly web

Type III. Associated with metatarsal and metacarpal fusion

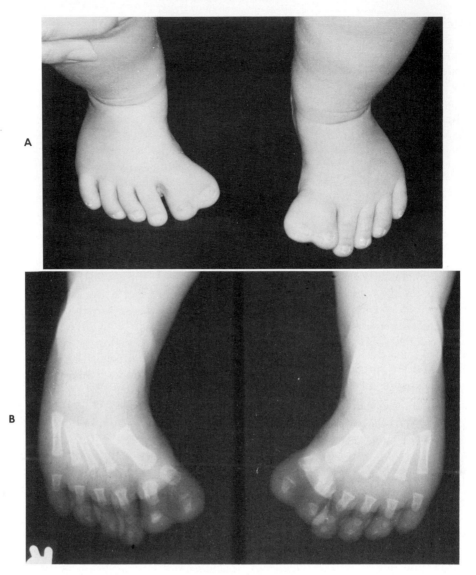

Fig. 4-21. Bilateral duplication and syndactyly of the hallux. The tibialmost toe should be removed and the abductor hallucis reattached to the remaining proximal phalanx. If the abductor hallucis is lengthened, the metatarsus adductus will resolve.

Surgical intervention for simple syndactyly of the foot is rarely indicated. The deformity is functionally insignificant and rarely becomes symptomatic. When surgery for cosmetic reasons is necessary, techniques of syndactyly release for the fingers apply as well to the toes.

The basic surgical technique involves outlining dorsal and volar skin flaps, based proximally. Flaps are incised, and this skin is utilized to close the cleft and reconstruct the web by suturing the flaps side to side. Opposing surfaces of the toes are then covered with free split-thickness skin grafts as required. Attempts to close flaps without using skin grafts leads to inevitable contracture and deformity.

Macrodactyly. Usually seen as a manifestation of a generalized problem (neurofibromatosis, arteriovenous fistula, hemangioma),

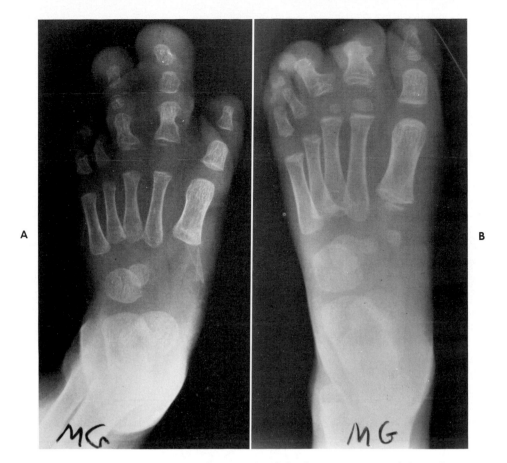

Fig. 4-22. A, Macrodactyly involving the second and third toes. Digits are adult sized at 2 years of age. **B,** Initial procedure included epiphysiodesis and soft tissue resection. Three years later interphalangeal resection and fusion with further soft tissue removal resulted in better cosmesis and shoe fit. (Courtesy Dr. Semour Zimbler, San Mateo, Calif.)

gigantism of a toe can result in significant functional as well as cosmetic problems (Fig. 4-22). Both gait abnormalities and difficulty with footwear occur, making surgery necessary. The toe may be reduced in length by a partial or total proximal or middle phalangectomy. Circumference of a toe can be reduced by staged defatting procedures. If the third or fourth toe is involved, amputation may be acceptable. However, amputation of a gigantic second toe can result in progressive hallux valgus deformity. Tachdjian (1972) has recommended syndactyly of the second to the fourth toes if a gigantic third toe is amputated. Overgrowth of the metatarsal may be managed by epiphysiodesis at an appropriate time.

Congenital hammertoe. A rare congenital deformity, hammertoe is recognized as a flexion contracture of the proximal interphalangeal joint with or without fixed deformity of the distal interphalangeal joint. With ambulation and footwear the metatarsophalangeal joint eventually becomes hyperextended. Like syndactyly and polydactyly, hammertoe is frequently a familial problem, most often involving the middle toes. With shoe wear, callus formation over the dorsal aspect of the proximal interphalangeal joint can result in symptoms.

Because the deformity usually eventually becomes symptomatic, early treatment is indicated. In infancy, adhesive strapping combined with stretching of the contracted volar capsule of the proximal interphalangeal joint if often effective. Early surgical treatment is usually not necessary since the deformity does not become symptomatic until early adolescence. After the foot has reached an appropriate size, correction can easily be obtained surgically by partial phalangectomy and interphalangeal fusion. If contracture of the dorsal metatarsophalangeal joint capsule has occurred, capsulotomy must also be carried out. Specifics of surgical treatment are described in Chapter 20.

Overlapping toes. Often familial, overriding is most commonly seen as the fifth toe overlapping the fourth. There is dorsiflexion of the metatarsophalangeal joint with adduction and external rotation of the digit. The condition is usually bilateral and, in about 50% of the cases, causes disabling symptoms (Cockin, 1968). Discomfort is aggravated by shoe wear and accompanying callus formation over the dorsal aspect of the proximal interphalangeal joint.

Because, as in hammertoe, symptoms are likely to develop later in life, early treatment may be of some benefit. In infancy, stretching the medial collateral ligament structure and dorsal medial capsule with adhesive taping into the correct position may be of some benefit. In most cases, surgical correction can be carried out without bone resection or interference with growth; therefore treatment in early childhood is possible.

Treatment. Most described procedures involve tenotomy of the extensor digitorum communis to the fifth toe as well as capsulotomy of the dorsal medial metatarsophalangeal joint.

Lapidus (1942) did the extensor tenotomy at the midtarsal level and rerouted the distal tendon stump plantarward around the medial side of the small toe, inserting the stump into the abductor digiti minimi. Butler's operation (Cockin, 1968) frees the entire toe via a racquet incision at its base with proximal extensions dorsally and at the plantar lateral margin. After extensor tenotomy and dorsal capsulotomy the plantar capsule, if adherent, is freed from the metatarsal head. Closure of the skin is then completed with the toe in the corrected position; no postoperative cast is necessary.

Syndactylization of the fifth to the fourth toe is advocated by Scrase (1954) and Kelikian et al. (1961). A double U-incision between the fourth and fifth toes with excision of the intervening skin permits the syndactyly. Correction via capsulotomy and extensor digitorum tenotomy can be accompanied by removal of enough proximal phalanx to correct the deformity (Leonard and Rising, 1965). Amputation for overlapping fifth toe generally results in pain and pressure at the head of the fifth metatarsal and therefore is not recommended. If the deformity is too severe, attempted correction without bony resection can result in vascular compromise. For this reason procedures restricted to soft tissues tend to be more applicable to children and adolescents than to adults (p. 597).

Congenital underlapping toes (congenital curly toe). This common familial deformity is most often seen in the lateral three toes. It presents as a combination of flexion, abduction, and external rotation primarily at the distal interphalangeal joint. In severe cases the proximal interphalangeal joint is also rotated and the toenail pointed laterally.

Unlike congenital overlapping toes, the congenital curly toe rarely becomes symptomatic. Early conservative treatment is not of benefit in correcting curly toe deformity.

Sweetman (1958) evaluated the long-term results of fifty cases: twenty-one patients treated and twenty-nine untreated. In no patient, either treated or untreated, did the deformity progress; 25% improved whether treated or not. Even though the deformity persisted in many cases, most patients had forgotten that it was present.

If surgery is required because of symptoms, syndactylization of the curly toe to its neighbor seems most appropriate. Correction may be obtained by excising an appropriate wedge from the superolateral aspect of the distal interphalangeal joint. Sharrard (1963) recommended transfer of the extensor digitorum longus of the affected toe to the dorsolateral aspect of the extensor hood. He found that this was of benefit, particularly if the deformity was not too severe.

REFERENCES
Embryology and genetics

Blechschmidt, E.: The stages of human development before birth, Philadelphia, 1961, W. B. Saunders Co.

Fuller, D. J., and Duthie, R. B.: The timed appearance of some congenital malformations and orthopaedic abnormalities. In American Academy of Orthopaedic Surgeons, Instructional Course Lectures, vol. 23, St. Louis, 1974, The C. V. Mosby Co.

Gardner, E., Gray, D. J., and O'Rahilly, R.: The prenatal development of the skeleton and joints of the human foot, J. Bone Joint Surg. 41A:847, 1959.

McKusick, V. A.: Mendelian inheritance in man, ed. 4, Baltimore, 1975, Johns Hopkins University Press.

Zimbler, S., and Craig, C.: Foot deformities, Orthop. Clin. North Am. 7:331, 1976.

Clubfoot (talipes equinovarus)

Abrams, R. C.: Relapsed clubfoot. The early results of an evaluation of the Dillwyn Evans operation, J. Bone Joint Surg. 51A:270, 1969.

Bohm, M.: The embryologic origin of clubfoot, J. Bone Joint Surg. 11:229, 1929.

Brockman, E. P.: Congenital clubfoot, London, 1930, John Wright & Sons, Ltd.

Denham, P. A.: Congenital talipes equinovarus, J. Bone Joint Surg. 40B:583, 1967.

Dunn, H. K., and Samuelson, K. M.: Flat topped talus. A long term report of 20 clubfeet, J. Bone Joint Surg. 56A:57, 1974.

Dwyer, F. C.: The treatment of relapsed clubfoot by insertion of a wedge into the calcaneum, J. Bone Joint Surg. 45B:67, 1963.

Evans, D.: Relapsed clubfoot, J. Bone Joint Surg. 43B:722, 1961.

Fisher, R. L., and Shaffer, S. R.: An evaluation of calcaneal osteotomy in congenital clubfoot and other disorders, Clin. Orthop. 70:141, 1970.

Fried, A.: Recurrent congenital clubfoot, J. Bone Joint Surg. 41A:242, 1959.

Gardner, E.: Osteogenesis in the human embryo and foetus. In Bourne, G. editor: Biochemistry and physiology of bone, Chapter 13, New York, 1956, Academic Press, Inc.

Heywood, A. W. B.: The mechanics of the hindfoot in clubfoot as demonstrated radiographically, J. Bone Joint Surg. 46B:105, 1964.

Irani, R. N., and Sherman, M. S.: The pathological anatomy of clubfoot, J. Bone Joint Surg. 45A:45, 1963.

Keim, H. A., and Ritchie, G. W.: Nutcracker treatment of clubfoot, J.A.M.A. 189:613, 1964.

Johanning, K.: Excochleatio ossis cuboidei in the treatment of pes equino varus, Acta Orthop. Scand. 27:310, 1958.

Kite, J. H.: The non-operative treatment of congenital clubfoot, South. Med. J. 23:337, 1930.

Lloyd-Roberts, G. C.: Congenital clubfoot, J. Bone Joint Surg. 46B:369, 1964.

Lowe, L. W., and Hannon, M. A.: Residual adduction of the forefoot in treated congenital club foot, J. Bone Joint Surg. 55B:809, 1973.

Paturet, G.: Traite d' anatomie humaine, vol. 2, Paris, 1951, Masson & Cie.

Ponseti, I. V., and Smoley, E. N.: Congenital clubfoot: the results of treatment, J. Bone Joint Surg. 45A:261, 1963.

Settle, G. W.: The anatomy of congenital clubfoot talipes equinovarus: sixteen dissected specimens, J. Bone Joint Surg. 45A:1341, 1963.

Smith, W. A., Campbell, P., and Bonnett, C.: Early posterior ankle release in treatment of congenital clubfoot, Orthop. Clin. North Am. 7:889, 1976.

Swann, M., Lloyd-Roberts, G. C., and Catterall, A.: The anatomy of uncorrected club feet, J. Bone Joint Surg. 51B:263, 1969.

Turco, V. J.: Surgical correction of the resistant clubfoot, J. Bone Joint Surg. 53A:477, 1971.

Turco, V. J.: Resistant congenital clubfoot. In American Academy of Orthopaedic Surgeons Instructional Course Lectures, vol. 24, St. Louis, 1975, The C. V. Mosby Co.

Waisbrod, H.: Congenital clubfoot: an anatomical study, J. Bone Joint Surg. 55B:796, 1973.

Wiley, A. M.: Club foot—an anatomical and experimental study of muscle growth, J. Bone Joint Surg. 41B:821, 1959.

Wynne-Davies, R.: Family studies and the cause of congenital club foot, J. Bone Joint Surg. 46B:445, 1964.

Metatarsus adductus and metatarsus varus

Berman, A., and Gartland, J. J.: Metatarsal osteotomy for the correction of adduction of the fore past of the foot in children, J. Bone Joint Surg. 53A:498, 1971.

Bleck, E. E., and Minaire, P.: Persistent medial deviation of the talar neck: a common cause of intoeing in children. Presented at the annual meeting of the American Academy of Orthopaedic Surgeons, New Orleans, 1976.

Fowler, B., Brooks, A. L., and Parrish, T. F.: The cavovarus foot, J. Bone Joint Surg. 41A:757, 1959.

Helbing, C.: Ueber den Metatarsus varus, Dtsh. Med. Wochenschr. 21:1312, 1905.

Heyman, C. H., Herndon, C. H., and Strong, J. M.: Mobilization of the tarsometatarsal and intermetatarsal joints for the correction of resistant adduction of the fore part of the foot in congenital clubfoot and congenital metatarsus varus, J. Bone Joint Surg. 40A:299, 1958.

Kendrick, R. E., Sharma, N. K., Hassler, W. E., and Herndon, C. H.: Tarsometatarsal mobilization for resistant adduction deformity of the fore part of the foot: a follow-up study, J. Bone Joint Surg. 52A:61, 1970.

Kite, J. H.: Congenital metatarsus varus, J. Bone Joint Surg. 32A:500, 1950.

Kite, J. H.: Congenital metatarsus varus, J. Bone Joint Surg. 49A:388, 1967.

Lichtblau, S.: Section of the abductor hallucis tendon for correction of metatarsus varus deformity, Clin. Orthop. 110:227, 1975.

Lincoln, C. R., Wood, K. E., and Bugg, E. I.: Metatarsus varus corrected by open wedge osteotomy of the first cuneiform bone, Orthop. Clin. North Am. **7:**795, 1976.

Lloyd-Roberts, G. C., and Clark, C. R.: Ball and socket joint in metatarsus adductus varus, J. Bone Joint Surg. **55B:**193, 1973.

McCormick, D. W., and Blount, W. P.: Metatarsus adductovarus—"skewfoot," J.A.M.A. **141:**449, 1949.

Peabody, C. W., and Muro, F.: Congenital metatarsus varus, J. Bone Joint Surg. **15:**171, 1933.

Ponseti, I. V., and Becker, J. R.: Congenital metatarsus adductus: the results of treatment, J. Bone Joint Surg. **48A:**702, 1966.

Reimann, I.: Congenital metatarsus varus. On the advantages of early treatment, Acta Orthop. Scand. **46:**857, 1975.

Reimann, I., and Werner, H. H.: Congenital metatarsus varus, Clin. Orthop. **110:**223, l975.

Specht, E. E.: In DuVries, H.: Surgery of the foot, ed. 3, St. Louis, 1973, The C. V. Mosby Co.

Wynne-Davies, R.: Family studies and the cause of congenital club foot—talipes equinovarus, talipes calcaneovalgus and metatarsus varus, J. Bone Joint Surg. **46B:**445, 1964.

Flat feet

Bleck, E. E.: The shoeing of children—sham or science? Develop. Med. Child Neurol. **13:**188, 1971.

Bleck, E. E., and Berzins, U. E.: Conservative management of pes valgus with plantar flexed talus, flexible, Clin. Orthop. **122:**85, 1977.

Chambers, E. F. S.: An operation for the correction of flexible flatfoot of adolescents, Surg. Gynecol. Obstet. **54:**77, 1946.

Harris, R. I., and Beath, T.: Hypermobile flat-foot with short tendo achillis, J. Bone Joint Surg. **30A:**116, 1948.

Helfet, A. J.: A new way of treating flat feet in children, Lancet **1:**262, 1956.

Henderson, W. H., and Campbell, J. W.: UCBL shoe insert: casting and fabrication, Biomechanics Laboratory, University of California, Berkeley, Techn. Rep. 53, 1967.

Hoke, M.: An operation for the correction of extremely relaxed flat feet, J. Bone Joint Surg. **13:**773, 1931.

Jack, E. A.: Naviculo-cuneiform fusion in the treatment of flat foot, Am. J. Roentgenol. Radium Ther. Nucl. Med. **35B:**75, 1953.

Kidner, F. C.: The prehallux (accessory scaphoid) in its relation to flatfoot, J. Bone Joint Surg. **11:**831, 1929.

Lusted, L. B., and Keats, T. E.: Atlas of roentgenographic measurements, ed. 2, Chicago, 1967, Year Book Medical Publishers, Inc.

Miller, G. R.: Hypermobile flatfeet in children, Clin. Orthop. **122:**95, 1977.

Miller, O. L.: A plastic foot operation, J. Bone Joint Surg,. **9:**84, 1927.

Rose, G. K.: Correction of the pronated foot, J. Bone Joint Surg. **44B:**642, 1962.

Semour, N.: The late results of naviculo-cuneiform fusion, J. Bone Joint Surg. **49B:**558, 1967.

Templeton, A. W., McAlister, W. H., and Zim, I. D.: Standardization of terminology and evaluation of osseous relationships in congenitally abnormal feet, Am. J. Roentgenol. Radium Ther. Nucl. Med. **93:**374, 1965.

Young, C. S.: Operative treatment of pes planus, Surg. Gynecol. Obstet. **68:**1099, 1939.

Zadek, I.: The accessory tarsal scaphoid, J. Bone Joint Surg. **30A:**957, 1948.

Peroneal spastic flatfoot (tarsal coalition.)

Badgley, C. E.: Coalition of the calcaneus and navicular, Arch. Surg. **15:**75, 1927.

Conway, J. J., and Cowell, H. R.: Tarsal coalition: clinical significance and roentgenographic demonstration, Radiology **92:**799, 1969.

Cowell, H. R.: Talocalcaneal coalition and new causes of peroneal spastic flatfoot, Clin. Orthop. **85:**16, 1972.

Cowell, H. R.: Diagnosis and management of peroneal spastic flatfoot. In American Academy of Orthopaedic Surgeons, Instructional Course Lectures, vol. 24, St. Louis, 1975, The C. V. Mosby Co.

Harris, R. I.: Rigid valgus foot due to talocalcaneal bridge, J. Bone Joint Surg. **37A:**169, 1955.

Harris, R. I., and Beath, T.: Etiology of peroneal spastic flatfoot, J. Bone Joint Surg. **30B:**624, 1948.

Jayakumar, S., and Cowell, H. R.: Rigid flatfoot, Clin. Orthop. **122:**77, 1977.

Korvin, H.: Coalitio talocalcanea, Z. Orthop. Chir. **60:**105, 1934.

Leonard, M.: The inheritance of tarsal fusion and the relationship to spastic flatfoot. Presented at British Orthopaedic Research Society, 1972.

Outland, T., and Murphy, I. D.: The pathomechanics of peroneal spastic flat foot, Clin. Orthop. **16:**64, 1960.

Slomann, H. C.: On coalitio calcaneo-navicularis, J. Orthop. Surg. **3:**586, 1921.

Wray, J. B., and Herndon, C. H.: Hereditary transmission of congenital coalition of the calcaneus to the navicular, J. Bone Joint Surg. **45A:**365, 1963.

Congenital convex pes valgus (congenital vertical talus)

Becker-Anderson, H., and Reimann, I.: Congenital vertical talus, Acta Orthop. Scand. **45:**130, 1974.

Colton, C. L.: The surgical management of congenital vertical talus, J. Bone Joint Surg. **55B:**566, 1973.

Coleman, S. S., and Jarrett, J.: Congenital vertical talus: pathomechanics and treatment, J. Bone Joint Surg. **48A:**1026, 1966.

Coleman, S. S., Stelling, F. H. and Jarrett, J.: Pathomechanics and treatment of congenital vertical talus, Clin. Orthop. **70:**62, 1970.

Drennan, J. C., and Sharrard, W. J.: The pathological anatomy of convex pes valgus, "Persian slipper foot," J. Bone Joint Surg. **53B:**455, 1971.

Eyre-Brook, A. L.: Congenital vertical talus, J. Bone Joint Surg. **49B:**618, 1950.

Hark, F. W.: Rocker bottom foot due to congenital subluxation of the talus, J. Bone Joint Surg. **32A:**344, 1950.

Herndon, C. H., and Heyman, C. H.: Problems in the recognition and treatment of congenital convex pes valgus, J. Bone Joint Surg. **45A:**413, 1963.

Jayakumar, S., and Ramsey, P.: Vertical and oblique talus: a diagnostic dilemma. Scientific exhibit at the annual meeting of the American Academy of Orthopaedic Surgeons, Las Vegas, 1977.

Lamy, L., and Weissman, L.: Congenital convex pes valgus, J. Bone Joint Surg. **21:**79, 1939.

Lloyd-Roberts, G. C., and Spence, A. J: Congenital vertical talus, J. Bone Joint Surg. **40B:**33, 1958.

Patterson, W. R., Fritz, D. A., and Smith, W. S.: The pathologic anatomy of congenital convex pes valgus, J. Bone Joint Surg. **50A:**458, 1968.

Osmond-Clarke, H.: Congenital vertical talus in infancy, J. Bone Joint Surg. **48B:**578, 1966.

Arthrogryposis multiplex congenita

Adams, R. C., Denny-Brown, D., and Pearson, C. M.: Diseases of muscle; a study in pathology, ed. 2, New York, 1953, Harper & Brothers, Hoeber Medical Division. 1953.

Banker, B. Q., Victor, M., and Adams, R. D.: Arthrogryposis multiplex congenita due to congenital muscular dystrophy, Brain **80:**319, 1957.

Carmack, J. C., and Hallock, H.: Tibiotarsal arthrodesis after astragalectomy. a report of eight cases, J. Bone Joint Surg. **29:**476, 1947.

Drachman, D. B., and Banker, B. Q.: Arthrogryposis multiplex congenita, Arch. Neurol. **5:**77, 1961.

Drachman, D. B., and Coulombre, A. J.: Experimental clubfoot and arthrogryposis multiplex congenita, Lancet **2:**523, 1962.

Drummond, D., Siller, T. N., and Cruess, R. L.: Management of arthrogryposis multiplex congenita. In American Academy of Orthopaedic Surgeons, Instructional Course Lectures, vol. 23, St. Louis, 1974, The C. V. Mosby Co.

Gibson, D. A., and Urs, N, D. K.: Arthrogryposis multiplex congenita, J. Bone Joint Surg. **52B:**483, 1970.

Lloyd-Roberts, G. C., and Lettin, A. W. F.: Arthrogryposis multiplex congenita, J. Bone Joint Surg. **52B:**494, 1970.

Mead, N. L., Lithgow, W. C., and Sweeney, H. J.: Arthrogryposis multiplex congenita, J. Bone Joint Surg. **40A:**1285, 1958.

Middleton, D. E.: Studies on prenatal lesions of skeletal muscle as a cause of congenital deformity. I. Congenital tibial kyphosis. II. Congenital high shoulder. III. Myodystrophia foetalis, Edinburgh Med. J. **41:**401, 1934.

Menelaus, M. B.: Talectomy for equinovarus deformity in arthrogryposis and spina bifida, J. Bone Joint Surg. **53B:**468, 1971.

Oh, W. H.: Arthrogryposis multiplex congenita of the lower extremities; report of two siblings, Orthop. Clin. North Am. **7:**511, 1976.

Sheldon, W.: Amyoplasia congenita, Arch. Dis. Child. **7:**117, 1932.

Tompkins, S. F., Miller, R. J., and O'Donoghue, D. H.: An evaluation of astragalectomy, South. Med. J. **49:**1128, 1956.

Talipes calaneovalgus

Larsen, B., Reimann, I., and Becker-Anderson, H.: Congenital calcaneovalgus with special reference to its treatment and its relation to other foot deformities, Acta Orthop. Scand. **45:**145, 1974.

Wetzenstein, H.: Prognosis of pes calcaneovalgus congenita, Acta Orthop. Scand. **41:**122, 1970.

Abnormalities of the toes

Cockin, J.: Butler's operation for an overriding fifth toe, J. Bone Joint Surg. **50B:**78, 1968.

Farmer, A. W.: Congenital hallux varus, Am. J. Surg. **95:**274, 1958.

Frazier, T. M.: A note on race specific congenital malformation rates, Am. J. Obstet. Gynecol. **84:**184, 1960.

Kelikian, H., Clayton, L., and Loseff, H.: Surgical syndactylia of the toes, Clin. Orthop. **19:**208, 1961.

Kessel, L., and Bonney, G.: Hallux rigidus in the adolescent, J. Bone Joint Surg. **40B:**668, 1958.

Kirtland, L. R., and Russell, R. O.. Polydactyly, report of a large kindred, South. Med. J. **69:**436, 1976.

Lapidus, P. W.: Transplantation of the extensor tendon for correction of the overlapping fifth toe, J. Bone Joint Surg. **24:**555, 1942.

Leonard, M. H., and Rising, E. H.: Syndactylization to maintain correction of overlapping 5th toe, Clin. Orthop. **43:**241, 1965.

McElvenny, R. T.: Hallux varus, Q. Bull. Northwestern Univ. Med. Sch. **15:**277, 1941.

McCusick, V. A.: Mendelian inheritance in man: catalogues of autosomal dominant, autosomal recessive, and X-linked phenotypes, ed. 2, Baltimore, 1968, Johns Hopkins Press.

Nathan, P. A., and Keniston, R. C.: Crossed polydactyly. Case report and review of the literature, J. Bone Joint Surg. **57A:**847, 1975.

Scrase, W. H.: The treatment of dorsal adduction deformities of the fifth toe, J. Bone Joint Surg. **36B:**146, 1954.

Sharrard, W. J. W.: The surgery of deformed toes in children, Br. J. Clin. Pract. **17:**263, 1963.

Sweetnam, R.: Congenital curley toe: an investigation into the value of treatment, Lancet **2:**398, 1958.

Tachdjian, M. O.: Pediatric orthopaedics, Philadelphia, 1972, W. B. Saunders Co.

Thompson, S. A.: Hallux varus and metatarsus varus, Clin. Orthop. **16:**109, 1960.

Zimbler, S., Craig, C., Oh, W. H., and Iacono, V.: Exhibit presented at the annual meeting of the American Academy of Orthopaedic Surgeons, Las Vegas, 1977.

5

BONES OF THE FOOT AND THEIR AFFLICTIONS

Donald E. Baxter and Roger A. Mann

ACCESSORY BONES

Both Trolle (1948) and O'Rahilly (1953) have studied accessory bones. Trolle (1948) studied serial microscopic sections from the 508 feet of 254 embryos between 6 and 27 weeks of fetal age and found that in nearly 80% accessory bones preformed in hyaline cartilage were present. The high incidence of such bones in embryonic feet did not correlate well with their incidence in adult feet. Trolle was unable to find an os trigonum in any of the embryonic feet he studied, although it occurs frequently in adults. Conversely, in 13% of the embryonic feet he found anlagen of the os paracuneiforme, in spite of a much lower incidence in adult feet. He concluded that accessory bones may (1) develop from an independent element preformed in hyaline cartilage, (2) develop from an inconstant ossification center, (3) be explained as tendon bones, (4) be due to unrecognized pathologic lesions. Thus it would seem that there are several explanations for the presence of these abnormalities. O'Rahilly (1953) catalogued thirty-eight tarsal and sesamoid bones (*ossa tarsalia et sesamoidea*) and stated that the bones may have been incomplete fusions, accessoria, or bipartitions. Henderson (1963) and Wildervanck et al. (1967) have shown hereditary causation of accessory bones in some in-

stances. From the clinical standpoint only two ossicles, the os trigonum and the accessory navicular (prehallux), become symptomatic with any frequency.

Os trigonum

The os trigonum varies greatly in size and shape and appears at the posterior process of the talus. It may be an actual part of the body of the talus (Fig. 5-1, *A*) or a separate bone that may or may not adhere to the talus by a cartilaginous plate (Fig. 5-2). The ossicle is usually asymptomatic and detected only during routine radiography. It has been mistaken for fracture of the posterior process of the talus. It arises from a separate ossification center and appears between 8 and 11 years of age (McDougall, 1955). It is present in 7% of radiographs of normal feet (Bizarro, 1921). Ossicles that are separated from the talus may become loose, producing pain on plantar flexion of the foot; those that are part of the talus may be fractured.

Diagnosis. The os trigonum may cause pain in the retrocalcaneal space which is aggravated on walking, especially when the foot is in plantar flexion. When pressure is applied with the thumb and index finger against the posterior lip of the talus, pain is sharp. Except in sudden fracture of an attached os trigonum,

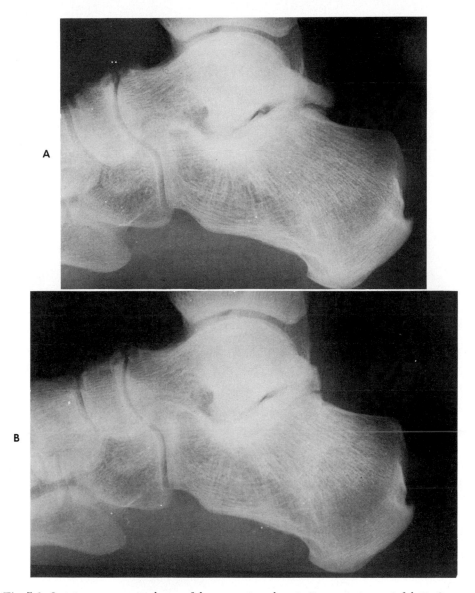

Fig. 5-1. Os trigonum as actual part of the posterior talus. **A,** Preoperative; painful. **B,** One year postoperative; completely asymptomatic.

the onset of symptoms is gradual. The symptoms become progressively worse, and the condition must be differentiated from retrocalcaneal bursitis. In bursitis the symptoms are acute, generally with swelling and tenderness over the retrocalcaneal space, usually posteriorly and just above the insertion of the tendo Achillis instead of at the anterior part of the retrocalcaneal space. Symptomatic cases require surgical removal of the os trigonum.

Procedure for removal of os trigonum. By the procedure for removal of the os trigonum outlined, weight bearing may begin as tolerated in several days. Healing is uneventful in most cases (Fig. 5-1, *B*).

1. Make a linear incision, about 8 cm long, over the retrocalcaneal space posterior to the lower end of the fibula.

2. Retract the skin and make a similar incision in the fascia. The anterior margin of the fascia will be contiguous with the sheath of the peroneal tendons, which are readily retracted to expose the retrocalcaneal space.

3. Denude the os trigonum of all attachments. The separated os trigonum can usually be brought out of the wound. The ossified type may be amputated by means of an osteotome.

4. Smooth the cut surface with a rasp.

5. Suture the fascia and skin in layers.

Accessory navicular (tarsal scaphoid)

Accessory navicular is a congenital anomaly wherein the tuberosity develops from a second center of ossification. Geist (1925) reported a 14% incidence of this ossicle in supposedly normal feet, and Harris and Beath

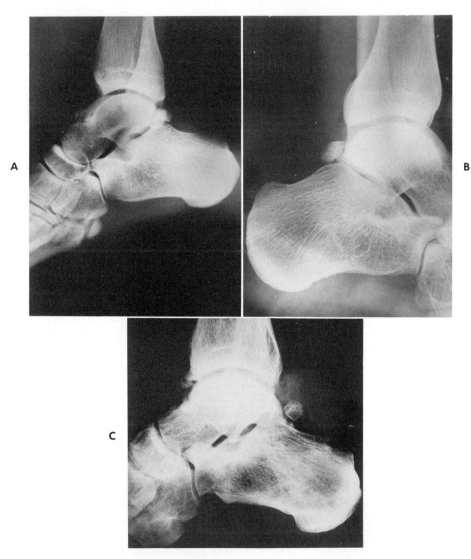

Fig. 5-2. Os trigonum. **A** and **B**, Attached to the talus by a cartilaginous plate. (In **A**, note the os vesalianum at the base of the fifth metatarsal.) **C**, Completely detached from the body of the talus.

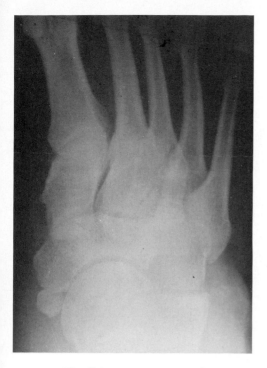

Fig. 5-3. Accessory navicular.

(1947) reported a 4% incidence in young men. McKusick (1968) lists the ossicle with those that are inherited as an autosomal dominant trait and reports an incidence of 5%.

There are two distinct types of accessory navicular. One is a typical, usually small, accessory bone without attachment to the body of the navicular but with a well-defined round or oval outline of demarcation (Fig. 5-3). The other type is a definite part of the body of the navicular, but the tuberosity is separated by a fibrocartilaginous plate of irregular outline (Figs. 5-4 to 5-6). The first type is the true os tibiale externum or naviculare secundarium, which seldom produces symptoms. The second type often has an elongated neck articulating with the tibial side of the head of the talus and fits the description of prehallux or bifurcated navicular. It may become symptomatic and occasionally is mistaken for fracture of the tuberosity of the navicular. The ensuing discussion concerns this second type.

Zadek (1926) studied fourteen cases of symptomatic accessory navicular. Radio-

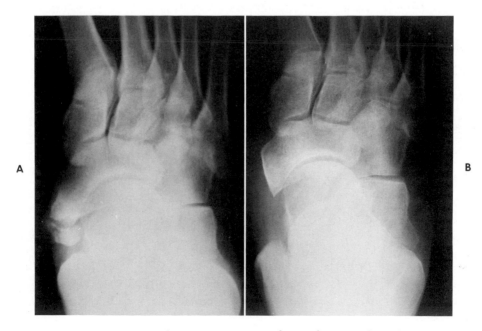

Fig. 5-4. Large accessory navicular. A, Preoperative. The cartilaginous plate is loose and painful. B, One year postoperative.

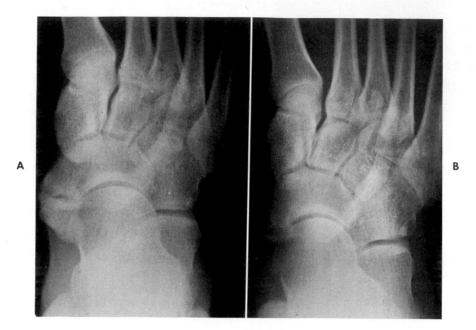

Fig. 5-5. Accessory navicular. A, Preoperative; B, postoperative.

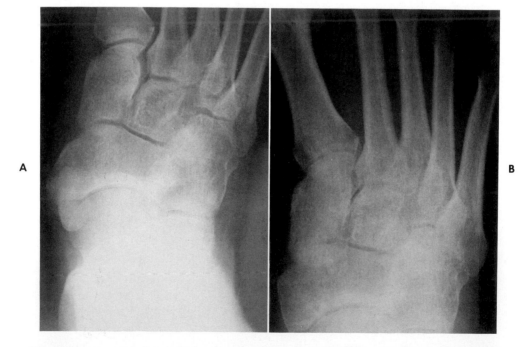

Fig. 5-6. Large accessory navicular extending under the body of the navicular. A, Preoperative; causing abduction of the forefoot. B, Two years postoperative.

graphically he observed definite fusion with the body of the navicular in five cases; there was partial fusion in three, and complete separation in six. In 1948 Zadek and Gold studied microscopically the structures connecting the accessory bone to the body of the navicular. They recorded that these structures were variously composed of a soft tissue plate of hyaline cartilage, dense fibrocartilage, or both and sometimes showed ossification as well.

Kidner (1929) discussed the relationship of flatfoot in the presence of a prehallux and theorized that the etiology of the flatfoot deformity was due to the following:

1. Alteration of the line of pull of the posterior tibial tendon due to the prominence created by the presence of the prehallux
2. The forcing of the posterior tibial tendon by the prehallux to become more an adductor than a supinator of the forefoot, thereby decreasing the support of the longitudinal arch
3. The impingement of the prehallux against the medial malleolus as the foot adducts, which tends to keep the foot reflexly in an abducted position and also partially flattens the longitudinal arch

In a study of twenty patients between the ages of 7 and 40 years, all of whom had accessory navicular ossicles, Chater (1962) supported Kidner's contention. Twelve patients were cured by nonoperative treatment; of the eight remaining, six (children) had excision of the ossicles and two (adults) had the Kidner operation. According to Chater (1962) the Kidner technique appeared to have two advantages over simple excision: it reinforced the buttress mechanism of the spring ligament, and it helped counteract and correct talonavicular sag. Leonard (1965) reported thirteen patients (twenty-five feet) who had prehallux associated with pes planovalgus in whom the Kidner operation was performed for correction of the deformity. They reported satisfactory results in restoring the longitudinal arch and correcting heel valgus.

Giannestras (1973), on the other hand, has stated that in his experience only occasionally is the accessory navicular associated with pes planovalgus. He advocates simple excision if pressure symptoms occur.

In radiographic examination Harris and Beath (1947) found accessory tarsal navicular in the feet of 4% of 3,619 recruits of the Canadian army. Moreover, the results of a follow-up study of seventy-seven men throughout training showed that only four developed symptoms after prolonged marching. The authors concluded that except in rare instances neither accessory bones nor prominence of the navicular tuberosity produce significant symptoms.

Symptoms. An accessory navicular can become symptomatic in childhood or early adulthood. In children the symptoms are usually caused by pressure of the accessory bone against the shoe. At times the condition is associated with progressive flattening of the longitudinal arch. In adults it usually becomes symptomatic after trauma to the foot, often in the nature of a twisting injury. Physical examination will reveal a prominence over the medial side of the tarsal navicular which is rather tender to deep palpation. At times the examiner gets the impression that the ossicle is moving beneath his fingers. The radiographs verify the diagnosis.

Treatment. In the asymptomatic case reassurance as to the nature of the problem is usually adequate. In cases which have become acutely symptomatic following an injury, immobilization in a short-leg walking cast followed by an adequate arch support is indicated. When the symptoms are due to pressure over the navicular, a shoe should be obtained that will not place pressure on the accessory navicular. Occasionally an injection of corticosteroids into the tender area will be beneficial. Sometimes the disability becomes intractable; then surgical intervention may be necessary.

The Kidner procedure is generally quite successful in alleviating the symptoms.

1. Make a slightly curved incision convex dorsally and centered over the talonavicular joint starting 1 cm anterior and below the medial malleolus to the medial cuneiform.
2. Incise the ligament and fascia along the anterior border of the tibialis posterior tendon

throughout the length of the incision. By sharp subperiosteal dissection, create and reflect an anterior fascial periosteal flap and an inferior ligamentous tendinous flap, thereby exposing the accessory bone and the body of the navicular.

3. Detach only the navicular insertion of the posterior tibial tendon along with a button of bone.

4. Excise the accessory navicular. The plane of excision can be detected by manual motion of the accessory bone.

5. Remove the enlarged irregular medial tuberosity of the navicular using an osteotome.

6. Transpose the tendon and button of bone downward and laterally along the plantar surface of the navicular while the foot is held in supination. Secure the tendon and bone to the plantar aspect of the navicular, utilizing pins or heavy sutures through drill holes.

7. Close periosteum, fascia, and skin in layers, and apply a supportive compression dressing.

8. Do not permit weight bearing for 7 to 10 days, at which time remove sutures and apply a short-leg walking cast with the forefoot slightly adducted and inverted.

9. Maintain the extremity in a short-leg walking cast in the corrected position for 5 weeks, after which time instruct the patient to wear a well-fitted oxford with an extended counter for 6 months.

Uncommon accessory ossicles; bifurcated medial cuneiform

The rare accessory medial cuneiform (os paracuneiforme) may present a problem. The procedure for removal of this bone is comparable to that described for removal of an accessory navicular.

Henderson (1963) reported four cases of os intermetatarseum between the first and second metatarsal heads bilaterally. All were associated with hallux valgus; three were familial.

Harris (1965) implicated the os sustentaculare and the os calcaneus secundarius in tarsal coalition and peroneal spastic flatfoot. Wilder-

vanck et al. (1967) reported a family with eight members in three generations who had os tibiale, os paranaviculare, tarsal coalition, and proximal symphalangism of the fingers.

Osteochondritis dissecans of any of the accessory ossicles may rarely be encountered (Fig. 5-7).

Any of the uncommon accessory ossicles may become diseased and produce symptoms. Horizontal bifurcation of the medial cuneiform is rare. Fig. 5-8 shows an asymptomatic case. Fig. 5-9 shows an asymptomatic anomalous medial cuneiform.

ABNORMALITIES OF THE METATARSALS
Metatarsus primus varus

In this deformity the first metatarsal is excessively adducted relative to the lateral four metatarsals, which positioning may be responsible for the development of hallux valgus in later life.

Harris and Beth (1947) concluded, on the basis of a radiographic study of the feet of over 3,000 young men, that the mean angle of divergence between the longitudinal axes of the first and second metatarsals was 7.5° whereas the mean angle in cases of severe hallux valgus was 11.3°. Some hallux valgus was present in over 40% of feet in which this angle was more than 14.5°. They were unable, however, to demonstrate that increased medial obliquity of the first metatarsocuneiform joint was associated with hallux valgus.

During childhood the deformity responds to plaster cast correction and sometimes to soft tissue stretching by manipulation. For adults with significant symptoms, corrective osteotomy is necessary. Tachdjian (1967) expressed the belief that during infancy this condition should be treated similarly to congenital metatarsus varus, with serial plaster casts.

Metatarsal fusion

Metatarsal fusion may occur as part of a syndrome described by Nievergelt (1944) in which there are dominantly transmitted multiple synostoses of the hands and feet, including tarsal and carpal coalitions and radial head

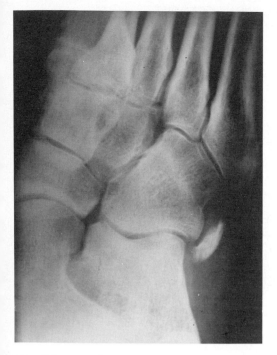

Fig. 5-7. Osteochondritis dissecans of the os peroneum.

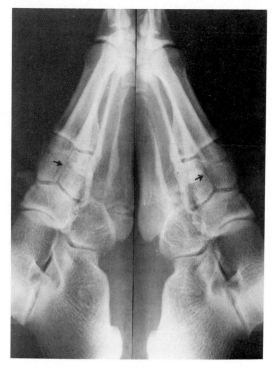

Fig. 5-8. Horizontal bifurcation of the medial cuneiform.

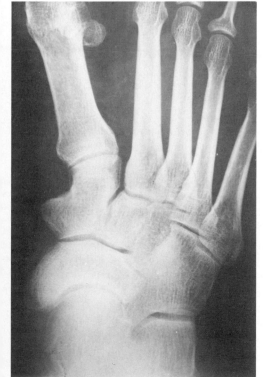

Fig. 5-9. Anomalous medial cuneiform; asymptomatic.

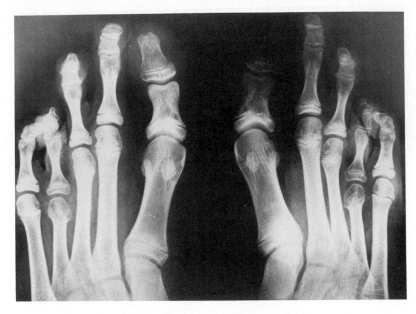

Fig. 5-10. Bilateral congenital short fourth metatarsal.

subluxations (Pearlman et al., 1964). Metatarsal and metacarpal fusion, most commonly of the fourth and fifth or third and fourth rays and associated with soft tissue syndactyly of both fingers and toes, has also been reported in five generations of one family (Kemp and Ravn, 1932).

Congenital short metatarsals

Shortness of the first metatarsal, posterior displacement of the sesamoids, and hypertrophy of the shaft of the second metatarsal were described by Morton (1935) as a syndrome causing pain at the base of the second metatarsal and calluses under the second and third metatarsal heads. He attributed this syndrome to atavistic regression of the human foot to a more primitive form. Since that time numerous authors have supported Morton's contention. Subsequent studies would indicate, however, the relative shortness of the first metatarsal should not be considered an abnormality; such shortnesss is hereditarily determined and probably is not connected with significant foot symptoms.

Harris and Beath (1947) studied shortness of the first metatarsal (defined as being at least 1 mm shorter than the second) and found that 33% of 3,619 Canadian recruits had relatively short first segments. However, even when the first metatarsal was markedly shorter than the second, there was no resultant functional incapacity. The hereditary aspects of relative lengths of the great and second toes in Caucasian twins were studied by Kaplan (1964), who concluded that the gene for a longer hallux (than the second toe) is recessive but has a greater gene frequency (87% for longer hallux, 13% for longer second toe). Therefore a longer second toe, although dominant, has a lesser frequency and occurred in only 24% of phenotypes in the population studied.

Shortness of other metatarsals (brachymetapody) may occur, and occasionally this condition results in excessive loading of the adjacent segments, with consequent plantar callus. Most cases are probably nonhereditary; but shortness of the first and fifth metatarsals was reported in persons with pseudohypoparathyroidism, and Steggerda (1942) reported the case of a family with apparently dominant transmission. One or many of the metatarsals may be congenitally short (Figs. 5-10 to 5-12) and may produce disability. Therapy cannot be standardized.

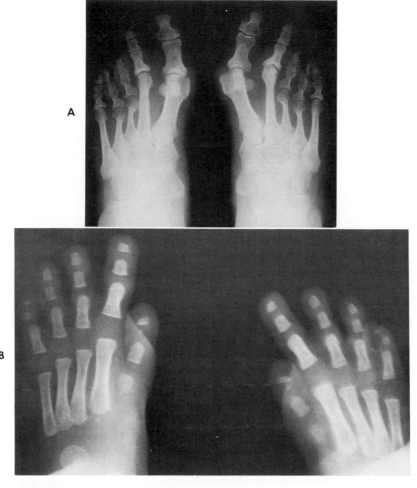

Fig. 5-11. A, Bilateral congenital short third and fourth metatarsals. **B,** Bilateral congenital underdevelopment of the first metatarsal.

Metatarsus proximus

Normally the second and third metatarsal heads are adjacent to each other, with little space between. They are occasionally situated so close to each other that the wearing of ordinary shoes squeezes them together and causes pain from friction, which may necessitate excision of the side of one of the heads (Fig. 5-13).

ABNORMALITIES OF THE SESAMOIDS
Distortion and hypertrophy

The sesamoids vary widely in size and shape. Some have projections that become weight-bearing points, thereby producing a deep-seated callus, usually under the tibial sesamoid.

Congenital variations of the sesamoids become a problem if the whole or part of the plantar surface of the sesamoid is not smooth or evenly shaped. The types of irregularities vary extensively. Sesamoids can be extraordinarily large or thick and may have a sharp projection on the plantar surface. Acquired irregularities may be secondary to a congenitally anomalously shaped sesamoid or to rotation of the sesamoid consequent to deformity of the great toe joint. Because the sesamoids normally fit into a groove on the plantar surface of the first metatarsal head, any rotation or abduction of the first metatarsal tends to rotate

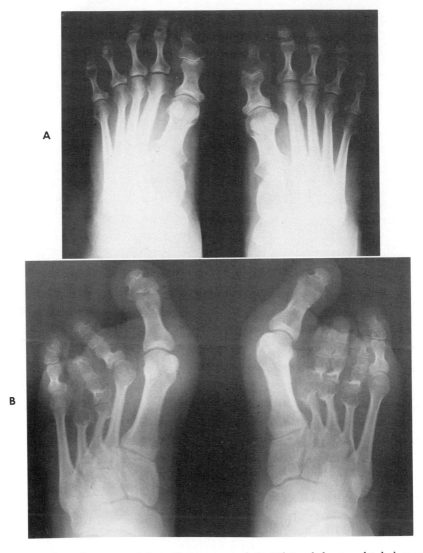

Fig. 5-12. A, Bilateral congenital short first metatarsal. **B,** Bilateral short multiple lesser metatarsals.

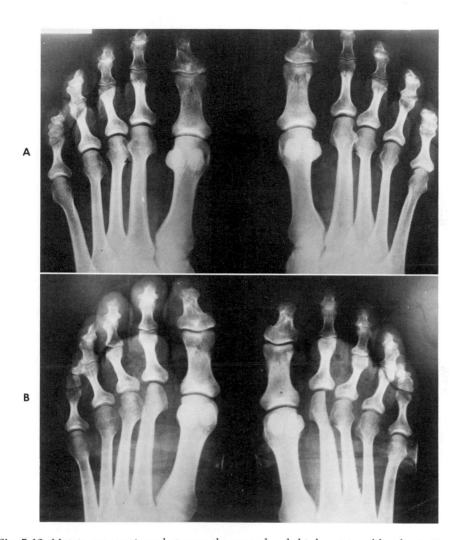

Fig. 5-13. Metatarsus proximus between the second and third metatarsal heads. **A,** Preoperative; **B,** postoperative.

the sesamoids. Their distorted shape also may be the result of hypertrophy. If hypertrophy is plantarward, the excess bone will induce a deep-seated callus and ultimately may ulcerate the soft tissue beneath it because of the pressure of weight bearing (Figs. 5-14 and 5-15).

Symptoms. Constant pain on weight bearing is the symptom that makes the patient seek relief. A deep-seated callus is typically present under the pivotal area. It may be mistaken for a verruca plantaris. The soft tissue under the sesamoid, debilitated by chronic irritation, may ulcerate and resist all palliative treatment. Misshapen or hypertro-

phied fibular sesamoids seldom produce keratotic changes of the skin, because normally they do not bear weight. The pain experienced between the first and second metatarsal heads may be due to irritation (Fig. 5-16). Occasionally an exostosis develops on the fibular sesamoid (Fig. 5-17).

Treatment. In mild cases proper weight distribution alleviates symptoms. In protracted cases sesamoidectomy is indicated.

Congenital absence of the tibial sesamoid

Two cases of congenital absence of the tibial sesamoid, in each case on one foot only, were

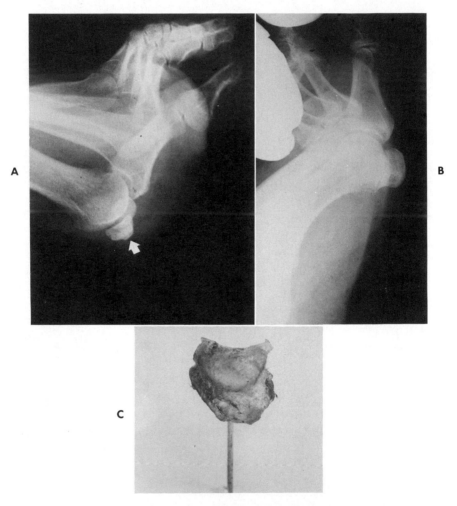

Fig. 5-14. A, Hypertrophic ridge on the plantar surface of the tibial sesamoid; produced a hyperkeratotic skin lesion (arrow). **B,** Unusually thick tibial sesamoid; induced a deep-seated callus beneath. **C,** Extensive hypertrophy of an excised sesamoid; caused a chronic ulcer under the first metatarsal head.

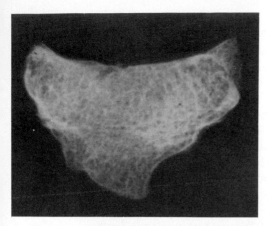

Fig. 5-15. Medial view of the tibial sesamoid after removal. Exostotic enlargement on its plantar aspect caused a keratotic lesion and chronic ulcer on the foot of 15 years' duration.

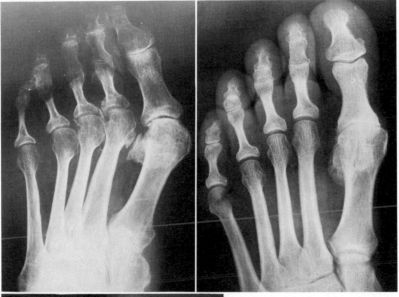

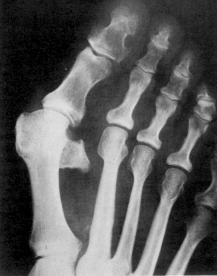

Fig. 5-16. Hypertrophic changes of the fibular sesamoid; pain in the first metatarsal interspace.

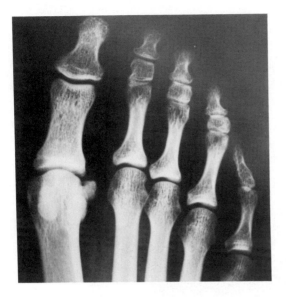

Fig. 5-17. Exostosis of the fibular sesamoid.

reported by Inge (1936). The anomaly is probably more prevalent than is realized and goes unnoticed because ordinarily it is symptomless. Such an anomaly, however, can produce a painful callus under the first metatarsal head when there is a hammertoe deformity of the great toe. The absence of the sesamoid weakens the flexor hallucis brevis and predisposes the great toe to a clawed shape. Bilateral absence of the tibial sesamoid also may produce such deformity and intractable callus under the first metatarsal head as to require reduction of the hammertoe with lengthening of the extensor hallucis longus for relief of symptoms (Fig. 5-18).

Inconstant sesamoids

Accessory, or inconstant, sesamoids may occur under any weight-bearing surface of the foot (Figs. 5-19 to 5-21), especially under the heads of the lesser metatarsals (Fig. 5-22) or any of the phalanges and at times under all the metatarsal heads. Patterson (1937) and Lapidus (1940) each reported such a case. The accessory sesamoids vary widely in size and shape. Ordinarily they are asymptomatic but can become painful when the ossicle is unusually large or when the metatarsal above it

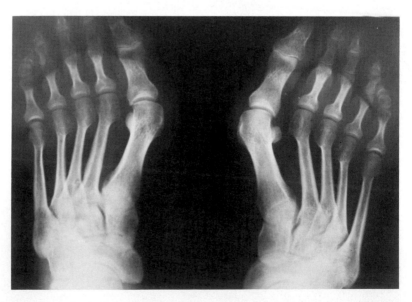

Fig. 5-18. Congenital absence of both tibial sesamoids. Hammered great toe with resulting pain under the first metatarsal head occurred.

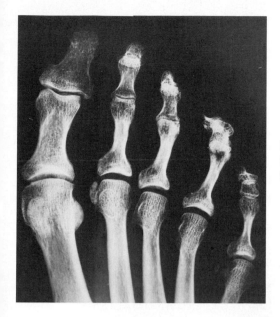

Fig. 5-19. Accessory sesamoid in the short flexor of the second toe. It had rotated into the first metatarsal interspace and caused chronic pain.

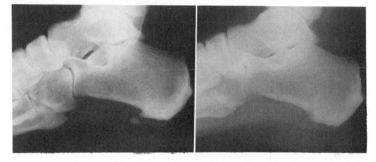

Fig. 5-20. Pain under the calcaneal tuberosity caused by an accessory sesamoid in the plantar fascia. Symptoms were relieved by excision of the sesamoid.

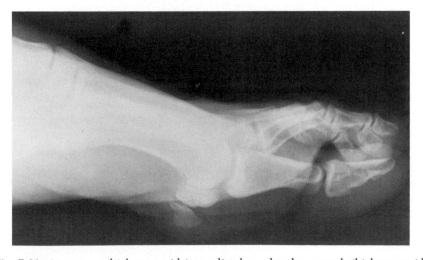

Fig. 5-21. Accessory tibial sesamoid immediately under the normal tibial sesamoid.

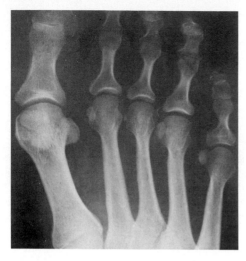

Fig. 5-22. Inconstant sesamoids under the lesser metatarsals.

rotates. They are more likely to produce symptoms under the second or fifth metatarsal head. Sesamoids under the second metatarsal head can be excised through an incision over the first metatarsal interspace. Under the fifth metatarsal head they are best excised through an incision along the lateral plantar border of the fifth metatarsophalangeal joint.

Subhallux sesamoid

A sesamoid may occur as an accessory bone under the interphalangeal joint of the great toe. This accessory has been called a subhallux sesamoid. When a subhallux sesamoid is unusually large, it can act as a pivot point and in time may become quite disabling.

Characteristics. The patient usually presents for treatment because of a large, midline, deep-seated callus on the plantar aspect of the interphalangeal joint of the great toe. At times a chronic ulcer is associated with the condition. A lateral projection of the great toe will confirm the clinical suspicion of a subhallux sesamoid (Fig. 5-23).

Treatment. The treatment of choice consists of debridement of the callus and adequate padding. If ulceration is present, protection of the area from weight bearing and multiple reductions of the callus will permit the ulcer to heal.

If the callosity remains symptomatic, exci-

sion of the subhallux sesamoid is indicated.

1. Make a midline medial incision centered over the interphalangeal joint of the great toe.

2. Deepen the incision to expose the sheath of the flexor hallucis longus tendon.

3. Open the tendon sheath and note the sesamoid between the interphalangeal joint and the flexor hallucis longus tendon.

4. Excise the subhallux sesamoid, being careful not to detach the insertion of the flexor hallucis longus tendon.

5. Close the wound in a routine manner. The patient may ambulate the following day in a wooden shoe, which should be worn for approximately 3 weeks.

MISCELLANEOUS MINOR CONGENITAL ANOMALIES
High dorsum of base of first metatarsal–first cuneiform joint

Congenital enlargement of the dorsum of the first metatarsal–first cuneiform joint is common (Fig. 5-24). It becomes symptomatic only from friction and pressure of the shoe, usually in early adult life and mostly in women. Resulting problems include the following: (1) acute cellulitis over the dorsum of the joint, which may or may not extend down to the bone, producing osteomyelitis (the infection enters through a hair follicle in the skin over the bony prominence), (2) tenosynovitis of the extensor hallucis longus tendon, which lies immediately over this enlargement, (3) constant friction and pressure over the area, gradually producing a fibrotic mass that may break down to form a chronic draining sinus, and (4) osteophytic changes in the form of lipping at the base of the first metatarsal and medial cuneiform.

Treatment. In moderate cases avoidance of shoes that exert pressure and friction over the area ameliorates symptoms. In protracted cases, especially when lipping has formed, removal of the bony prominence is indicated.

The following technique makes ambulation possible in 48 hours. Healing is usually uneventful and complete in from 6 to 8 weeks.

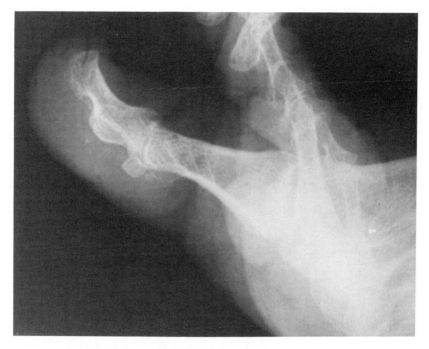

Fig. 5-23. Large subhallux sesamoid under the interphalangeal joint; resulted in a chronic ulcer beneath.

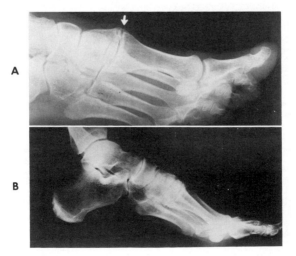

Fig. 5-24. High dorsum of the base of the first metatarsal–first cuneiform articulation. **A,** Preoperative; **B,** postoperative.

1. Make a longitudinal incision along the dorsomedial aspect of the base of the first metatarsal–first cuneiform.

2. Retract the lateral skin margin and make a longitudinal incision in the ligaments and capsule over the middle of the joint. This will obviate having two lines of sutures in the same plane.

3. Retract the periosteal margins to expose the bony prominence. Remove the prominence with an osteotome. Smooth with a rasp and cover with bone wax.

4. Close the fascia and skin in layers and apply a compression bandage.

Rare minor anomalies

Some rare anomalies are illustrated in Figs. 5-25 to 5-30. These include (1) adaptive changes in the base of the second metatarsal as a result of grating of the base of the first metatarsal into the second, (2) a bifurcated first cuneiform with an abnormal hallux and proximal phalanges, (3) synostosis of the shafts of the left second and third metatarsals, (4) polydactyly, syndactyly, and anomalous lesser metatarsals in the same foot, (5) syndactyly of both feet with symphalangism of the left third toe and absence of all of the right third toe except for the epiphysis of the proximal phalanx, and (6) an old untreated congenital vertical talus.

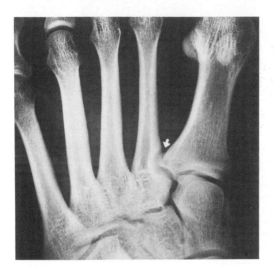

Fig. 5-25. Base of the first metatarsal eroding into the base of the second metatarsal. Note the secondary bony reaction in the base of the second metatarsal.

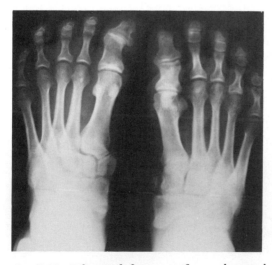

Fig. 5-26. Bifurcated first cuneiform; abnormal hallux and proximal phalanges.

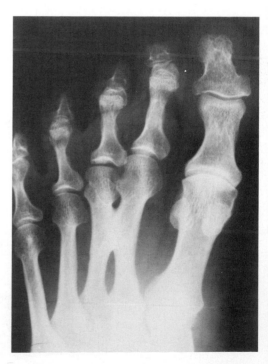

Fig. 5-27. Asymptomatic synostosis of the shafts of the left second and third metatarsals.

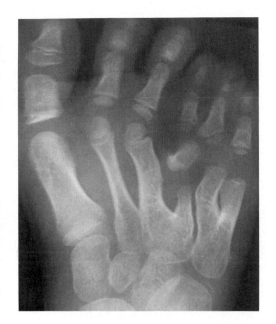

Fig. 5-28. Polydactyly, syndactyly, and anomalous lesser metatarsals in the same foot.

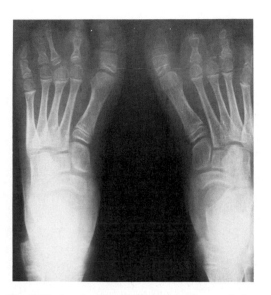

Fig. 5-29. Syndactyly of both feet with symphalangism of the left third toe and absence of all the right third toe except for the epiphysis of the proximal phalanx. This child had a hypoplastic external ear and hypoplastic thumbs and was also mentally retarded.

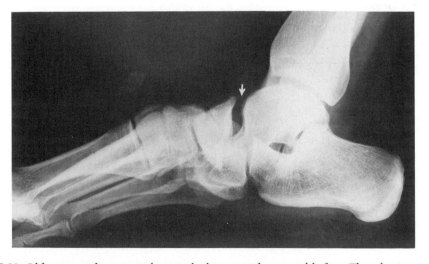

Fig. 5-30. Old untreated congenital vertical talus; caused an unstable foot. The talus is vertically aligned, and the talonavicular findings represent adaptive changes.

DISEASES OF THE SESAMOIDS

The medial and lateral sesamoids under the first metatarsal are the most constant of the foot. They may be congenitally absent, or additional sesamoids may occur in the lesser toes (p. 111).

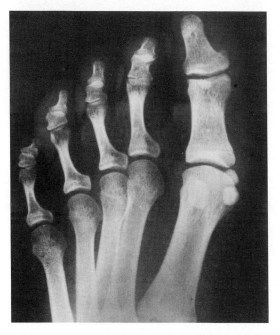

Fig. 5-31. Dorsoplantar view of dislocation of the distal half of a bipartite sesamoid into the first metatarsophalangeal joint.

Sesamoids, named for their similarity in appearance to sesame seeds, do not contain periosteum. They are intimately related to the fibrous tissue of the tendon. The superior (dorsal) surface of the sesamoid is composed of cartilage which articulates with the cartilaginous projection of the metatarsophalangeal joint. The plantar surface of the sesamoid is covered by thick fibrous tissue (the plantar aponeurosis). The medial (tibial) sesamoid is larger than the lateral and lies more directly under the metatarsal head. The smaller (lateral) sesamoid articulates with the outer (fibular) side of the distal first metatarsal (Colwill, 1969).

Bipartite and multipartite sesamoids (Fig. 5-31) occur in approximately 10% of all feet; the tibial sesamoid is more often the divided one. Three fourths of bipartite sesamoids are unilateral. Most bilateral sesamoids are symmetric; thus the differentiation between a fractured sesamoid and a multipartite sesamoid may not be confirmed by comparison with the sesamoid of the opposite member (Colwill, 1969). Fractures are confirmed by healing and decreased pain (Devas, 1963).

Simple sesamoiditis

Sesamoiditis is a painful condition that may be acute or chronic in nature. The acute form

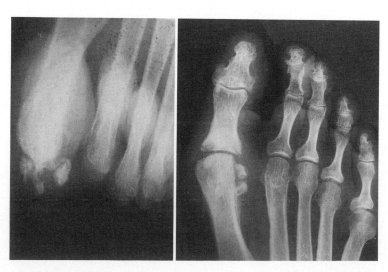

Fig. 5-32. Nonpyogenic osteomyelitis of both sesamoids of 5 months' duration with complete disorganization.

is usually secondary to trauma—e.g., jumping from a height, stepping on a rock, and rarely a fracture or osteomyelitis (Figs. 5-32 and 5-33). The chronic form is usually secondary to repeated small traumas—e.g., jogging on hard surfaces, prolonged standing on hard surfaces with leather soles, or a plastic shoe insert which ends just at the proximal edge of the sesamoid.

The symptoms consist mainly of pain local-

ized under the first metatarsophalangeal joint which is aggravated with weight bearing. In some cases any active motion of the metatarsophalangeal joint will cause pain.

The physical findings consist of tenderness over the involved sesamoid when it is palpated. The tibial sesamoid seems to be more involved than the fibular. Passive dorsiflexion of the metatarsophalangeal joint often causes significant pain. Occasionally an enlargement

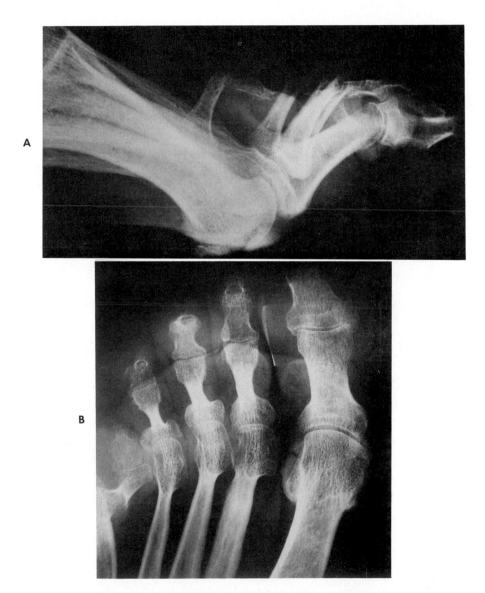

Fig. 5-33. **A,** Medial view. Avascular necrosis of the tibial sesamoid secondary to diabetes mellitus. **B,** Dorsoplantar view. Degenerative changes of the fibular sesamoid.

of a sesamoid is noted. At times slight plantar flexion of the first ray or a mild cavus foot is observed with the chronic type of sesamoiditis.

The routine radiographic evaluation of the sesamoids should include tangential views. Treatment is directed toward relieving weight bearing by the sesamoids as well as keeping the metatarsophalangeal joint from dorsiflexing. Relief of pressure on the sesamoids can be achieved by having the patient rest and use crutches, by placing a pad in the shoe to relieve pressure on the sesamoids, by taping the great toe into slight plantar flexion and using a wooden shoe to decrease dorsiflexion at the metatarsophalangeal joint, and if necessary, by applying a short-leg cast to prevent dorsiflexion. The systemic treatment for sesamoiditis includes antiinflammatory medications; local treatment includes an occasional injection of corticosteroids.

Osteochondritis deformans juvenilis, chondromalacia, and avascular necrosis of the sesamoids. These disorders are varieties of so-called sesamoiditis.

Osteochondritis deformans juvenilis usually affects adolescents and young adults. Radiographically fragmentation and changes similar to those that occur in osteochondritis deformans juvenilis of any other bone may be seen. The pain caused by this condition is treated by means of protective padding until it subsides. Repair and secondary bone changes may lead to a breaking of the sesamoid or cause other deformities. Osteochondritis may also occur in accessory bones (Fig. 5-34).

Chondromalacia is thought to be another cause of simple sesamoiditis. No abnormality or displacement exists in this disorder, but local tenderness persists over the articular surface. Degeneration of the sesamoid may produce hallux rigidus; the metatarsophalangeal joint appears normal but the metatarsal joint, which articulates with the sesamoid, shows the abnormality (Gervis, 1960).

Avascular necrosis of the sesamoids can

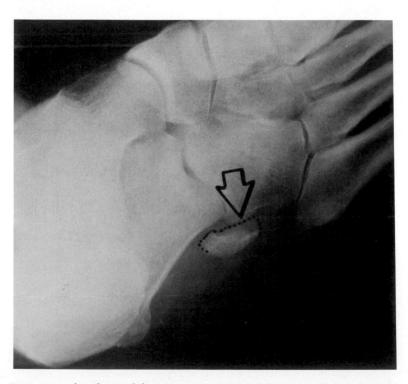

Fig. 5-34. Osteochondritis of the os peroneum; painful. Excision was necessary.

occur after an acute osteomyelitis or may be a presenting feature of developmental vascular change (Fig. 5-33). If the deformity is severe and the symptoms persist after conservative treatment has been carried out, excision may be necessary (Golding, 1960).

VASCULAR DISORDERS

Before describing particular vascular afflictions or dysfunctions, we shall attempt to clarify the terms as they are presented here. *Aseptic necrosis* signifies bone death without infection. An *infarct* is an area of necrosis caused by local anemia due to an obstruction of circulation (of any origin) to that particular region. *Epiphysitis* is an inflammatory response of the epiphyseal bone. *Apophysitis* is an inflammatory response of a bony process attached to a bone. *Osteochondrosis* signifies a disease (degeneration, necrosis) of the growth ossification centers, after which regeneration or recalcification occurs. *Osteochondritis* is an inflammatory response of bone and cartilage that can occur at any age. *Osteochondritis deformans juvenilis* implies a growth center and is an osteochondrosis; *juvenile deforming tarsal osteochondritis* is an osteochondritis of the developing tarsal navicular. The foregoing terms are often interchangeable.

Present thinking implies a vascular etiology of these disorders; aseptic necrosis of the tarsal navicular may be the same entity as osteochrondrosis or osteochondritis deformans juvenilis.

The osteochondroses

Because of the locomotor and weight-bearing functions of the foot, forces acting on the growing bones often play a part in the disruption of the blood supply to the various primary and secondary growth centers. These particular changes have been given eponyms after the men who first observed and reported them.

Osteochondrosis of the tarsal navicular (Köhler's disease). The average age of onset of this affection of the developing navicular is 5 years. It is an avascular necrosis that is related to the peculiar circinate blood supply of the

growing navicular (Waugh, 1958). Current opinion holds that compression induces abnormal ossification at a critical stage in development (Fig. 5-35). Further compression from the formation of this additional bone results in the development of ischemia.

Radiographs demonstrate sclerotic bone which resembles a coin or pancake. Reactive hyperemia follows sequentially, along with pain, tenderness, and swelling. Because of the abundant blood supply, the regeneration of bone produces a normal adult tarsal navicular. Reports of the persistence of deformity are rare.

The treatment of osteochondrosis of the tarsal navicular is supportive. Some children experience intense pain; others have only vague discomfort. Pain may be reduced by means of plaster immobilization or a regimen of decreased weight bearing. As has been indicated, the disease is self-limited.

Osteochondrosis of the metatarsal head (Freiberg's infraction). Infraction, meaning incomplete fracture, is not truly an applicable term for this disorder, which is also called Köhler's second disease and, in Europe, Panner's disease. It usually occurs in the head of the second metatarsal and is also an avascular necrosis. Freiberg's infraction most often appears in the second decade of life and is characterized by local tenderness and pain in the area adjacent to the affected bone.

As with other osteochondroses, incidental trauma to the primary growth center at a significant stage of development is thought to cause vascular deprivation and secondary changes. Because the second toe is usually the longest one, it is subject to pressure on its long axis from the wearing of shoes. If the pressure occurs during a critical phase of epiphyseal maturation, an osteochondrosis of this epiphysis may result (Braddock, 1959).

The diagnosis of Freiberg's infraction, which must be differentiated from a stress fracture, is made radiographically (Figs. 5-36 and 5-37). The radiograph will show osteosclerosis in the early stages and osteolysis in later stages. Symptoms may vary widely.

The treatment of the disease is directed toward protection and the alleviation of dis-

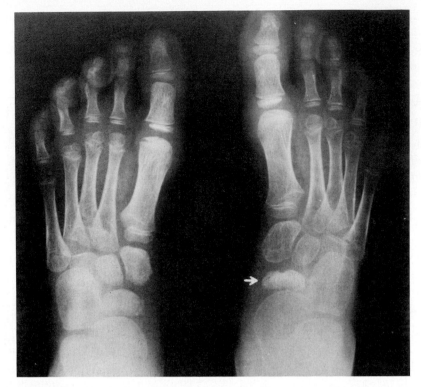

Fig. 5-35. Osteochondrosis of the right navicular (Köhler's disease).

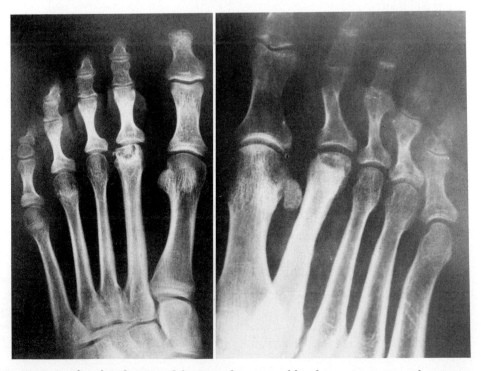

Fig. 5-36. Freiberg's infraction of the second metatarsal head in active state, with sequestration.

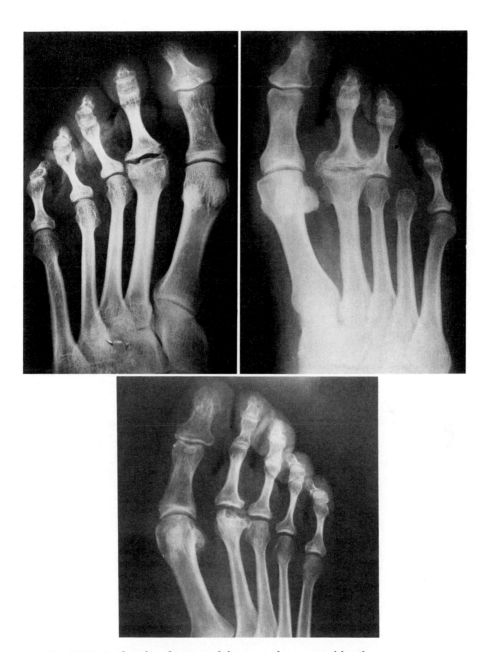

Fig. 5-37. Freiberg's infraction of the second metatarsal head in static state.

comfort by various means, including the limitation of activity and the use of a plaster walking cast. In response to healing, excessive bone may develop on the plantar surface of the involved metatarsal head. Instances of surgical intervention to alleviate secondary bone overgrowth have been reported. Adults who have persistent pain in the second metatarsophalangeal joint as a result of Freiberg's infraction may require an arthroplasty of the joint in which the metatarsal head is debrided of the loose fragment and reshaped. Excision of the metatarsal head should be avoided.

Osteochondrosis of the calcaneal apophysis (Sever's disease). This disease is an apophysitis or avascular necrosis of the traction apophysis of the heel (Fig. 5-38). Again, direct trauma from weight bearing and the pull of the tendo Achillis insertion are thought to be causative factors. It occurs in school-age children bilaterally at times. Its clinical manifestations are progressive heel pain, local tenderness, and painful gait.

An initial radiograph of the involved apophysis will demonstrate sclerosis and fragmentation. Radiography after resolution of the condition will show decreased bone density and atrophy. The epiphyseal line will be irregular. Some patients without this disorder manifest similar radiographic changes but have no symptoms.

Treatment is directed toward protection and the relief of pain and may include decreased physical activity, the wearing of sandals, or rigid immobilization. Often a heel lift to hold the foot in equinus is used.

Osteochondrosis of the fifth metatarsal head, the tibial sesamoid of the first metatarsal, the cuboid, the cuneiform, and the talus occurs less commonly (Fig. 5-39). In these sites the clinical findings and the aims of treatment are similar.

Avascular necrosis; bone infarct

Avascular necrosis is a process of bone death without infection. If avascular necrosis occurs in a solitary primary growth center, it is classified as an osteochondrosis.

At the time of onset, the involved bone exhibits decreased vascularity, marrow necrosis, and perhaps calcific deposit on the medullary interstices. The bone becomes radiographically dense (with or without fragmentation) in contrast to the remaining

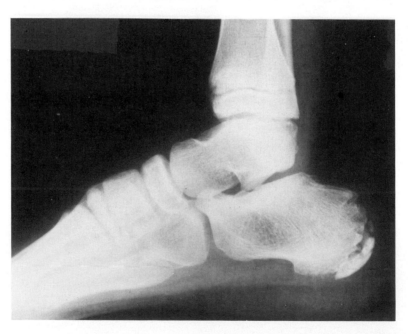

Fig. 5-38. Osteochondrosis of the calcaneal apophysis in a 14-year-old boy; increased density of the apophysis as well as fragmentation.

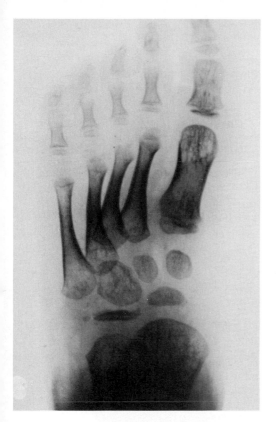

Fig. 5-39. Osteochondrosis of the cuboid. (From Khoo, F. Y.: J. Bone Joint Surg. **32B:**230, 1950.)

bones, which may show signs of osteoporosis of disuse (Aegerter and Kirkpatrick, 1975). With a return of reparative vascular invasion and new bone apposition, the radiographic picture changes. Whereas the affected bone has a moth-eaten appearance and becomes atrophic with the invasion of granulation tissue, the new bone apposition manifests greater density (Bobechko and Harris, 1960). In the event that many bones are affected with avascular necrosis, a complete metabolic investigation must be performed to rule out the presence of systemic disease. Care must be taken not to mistake avascular necrosis for a tumor.

Avascular necrosis of the bones of the foot may occur secondary to trauma, particularly if fracture or dislocation has occurred and the blood supply has been interrupted (Fig. 5-40). The fractured talus is especially vulnerable to avascular necrosis. (See Chapter 6.)

In cases of avascular necrosis that cannot be ascribed to metabolic, infectious, or traumatic causes, congenital factors have been cited as etiologic agents. Shaw (1954) reported a particular case of avascular necrosis in which progressive destruction of one or more pha-

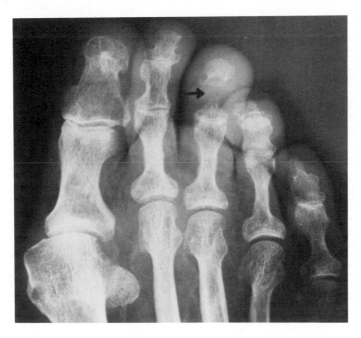

Fig. 5-40. Avascular necrosis of the third middle phalanx.

langes occurred in six generations of one family. "Idiopathic" avascular necrosis of the metatarsal heads and tarsal bones has been encountered, but reports of such cases are are (Fig. 5-41).

No rationale exists to explain the arrest of this condition. Except for the uncommon case in which destruction is permanent, treatment by supportive measures is indicated.

The term "bone infarct" designates a region of circulatory deprivation of bone that can occur in the metaphyseal or diaphyseal region of a tubular bone and may by asymptomatic. Both bone infarct and aseptic necrosis may describe the same condition.

Osteochondritis

Osteochondritis indicates disruption of the blood supply to mature bone adjacent to cartilage. Trauma, caisson disease, embolism, arteritis obliterans, and heritable predisposing factors may be implicated as causes of osteochondritis (Figs. 5-42 and 5-43). In the event that conditions of osteochondritis cause disruption of the normal continuity of the adjacent convex articular surface of subchondral bone, an osteochondritis dissecans develops (Stillman, 1966).

The talus is the bone of the foot which is most vulnerable to osteochondritis (Figs. 5-44 and 5-45). According to Berndt and Harty

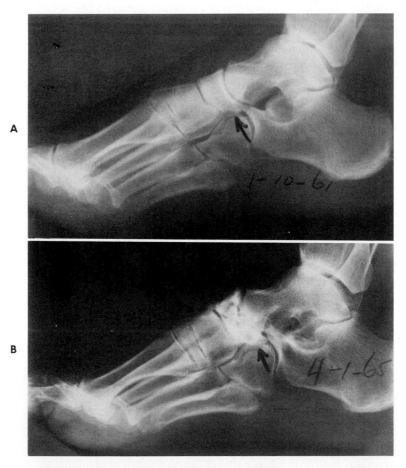

Fig. 5-41. Avascular necrosis of the navicular in a 42-year-old woman; pain in the talonavicular joint. **A,** 1961, No osseous changes. **B,** 1965, Extensive dissolution of this bone; no underlying cause could be found.

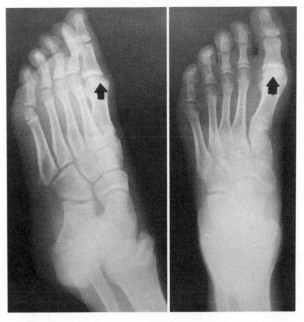

Fig. 5-42. Osteochondritis of the left first metatarsal head in a 13-year-old girl. Her parents had forced her to toe-dance for the three previous years.

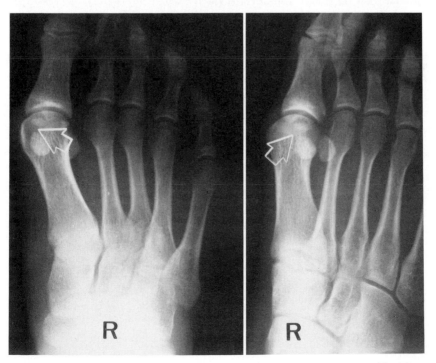

Fig. 5-43. Osteochondritis of the first metatarsal head in a 15-year-old girl.

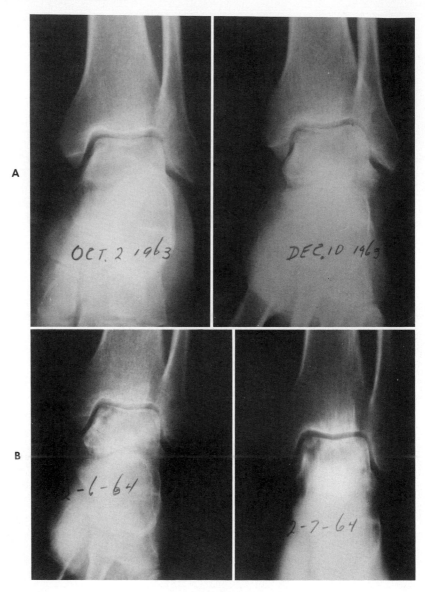

Fig. 5-44. In an accident the right foot of this 44-year-old man was caught, and there was complete inversion. ("The bottom of my foot was parallel to my inner ankle, and I twisted it back in place.") The injury was a medial dislocation of the talus with disruption of the lateral collateral ligaments. **A,** left, Negative findings; right, definite evidence of a crushing injury to the trochlear surface of the talus at the medial malleolus. **B,** left, Obvious osteochondritis dissecans; right, tomogram of the area.

(1959), in a summary of 183 cases, osteochondritis dissecans of the talus (Fig. 5-44, *B*) most often occurs after transchondral fracture that has been initially misdiagnosed or unrecognized or has not immediately appeared radiographically. Vascular impairment is believed

to be perpetuated by the constant shearing of joint action. The ensuing capillary fracture, with failure to revascularize, impedes the normal process of healing. The ultimate result of an unhealed transchondral fracture fragment of the talus is chronic synovitis, which in

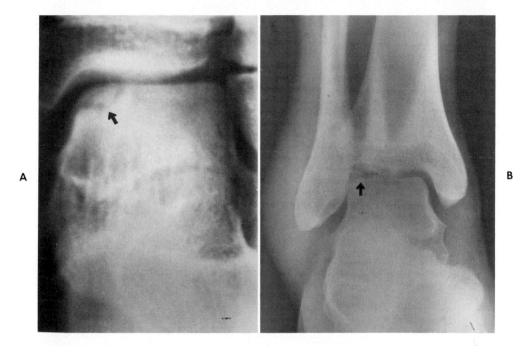

Fig. 5-45. Osteochondritis of the trochlear surface of the talus in a 13-year-old girl. **A,** On the tibial side, note the complete separation of the bone fragment (arrow). **B,** Osteochondritis of the trochlear surface of the talus (arrow). Note the widening of the overlying ankle joint secondary to the reparative process. **B,** On the fibular side, note the resulting edema (arrow).

time can result in degenerative arthritis of the ankle joint.

Radiographic examination, along with the patient's history of recurrent ankle sprain and previous symptoms, confirms the diagnosis. In view of the poor results obtained from conservative measures, treatment of this disorder should be surgical. Even for children surgical extirpation or replacement and fixation of the fragment are advised.

ARTHRITIDES

Degenerative arthritis or osteoarthritis is a process occurring in middle-aged and elderly persons. The most common sites in the foot are the first metatarsocuneiform joint and the first metatarsophalangeal joint. However, it can occur within any joint of the foot (Fig. 5-46). As the degenerative process continues, structural changes occur in the joint which over a period of time result in functional loss. This functional loss, in turn, places stress on other areas of the foot, causing further pain due to the abnormal use of the foot.

The etiology of degenerative arthritis is still controversial, but biochemical changes occur within the articular cartilage along with proliferation of bone about the joint and subsequent distortion of the joint.

The foot is unique insofar as it is constantly under stress during gait; consequently any abnormality within the foot that causes pain will cause the person to alter his gait pattern. This results in further discomfort which may be manifest in the other joints of the lower extremity and back.

The typical history given is somewhat dependent on the joint or joints of the foot involved. Generally, however, the symptoms are worse in the mornings until the person has had a chance to "loosen up"; but symptoms are also aggravated by prolonged walking and standing. Changes in the weather often bring about increased pain in arthritic joints.

Physical examination demonstrates that the affected joint is tender and may be warmer than usual. Motion of the joint often causes discomfort. Bony proliferation around the

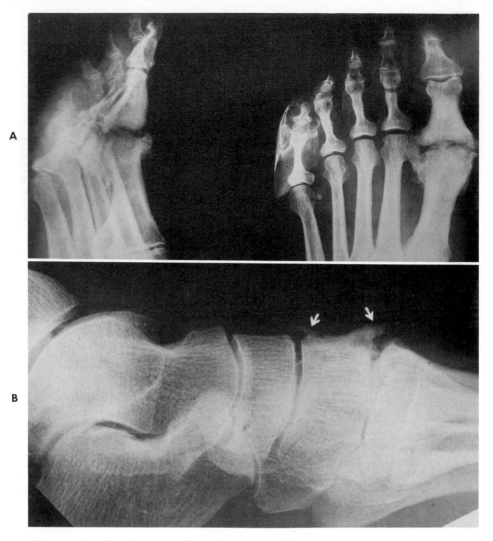

Fig. 5-46. A, Degenerative arthritis of the first metatarsophalangeal joint (hallux rigidus); extensive reactive bone proliferation. **B,** Degenerative arthritis of the first metatarsocuneiform articulation.

margin of the affected joint is often seen.

Radiographic examination demonstrates a decrease in the joint space, sclerotic joint margins, and proliferative bone about the periphery of the joint.

Treatment. In general, initially conservative treatment should be provided. Anti-inflammatory medications can be given either systemically or through local injections. Proper-fitting shoes should be prescribed. Orthotics which will remove stress from the

rigid and painful area may be useful. (See Chapter 17.)

Orthotic devices could include a molded leather ankle brace for ankle and midtarsal dysfunction or a rocker-bottom shoe that would help take the stress off the proximal and distal joints of the foot. A rocker-bottom shoe causes a rolling motion which in turn reduces stress on the foot.

If conservative measures fail, surgical intervention may be indicated: for degenerative

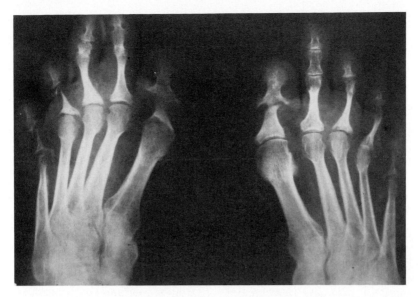

Fig. 5-47. Psoriatic arthritis; extensive destruction of some of the proximal phalanges.

arthritis of the first metatarsophalangeal joint, see p. 584; for degenerative arthritis of the metatarsocuneiform joints, see Chapter 19.

Psoriatic arthritis

Patients with psoriasis have a greater incidence of arthritis than does the population in general. There is a striking involvement of the distal interphalangeal joint associated with marked destruction and psoriatic changes in the adjacent nails. Frequently destruction of the proximal phalanges occurs and the bone atrophies to needle points (Fig. 5-47). Many of the cases resemble rheumatoid arthritis. The psoriasis usually antedates the arthritis by months or years; but the conditions can appear simultaneously. The arthritis infrequently appears first. The details and management are similar to those for rheumatoid arthritis.

Gouty arthritis

Gout has been known since antiquity and is secondary to an alteration in purine metabolism. It occurs more frequently in males than in females and exhibits a definite inheritance pattern. Approximately 50% to 75% of initial attacks involve the great toe. Ninety percent of patients with gout experience one or more acute attacks in the toes during their lifetime (Stanbury et al., 1972). Gout can also present as an acute periarthritis of the great toe joint, often referred to as gouty bursitis.

The onset of an acute gouty attack is sudden; the great toe joint becomes swollen and excruciatingly painful. The attack is self-limiting but tends to recur at intervals. Gout can also occur in the plantar fascia as a plantar fasciitis or a tenosynovitis or occasionally in any of the joints of the foot. Acute attacks often occur after the stress of a surgical procedure. The patient with postoperative pain in the foot should be evaluated for possible gout. When an acute attack occurs, it can last from several days to weeks.

Chronic gouty arthritis with its tophaceous deposits is rare today, probably because of the excellent medical management of most patients who have gouty arthritis; however, 10% of untreated gout patients develop chronic tophaceous deposits in the soft tissues followed by invasion and destruction of joints and bones. The diagnosis of gouty arthritis is made by obtaining a serum uric acid report of more than 7 mg/100 ml. Sodium urate crystals are consistently and uniquely present in the joint aspirates of patients with acute gouty arthritis. Patients with primary gout, who have sodium urate levels of 9 mg/100 ml or less, usually do not develop visible tophi, even if left untreated. When the serum urate level exceeds 11 mg/100 ml, tophaceous deposits are inevitable and, unless preventive measures are taken, are likely to occur within a few years of the initial acute attack.

Radiographic examination of patients with joint involvement reveals a characteristic periarticular erosion just proximal to the joint, often on both the tibial and the fibular aspects of the first metatarsal head (Fig. 5-48). A feature that distinguishes gouty arthritis from other arthritides is the presence of destructive lesions in bones remote from the articular surface. Many of the lesions are expansile with overhanging margins displaced away from the axis of the bone and secondary calcifications within the tophi or degenerative tissue. There may be tophaceous deposits below the deep fascia which can encircle and invade tendons, but the nerves and blood vessels are spared although surrounded by the tophaceus material.

Treatment. The treatments of acute and chronic cases of gouty arthritis are different.

In patients with acute tophaceous gout, elevation and rest of the foot accompanied by therapeutic doses of colchicine, phenylbutazone, or cortisone are used to relieve pain. To prevent subsequent acute episodes, the patient should have the regular supervision of an internist.

In patients with chronic tophaceous gout, removal of the tophaceous material by curetting usually prevents the return of deforming overgrowth (Woughter, 1959). Kurtz (1965) has emphasized that (1) amputation is rarely indicated; (2) in cases of draining sinuses over tophi, local curettement of as much of the deposit as possible followed by application of wet dressings will promote healing; and (3) if the skin sloughs and a surgical wound exudes urates, treatment with wet dressings and antibiotics will result in healing with surprisingly little scarring.

Rheumatoid arthritis

Rheumatoid arthritis is a systemic disease of unknowm etiology that affects primarily the synovial tissues.

Joint inflammation is the dominant clinical feature. The disease, which affects women

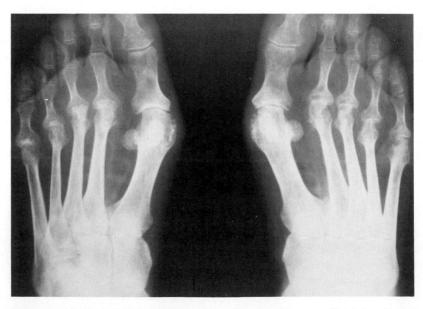

Fig. 5-48. Gouty arthritis in a 65-year-old woman with a long history of high levels of uric acid and tophi in other parts of her body.

three times as frequently as men, is said to occur in 2% to 3% of people over 55 years of age. No clear-cut racial or occupational predisposition is evident. There are geographic aggregations of people with rheumatoid arthritis, but whether these clusters appear because of genetic or environmental influences is unclear.

In most patients acute rheumatoid arthritis runs a variable course. It often assumes a chronic form, which leads to progressive joint destruction. Although all joints may be involved, the metacarpophalangeal and the metatarsophalangeal joints are usually affected. Careful questioning reveals that the disease begins as frequently in the feet as in the hands.

A diagnosis of rheumatoid arthritis is based on clinical, laboratory, and radiographic findings. Although the disease commonly begins insidiously, an acute onset is not by any means rare. X-ray studies and laboratory tests give little diagnostic help during the acute stage. Generally the diagnosis must be tentative for several weeks until the disease has progressed and its true nature become apparent. With progression to a subacute or chronic arthritis, symmetric involvement usually occurs. Although not common, the condition may also begin asymmetrically. Swelling is chiefly intra-articular with effusion, but periarticular soft tissue swelling is often present. Involvement of the proximal interphalangeal and metatarsophalangeal joints is particularly suggestive. Radiographic examination may reveal only soft tissue swelling and juxta-articular osteoporosis; but in the more advanced disease, cartilaginous thinning, bony erosion, and dislocations may be seen (Fig. 5-49). Laboratory studies reveal a moderately to markedly increased sedimentation rate. A test for rheumatoid factor is frequently positive, although a negative result does not in any way preclude the diagnosis.

Even when all the joints of the foot and ankle are involved in the rheumatoid process, the metatarsophalangeal, proximal interphalangeal ankle, and subtalar joints are what produce the most disability. Rheumatoid arthritis begins in the feet in approximately 17%

of reported cases. The forefoot is more commonly involved than the hindfoot.

The destruction and deformity of the joints are preceded by noticeable swelling. Initially there is swelling with tenderness accompanied by increased skin temperature and erythema over the involved joint. Later, the characteristic deformities with dorsal subluxation of the metatarsophalangeal joint appear and are followed by complete dislocation, which pulls the plantar fat pad distally into an ineffective position. The plantar aponeurosis and all the flexor tendons are likewise drawn up on top of the metatarsal head, thereby holding the metatarsal head down in a plantar-flexed position. The metatarsal heads are palpable, lying just beneath the plantar skin.

The end-state malformations seen in the forefoot are (1) hallux valgus, (2) marked claw-toe and hammertoe deformities associated with dorsal dislocation of the metatarsophalangeal joint, (3) loss of the plantar fat pad, (4) plantar callosities under the heads of the metatarsals, (5) dorsal callosities over the interphalangeal joint caused by shoe pressure, and (6) terminal callosities at the tips of

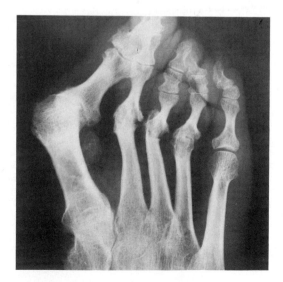

Fig. 5-49. Rheumatoid arthritis of the first four metatarsophalangeal joints; atrophic changes of the articular surfaces of these joints.

the toes caused by direct pressure secondary to their flexed position.

Involvement of the hindfoot, most notably the subtalar and talonavicular joints, leads to a progressive valgus deformity of the calcaneus and secondarily causes loss of the longitudinal arch. Rupture of the posterior tibial tendon, which is more common in rheumatoid arthritis, can also occur and leads to loss of the longitudinal arch with progressive valgus of the hindfoot. If the ankle joint is also involved, marked instability of the entire foot-ankle complex results (Fig. 5-50).

Rheumatoid arthritis can be divided into four stages (Fig. 5-51).

Stage 1. In the first stage there is no bony deformity, and no surgery is indicated.

Stage 2. In this stage there is early involvement without fixed deformity. Radiographs show minimal erosive changes. Synovectomy as a prophylactic and therapeutic measure may be employed if there has been unremitting synovitis despite adequate nonsurgical measures for a period of not less than 6 months and if the patient has had the disease for not less than one year. The ankle, metatarsophalangeal, and interphalangeal joints lend themselves to synovectomy.

Stage 3. At this stage of involvement, soft tissue deformity has occurred but there have been no significant erosive changes. Under these circumstances synovectomy, tendon transfer, and repair and release are indicated as well as capsulotomy.

Stage 4. Deformity and articular destruction have occurred at this stage, and reconstructive surgical procedures such as arthroplasties or arthrodeses are required.

Treatment. An appreciation of the clinical course of the disease is essential for the proper planning of a treatment program. Treatment is directed toward (1) relief of pain, (2) prevention of deformity, (3) correction of deformity, (4) restoration of function, and (5) preservation of function.

Medical management should be continued throughout all stages of the disease and may be the only treatment necessary during the early phases. Treatment should include antiinflammatory medication and orthopaedic appliances.

Drug therapy. Agents that reduce inflammation and relieve pain are recommended. Salicylates are prescribed as the first line of defense and may be the only drug needed, though other antiinflammatory medications

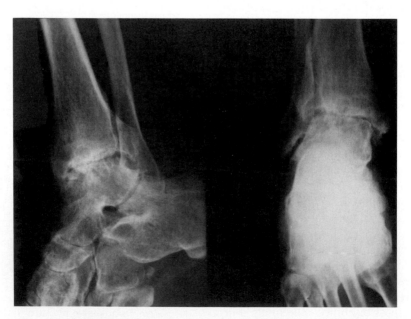

Fig. 5-50. Rheumatoid arthritis of the tarsus and ankle joints.

can be used. Steroid injections into the ankle and the subtalar joint are occasionally beneficial, but restraint should be exercised.

Conservative treatment. The proper balance of rest and exercise is essential to help prevent loss of motion in the joints and to preserve muscle power. A well-fitted splint such as the UCBL insert (Fig. 16-10) can maintain the tarsal joints in a balanced position, provided a fixed deformity is not present.

The UCBL insert may sufficiently relieve the pain that arises from the subtalar and transverse tarsal joints, as well as the plantar fascia, to allow the patient to be ambulatory. The orthotic should be left in place as long as necessary, depending on the activity of the disease process, and should be removed at least once (and preferably several times) a day for the patient to carry out active and passive range of motion exercises. If the deformity is fixed or the pain is not relieved by such an insert, the patient should be fitted with a short-leg double upright brace with a free ankle. If the pain still persists, consideration should be given to immobilization by a molded leather ankle brace with metal stays. For relief of forefoot pain, a metatarsal pad and crepe soled shoe often will help reduce excessive plantar pressure.

Surgical treatment. Although medical management should continue throughout the progression of the disease, surgical procedures are indicated in the later phases.

Hindfoot and ankle deformity. Rheumatoid involvement of the hindfoot usually is more clinically apparent as an affliction of the subtalar joint. The ankle joint is frequently spared. If significant involvement of the subtalar joint has failed to respond to nonsurgical measures (including an orthotic and/or short leg brace) and if the ankle joint is only minimally involved, a subtalar arthrodesis is indicated.

For rheumatoid involvement of the subtalar as well as the ankle joint, Adam and Ranawat (1976) have reported on six patients who underwent pantalar arthrodesis. In each case complete solid fusion occurred, and the authors expressed satisfaction with their results.

Elbaor et al. (1976) have reported on talonavicular arthrodesis for rheumatoid arthritis of the hindfoot. They described thirty-five talonavicular fusions in thirty-one patients. In more than 85% of their cases, there was complete relief of pain and improvement in ambulatory status. They believe that their relatively simple talonavicular fusion of the passively correctable rheumatoid foot, before

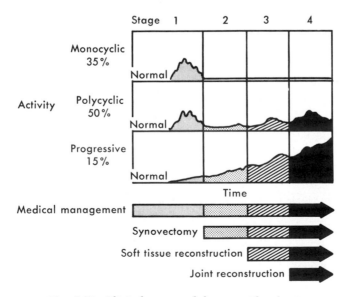

Fig. 5-51. Clinical course of rheumatoid arthritis.

it reaches the stage of a fixed valgus deformity, arrested the natural course of the disease and, in addition, eliminated the need for more elaborate corrective surgery.

Forefoot deformity. The typical forefoot deformities are hallux valgus, subluxation or dislocation of the metatarsophalangeal joints, and flexion of the interphalangeal joints of the lesser toes. There is a loss of effectiveness of the plantar fat pad which causes painful plantar callosities under the metatarsal head.

When conservative treatment fails, surgical treatment must be directed toward reestablishing the alignment of the metatarsals and phalanges, restoring adequate padding on the plantar surface of the foot, and correcting the deformed position of the interphalangeal joints. Surgical procedures of the forefoot and rheumatoid arthritis are discussed in Part 3.

In 1974, Watson reported a long-term follow-up of forefoot arthroplasties, stating that the chief aim of the operation was the relief of pain. In the long-term study he concluded that arthrodesis of the metatarsophalangeal joint of the great toe resulted in the highest proportion of painless feet. After a Keller operation he observed that the natural valgus of the flail great toe was not supported by the abnormal lesser toes. Consequently, during the takeoff phase of gait, the great toe and the lateral toes were displaced dorsally and laterally. As the toes migrated laterally and dorsally, the brunt of the patient's weight was shifted onto the metatarsal ends, causing callosities to develop once again at the distal ends of the remaining metatarsal shafts. When the first metatarsophalangeal joint was fused, it prevented the great toe from pushing the lesser toes laterally.

REFERENCES
General

American Rheumatism Association: Primer on the rheumatic diseases, New York, 1964, The Arthritis Foundation.

Giannestras, N. J.: Foot disorders: medical and surgical management, Philadelphia, 1973, Lea & Febiger.

Harris, R. I.: Retrospect—peroneal spastic flat foot (rigid valgus foot), J. Bone Joint Surg. **47A:**1657, 1965.

Harris, R. I., and Beath, T.: Army foot survey: an investigation of foot ailments in Canadian soldiers (forms no. 1574, Rep. Nat. Res. Counc., Canada), Ottawa, 1947.

Leonard, M. H., Gonzales, S., Breck, L. W., Basom, C., Palafox, M., and Kosicki, Z. W.: Lateral transfer of the posterior tibial tendon in certain selected cases of pes plano valgus (Kidner operation), Clin. Orthop. **40:**139, 1965.

McKusick, V. A.: Mendelian inheritance in man: catalogues of autosomal dominant, autosomal recessive, and X-linked phenotypes, ed. 2, Baltimore, 1968, Johns Hopkins Press.

Accessory bones

Bizarro, A. H.: On sesamoid and supernumerary bones of the limbs, J. Anat. **55:**256, 1921.

Chater, E. H.: Foot pain and the accessory navicular bone, Irish J. Med. Sci. **442:**471, 1962.

Geist, E. S.: The accessory scaphoid bone, J. Bone Joint Surg. **7:**570, 1925.

Giannestras, N. J.: Foot disorders: medical and surgical management, Philadelphia, 1973, Lea & Febiger.

Harris, R. I.: Retrospect-peroneal spastic flat foot (rigid valgus foot), J. Bone Joint Surg. **47A:**1657, 1965.

Harris, R. I., and Beath, T.: Army foot survey: an investigation of foot ailments in Canadian soldiers (forms no. 1574, Rep. Nat. Res. Counc., Canada), Ottawa, 1947.

Henderson, R. S.: Os intermetatarseum and a possible relationship to hallux valgus, J. Bone Joint Surg. **45B:**117, 1963.

Kidner, F. C.: The prehalux (accessory scaphoid) in its relation to flat-foot, J. Bone Joint Surg. **11:**831, 1929.

Leonard, M. H., Gonzales, S., Breck, L. W., Bason, C., Palafox, M., and Kosicki, Z. W.: Lateral transfer of the posterior tibial tendon in certain selected cases of pes plano valgus (Kidner operation), Clin. Orthop. **40:**139, 1965.

McDougall, A.: The os trigonum. J. Bone Joint Surg. **37B:**257, 1955.

McKusick, V. A.: Mendelian inheritance in man: catalogues of autosomal dominant, autosomal recessive, and X-linked phenotypes, ed. 2, Baltimore, 1968, Johns Hopkins Press.

O'Rahilly, R.: A survey of carpal and tarsal anomalies, J. Bone Joint Surg. **35A:**626, 1953.

Trolle, D.: Accessory bones of the human foot (translated by E. Aagesen) Copenhagen, 1948, Munksgaard.

Wildervanck, L. S., Geodhard, G., and Meiier, S.: Proximal symphalangism of fingers associated with fusion of os naviculare and talus and occurrence of two accessory bones in the feet (os paranaviculare and os tibiale externum) in an European-Indonesian-Chinese family, Acta Genet. **17:**166, l967.

Zadek, I.: The significance of the accessory tarsal scaphoid, J. Bone Joint Surg. **8:**618, 1926.

Zadek, I., and Gold, A. M.: Accessory tarsal scaphoid, J. Bone Joint Surg. **30A:**957, 1948.

Abnormalities of the metatarsals

Harris, R. I., and Beath, T.: Army foot survey: an investigation of foot ailments in Canadian soldiers (forms no.

1574, Rep. Nat. Res. Counc., Canada), Ottawa, 1947.

Kaplan, A. R.: Genetics of relative toe lengths, Acta Genet. Med. Gemellol. 13:295, 1964.

Kemp, T., and Ravn, J.: Ueber erbliche Hand- und Fussdeformitäten in einem 140-köpfigen Geschlecht, nebst einigen Bemerkungen über Poly- und Syndaktylie beim Menschen, Acta Psychiatr. Neurol. 7:275, 1932.

Morton, D. J.: The human foot: its evolution, physiology, and functional disorders, New York, 1935, Columbia University Press.

Nievergelt, K.: Positiver Väterschaftsnachweis auf Grund erblicher Missbildungen der Extremitäten, Arch. Julius Klaus Stift. Vererbungs-Forsh. 19:157, 1944.

Pearlman, H. S., Edkin, R. E., and Warren, R. F.: Familial tarsal and carpal synostosis with radial-head subluxation (Nievergelt's syndrome), J. Bone Joint Surg. 46A:585, 1964.

Steggerda, M.: Inheritance of short metatarsals, J. Hered. 33:233 1942.

Tachdjian, M. O.: Diagnosis and treatment of congenital deformities in the musculoskeletal system in the newborn and the infant, Pediatr. Clin. North Am. 14:307, 1967.

Abnormalities of the sesamoids

Colwill, M.: Osteomyelitis of the metatarsal sesamoids, J. Bone Joint Surg. 51B464, 1969.

Devas, M. B.: Stress fractures in children, J. Bone Joint Surg. 45B:528, 1963.

Gervis, W. H.: Hallux valgus and hallux rigidus, J. Bone Joint Surg. 42B:158, 1960.

Golding, C.: Museum pages. V. Sesamoids of the hallux, J. Bone Joint Surg. 42B:840, 1960.

Inge, G. A. L.: Congenital absence of the medial sesamoid bone of the great toe: a report of two cases, J. Bone Joint Surg. 18:188, 1936.

Lapidus, P. W.: Sesamoids beneath all the metatarsal heads of both feet, J. Bone Joint Surg. 22:1059, 1940.

Patterson, R. F.: Multiple sesamoids of the hands and the feet, J. Bone Joint Surg. 19:531, 1937.

Vascular disorders

Aegerter, E., and Kirkpatrick, J. A., Jr.: Orthopedic diseases, ed. 4, Philadelphia, 1975, W. B. Saunders Co.

Berndt, A. L., and Harty, M.: Transchondral fractures (osteochondritis dissecans) of the talus, J. Bone Joint Surg. 41A:991, 1959.

Bobechko, W. P., and Harris, W. R.: The radiographic density of avascular bone, J. Bone Joint Surg. 42B:626, 1960.

Braddock, G. I. F.: Experimental epiphysial injury and Freiberg's disease, J. Bone Joint Surg. 41B:154, 1959.

Shaw, E. W.: Avascular necrosis of the phalanges of the hands (Thiemann's disease), J.A.M.A. 156:711, 1954.

Stillman, B. C.: Osteochondritis dissecans and coxa plana: review of the literature, J. Bone Joint Surg. 48B:64, 1966.

Waugh, W.: The ossification and vascularisation of the tarsal navicular and their relation to Köhler's disease, J. Bone Joint Surg. 40B:765, 1958.

Gouty arthritis

Kurtz, J. F.: Surgery of tophaceous gout in the lower extremity, Surg. Clin. North Am. 45:217, 1965.

Stanbury, J. B., Wyngaarden, J. B., and Fredrickson, D. S., editors: The metabolic basis of inherited disease, ed. 3, New York, 1972, McGraw-Hill Book Co.

Woughter, H. W.: Surgery of tophaceous gout: a case report, J. Bone Joint Surg. 41A:116, 1959.

Rheumatoid arthritis

Adam, W., and Ranawat, C.: Arthrodesis of the hindfoot in rheumatoid arthritis, Orthop. Clin. North Am. 7:827, 1976.

Elbaor, J. E., Thomas, W., Weinfeld, M. and Potter, T.: Talonavicular arthrodesis for rheumatoid arthritis of the hindfoot, Orthop. Clin. North Am. 7:821, 1976.

Watson, M. S.: A long-term follow-up of forefoot arthroplasty, J. Bone Joint Surg. 56B:527, 1974.

6

FRACTURES AND FRACTURE-DISLOCATIONS OF THE ANKLE AND FOOT

Michael W. Chapman

Criteria for treatment

For best functional results in the treatment of all fractures, particularly those involving joints, four criteria must be fulfilled:

1. *Dislocations and fractures should be reduced as soon as possible.* Fractures are most easily reduced early. Reduction is easier to obtain before swelling occurs and before the fracture hematoma between the fragments organizes. Furthermore, gross displacement—particularly in the ankle, subtalar, and midfoot joints—results in considerable distortion of the soft tissues and can lead to impairment of peripheral circulation, neuropraxias, and loss of skin. Early reduction minimizes these complications.

2. *All joint surfaces must be precisely reconstituted.* Nonanatomic reduction may lead to joint instability and/or joint surface incongruity which predisposes to the development of arthritic changes.

3. *Reduction of the fracture must be maintained during the period of healing.* Once anatomic reduction has been achieved, it must be held until bone union and ligament repair have occurred. This can be accomplished by external immobilization with a plaster cast or splints or by internal fixation.

External immobilization, however, has definite deleterious effects on the soft tissue components of the injured part. The extent of these undesirable effects is largely dependent on the age of the patient; the older the patient, the more adverse the effects of long-term immobilization. In addition, holding fractures anatomically by external means is difficult and late loss of reduction in plaster is all too common.

An appreciation of the problems associated with external immobilization has prompted many surgeons, in spite of the possible risk of infection, to employ open reduction, rigid internal fixation, and early mobilization as their treatment of choice.

4. *Motion of joints should be instituted as early as possible.* To maintain itself in a state of health, obviously any organ or organ system must be used. Suppression of the normal functioning of the musculoskeletal system by immobilization of any of its parts is attended by numerous undesirable sequelae—including muscular atrophy, myostatic contracture, decreased joint motion, increased acidity of the synovial fluid, proliferation of the connective tissue in the capsular structures, internal synovial adhesions, cartilaginous degenera-

tion, and bone atrophy. Furthermore, vascular changes occur during the period of immobilization and these often result in edema after the external support is removed. Early mobilization obviates or decreases the possible occurrence of these abnormal processes.

The most ardent protagonist for early motion after the reduction of fracture was Lucas-Championnière (1910), who based his beliefs on clinical experience. Subsequent experimental evidence has gradually appeared in the medical literature to support his contentions (1910 to 1971).

FRACTURES AND FRACTURE-DISLOCATIONS OF THE ANKLE JOINT
Classification

Many classification systems for fractures and fracture-dislocations about the ankle joint exist, based for the most part, on the mechanism of injury.* Knowledge of a classification system enables the surgeon to offer better treatment through the understanding it provides of the interrelationship between the mechanism of injury and the pathologic anatomy. Occult ligamentous injury will be detected, and the optimal position of the limb in a closed reduction can be determined.

Lauge-Hansen (1948, 1950, 1952, 1954) has provided the most useful and comprehensive classification of ankle injuries; and in spite of the complex variety of ankle fractures, 98% to 99% can be fitted into his system. Most important, he emphasizes the role of the ligaments in these injuries. Students of ankle injuries are strongly advised to read the articles of Lauge-Hansen cited in the bibliography. The Lauge-Hansen system is quite complex, however, so from a practical point of view one can look at ankle fractures in a more simplified way—as advocated by Jergesen (1959).

When assessing fractures about the ankle within a functional framework, the practitioner should consider two concepts: (1) Anatomic reduction is desirable because the restoration of normal anatomy to a weight-bearing joint is of primary importance. (2) Stability of the ankle is related to the integrity of the malleolar and syndesmosis ligaments.

The foot is securely bound to the leg by two osseous ligamentous shrouds consisting of (on the one side) the medial malleolus and the corresponding medial collateral ligament and (on the other) the lateral malleolus and the lateral collateral ligaments. In addition, the intermalleolar space is maintained by the tibiofibular syndesmosis ligaments (Fig. 6-1). Any number of fracture and ligamentous disruption combinations can occur that may destroy the normal stability of the ankle. If we speak of the foot in relation to the leg, the basic mechanisms of injury can be thought of as (1) external rotation–eversion or abduction, (2) inversion-adduction, and (3) vertical loading.

Ankle injuries result from abnormal motion of the talus within the ankle mortise. Fractures of the malleoli can result from the impact of the talus. Fractures can also occur in tension, and the malleoli can be avulsed due to the pull exerted by the intact collateral ligaments attached to the talus.

Impact fractures tend to be spiral or oblique. Avulsion fractures tend to be at right angles to the line of pull of the ligament. Ligament failure rather than fracture may occur, so instability in any given injury can be due to a combination of fracture and ligament rupture. Fig. 6-2 illustrates the difference between these two mechanisms.

Fig. 6-3 is four radiographs showing some of the combinations of injuries seen in external rotation–eversion and abduction-type fractures. The possible varieties of injury include the following:

1. External rotation–eversion and abduction injuries
   a. Medial side
      (1) Transverse avulsion fracture of medial malleolus
      (2) Ruptured deltoid ligament
   b. Lateral side
      (1) Spiral fracture of lateral malleolus with fracture line proceeding from distal anterior to proximal posterior (external rotation)

*Ashhurst and Bromer, 1922; Bonnin, 1950; Lauge-Hansen, 1948, 1950, 1952, 1954; Mayer and Pohlidal, 1953; Kleiger, 1956.

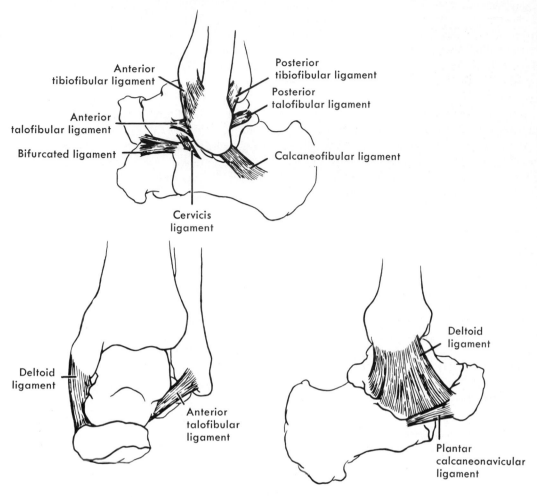

Fig. 6-1. Anatomy of the ankle. (From Chapman, M. W. In Instructional Course Lectures, American Academy of Orthopaedic Surgeons, vol. 24, St. Louis, 1975, The C. V. Mosby Co.)

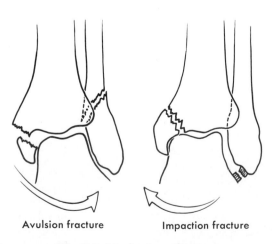

Avulsion fracture   Impaction fracture

Fig. 6-2. Mechanism of injury.

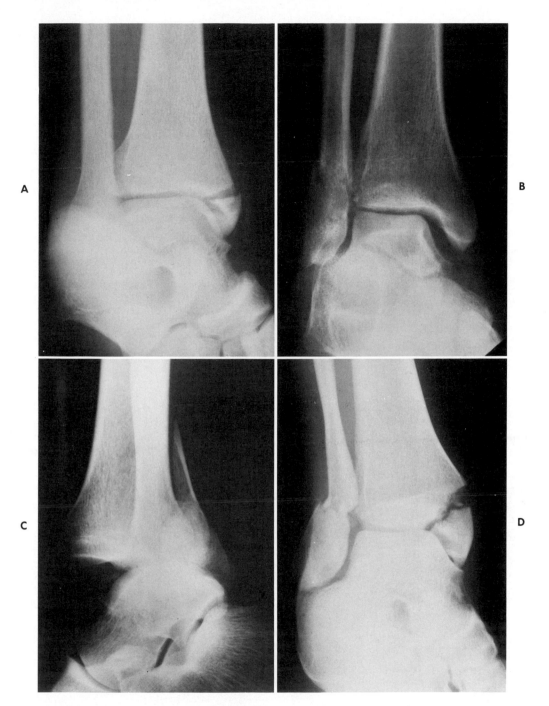

Fig. 6-3. External rotation–eversion and abduction injuries. **A,** External rotation–eversion. Transverse avulsion fracture of the medial malleolus. Look for associated syndesmosis ligament ruptures and/or a high proximal fracture of the fibula. **B,** External rotation–eversion. Short spiral-oblique fracture of the lateral malleolus with deltoid ligament rupture. **C,** External rotation–eversion. Spiral fracture of the lateral malleolus with avulsion fracture of the posterior malleolus. **D,** Abduction. The transverse comminuted fracture of the fibula is fairly typical. The avulsion fracture of the medial malleolus is usually more transverse.

(2) Spiral fracture of shaft of fibula above syndesmosis, usually associated with disruption of syndesmosis (external rotation)

(3) Short oblique fracture of fibula in mediolateral plane below or above syndesmosis, often with small lateral butterfly fragment at fracture (abduction)

c. Syndesmosis
(1) Torn anterior tibiofibular ligament (external rotation) through complete syndesmosis rupture (more common abduction mechanism)

(2) Avulsion fracture of posterior malleolus (external rotation)

Fig. 6-4 is a radiograph of an adduction-inversion injury. The possible varieties of such an injury include the following:

2. Adduction-inversion injuries
a. Medial side
(1) Oblique fracture of medial malleolus extending from corner of ankle mortise proximally and medially

b. Lateral side
(1) Transverse avulsion of lateral malleolus below syndesmosis
(2) Rupture of lateral collateral ligaments
c. Syndesmosis
(1) As part of fibular fracture, torn inferior fibers rare in adduction injuries
d. Posterior malleolus
(1) With posterior medial dislocation, occasional fracture of posterior and medial malleoli

Vertical compression fractures are typically due to falls from a height or deceleration motor vehicle injuries. The configuration of these fractures is quite variable. The usual fracture is accompanied by hyperdorsiflexion of the ankle, producing a vertical shear fracture of the anterior tibial plafond. This injury is usually accompanied by upward impaction of the tibial plafond, compressing the metaphyseal cancellous bone. With severe compression, an explosion-type fracture occurs in

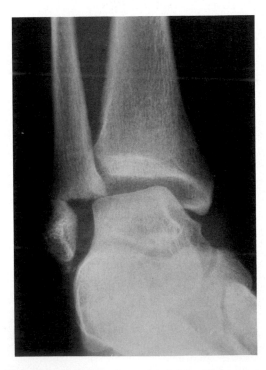

Fig. 6-4. Adduction-inversion injury. Transverse avulsion fracture of the lateral malleolus below the level of the syndesmosis. The talus is hinging on an intact deltoid ligament.

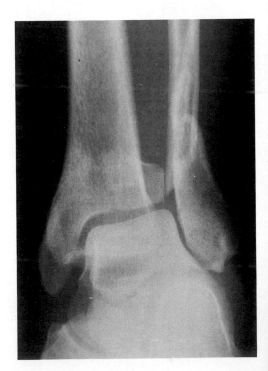

Fig. 6-5. Vertical loading–type fracture of the ankle. The fibular shaft is comminuted. The tibial plafond is driven proximally, resulting in crush fracture of the cancellous bone of the distal tibia.

which the malleoli are displaced outward as the talus drives into the central plafond of the tibia (Fig. 6-5).

Lauge-Hansen pointed out that these fractures occur in stages, with the sequence of fractures and ligament ruptures depending on the position of the foot at the time of injury.

Initial evaluation and emergency treatment

History. Most patients are unable to relate the exact mechanism of injury beyond the type of force involved. With a fall from a height or following a motor vehicle deceleration injury, the surgeon should look for occult impaction of the tibial plafond. The patient may describe complete dislocation of the foot on the leg with spontaneous relocation. This history, of course, would indicate a grossly unstable ankle with probable severe associated soft tissue injuries. Pedestrians hit by motor vehicles frequently have unstable adduction or abduction fractures. Weight-bearing twisting injuries are usually of the external rotation–eversion type, which makes up about 60% of all ankle fractures (Ashhurst and Bromer, 1922). Knee pain over the head of the fibula may suggest an unstable ankle with a high fibula fracture (Maisonneuve, 1840).

Physical diagnosis. The physical diagnosis is important in determining the degree of soft tissue injury, in ascertaining the presence of ligamentous injuries not evident at x-ray examination by assessing joint stability, and in determining the neurovascular status of the foot. Radiographs will reveal the extent of bony injury. Careful systematic palpation to identify areas of tenderness and swelling will help localize disruptions in the structures about the ankle and the interosseous area; the full length of the fibula should be so examined.

The location of findings, plus crepitus, will usually indicate a fracture. In minor seemingly stable injuries, such as an isolated undisplaced fracture of the lateral malleolus, one should look carefully for evidence of deltoid ligament injury. Stability of the ankle should be gently tested in varus, valgus, and particularly external rotation. Premedication and local anesthetics may be necessary. Anterior instability of the talus in the mortise is helpful in detecting unstable ligament injuries. Peroneal muscle spasm may hide lateral instability. If there is a question in the examiner's mind, examination with stress radiographs under anesthesia may be indicated. The neurovascular status of the foot should be carefully assessed. In particular, one should look for partial or complete common peroneal nerve paralysis.

Radiographic findings. Anteroposterior, lateral, and mortise views (the last, an oblique view with the foot internally rotated 15° to 20°) should be obtained. Fractures involving the plafond may require multiple oblique projections and biplane tomograms for full delineation. After correlation of the physical examination findings with the initial x-ray findings, further assessment of the fracture with evaluation of the integrity of the ankle mortise and the tibiofibular syndesmosis is of paramount importance.

The integrity of the syndesmosis is best assessed on the AP projection, as is well described by McDade (1975) (based on Bonnin, 1950), since complete disruption, if undisplaced, will appear normal. The rotatory malalignment that occurs when only the anterior inferior tibiofibular ligament is torn is subtle; the syndesmosis clear space, which represents the posterior tibiofibular joint, does not change as the fibula rotates outward. One must look instead at the extent of overlap of the fibula by the anterior tibial tubercle. Comparison views are often necessary because there is considerable anatomic variation (Fig. 6-6).

On a good mortise view the superior articular surface of the talus should be fully congruous with the tibial plafond. The medial and lateral joint spaces should be equal and comparable to the superior joint space. A line extending distally from the posterior syndesmosis of the tibia should pass lateral to the talus (*a-a* in Fig. 6-7). On lateral views the talar dome should be concentric with the tibial plafond (*b-b*).

Emergency treatment. Excessive swelling can so compromise treatment of even minor

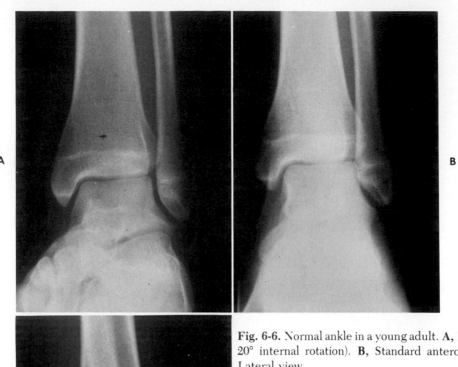

Fig. 6-6. Normal ankle in a young adult. **A,** Mortise view (15° to 20° internal rotation). **B,** Standard anteroposterior view. **C,** Lateral view.

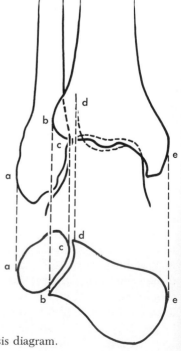

Fig. 6-7. Syndesmosis diagram.

ankle sprains that patients should all have their lower extremities elevated higher than their heart while undergoing initial evaluation and treatment. This usually requires that they be placed on a gurney.

Wounds and abrasions should be cleansed and sterily dressed. A soft compression dressing and radiolucent long leg splint should be applied prior to x-ray examination.

Grossly distorted ankles with severe skin distortion should be reduced immediately in the emergency room to avoid skin necrosis and also to eliminate tension on the neurovascular structures.

Treatment

Soft tissue considerations. Whether treatment of these fractures is by closed or open reduction, ultimate success depends on proper assessment and management of the associated soft tissue trauma.

Abrasions should be carefully cleansed and sterily dressed. Abrasions into the dermis quickly become colonized by skin bacteria; therefore any surgery planned should be done within a few hours. After 12 to 24 hours, depending on how dirty it is, a deep abrasion may contraindicate surgery for 3 weeks or more. Neglected abrasions can lead to local cellulitis with possible infection of the fracture hematoma.

Early closed reduction and elevation with a good compression dressing and splints or a cast are important to preventing edema. Ankle and foot edema can be severe, causing fracture blisters. Gross edema may contraindicate surgery and lead to loss of the initial closed reduction. Surgeons should avoid early surgery on the tensely swollen shiny-skinned "watermelon" ankle since skin closure may be impossible and marginal wound necrosis can occur.

One should always be alert for a compartment syndrome in the leg and foot. The physical findings that should alert the clinician are tenseness in the calf, leg pain with passive stretch of the muscles, and paresis of the deep peroneal nerve.

Closed versus open treatment. Undisplaced fractures without disruption of the ankle mortise are treated with cast immobilization. Undisplaced stable fractures of the lateral malleolus and distal medial malleolus can begin immediate weight bearing in a short-leg walking cast, which should be left in place for 6 weeks. Other stable injuries should be placed in a long-leg cast with the knee flexed 15°. The cast must be molded to assure the maintenance of position. Weekly radiographs for at least 4 weeks are usually necessary to ensure that these fractures do not displace. Depending on the surgeon's judgment about the stability of the ankle, weight bearing can begin in either a short or a long leg cast at 4 or 6 weeks. Any fracture, whether treated closed or open, if treated in a non–weight-bearing cast, will rehabilitate more quickly and easily if given 2 weeks in a short-leg walking cast prior to complete cast removal.

Displaced fractures or fracture-dislocations may be treated by closed reduction and cast immobilization or by open reduction and internal fixation. Open reduction and internal fixation are almost always indicated if anatomic reduction cannot be achieved. If anatomic reduction is achieved closed, it is often impossible to maintain and late displacement is frequent. In closed treatment interposition of the periosteum or other soft tissues, particularly when the medial malleolus is fractured, can prevent good fracture apposition and thereby lead to nonunion or fibrous union.

Open reduction and internal fixation are generally indicated if ankle fractures are displaced, particularly if the talus is subluxated in the ankle mortise. Closed treatment of displaced fractures may be indicated when (1) the condition of the soft tissues contraindicates surgery, (2) the patient is nonambulatory (paraplegic), (3) the patient is elderly and sedentary, and (4) the patient has undergone multiple trauma and surgery is contraindicated.

Closed reduction

External rotation–eversion and abduction. The mechanisms of these injuries are accompanied by posterolateral subluxation or dislocation of the foot on the leg; the foot is usually externally rotated with reference to the leg.

For reduction to be achieved, the foot must be brought anteriorly and medially into position and must be internally rotated on the tibia.

The malleoli are attached to the foot by the collateral ligaments; the "distal fragment" is, in reality, the foot with the attached malleoli. Hence reduction entails regaining the proper relationship of the foot to the tibia. If the deltoid ligament rather than the medial malleolus is disrupted or if the medial malleolar fragment is small, a shoulder or buttress exists medially against which the foot (talus) can be reduced. If the medial malleolar fragment is large, internal fixation of the medial malleolus may be necessary to produce stability of the joint.

A convenient way to carry out manipulative reduction, if an assistant is available, is to flex the patient's hip and knee approximately 30° to allow the extremity to rotate externally approximately 30°. The assistant holds the limb in this position by supporting the thigh with one hand and holding the first two toes with the other hand, thereby maintaining the foot in a vertical plane. Gravity produces medial and anterior replacement of the foot; and with the foot held in a vertical position, an attitude of internal rotation of the foot relative to the leg is achieved. A cast employing the principles of three-point molding can then be applied. The knee should be flexed only 15° in the cast. Rotational control is gained through molding rather than knee flexion. These principles are embodied in the cast shown in Fig. 6-8.

Adduction-inversion mechanisms. In these injuries the reverse of the maneuvers described for the abduction–external rotation injury is required. There is less often a lateral buttress against which to reduce the joint, and the medial malleolar fracture line frequently runs proximally from the level of the joint.

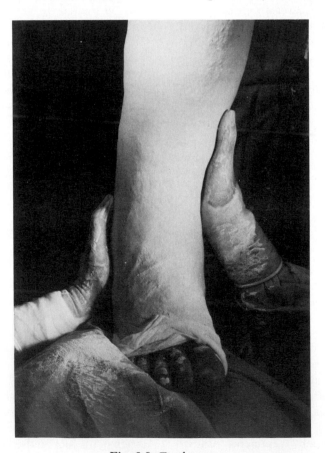

Fig. 6-8. Final cast.

Anterior lip fractures. It is difficult to avoid anterior subluxation in this injury when the patient is recumbent with his limb supported in the usual fashion at the foot and knee. Again the force of gravity can be used to assist the surgeon in reducing the fracture.

Suspend the leg over the end of the treatment table, where an assistant can carry out a posterior thrust of the foot against the leg. Or, more simply, have the patient lie prone on the table with his knee on the injured side flexed approximately 60°. An assistant supports the foot in this position, which permits the weight of the leg against the supported foot to reduce the subluxation. Reduction is maintained in this position while the surgeon applies the cast.

Vertical compression fractures. In stable impacted fractures with minimal displacement, immobilization in a neutral position with careful molding of the cast about the malleoli usually suffices. Unstable comminuted fractures present unique problems (p. 160).

Open reduction with internal fixation. Early surgery is usually best for optimal results. It is best carried out on the day of injury, before edema occurs. Open reduction within 7 days of injury is little different from that achieved on the day of injury. Between 7 and 14 days, the hematoma organizes and extensive debriding of the fracture fragments is necessary to achieve reduction; anatomic reduction can usually be achieved, however. Between 14 and 21 days, callus formation, soft tissue scarring, resorption, and osteoporosis of the fractured bone ends create technical problems which compromise reduction. After 21 days, anatomic reduction is frequently impossible to achieve and closed treatment is often indicated.

Bivalving of the cast and surgical preparation of the skin the evening before surgery are unwise, for an accidental nick of the skin may necessitate postponement of surgery.

Unless contraindicated, a tourniquet should be employed. Unexpected comminution is often encountered, so the surgeon should have a full armamentarium of bone instruments and fixation devices available. In addition to screws, Kirschner wires, small fragment screws, small plates, malleable wire, Steinmann pins, and Rush rods or Knowles pins may be useful. We no longer use Leinbach screws since they frequently break. One should be prepared to take an iliac bone graft in vertical compression fractures.

Repair of ligament ruptures. Ligamentous injuries associated with fractures are the subject of controversy in the literature and are discussed in more detail in Chapter 7.

The primary indication for repair is ligament interposition in the joint space, where exploration is necessary to achieve anatomic reduction (Coonrad and Bugg, 1954). If early mobilization is anticipated, ligament repair will be necessary to assure stability. Ligament repair is not necessary when anatomic reduction has been achieved and protection in a plaster cast for 6 weeks is planned. These injuries will require, at most, a short-leg walking cast to be worn for 6 weeks.

Fractures of one malleolus. A fracture of one malleolus without involvement of its ligamentous component or the opposite malleolus permits using the uninjured side as a buttress to immobilize the part until healing takes place (Fig. 6-3). If only the malleolar tip is injured, simple protection from forced inversion (in the case of a lateral malleolus) or eversion (in the case of a medial malleolus) suffices. These are actually third-degree sprains with a small bone chip attached to the fragment.

Radiographic evidence of fracture of just one malleolus does not guarantee stability; therefore clinical evaluation of the ligamentous structures at the distal tibiofibular junction and on the opposite side of the ankle is necessary to assess the stability of the injury. Except for avulsion fracture of the lateral malleolar tip, the most common isolated fracture of the lateral malleolus is a spiral fracture in the distal portion. Controversy exists over the indications for open reduction of these fractures. If the patient is young or middle aged, inability to achieve and hold a satisfactory reduction is the indication for surgery.

What is a satisfactory reduction? Since the talus follows the lateral malleolus even in the presence of an intact deltoid ligament, small persistent displacement of the fracture can lead to talotibial incongruity. For this reason, assuming that the talus is anatomically reduced in the ankle mortise, I would accept 1 mm or less of shortening or widening. Over 2 mm of displacement is an indication for open reduction. Between 1 and 2 mm requires consideration of the patient's age, activity level, etc.; but, in general, I would lean toward open reduction.

Isolated fractures of the lateral malleolus per se are seldom associated with nonunion although small avulsed fragments frequently do not unite.

Fractures of the medial malleolus, particularly those occurring below the level of the superior surface of the talus, may be asymptomatic even though they heal with fibrous union. Portis and Mendelsohn (1953) and Aufranc (1960) found little evidence to suggest that the isolated malleolar fracture, if not displaced, requires internal fixation. Fractures of the medial malleolus at the level of the plafond, however, result in complete functional loss of internal support provided by the medial collateral ligament. This fracture must be accurately reduced and internally fixed for the ankle to regain stability.

Bimalleolar fractures and fracture-dislocations. The terms bimalleolar fracture and fracture-dislocation are used to describe fractures of both malleoli, fractures of one malleolus plus complete disruption of the ligament on the opposite side, or fracture of the medial malleolus and rupture of the tibiofibular ligaments (Glick, 1964) associated with a fracture in the shaft of the fibula proximal to the tibiofibular ligament (Fig. 6-3).

Fibular fracture can occur at the proximal end of the fibula. If such a fracture is accompanied by ankle injury, one can assume that some disruption of the interosseous membrane has occurred anywhere from the distal tibiofibular syndesmosis to the level of the fibular fracture and that division of the distal tibiofibular ligaments has also taken place. Occasionally the injury will be manifested as a rupture of the deltoid ligament, with the line of dehiscence passing across the ankle capsule and continuing upward through the distal tibiofibular ligaments and interosseous membrane to the level of the proximal neck of the fibula. This particular combination is easy for the unwary examiner to miss since the ankle may be relocated when the technician positions it for radiographic examination. No fracture will be seen unless a full-length radiograph of the leg, including the upper end of the fibula, is taken.

Traditional teaching in English and American orthopaedics has held that with bimalleolar fractures, the majority of which are external rotation injuries, the key to reduction and stability of the ankle mortise is the medial malleolus. Fixation of the lateral side was not believed necessary because of the intact periosteal hinge (Charnley, 1963). This is now known to be not wholly true. McDade (1975) and more recently Yablon et al. (1977) have emphasized the key role of the lateral malleolus in determining the position of the talus in the mortise. With an intact medial osseous ligamentous bridge, subluxation of the talus in the presence of an external rotation fracture of the lateral malleolus can occur. Because the talus faithfully follows the lateral malleolus, anatomic reduction of the lateral malleolus is a must in bimalleolar fractures. Yablon et al. (1977) found that degenerative arthritis following displaced bimalleolar fractures is usually due to incomplete reduction of the lateral malleolus with residual talar tilt.

Reduction of the lateral malleolus can be difficult. Fixation of the medial side first may lock the distal lateral malleolar fragment behind the shaft and prevent reduction. It is best to open both sides simultaneously, inspect and cleanse the joint space and fracture site(s) of debris, and reduce and then fix either the lateral side first or the medial side.

Trimalleolar fractures and fracture-dislocations. Trimalleolar fractures and fracture-dislocations include all the combinations described for bimalleolar types of fracture and dislocation plus fractures of the posterior lip of the tibia.

The fragment may vary in size and may communicate with the medial malleolar fragment; or, if it is laterally placed, it may carry the posterior tibiofibular ligament with it. If the fragment carries one fourth or more of the articular surface of the tibia with it, a high risk of posterior subluxation of the talus exists unless the fracture is internally fixed (Fig. 6-3).

Fortunately most posterior lip fragments are small and do not, in themselves, compromise the stability of the ankle (Aufranc, 1960). In ankles with a posterior fragment involving more than 25% of the articular surface, open treatment is associated with better results than closed treatment (McDaniel and Wilson, 1977).

Fractures of anterior lip of distal tibia. Fracture of the anterior lip of the distal tibia may accompany malleolar fracture as a mirror image of the posterior trimalleolar fracture-dislocation; occasionally it occurs as an isolated injury.

It is generally the result of a vertical loading injury and therefore is not usually associated with fracture of the fibular shaft or disruption of the distal tibiofibular ligaments. The anterior lip of the tibia is more often comminuted than is the posterior lip; thus internal fixation techniques may be compromised.

Open reduction and fixation are indicated when the fracture is large enough to cause talar instability (25% to 35% of the articular surface) or is a component of a comminuted fracture that is amenable to open reduction.

Fractures with severe comminution and instability. It may not be possible to reduce and internally fix closed severely comminuted fractures of the ankle. Such injuries can usually be managed with external skeletal traction through the calcaneus or, following manipulation, with fixed traction produced by placing a pin in the calcaneus and one in the tibia proximally.

Early motion in these fractures is important to preserve ankle function and help mold the fracture surfaces. This can be achieved by performing a closed reduction with a Steinmann traction pin in the os calcis and then applying a bulky dressing or Delbet cast and placing the limb in traction on a Böhler-Braun frame. The traction will help maintain the reduction, and ankle motion can begin.

Occasionally both comminution and a complex-compound wound about the ankle create a situation in which it is impossible to employ the usual methods of malleolar fixation; yet to assure the survival of the foot and permit management of the surrounding soft tissue, stability must be achieved. In this situation the technique of driving a vertical Steinmann pin through the calcaneus and the talus into the distal tibia (Fig. 6-9) can be used to preserve the foot (Dieterlé, 1935; Childress, 1965).

Fractures of lateral malleolus with posterior displacement of proximal fibular fragment. Bosworth (1947), Fleming and Smith (1954), and Meyers (1957) all described bimalleolar types of fracture accompanied by displacement of the proximal fibula at the fracture site posteriorly on the tibia in a position

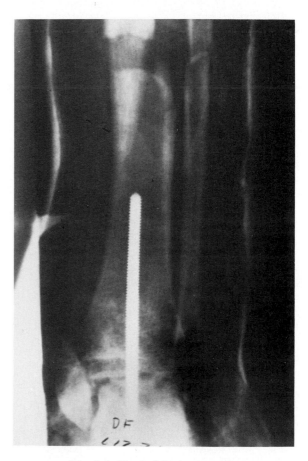

Fig. 6-9. Vertical Steinmann pin.

that usually makes reduction by closed manipulation impossible. The ligamentous support of the syndesmosis apparently remains intact and holds the fibula in its dislocated position. In these types of fracture, open reduction is necessary and a posterolateral approach is appropriate (Figs. 6-10 and 6-11).

Open fractures and fracture-dislocations of ankle. The same principles of meticulous debridement, copious irrigation, and use of systemic and local bactericidal antibiotics apply to open fractures of the ankle as apply to open fractures and injuries elsewhere in the body.

Wounds in this area almost always communicate with the ankle joint. The ankle joint must be explored. Although not essential, the ankle joint capsule is usually closed primarily; if this is done, a closed suction tube–irrigation system should be left in place to permit drainage Joint closure, as either a primary or a delayed primary procedure, is essential (Jer-

gesen, 1959). The skin wound can be closed by primary closure, delayed primary closure, or secondary closure—depending on the degree of soft tissue damage and contamination and on the amount of elapsed time since occurrence of the injury. The safest procedure, however, is to leave the wound above the joint capsule open and carry out a delayed primary closure.

Infection is the major complication to be avoided and can be related directly to the type of wound. Gustilo and Anderson (1976) classified wounds as type I, II, or III, with type I being a wound less than 1 cm long and clean and type III having extensive soft tissue damage. In their review of open fractures Chapman and Mahoney (1977) noted that 60% of open ankle injuries had type I wounds and only 10% had type III wounds. In their series of open fractures in which immediate fixation was achieved, the infection rate in type I wounds was 2%, in type II wounds 8%, and in

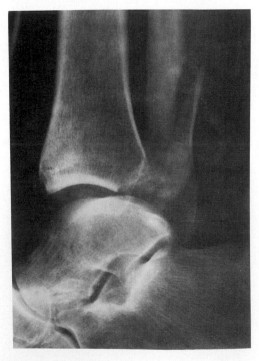

Fig. 6-10. Bosworth fracture with characteristic posterior displacement of the proximal fibula.

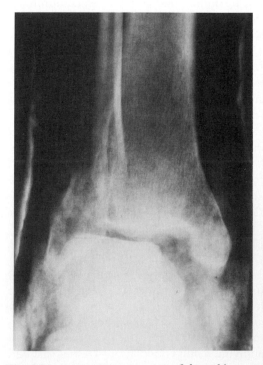

Fig. 6-11. Anteroposterior view of the ankle mortise in Fig. 6-10 showing lateral subluxation of the talus.

type III wounds 29%. This is significant insofar as it means that immediate internal fixation of ankles with type I wounds can be performed without an infection rate greater than that seen in closed fractures. The risk of infection in type II and type III wounds is substantial.

In the most commonly seen open fracture-dislocation about the ankle, a transverse wound occurs at the level of the medial malleolus centered on the medial side of the leg. The foot is dislocated posterolaterally; frequently the proximal surface of the avulsed medial malleolus and the articular surface of the tibia appear in the wound. In these injuries the wound is so close to the surface of the fracture and to the joint that rigid internal fixation is necessary to protect the overlying soft tissues from pressure and recurrent tension. Since the open wound lies directly over the medial malleolus, internal fixation of the medial malleolar side can usually be accomplished with one screw; little if any additional dissection is necessary after the wound has been debrided and irrigated and the dislocation has been reduced.

It is unlikely that the minimal surgery required to place a medial malleolar screw will increase the risk of infection; and, in fact, the opposite may be true since the stability achieved allows optimal treatment of the soft tissues. Again, by way of emphasis, the wounds should be closed by delayed primary closure (Fig. 6-12).

Surgical technique

Medial malleolus. The skin incision should be vertical, parallel with the long axis of the tibia, and placed directly over the malleolus. Dissection is carried sharply to bone, and any undermining necessary should take place at the level of the periosteum. The incision must be long enough to offer good exposure without excessive retraction. It has the advantages of being extensible, being optimally located for the insertion of a screw, and avoiding significant undermining or flaps. I have never had a patient complain of a tender scar in this location. The J-shaped incision posterior or anterior and distal to the malleolus has the disadvantages of not being easily extended distally, therefore frequently compromising the exposure needed for screw insertion, and requiring undermining (which leads to an increased incidence of marginal wound slough).

1. Elevate the periosteum from the edges of the fracture line for a distance of 2 to 3 mm with a no. 15 scalpel blade used edge on. The full anterior and posterior extents of the fracture must be seen to assure accurate reduction.

2. Lightly curette and irrigate the fracture surfaces to remove all organized hematoma.

3. Explore the joint through the fracture site to detect occult chondral and osteochondral fractures of the talus and to debride and irrigate the joint as needed.

4. Anatomically reduce the fracture by grasping the malleolus transversely in a towel clip and guiding it into place with a periosteal elevator in the other hand. The reduction should be securely maintained by mechanical means while the internal fixation is inserted. The best method I have found is to use two A-O towel clip–type bone clamps or two towel

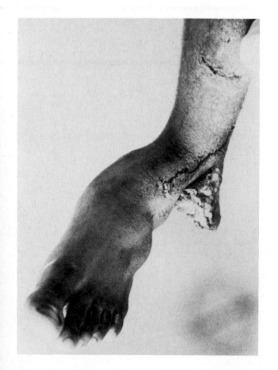

Fig. 6-12. Typical open fracture of the ankle.

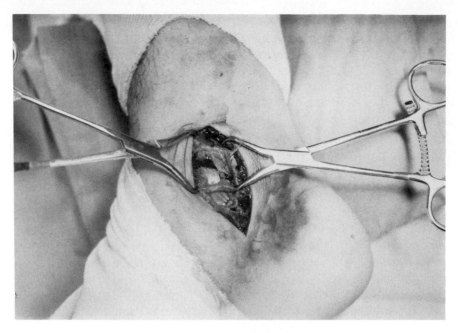

Fig. 6-13. Towel clips to hold a fracture.

clips across the fracture at its anterior and posterior borders. The towel clips are held with 4 × 8's tied through their handles (Fig. 6-13). A Bishop clamp can also be used, but I find them heavy and they often interfere with hardware placement. The towel clip method does not interfere with hardware placement, and the clips prevent slippage of the fracture.

The best fixation is usually provided by a lag screw placed at right angles to the fracture line and as vertical as possible. The screw should enter the distal tip of the malleolus; otherwise, comminution may occur and the screw head will be too prominent. The malleolar screws provided in the A-O equipment (*Arbeitsgemeinschaft für Osteosynthese*, Swiss association for study of internal fixation) are ideal although lag technique can be used with a standard bone screw (Fig. 6-14). Small or comminuted fragments not amenable to screw fixation are best fixed with

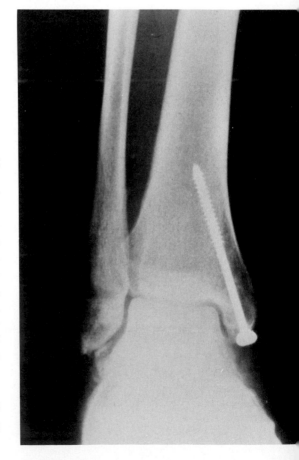

Fig. 6-14. A-O malleolar screw fixing a fracture of the medial malleolus employing the principle of lag fixation.

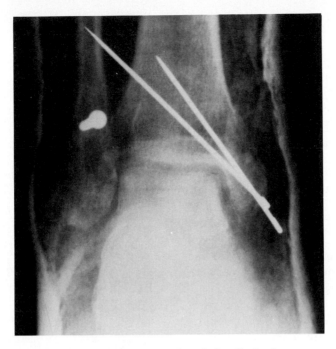

Fig. 6-15. Kirschner wire fixation of a comminuted medial malleolar fracture. Note that one wire was left excessively long.

two or more Kirschner wires (Fig. 6-15). I have had no experience with the Zuelzer hook plate (Zuelzer, 1958). Vertical adduction–type fractures tend to slip with a single screw. Fixation with two Kirschner wires as illustrated in Fig. 6-15 prior to insertion of the screw will prevent displacement.

Very small fragments may be excised and a repair of the deltoid ligament to a drill hole in the malleolus can be effected.

Lateral malleolus. The same principles of incision and exposure described for the medial malleolus are applicable. If syndesmosis repair is anticipated, the incision should be somewhat anterior; and if fixation of the posterior malleolus through the same incision is planned, the incision should be placed somewhat posterior.

The configuration of the fracture determines the type of fixation to be employed. Ideal fixation provides interfragmentary compression and rotational control. Oblique and spiral fractures whose lengths are greater than one and one half times the diameter of the bone at the level of the fracture are best fixed with interfragmentary lag screws as in Fig. 6-16. Standard bone screws are often too large.

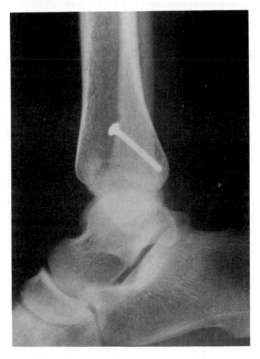

Fig. 6-16. Screw used to provide interfragmentary fixation of an oblique fracture of the lateral malleolus.

The 3.5 mm screws in the A-O set are ideal (and are best placed from anterior to posterior through an anterior stab wound). Transverse or short oblique fractures above the syndesmosis are fixed with a 4- or 6-hole plate, depending on the degree of stability desired (Fig. 6-17). These plates must be fairly malleable and small to fit well.

We prefer the semitubular A-O plates but have also found Acme plates to work well. Intramedullary fixation with a Rush rod or Steinmann pin works well (Fig. 6-18); but if the fracture is rotationally unstable, an oblique Kirschner wire should be placed across the fracture. The A-O tension-band wire technique is useful for transverse fractures at or below the syndesmosis and comminuted fractures (Fig. 6-19).

Posterior malleolus. Injuries to the posterior malleolus are usually posterolateral and are best fixed through a posterolateral approach with the patient prone. The lateral and medial malleoli can easily be repaired with the patient prone. Preoperative radiographs should be carefully assessed. Occasionally a posterior malleolar fracture is an extension of a medial malleolar fracture and should be approached medially.

Because of limited exposure, posterior malleolar fractures can be difficult to fix internally. Since the intra-articular component of the fracture cannot be seen when reduced, the entire extra-articular portion of the fracture should be visualized to ensure the accuracy of reduction. Fixation with two Kirschner wires while the malleolus is held in place ensures that reduction will not be lost during screw placement. To guarantee optimal closure of the intra-articular component, the screw should be at right angles to the fracture and just above the tibial plafond.

If the screw cannot easily be placed from posterior to anterior, it can be placed from anterior to posterior through a small stab wound (Fig. 6-20).

Syndesmosis separations. Syndesmosis separations which are unstable should be stabilized. Occasionally stabilization of an associated fibular fracture provides adequate stability, and fixation across the syndesmosis

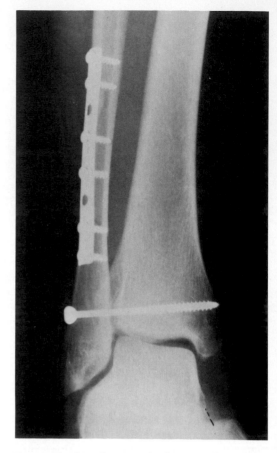

Fig. 6-17. Plate fixation of a fracture of the fibula.

can be avoided. With fibular fractures above a syndesmosis separation, some surgeons elect to treat only the syndesmosis separation. This is acceptable; but great care must be exercised to avoid residual external rotational deformity of the distal fragment and avoid overtightening the syndesmosis screw, which can produce a valgus malposition of the lateral malleolus. Proximal migration of the lateral malleolus should be avoided by making certain that shortening at the fracture site has not occurred. It is usually best to stabilize the fibula first and then the syndesmosis.

When transfixing the syndesmosis, the surgeon should take care to ensure that the fibula is reduced posteriorly into the tibial sulcus. Fixation can be obtained with a lag screw or Steinmann pin (Fig. 6-21). Screws should employ the lag principle and be at

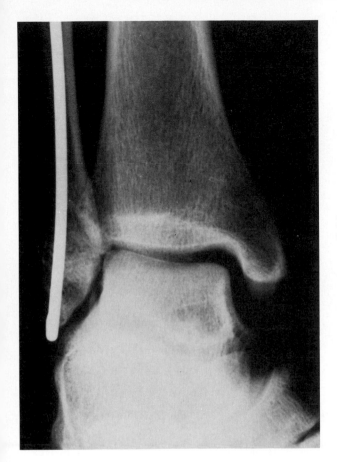

Fig. 6-18. Rush rod fixation of a fracture of the fibula.

Fig. 6-19. Intramedullary Kirschner wires and a tension band figure-eight wire used to fix a fracture of the lateral malleolus.

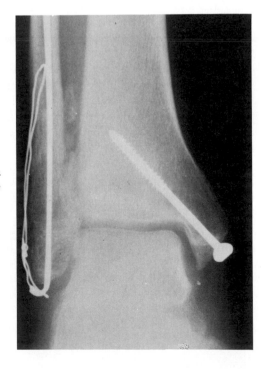

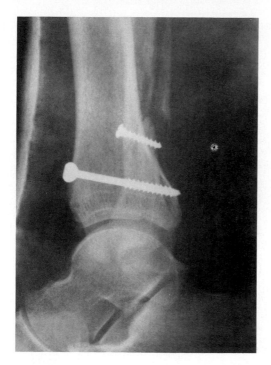

Fig. 6-20. Fracture of the posterior malleolus fixed with an interfragmentary malleolar screw placed through an anterior stab wound. Due to comminution there is a small defect in the articular surface of the tibial plafond.

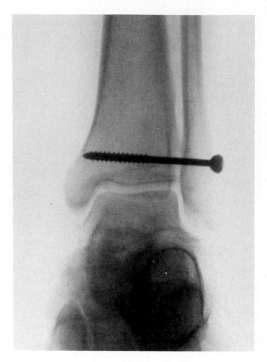

Fig. 6-21. Syndesmosis rupture fixed with a malleolar screw.

right angles to the distal tibiofibular joint, passing from the posterolateral border of the fibula anteromedially into the tibia.

These screws must be removed at 6 weeks in most patients before unprotected weight bearing is allowed, for the dynamic function of the fibula (McMaster and Scranton, 1975; Scranton et al., 1976) may lead to screw fracture.

Comminuted fractures. A comminuted fracture of the ankle is usually due to vertical loading that produces compression of the cancellous bone above the tibial plafond. An unstable fracture of the distal shafts of the tibia and fibula may be associated. Because the degree of comminution may make internal fixation impossible, closed treatment is often indicated. The surgeon must weigh the goals of surgery against such risks as increased soft tissue trauma from multiple or larger incisions and the ill effects of prolonged surgery. Resto-

ration of the joint surface and treatment of the remainder of the fracture with a cast are often necessary.

Some authors advocate total reconstruction of comminuted fractures with multiple fixation devices, including large buttress plates, to stabilize the shaft component (Müller et al., 1970) and permit early mobilization in the absence of external fixation. This type of reconstruction is usually possible only with the A-O type of equipment. The procedures are difficult and should be undertaken only by surgeons who are intimately familiar with the method and do more than an occasional fracture of this type.

My preference is to restore the joint surface using multiple Kirschner wires and occasional interfragmentary screws combined with cast immobilization. I frequently plate the fibula but rarely the tibia (Fig. 6-22).

In the presence of a fractured fibula, it is wise first to internally fix the bone to restore length; this will serve as a guide to the proper position for the tibial fragments. The tibial

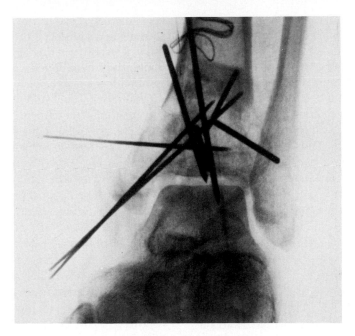

Fig. 6-22. Comminuted fracture of distal tibia and fibula fixed with multiple K-wires.

fracture is best approached by a long midline anterior incision between the extensor hallucis longus and the neurovascular bundle. Periosteal attachments to the bone fragments should be preserved. The tibial plafond is often fractured into four major fragments with a central area of bone compression. Restoration of length usually leaves a gap in the metaphysis, which should be packed with cancellous bone from the ilium.

Although not as versatile as the direct anterior approach, the transfibular approach can be useful particularly when the fibula is fractured and the syndesmosis disrupted (Wiggins, 1975).

Postoperative care. In the immediate postoperative period the most frequent problem is swelling, which can be controlled by bed rest and elevation. All circumferential casts should be univalved, and the underlying padding should be split.

Fractures that are unstable after fixation usually require a long-leg non–weight-bearing cast for 6 weeks followed by 2 weeks in a short-leg walking cast.

Stable fractures can be treated according to

the need for early joint mobilization and the surgeon's confidence in his repair.

In their series of patients in whom a stable situation was produced at the time of internal fixation, Burwell and Charnley (1965) described a minor modification of the usual postoperative care for internal fixation of ankle fractures. In the early postoperative period, the injured limb was removed from the protective plaster cast for active non–weight-bearing exercise and a long leg cast was replaced by a short leg plaster cast. The authors reported an early recovery of maximum range of motion in patients thus treated.

Ankle fractures in children. These are rare. If the skeleton proper is affected, trauma in this region usually produces epiphyseal separation. Treatment is the same as for epiphyseal separation injuries of the long bones.

FRACTURES AND FRACTURE-DISLOCATIONS OF THE TALUS

Although the literature on fractures and fracture-dislocations of the talus is relatively extensive, major fractures of this bone are encountered infrequently. Davidson et al. (1967), in a statistical review of 25,000 fractures, found only fifty-six involving the talus. Because fractures and fracture-dislocations of this bone are uncommon, a series of cases reported in a single article is apt to be small. Furthermore, these series often include a variety of fractures, each requiring a different therapeutic approach. Thus it is impossible to enunciate standardized and universally applicable procedures for all fractures of the talus.

Excellent reviews of talar fractures and fracture-dislocations—including classifications, discussions about mechanism of injury, and reports of the results of treatment—are contained in the literature.*

Vascular supply and avascular necrosis

Three fifths of the talus is covered by articular cartilage; but in spite of this, the blood supply is copious with extensive anastomoses. Mulfinger and Trueta (1970), in a classic work, described the extraosseus and intraosseus blood supply of the talus. Other studies have been those of Sneed (1925), Wildernauer (1950), Haliburton et al. (1958), and Kelly and Sullivan (1964). There are three major extraosseus sources of blood: the posterior tibial artery provides vessels medially; the dorsalis pedis provides anterior dorsal vessels; and the peroneal artery, anastomosing with the dorsalis pedis, enters laterally through the subtalar joint.

The major blood supply to the body of the talus is from the artery of the tarsal canal, derived from the posterior tibial artery. This artery enters medially via the interosseus ligament in the tarsal canal and anastomoses with the artery of the tarsal sinus. The second most important blood supply comes through the deltoid ligament from the posterior tibial artery. Surgical approaches to the talus medially therefore should osteotomize the malleolus rather than cut the deltoid ligament. A

secondary system is the arteries from the dorsalis pedis entering the dorsal neck of the talus. The artery of the tarsal sinus is not itself a major source of blood, as evidenced by the low incidence (6%) of avascular necrosis of the talus after triple and subtalar arthrodeses. The capsular branches entering through the posterior tubercle of the talus provide local blood supply only and do not anastomose with the other vessels. Such extensive anastomoses take place within the talus that interruption of two of the three major sources of blood supply is necessary for avascular necrosis to occur.

Fractures of the talar neck have only a 6% incidence of avascular necrosis; but in that 6% occult subtalar dislocation is possible. Fractures of the neck of the talus combined with subtalar dislocation, thus interrupting two of the three sources of blood supply, have a reported incidence of avascular necrosis from 18% (Mindell et al., 1963) to 76% (Dunn et al., 1966). Fractures of the talar neck with dislocation of the ankle and subtalar joints have an incidence of 62% (Mindell et al., 1963) to 100% (Pantazopoulos et al., 1974).

Multiple articular surfaces

The talus, in its articulation with contiguous structures, possesses eight well-defined articular facets. Smooth and precise motion over each of these articular surfaces is necessary for normal functioning of the ankle, subtalar, and talonavicular articulations. It appears obvious that if arthritic changes are to be avoided the articular surfaces must be preserved and the correct anatomic relationships between them must be restored.

In treating fractures of the talus, the surgeon should have as his objective the precise repositioning of the parts. Boyd and Knight (1942), Taylor (1962), and McKeever (1963) concur that open reduction and internal fixation may be the best method of treatment for achieving these objectives.

Classification

Fractures of the talus may be classfied as follows:
1. Fractures of head
2. Fractures of neck (Hawkins)

---

*Anderson, 1919; Coltart, 1952; Watson-Jones, 1955; Mindell et al., 1963; Pennal, 1963; Dunn et al., 1966; Hawkins, 1970; Kenwright and Taylor, 1970; Pantazopoulos et al., 1974.

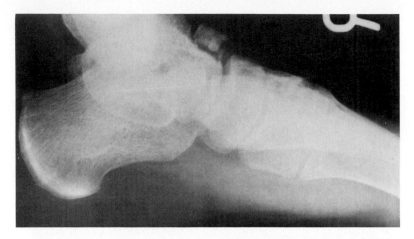

Fig. 6-23. Completely detached fragment of bone from the dorsum at the head of the talus.

a. Undisplaced
b. Displaced with subtalar luxation
c. Displaced with subtalar and ankle dislocation
3. Fractures of body
4. Osteochondral fractures
5. Lateral process fractures

Fractures of the *head* of the talus (Figs. 6-23 and 6-24) are less common than fractures of the neck. Both may occur when force is transmitted through the navicular—e.g., when a person falls from a height and lands on a plantar-flexed foot. The displacement is not usually marked; immobilization of the foot for 4 to 6 weeks in a well-molded walking cast and subsequent weight bearing without support are usually adequate to ensure the return of normal function.

Next to the small chip or avulsion fractures of the talar head, fractures through the *neck* of the talus occur most commonly (Fig. 6-25). In Coltart's (1952) review of over 200 cases, this fracture occurred twice as frequently as did fracture of the body of the talus. Ray (1967) reported a series of thirty-four fractures of the talus; seventeen of these were fractures of the neck. Talar neck fractures deserve particular attention since they have the potential of healing without disability but may lead to avascular necrosis of the body of the talus.

Hawkins (1970), in an excellent review of fifty-seven fractures of the neck of the talus, classified these fractures into three groups.

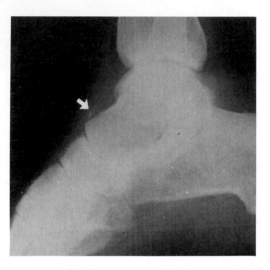

Fig. 6-24. Chip fracture over the dorsum of the head of the talus.

Group I consisted of six cases of linear vertical fractures that were undisplaced. In these cases the fracture entered the sinus tarsi between the middle and posterior facets. The body of the talus retained its normal position in the ankle and subtalar joints. Treatment consisted of simple immobilization. Aseptic necrosis did not occur in any of the six cases. Group II consisted of twenty-four cases in which the vertical fractures through the neck were displaced and the subtalar joint was luxated. The ankle joint remained normal. Open reduction was necessary in fourteen of

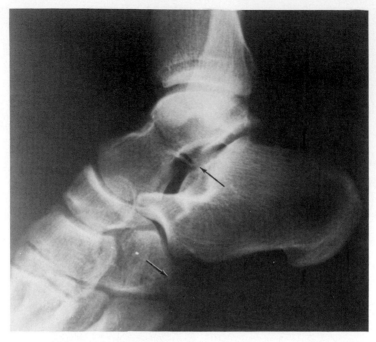

Fig. 6-25. Fracture at the neck of the talus in a 25-year-old man. Note the fractured cuboid. The patient was driving an automobile, his left foot on the clutch, at the time of a collision.

these cases. Avascular necrosis occurred in ten of the twenty-four cases. Group III included twenty-seven cases of displaced vertical fractures of the neck, complicated by dislocations of both subtalar and ankle joints. Primary talectomies were performed in five of the cases, and open reduction was necessary in twenty of them. Avascular necrosis occurred in twenty of the twenty-two cases.

Fractures of the *body* of the talus occur in varying degrees. Marginal fractures are easily overlooked but may produce disabling symptoms (Fig. 6-26). The prognosis in fractures of the body of the talus is not as good as in fractures of the neck. Frequently even a slight disruption of the congruity of the joint surface causes a step deformity and subsequent arthritis of the ankle joint. An equally severe disability occurs when the fracture causes incongruity of the subtalar joint with resulting subtalar motion that may necessitate subtalar arthrodesis. In these cases of fracture of the body of the talus, anatomic reduction should be attempted. Even though reduction is achieved, a good painless range of motion may

not be restored (Coltart, 1952). Massive comminuted and destructive fractures of the body, of course, require arthrodeses and reconstructive procedures.

Treatment

Avulsion fractures of the dorsum of the talar head and neck can be treated as third-degree sprains with 3 to 6 weeks' immobilization in a short-leg walking cast. A good result can be expected.

Undisplaced or slightly displaced fractures of the neck can likewise be treated with a short leg cast; but to prevent displacement, weight bearing should be delayed until radiologic union has occurred.

Neck fractures with subtalar joint subluxation often reduce in equinus. Anatomic reduction, however, must be achieved and maintained until radiographic union of the neck fracture occurs.

Closed reduction of talar neck fractures with subtalar subluxation or dislocation is rarely successful, especially if combined with ankle dislocation. In most cases open reduc-

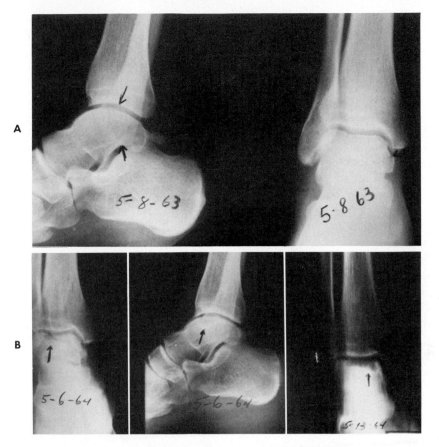

Fig. 6-26. Foot of a 30-year-old man who was driving an automobile with his foot on the brake at the time of collision. **A,** Anteroposterior and lateral views show a comminuted fracture of the body of the talus. **B,** One year later anteroposterior, lateral, and tomographic views show necrosis of part of the trochlear surface of the talus.

tion and internal fixation will be indicated.

Displaced fractures of the talar neck are best approached medially through an incision from proximal and anterior to the medial malleolus extending distally and plantarward to the tubercle of the navicular. Fixation can be obtained with multiple Kirschner wires or a lag screw placed across the fracture from distal to proximal entering on the medial side of the talar neck. If the fracture is unreducible or the subtalar joint remains subluxated, a separate lateral incision (of Ollier) may be necessary.

Undisplaced fractures of the body can be treated conservatively; however, displaced fractures should be anatomically restored by open reduction and internal fixation.

Primary subtalar joint arthodesis for some of Hawkins group II and all group III injuries was originally advised by Boyd and Knight (1942). Boyd and most other trauma surgeons have found that primary subtalar joint arthrodesis does not significantly alter the incidence of avascular necrosis of the talus. The added trauma of the arthrodesis is inadvisable in the acutely traumatized foot.

Primary talectomy has also been advised, but due to tibiocalcaneal pain the long-term results of this procedure have not been good.

On the Orthopedic Service at San Francisco General Hospital, we have found that, in spite of the high incidence of avascular necrosis in group II and group III injuries, union of the fracture usually does occur. Revascularization of the talus can take place (Fig. 6-27), and the clinical result can be satisfactory. We establish the prognosis early by looking for subchondral osteoporosis under the dome of the talus on an AP radiograph. This finding indicates preservation of the blood supply and is usually present 6 weeks after the injury as illustrated in Fig. 6-27, B.

The talus should be protected from weight bearing in a short leg cast until fracture union occurs. Further protection from weight bearing is not necessary because collapse due to avascular necrosis does not seem to be related to weight bearing.

For avascular necrosis of the talus with collapse, the tibiotalar fusion described by Blair (1943) excises the dead body and fuses the tibia with a sliding graft to the talar neck preserving the normal height of the foot. It is the fusion of choice.

Osteochondral fractures of talus. Osteochondral fractures of the talus occur along the corners of the dome of the talus as a component of severe sprains or fracture-dislocations of the ankle. They are frequently occult since bony involvement may be slight and the radiographic findings therefore minimal. Recurrent ankle pain and disability after seemingly minor sprains may be due to unsuspected osteochondral fractures.

In fracture-dislocations which are treated open, careful inspection of the talus is necessary. A major osteochondral fracture of the talus may be the main prognostic feature of the injury.

Rendu (1932) was the first to describe an intra-articular fracture of the dome of the talus. Since then numerous reports of this relatively rare injury have appeared.*

Berndt and Harty (1959) showed that the

*Marks, 1952; Berndt and Harty, 1959; Rosenberg, 1965; Davidson et al., 1967; Gustilo and Gordon, 1968; Davis, 1970; Mukherjee and Young, 1973; Yvars, 1976.

Fig. 6-27. A, Fracture of the talar neck with subtalar and ankle joint dislocation. **B,** Six weeks later, after open reduction and internal fixation; subchondral osteoporosis in the medial half of the talus but not in the lateral half.

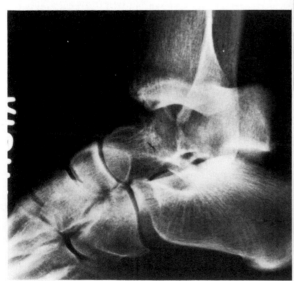

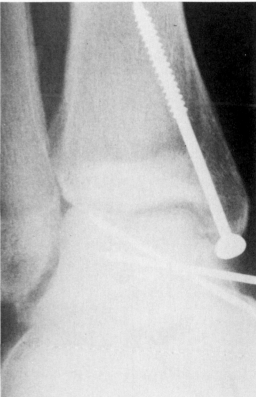

A

common denominator in this injury is inversion with dorsiflexion (producing lateral marginal fractures) and plantar flexion with rotation (producing medial fractures). They also staged the injuries according to displacement: stage I, a small area of compression of subchondral bone; stage II, a partially detached osteochondral fragment; stage III, a completely detached fragment remaining in place; and stage IV, a displaced osteochondral fragment.

Radiographic identification of these fractures is difficult, particularly early (Fig. 6-28, A). Mortise views of the talus in varying degrees of dorsiflexion and plantar flexion may reveal the fracture. AP tomograms are sometimes quite helpful (Fig. 6-28, B). Late fractures can present as loose bodies or osteochondritis dissecans (Mark, 1952).

I agree with Mukherjee and Young (1973) that large dome fractures with displacement should be accurately reduced by open reduction. Fixation, if necessary, can be achieved with a Smillie nail. Small fractures without displacement can be treated conservatively until radiographic union occurs. Small fragments with displacement are treated by early excision. Most lateral lesions can be reached through an anterolateral approach, particularly if the lateral collateral ligament is transected. Medial lesions often require osteotomy of the medial malleolus.

Lateral process fractures Fractures of the lateral process of the talus (Fig. 6-29) involve the posterior articulation of the subtalar joint and are relatively uncommon injuries, having an incidence of less than 1% among sprains and fractures in the ankle region (Mukherjee et al., 1974).

A large number of these fractures probably go unrecognized. Sprains with tenderness over the lateral process of the talus, just below

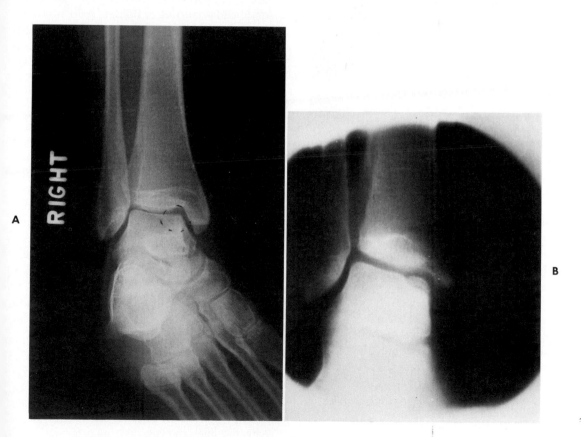

Fig. 6-28. Osteochondral fracture of the talus. **A,** AP radiograph; **B,** AP tomogram.

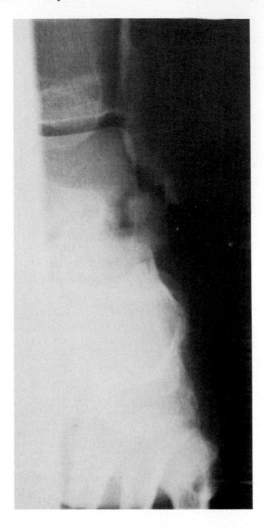

Fig. 6-29. Fracture of the lateral process of the talus. (Courtesy Dr. Paul Hazelrig.)

the tip of the lateral malleolus, require careful radiographic study. The fracture occurs from compression of the lateral process of the talus where the foot dorsiflexes and is inverted (Hawkins, 1965; Fjeldborg, 1968; Mukherjee, et al., 1974). The fracture fragments are frequently comminuted and displaced. Delay in diagnosis and treatment can only lead to subtalar joint arthritis. Treatment is conservative if the fracture is undisplaced, internal fixation if large enough and displaced, and excision if small or comminuted.

FRACTURES OF THE CALCANEUS

Fractures of the calcaneus are the most common fractures of the bones of the tarsus, comprising 60% of all fractures in this region of the foot. Since these fractures are usually caused by a fall from a considerable height, fractures of other skeletal parts may occur at the same time and frequently complicate treatment. One out of ten patients with fractures of the calcaneus also has fractures of the spine; one out of four has other fractures of the extremities.

Approximately 25% to 30% of fractures of the calcaneus, fortunately, do not involve the posterior facet of the subtalar joint; however, the possibility of this involvement should not be overlooked since it may be a source of residual disability.

Anatomy

The anatomy of the calcaneus is shown in Fig. 6-30. The superior surface of the calcaneus climbs upward from the front and back toward the middle. The angle between these two inclinations is referred to as the tuber angle and according to Böhler (1958) normally varies between 20° and 40°. Decrease in this angle relative to that of the normal opposite foot implies upper displacement of the tuberosity.

Classification

Clinical observations have led to various classifications of fractures of the calcaneus. The value of such classifications is greater than merely satisfying an academic interest. Since the types of therapeutic procedure employed and the types of fracture sustained are independent variables, final evaluation of any treatment will depend on the control of one of these variables. This control can be partially accomplished by classifying the types of fracture.

Over sixty years ago Cotton and Henderson (1916) described comminuted fractures of the calcaneus in these general terms:

What we see are *smashes* of the os calcis. . . . The lines of fracture, as sketched by the x-rays, are *not* uniform. In general, there is a smash below the weight-bearing vertical line of the tibia, running more or less (mostly less) vertically, and various radiating lines running down and forward, and backward. The heel is driven up and often is driven outward. The whole bone is compressed vertically and expanded laterally; there is often a pushing of fragments inward, under the ankle, and almost uniformly a considerable pushing outward of bone-fragments, capped by the usually intact outer lamelia of the calcis out under the external malleolus. This is *the* type lesions.*

Fig. 6-31 is a radiograph of a comminuted ("smash") fracture of the calcaneus.

Subsequently, more precise classifications have been proposed. We have used the classification suggested by Rowe et al. (1963), who combine their ideas with those of Warrick and Bremner (1953) and Watson-Jones (1955) (Fig. 6-32).

Type 1	A.	Fracture of the tuberosity
	B.	Fracture of the sustentaculum
	C.	Fracture of the anterior process
Type 2	A.	Beak fracture
	B.	Avulsion of the tendo Achillis insertion
Type 3		Oblique fracture not involving the subtalar joint
Type 4		Fracture involving the subtalar joint
Type 5		Central depression fracture with comminution

*Cotton, F. J., and Henderson, F. F.: Results of fracture of the os calcis, Am. J. Orthop. Surg. **14:**290, 1916.

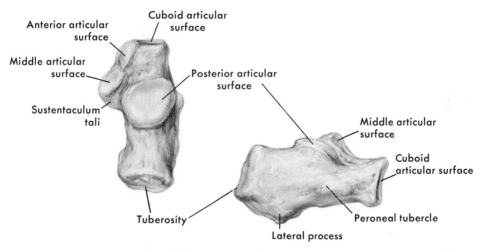

Fig. 6-30. Anatomy of the calcaneus.

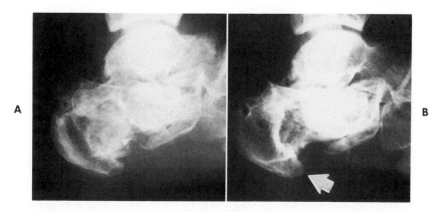

Fig. 6-31. Foot of a 30-year-old man with a comminuted ("smash") fracture of the calcaneus. Note the multiple vertical and horizontal breaks. The injury occurred on April 28, 1969. **A,** Lateral view taken Oct. 7, 1969. **B,** Lateral view one year later. The posterior part of the calcaneus has lifted dorsally. Arrow indicates a sharp prominence on the plantar tuberosity which is the only point of contact with the ground during weight bearing.

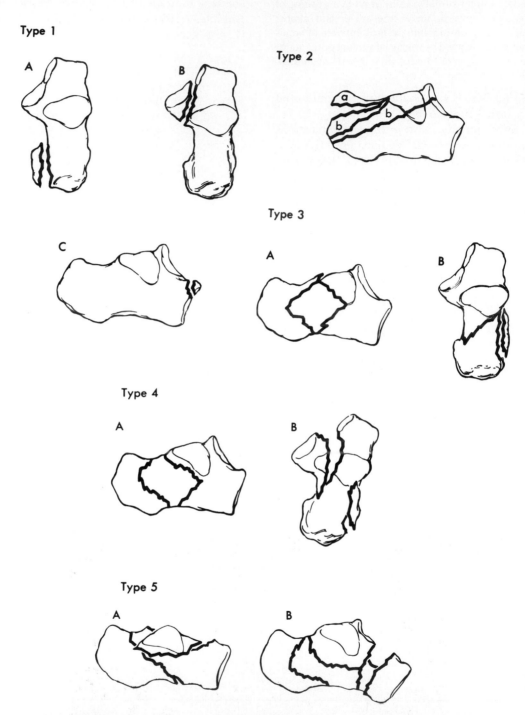

Fig. 6-32. Classification of Rowe et al. of calcaneal fractures. (From Rowe, C. R., et al.: J.A.M.A. 184:920, 1963.)

Fractures involving the upper part of the tuberosity, with displacement of the fragments, usually are not avulsion fractures because the fracture line is superior to the attachment of the tendo Achillis. The fracture can usually be approximated by manipulation. Should displacement recur, the fragments may be secured with a single screw.

Gellman (1951) believes that fracture of the anterior process of the calcaneus is commonly overlooked (Figs. 6-33 and 6-34). The mechanism of this injury is probably forceful adduction of the forepart of the foot in combination with plantar flexion. The bifurcate calcaneo-navicular-calcaneocuboid ligament may play a part in the avulsion of the anterior process of the calcaneus. Pain in the region of the calcaneocuboid joint warrants oblique radiographs

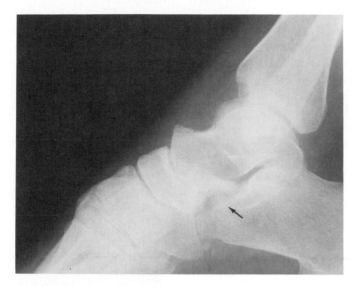

Fig. 6-33. Large fracture of the anterior process of the calcaneus in a 40-year-old woman. Conservative treatment produced good results.

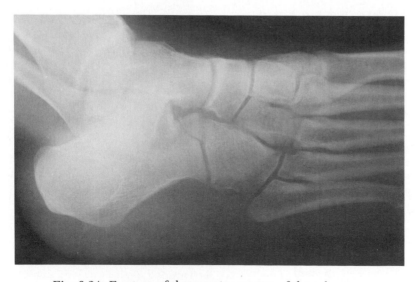

Fig. 6-34. Fracture of the anterior process of the calcaneus.

of the foot to rule out this fracture (Fig. 6-34).

If there is gross displacement, treatment is directed toward reduction of the fragment and immobilization for 4 to 6 weeks, after which physical therapy treatments should be given. In his four cases Gellman (1951) reported the average convalescence to be 13 weeks, with mild residual discomfort and swelling remaining at the end of that time. Piatt (1956) named the anterior process of the calcaneus the promontory of the calcaneus and described ten cases of fracture; one case of nonunion occurred with minimal residual disability. Hunt (1970) agreed with Gellman (1951) that the significance of this fracture has been underestimated. He stated that although not enough cases have been reported to set forth a definite program of therapy initial treatment should extend beyond simple immobilization.

Beak fractures may occur, with interruption of the bony attachment of the tendo Achillis to the distal fragment (Fig. 6-35). Failure to approximate the fragments may result in deformity and functional loss (Figs. 6-36 and 6-37). Avulsion of the tendo Achillis with minimal elevation of the periosteum may be overlooked on the radiograph.

Minimally displaced fractures should be treated conservatively. Interesting cases of avulsion fracture of the calcaneus have been reported by Mooney (1935) and Rothberg (1939).

Oblique fractures not involving the subtalar joint (Fig. 6-38) have the same mechanism of injury, e.g., landing on the heel after a fall or receiving a severe blow from below during standing, as do the more severe fractures which involve the joint. The oblique fracture that extends from the posteromedial aspect to the anterolateral aspect does not enter the joint. The problem of traumatic arthritis is therefore nonexistent, although soft tissue injury and the problems of associated thickening and broadening of the calcaneus can occur. In these cases, if the displacements are corrected by manipulation, a good functional recovery usually can be expected.

It appears that there is general agreement about the treatment of fractures of the anterior process, beak fractures, and minimally displaced fractures not entering the subtalar joint. For the treatment of comminuted fractures which enter the subtalar joint, however, no such agreement exists. This type has given fracture of the calcaneus a bad reputation, for it results in a significant rate of residual disability. Diverse methods of treatment exist, each having strong personal advocates. The literature is largely composed of reports of the results of different types of therapy and is so voluminous as to make analysis, evaluation, and summarization of all the therapeutic methods that have been proposed inadvisable.

Historical approach to treatment

A historical approach appears appropriate since it defines the problem and orients the practitioner to the origin of the various therapeutic procedures.

Prior to the improvement of radiographic techniques, the practitioner was able to do

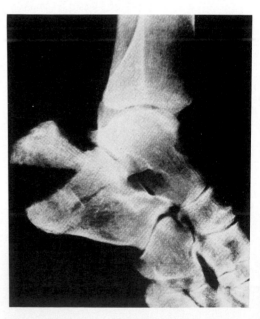

Fig. 6-35. Typical beak fracture of the calcaneus. (From Conwell, H. E., and Reynolds, F. D.: Key and Conwell's management of fractures, dislocations, and sprains, ed. 7, St. Louis, 1961, The C. V. Mosby Co., p. 1084.)

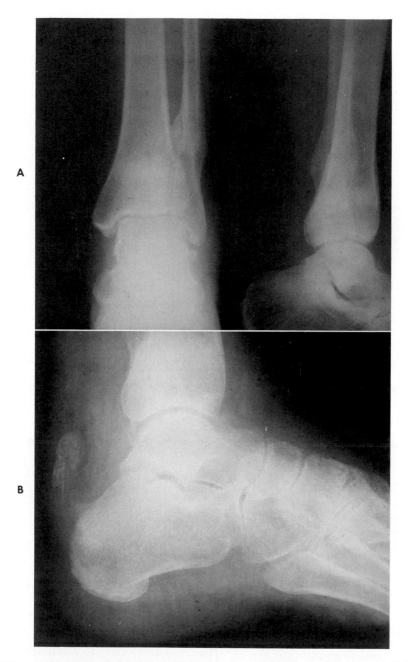

Fig. 6-36. Leg and foot of a 60-year-old woman who had taken a sudden step and the tendo Achillis pulled off a part of the calcaneus. **A,** The leg was immobilized in a short-leg walking cast because of pain from an old fracture of the fibula. **B,** After removal of the cast.

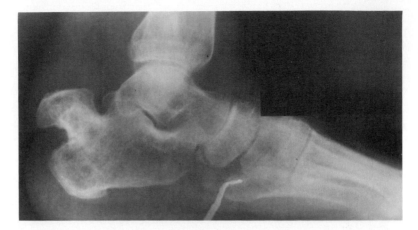

Fig. 6-37. Horizontal fracture of the posterior tuberosity of the calcaneus with rupture of the inserted portion of the tendo Achillis in a 48-year-old woman. Unsuccessful open reduction was performed 4 days after the injury. A radiograph taken 6 months later showed a dorsal fragment united with the body of the calcaneus and the tendo Achillis attached only to this fragment. (Courtesy Dr. R. J. Westwater.)

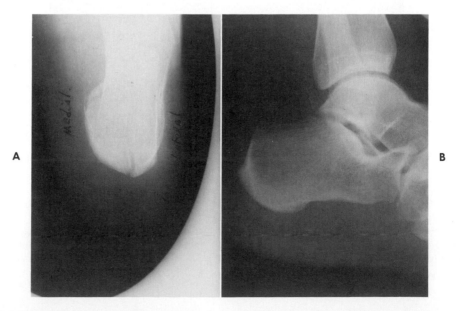

Fig. 6-38. A, Axial view of the calcaneus; horizontal fracture. **B,** Lateral view; fracture not visible.

little more for fractures of the calcaneus than prescribe bed rest, elevation, and immobilization. Cotton and Wilson (1908) pointed out that loss of subtalar motion appeared to be crucial in permanent residual disabilities from fracture of the calcaneus and insisted that attempts be made to manipulate the fragments into better alignment. These authors emphasized the need to compress the displaced lateral fragment from under the lateral malleolus, even if beating it with a mallet was necessary. A decade later, Cotton and Henderson (1916), in reviewing their cases, concluded that conservative treatment yielded incredibly poor results. Goff (1938) reviewed the status of the treatment of fractures of the calcaneus in a classic article. In pen-and-ink sketches he depicted forty-one methods of treatment that were being used at the time. Bankart (1942), in an introductory remark of an article, stated: "The results of the treatment of crush fractures of the os calcis are rotten."

During the past thirty-five years, clinicians have investigated the problem of fractures of the calcaneus. Using improved radiographic techniques, they have initiated experimental studies and have evaluated the results of treatment in many series of cases; however, unanimity of opinion as to the best method of treatment has not been reached over the years. Treatment is varied and each method has its proponents. Recommended procedures range from no reduction and immediate mobilization to open reduction, bone grafting, and plaster immobilization; a multitude of suggested procedures lie between these extremes.

As noted by O'Connell et al. (1972), however, the "literature reveals that the overwhelming enthusiasm for operatively treating intra-articular fractures of the os calcis which pervaded the 1950's has gradually given way in the last decade to a more conservative approach." Operative treatment, although resulting in good radiologic appearance, usually fails to preserve subtalar joint motion and, particularly if prolonged immobilization is used, may result in a painful stiff foot. The well-documented studies of Lindsay and

Dewar (1958), Lance et al. (1963), Rowe et al. (1963), and Barnard and Odegard (1970) have shown that closed reduction of the fracture, supportive dressing, and early motion offer results equal to and probably better than those achieved by open reduction and internal fixation.

Treatment

At present, there are four kinds of treatment of comminuted fractures of the calcaneus: (1) conservative treatment, (2) treatment with pins, traction, or both, (3) treatment by open reduction, and (4) treatment by primary arthrodesis. The surgeon should decide which method to employ, keeping in mind that the sole object of corrective treatment is to preserve motion in the disrupted joints and the ankle and forefoot. For the attainment of this goal, all procedures to reduce swelling, relieve pain, and obtain early motion should be used

Conservative treatment. Conservative treatment excludes reduction, the use of pins, skeletal traction, and surgical procedures (Fig. 6-39). Elevation of the foot, placement of ice packs around the heel, bed rest, massage, exercise, and medication for pain comprise the regimen. The techniques and results of conservative treatment of comminuted fractures of the calcaneus are reported by a number of investigators.*

Treatment with pins, traction, or both. The use of pins to improve anatomic relationships was pioneered by Böhler (1958), who found that treatment consisting of postreduction immobilization in plaster casts yielded unsatisfactory results. Reduction by traction, followed by early mobilization, has decreased residual disability (Gossett, 1969; Nosny et al., 1969).

A variation of the traction method developed by Essex-Lopresti in 1952 is closed reduction with a Gissane spike through the tuberosity of the os calcis followed by fabrication of a slipper cast incorporated into the cast to

---

*Bertelsen and Hasner, 1951; Carothers and Lyons, 1952; Essex-Lopresti, 1952; Dautry, 1961; Lance et al., 1963; Morretti and Piovani, 1967; Dragonetti, 1969; Nosny et al., 1969; Barnard and Odegard, 1970.

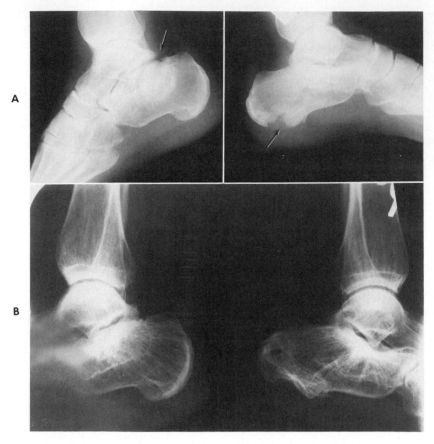

Fig. 6-39. Bilateral fractures of the calcaneus in a 40-year-old man who fell 15 feet from a telephone pole. The fractures were treated with elevation, enzymes, compression dressings, and early weight bearing in equinus casts. The patient returned to his job climbing poles in 6 months. **A,** At the time of the injury. **B,** One year later.

allow early ankle and subtalar motion. No sufficiently large comparative series has been published to evaluate this method.

The problem of frequent pin track infection and no significant improvement in results over conservative methods led surgeons to open reduction.

Treatment by open reduction. The current method of open reduction that is widely used was described by Palmer (1948) and extended by Widén (1954). Maxfield and McDermott (1955) and Maxfield (1963) reported favorably on their use of open reduction and grafting. These authors immobilized patients' limbs in plaster casts for 8 weeks. Vestad (1968) and Hazlett (1969) reported improved results after

using open reduction, maintaining the reduction by bone grafts or metallic fixation. It should be noted that Hazlett, in his treatment of fractures, avoided postoperative immobilization and encouraged immediate motion of the ankle and subtalar joints and the toes.

In Palmer's (1948) method, open reduction is done as soon as possible after injury. Reduction is assisted by traction on a Kirschner wire placed through the tuberosity. A lateral approach is used, and the usually intact lateral wall of the os calcis is turned down with the attached soft tissues. The depressed fragments of the subtalar joint are then elevated under direct vision and the resulting bony defect in the body of the os calcis is packed with iliac cancellous bone. Some surgeons prefer to augment fixation with multiple Kirschner wires. Due to instability these fractures should be kept non–weight bearing in a short leg cast for 6 to 8 weeks followed by a walking cast for 2 weeks.

The series of Maxfield and McDermott (1955) and Leonard (1957) indicate that about 70% good results can be expected, "good" being defined as return to work with few subjective complaints.

Treatment by primary arthrodesis. Based on the assumption that comminuted fractures involving the articular surfaces cause irreparable damage and that a painless rigid foot is preferable to a painful movable one, many surgeons have advocated primary subtalar or triple arthrodesis.

Leriche (1922) reported having obtained a satisfactory result in a single case; Wilson (1927) strongly advocated immediate arthrodesis; and Kiaer and Anthonsen (1942) reported obtaining "satisfactory" results in eighteen of twenty-two patients. A number of investigators* have reported results of treatment of severe fractures of the calcaneus by immediate arthrodesis; however, these results have not been as good as those following conservative treatment.

An excellent review of fractures of the os calcis by O'Connell et al. (1972) summarizes well the pros and cons of the various methods of treatment. I agree with their recommendations. Extra-articular fractures fare uniformly well with conservative care. Intra-articular fractures involving the subtalar joint also seem to do best with conservative care emphasizing early mobilization. Two years is generally required for maximum recovery although many patients can be back at work by 12 to 16 weeks after injury.

Late disability following calcaneal fractures occurs. The disability is usually caused by peroneal tendinitis secondary to impingement between the fibula and the laterally expanded calcaneus, ankle arthritis related to

---

*Gallie, 1943; Brattström, 1953; Moberg and Erfors, 1953; Thompson and Friesen, 1959; Hall and Pennal, 1960; Harris, 1963; Zagra and Bellistri, 1970.

unrecognized ankle trauma, heel spurs, or degenerative arthritis of the subtalar, calcaneocuboid, or talonavicular joints. Conservative treatment for this problem using a well-fitted molded leather ankle brace with lateral metal stays is often quite successful. If conservative treatment fails, late decompression of the peroneal tendons can be achieved as described by Deyerle (1973). Heel spurs on rare occasion can be excised. A subtalar arthrodesis may be performed for arthritis of the subtalar joint only, but a triple arthrodesis is indicated if other joints are involved.

At San Francisco General Hospital we treat in excess of 100 os calcis fractures per year by conservative means; we do only one or two operative procedures per year for late disability resulting from these fractures.

FRACTURES OF THE CUBOID

Isolated fractures of the cuboid are rare. Fractures of the cuboid accompanied by fractures of the adjacent cuneiforms or of the base of the lateral metatarsals or both are more common, but even these combinations are encountered infrequently.

Wilson (1933), in a series of approximately 5,000 fractures, found only ten cases of isolated fracture of the cuboid. Hermel and Gershon-Cohen (1953) reported five cases of compression fracture of the cuboid in which the cuboid was compressed between the fourth and fifth metatarsals and the calcaneus. Fig. 6-40, *A*, shows a comminuted compression fracture of the cuboid in a youth 21 years of age who fell asleep and drove his car into a tree. His fracture was treated during the acute phase by casting; he now wears a shoe insert and walks with minimal disability. Fig. 6-40, *B*, shows a comminuted fracture of the cuboid in a young man 17 years of age who fell from a motorcycle.

Watson-Jones (1955) does not discuss the problem of cuboid fracture; Böhler (1958) and Conwell and Reynolds (1961) both state that fractures of this bone rarely show major displacements and need be treated only by immobilization; and Jackson and Dickson (1965) report having seen only three cases of fracture of the cuboid (Fig. 6-41).

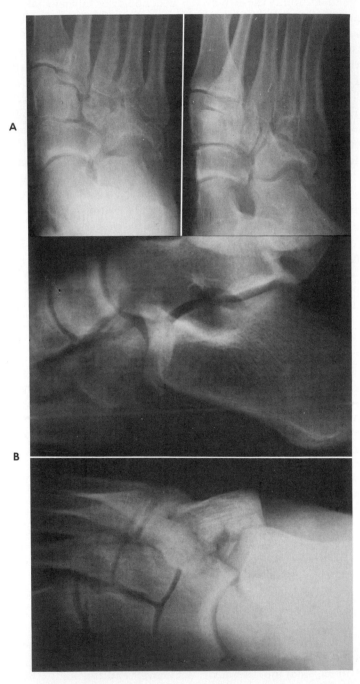

Fig. 6-40. **A,** Comminuted compression fracture of the cuboid in a youth 21 years of age. **B,** Comminuted fracture and dislocation of the left cuboid in a youth 17 years of age.

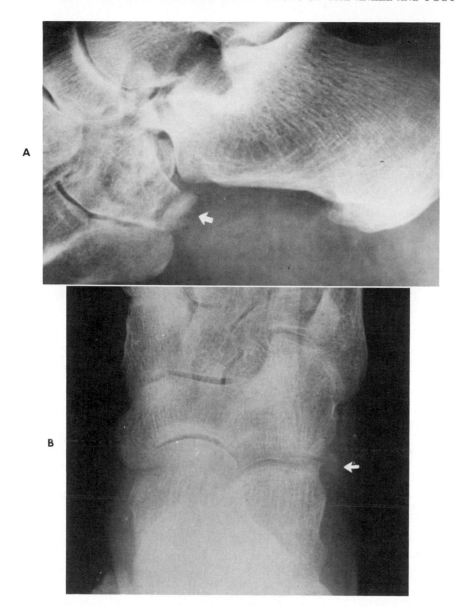

Fig. 6-41. A, Fracture and displacement of the plantar surface of the cuboid. **B,** Chip fracture of the lateral side of the cuboid.

FRACTURES OF THE NAVICULAR

Although fractures of the navicular occur twice as frequently as fractures of the cuboid (Wilson, 1933), they are still uncommon. Watson-Jones (1955) divides these fractures into three types: (1) fractures of the tuberosity, (2) chip fractures of the dorsal lip, and (3) transverse fractures, with or without sepa-

ration and displacement of the dorsal fragments.

Fracture of the tuberosity of the navicular must be distinguished from congenital os tibiale externum. The line of separation in os tibiale externum is usually smooth and regular, whereas in a fracture it is rough; and unlike the fracture, os tibiale externum com-

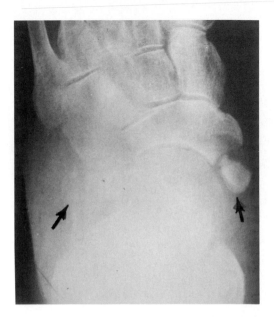

Fig. 6-42. Avulsion fracture of the neck of the navicular and fracture of the head of the calcaneus.

monly occurs bilaterally. Small persistently painful fractures that fail to heal with immobilization may require excision of the fragments (Figs. 6-42 and 6-43).

Dorsal chip fractures may be treated conservatively; only a short period of immobilization is required and usually little disability results. If pain persists, however, the fragment may be excised (Fig. 6-44).

Transverse fractures through the body of the navicular are more serious. The literature dealing with this type of fracture is not extensive and consists mainly of reports of single cases or small series of cases (1908 to 1970). No consensus as to preferred treatment seems to have been reached. In general, simple linear fractures without displacement may be treated conservatively; a good functional result is to be anticipated (Fig. 6-45). Displaced fractures should be reduced and fixed by pins or screws. If the articular surfaces are malaligned or destroyed (Fig. 6-46), degenerative changes are to be expected and some type of arthrodesis may be required at a later date.

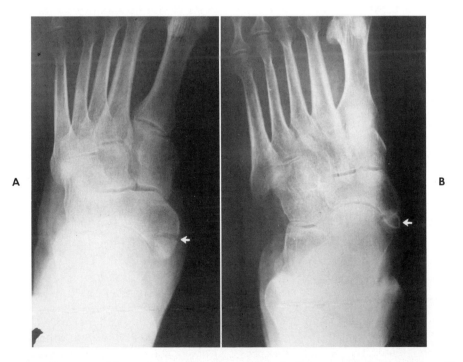

Fig. 6-43. A, Fracture of the neck of the navicular without displacement. **B,** One year later. The fractured fragment is tilted on its end, producing a peroneal spastic flatfoot. Note the rarefaction at the head of the talus.

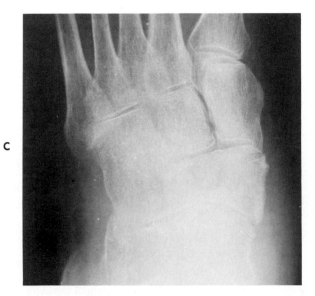

Fig. 6-43, cont'd. C, After removal of the fractured fragment. The peroneal spasm has disappeared.

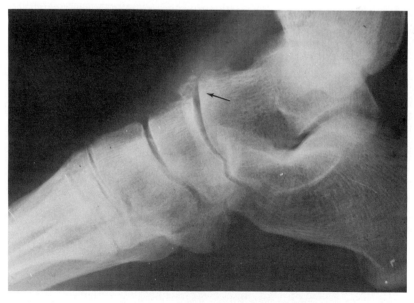

Fig. 6-44. Chip fracture over the dorsum of the navicular. The chip was removed to relieve pain.

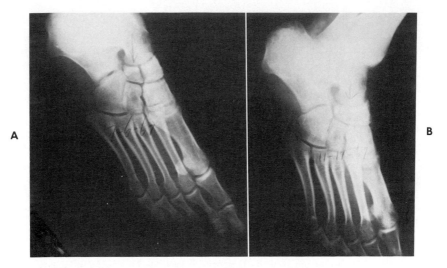

Fig. 6-45. Transverse fracture through the body of the navicular. It was treated conservatively with casting and non–weight bearing. **A,** At the time of the injury. **B,** One year later. The fracture has healed, resulting in minimal disability.

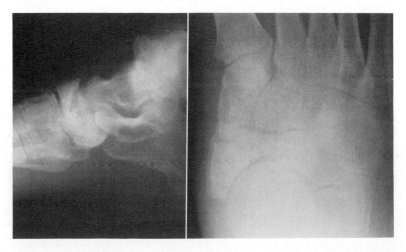

Fig. 6-46. Vertical and transverse views of a comminuted fracture of the navicular.

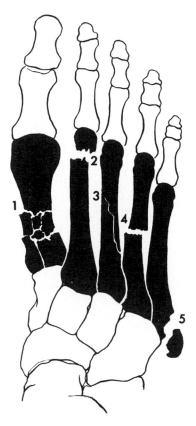

Fig. 6-47. Types of fractures of the metatarsals: *1*, comminuted; *2*, transverse with displacement; *3*, oblique or spiral; *4*, transverse; *5*, avulsion fracture of the tuberosity. (After Netter.)

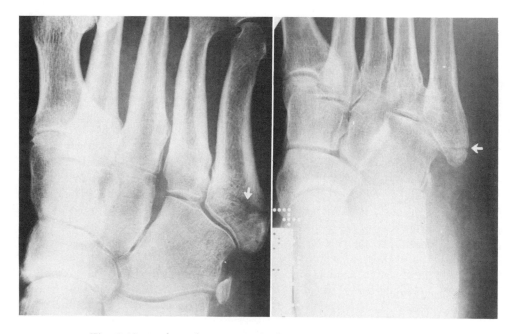

Fig. 6-48. Avulsion fractures at the base of the fifth metatarsal.

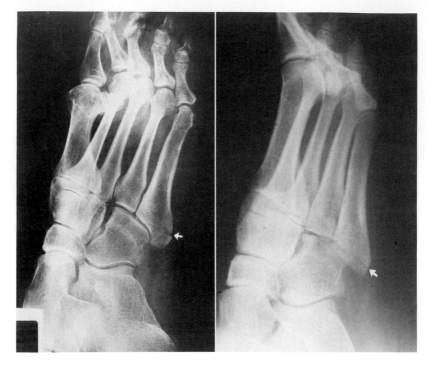

Fig. 6-49. Fractures of the tip of the fifth metatarsal base.

FRACTURES OF THE METATARSALS

The metatarsals are vulnerable to all types of fracture (Fig. 6-47) due to such causes as the dropping of heavy objects on the foot, muscle pull, and severe twists.

The base of the fifth metatarsal is a frequent site of fracture (Figs. 6-48 and 6-49), which can produce complications because the peroneus brevis inserts into it and the peroneus longus is held by it in the cuboid groove. Among children, fracture of the base of the fifth metatarsal must be differentiated from fracture of the epiphyseal line. Ordinarily there is no displacement.

The only treatment required in most undisplaced fractures of the base of the metatarsals is to strap the foot by binding the bases and heads of all metatarsals with adhesive tape. Usually little or no disability results (Fig. 6-51). Sometimes a walking cast is needed for about 6 weeks. In cases of severe avulsion of the broken fragment, open reduction may be required in which the fragment is pinned through the shaft and maintained while the patient wears a walking cast for 6 weeks.

Fractures of the lateral lesser metatarsals resulting from injury are, for the most part, multiple (Figs. 6-50 to 6-52) and usually occur at the neck, the weakest part of the metatarsal bones. Such fractures may be serious when displacement is plantarward and not reduced; disability may result because of abnormal pressures on weight bearing.

Fractures of the shafts of the metatarsals may require traction for reduction. At times, when manipulative reduction fails, it may be necessary to correct the displacement by open reduction and the use of pins or wire to maintain apposition

Fracture of the first metatarsal is rare because of the strength of this bone. When the bone does fracture, displacement is slight (Fig. 6-53); immobilization for 6 weeks suffices. Displacement can be reduced by closed reduction and, if necessary, maintained by a Kirschner wire.

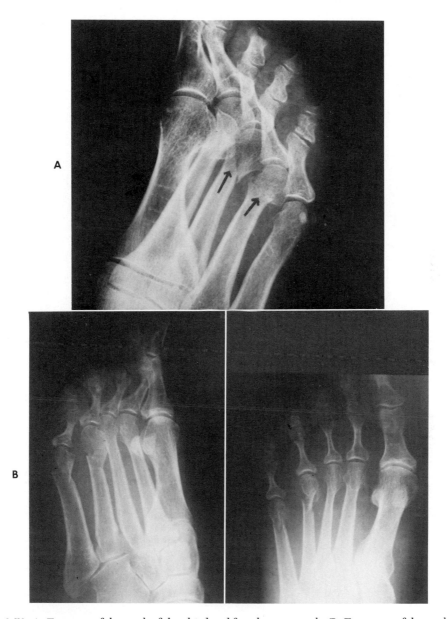

Fig. 6-50. A, Fracture of the neck of the third and fourth metatarsals. **B,** Fractures of the neck of the fourth and fifth metatarsals.

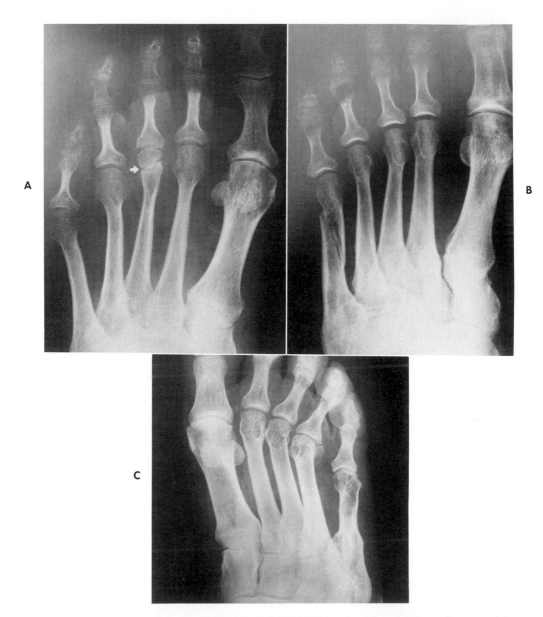

Fig. 6-51. **A,** Ununited fracture of the head of the third metatarsal. **B,** Oblique fracture of the fifth metatarsal shaft. **C,** Malunited fracture of the fifth metatarsal shaft.

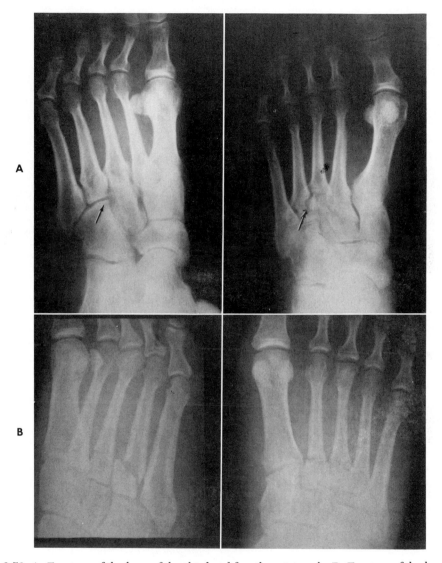

Fig. 6-52. A, Fracture of the base of the third and fourth metatarsals. **B,** Fracture of the base of the second, third, and fourth metatarsals treated by immobilization with a plaster boot.

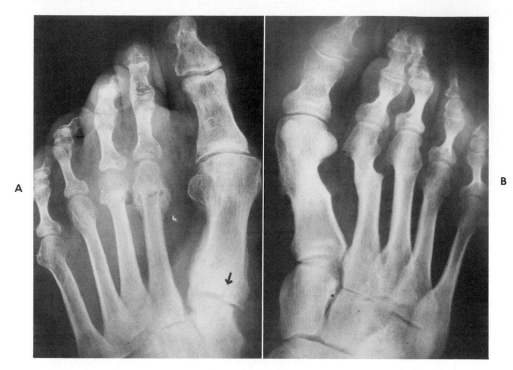

Fig. 6-53. **A,** Neglected fracture at the base of the first metatarsal; concomitant fracture of the neck of the second metatarsal. **B,** Old fracture of the first and second metatarsals.

FRACTURES OF THE PHALANGES
Fifth proximal phalanx

The most common fracture of the forefoot is that of the fifth proximal phalanx. Stubbing the fifth toe is the usual cause. Among children the fracture may be at the epiphyseal plate (Fig. 6-54, *A* and *B*); among adults it is likely to be at the base and neck (Fig. 6-54, *C* and *D*).

Phalanges of the middle toes

Fracture of any of the three middle toes is uncommon; when it does occur, usually the proximal phalanx, a relatively long bone, is broken. The middle and distal phalanges are seldom fractured.

Displacement is rare in fracture of the phalanges of the three middle toes; when it does occur, it can be readily reduced, often without an anesthetic.

The adjacent toes may serve as a splint. Adhesive tape, ½ inch wide, is wound around the fractured toe as well as around the two or three adjacent toes so none can move independently. Strips of adhesive tape wound around the metatarsophalangeal joints will limit motion. Immobilization is maintained for about 4 weeks. Ambulation is permitted immediately, provided the sole of the shoe is semirigid.

Hallux phalanges

Fractures of the hallux phalanges present a more difficult problem than do fractures of the other phalanges. The hallux phalanges are comparatively large, and their function is as important as that of all the other phalanges put together. The proximal phalanx of the hallux is broken most frequently (Fig. 6-55). The distal phalanx may be fractured, however, and when this occurs the fracture is often comminuted or dislocated (Figs. 6-56 and 6-57). A rare type of injury encountered frequently in the fingers but seldom in the toes is an avulsion fracture of the distal phalanx of the hallux (Fig. 6-58).

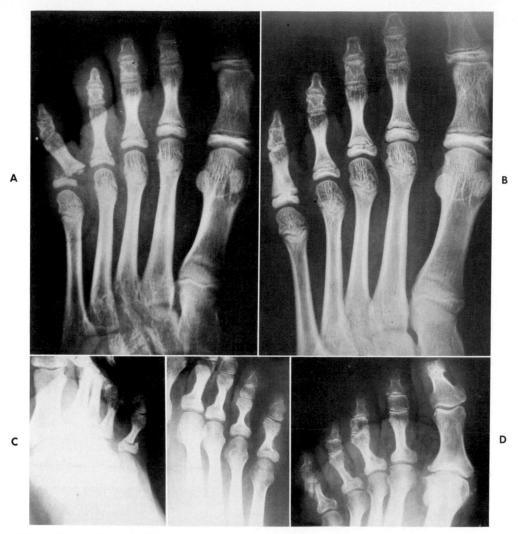

Fig. 6-54. A, Fracture-dislocation at the epiphyseal plate of the base of the fifth proximal phalanx. **B,** After closed reduction and healing. **C,** Fracture at the base of the fifth proximal phalanx. **D,** Fracture at the neck of the fifth proximal phalanx. Neglect resulted in nonunion.

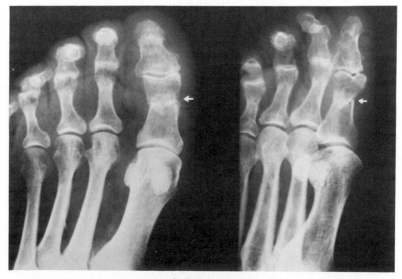

Fig. 6-55. Impacted fracture of the proximal phalanx of the hallux.

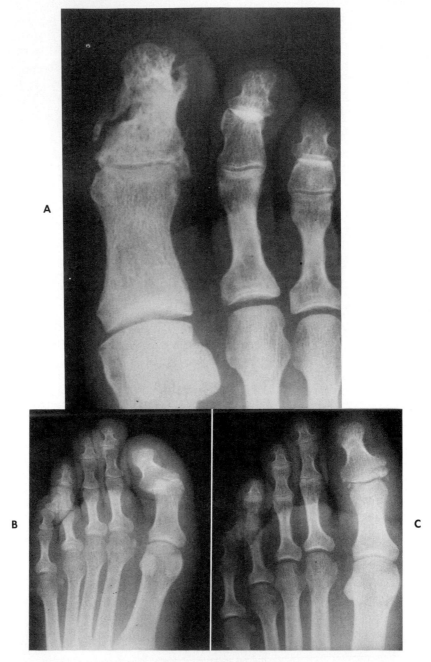

Fig. 6-56. A, Comminuted fracture of the distal phalanx of the great toe. Amputation was necessary because of nonhealing of the fragmentation. **B,** Dislocation of the hallux interphalangeal joint with chip fracture of the head of the proximal phalanx. **C,** After closed reduction of the fracture. Arthritis may develop in this joint, requiring arthrodesis.

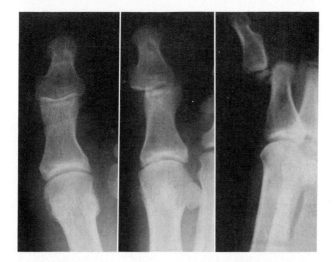

Fig. 6-57. Dislocation of the hallux interphalangeal joint and chip fracture of the head of the proximal phalanx. It was reduced by closed reduction.

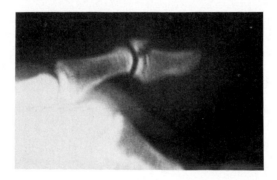

Fig. 6-58. Avulsion fracture of the distal phalanx of the hallux in a young man who stubbed his toe while walking barefoot along a city street.

If there is no displacement, the hallux should be bound to the two adjacent toes and a walking cast extending beyond the toes should be applied and maintained for 4 weeks. When displacement is present but cannot be reduced by manipulation, open reduction is indicated.

FRACTURES OF THE SESAMOIDS

The tibial sesamoid is more likely to fracture because normally it receives most of the weight transmitted by the first metatarsal. The fracture is usually transverse or comminuted (Fig. 6-59). The condition must always

be differentiated from a normal bifurcation: in a true fracture the line of division is jagged and irregular, whereas in bifurcation the outline is regular and the division is smooth. Fracture of the fibular sesamoid is rare (Fig. 6-60).

Direct trauma or injury incurred by jumping from heights or by excessive dancing of any type may cause the fracture. In rare instances fracture of the sesamoid is spontaneous.

The onset of symptoms is sudden, but the patient may not seek professional help for days or weeks after the accident. On palpation of the sesamoid, especially on dorsiflexion of

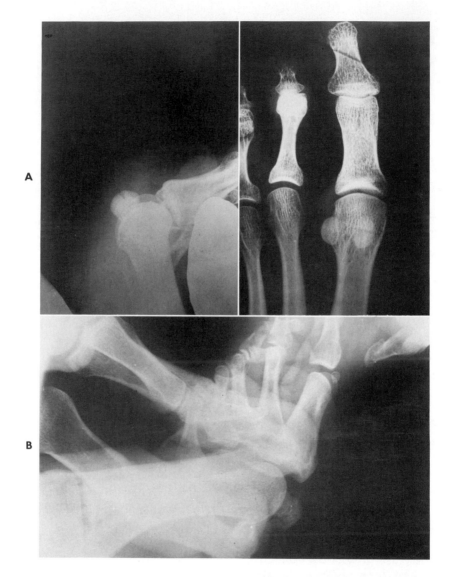

Fig. 6-59. A, Transverse fracture of the tibial sesamoid. **B,** Comminuted fracture of the tibial sesamoid.

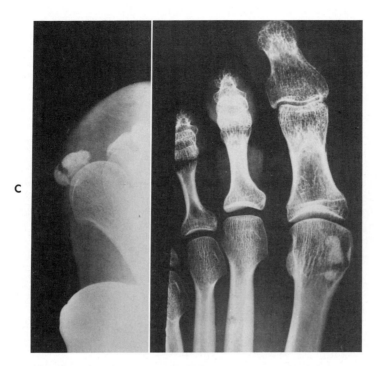

Fig. 6-59, cont'd. C, Fracture of the proximal portion of the tibial sesamoid.

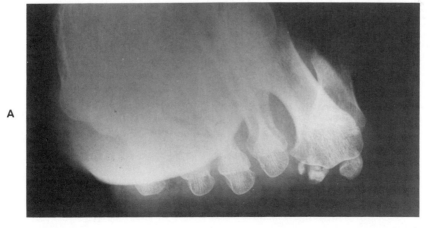

Continued.

Fig. 6-60. A and B, Comminuted fracture of the fibular sesamoid. C, Feet of a 20-year-old woman who had had pain in the left great toe joint for about a year. Routine radiographs did not give a definite explanation of pain. D, Tangential view showing an old fracture of the fibular sesamoid. Excision of the ossicle gave complete relief.

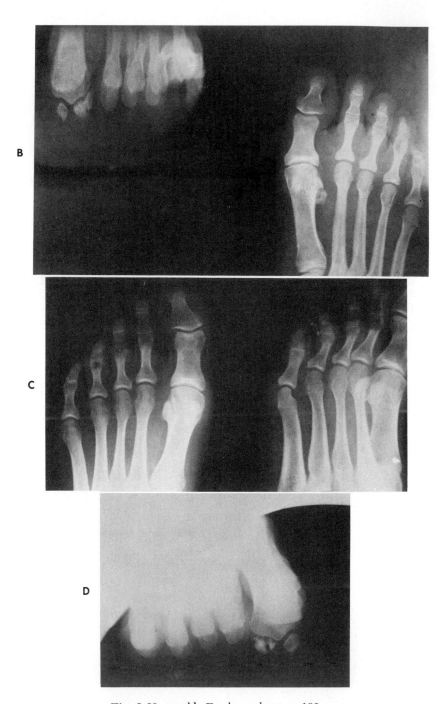

Fig. 6-60, cont'd. For legend see p. 193.

the great toe, pain is sharp. Sometimes pain is mild and gradually becomes severe. The periarticular structures on the plantar surface of the first metatarsophalangeal joint become swollen.

A recent fracture should be immobilized completely for 3 weeks with the metatarsophalangeal joint plantar flexed. In many cases palliative measures fail because of delayed treatment. Surgical removal of the sesamoid is then inevitable.

FATIGUE (MARCH, STRESS) FRACTURES

Fatigue fractures have been recognized by military surgeons for over a century, and the literature about them is voluminous. A critical review of this subject and an exhaustive bibliography may be found in the monograph by Morris and Blickenstaff (1967).

Since 80% of all fatigue fractures occur in the bones of the feet, a short discussion of them seems pertinent.

The metatarsals are the most frequently involved bones and account for more than 50% of all fatigue fractures. Of these, fractures of the second metatarsal occur most frequently (Fig. 6-61), followed by fractures of the third (Fig. 6-62, A) and then the fourth metatarsal (Fig. 6-62, B). The first metatarsal and the fifth metatarsal (Fig. 6-62, C) are rarely affected. The only other bone of the foot about which there are reports of fatigue fractures is the calcaneus (Fig. 6-63). Fracture of this bone occurs only half as frequently as fracture of the metatarsals.

The patient's history often provides diagnostic evidence of the condition. Fatigue fractures occur in people who subject the bones of their feet to prolonged, continued, cyclic stresses (e.g., athletes, joggers, and military personnel). History of specific trauma is lacking; insidious onset of pain is usual. Rest relieves the acute pain, but a residual dull ache occasionally persists. Activity increases the pain.

Examination reveals sharply localized tenderness that is restricted to the bone; there is no pain in the ligamentous structures. Swelling and increased local heat may occur over the site of fracture.

Radiographs obtained shortly after the on-

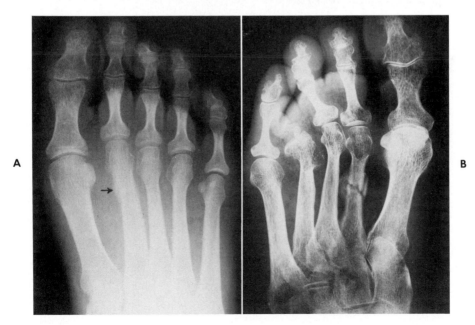

Fig. 6-61. A, Fatigue fracture at the neck of the second metatarsal. **B,** Fatigue fracture comminuted with extensive formation of callus and coincidental aseptic necrosis of the fourth digit.

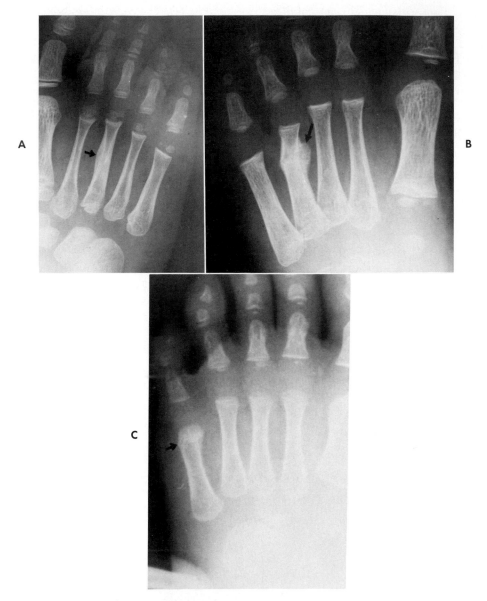

Fig. 6-62. A, Fatigue fracture of the third metatarsal in a child. **B,** Spontaneous fracture of the fourth metatarsal in a child. **C,** Spontaneous fracture of the neck of the fifth metatarsal in an infant. (**A** courtesy Dr. Jack Stern; **B** courtesy Dr. Frank Weinstein.)

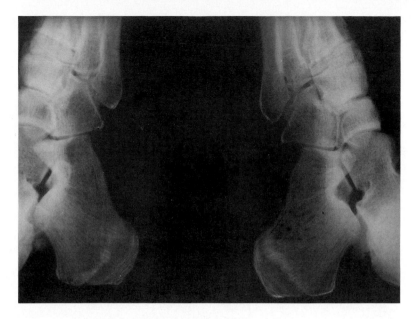

Fig. 6-63. Bilateral fatigue fractures of the calcaneus in a 22-year-old Army recruit. (Courtesy Dr. David A. Hunt, Fremont, Calif.)

set of symptoms may appear normal. A lapse of 2 or 3 weeks may be necessary before endosteal callus or periosteal callus or both are evident.

When a patient with this condition is seen promptly, the treatment is avoidance of those activities that produced the condition; if the symptoms are more acute, rest and immobilization may be required. If the activity that led to the onset of symptoms is continued, complete fracture with or without displacement may ensue. In such a situation, treatment is similar to that of any acute fracture.

DISLOCATIONS
Dislocations of the subtalar joint

A complete dislocation of the talus onto the calcaneus necessarily involves the talonavicular joint. Basically this uncommon type of injury may be described as a displacement of all the components of the foot from the talus.

Leitner (1952) researched the world literature thoroughly and found fewer than 300 reported cases of this type of dislocation. He added fifty-four cases of his own (forty-two were fresh injuries, twelve were old unreduced dislocations) for the review. These injuries comprised 1% of all the dislocations that were encountered over a twenty-five year period in his service for the treatment of traumatic injuries. Since Leitner's review, von Vogt (1959) has added three cases and Soustelle et al. (1964) have noted one additional case.

Since the articles of Leitner (1952, 1954) constitute the most comprehensive studies dealing with this injury, it seems appropriate to summarize them here:

Medial displacements of the foot on the talus occurred six to seven times more frequently than lateral displacements of the foot on the talus. Only one case of posterior displacement was reported. In fresh dislocations closed manipulative reduction was accomplished in 90% of cases. In 10% of cases, open reduction was necessary because of the interposition of soft tissue or the displacement of tendons.

Dislocations of the midtarsal (Chopart's) joint

Dislocations of the midtarsal joints (the talonavicular and calcaneocuboid articulations), unaccompanied by fractures, appear to be rare. Standard textbooks dealing with inju-

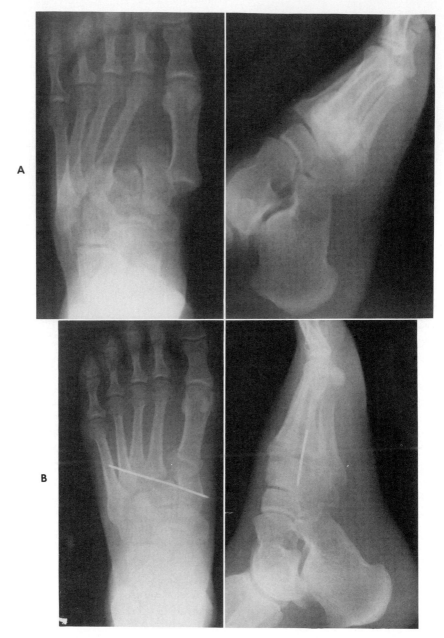

Fig. 6-64. A, Tarsometatarsal fracture-dislocation. **B,** After closed reduction and internal fixation with Kirschner wires.

ries to the skeletal system give them only a passing mention (Watson-Jones, 1955; Böhler, 1958; Conwell and Reynolds, 1961). Individual dislocations of the navicular or the cuboid occur more frequently, but the literature on these dislocations is also sparse. Reports of a few cases have been published intermittently and student theses have appeared in the French and German literature (Gilland, 1936; Willigens, 1936; Boidard, 1939; Weh, 1939).

Dewar and Evans (1968) reported several cases of subluxated cuboid that were first diagnosed as sprains and intimated that reduction was accomplished easily enough in cases which were seen promptly; however, in cases which were not promptly seen, open reduction and internal fixation or limited arthrodesis were necessary.

Dislocations of the cuboid

Drummond and Hastings (1969) reported one case of medical and inferior dislocation of the cuboid that was initially overlooked. They could find no similar case in the literature. The dislocation, treated by open reduction, was fixed by means of two cross wires, a wire to the calcaneus and one to the lateral cuneiform.

Dislocations of the tarsometatarsal (Lisfranc's) joint

Dislocations of the tarsometatarsal joint, with or without accompanying fractures between the tarsus and the metatarsus, constitute a special category of injuries to the foot (Fig. 6-64). Although these dislocations exhibit a wide range of individual variation, they share a similar general pattern and have many elements in common. They occur as a result of abrupt force applied to the forefoot, usually in falls from great heights or in automobile accidents. They have also been described as typical injuries sustained by motorcyclists (Detlefsen, 1968). These dislocations can be serious, since the disruption may be complicated by arterial injury, which results in the interruption of the blood supply to the distal portions of the foot.

Gissane (1951) reported three cases, and Groulier and Pinaud (1970) reported four others that required amputation. Fortunately this injury occurs relatively infrequently, but prompt diagnosis and reduction are essential.

Since the monumental study of Quénu and Küss (1909) of thirty-two dislocations of the tarsometatarsal joint, reports of small series of cases or single cases have appeared sporadically in the literature. Schiller and Ray (1970) reported a case of an unusual dislocation of the medial cuneiform bone, which could have been overlooked because of its deceptive radiographic appearance. Several comprehensive studies of these injuries—including case reports, descriptions of the mechanisms of injury, classification of the types of injury, descriptions of treatment, and evaluation of results—exist: Aitken and Poulson (1963), Cherkes-Zade (1969), Taussig et al. (1969), and Perriard et al. (1970). Groulier and Pinaud (1970) reviewed 120 cases in the literature, added ten of their own, and included an exhaustive bibliography in their article on this subject.

The importance of prompt realignment of the joints and reduction of fractures is emphasized in all these articles. If manipulation is carried out immediately, reduction may be accomplished easily; thereafter, only immobilization in plaster casts is necessary. Arenberg (1969) reported a case in which an excellent reduction was achieved by manipulation within 50 minutes after the initial injury occurred.

Often dislocations or fracture-dislocations or both are unstable; then several methods can be used to maintain alignment. Fitte and Garacotche (1940) employed traction with pins through the calcaneus and metatarsals. Collett et al. (1958) used toe traction and attached the toes to an outrigger type of appliance to maintain alignment. The majority of authors, however, report the need for open reduction and internal fixation. Huet and Lecoeur (1946) and Ballerio (1953) described the role of the peroneus longus in preventing successful treatment of these injuries by closed reduction and advocated treatment by open reduction. Geckeler (1949), del Sel (1955), Collett et al. (1958), Tondeur (1961), Taussig et al. (1969), and Groulier and Pinaud (1970) all advise open reduction, accurate alignment, and internal fixation with pins or staples.

I have found that most can be managed with closed reduction and percutaneous Kirschner wire stabilization. Anatomic reduction is important, and one should not hesitate to proceed with open reduction since malalignment can lead to late tarsometatarsal arthritis.

Dislocations of the metatarsophalangeal joints and the phalanges

Although dislocations of these joints (chronic, progressive, or sometimes both) are common deformities of the forefoot, acute traumatic dislocations are rare. The majority of chronic dislocations occur between the proximal phalanges and the metatarsals. Dislocation of the first metatarsophalangeal articulation (frequently compound) is the most common. In the usual deformity the phalanx is displaced onto the dorsum of the metatarsal. The diagnosis is readily made and manipulation will usually reduce the dislocation.

Traction, a frequent adjunct in the manipulative reduction of most dislocations, often fails to accomplish reduction in dislocations of the metatarsophalangeal articulations because of the peculiar arrangements of the connective tissue structures in the vicinity of these joints. The inferior capsule may be torn and lie against the metatarsal head, or the capsule may be torn and displaced around the metatarsal head like a buttonhole, or the flexor tendons may be displaced around the neck of the metatarsal. In these situations traction only tightens the soft tissues around the metatarsal, thus preventing reduction. To achieve reduction, the phalanx should be hyperextended and angled plantarward so the inferior edge of the articular surface contacts the superior aspect of the articular surface of the metatarsal head. Pressure (not traction) is applied and keeps the edge of the articular surface of the phalanx against the articular surface of the metatarsal. As the phalanx is replaced, its inferior edge wipes any soft tissue from the head of the metatarsal.

These dislocations are usually stable and require only minimal external fixation with strapping.

REFERENCES
Criteria for treatment

Akeson, W. H.: An experimental study of joint stiffness, J. Bone Joint Surg. 43A:1022, 1961.

Clark, D. D., and Weckesser, E. C.: The influence of triamcinolone acetonide on joint stiffness in the rat, J. Bone Joint Surg. 53A:1409, 1971.

Collins, D. H., and McElligott, T. F.: Sulphate ($^{35}SO_4$) uptake by chondrocytes in relation to histological changes in osteoarthritic human articular cartilage, Ann. Rheum. Dis. 19:318, 1960.

Davenport, H. K., and Ranson, S. W.: Contraction resulting from tenotomy, Arch. Surg. 21:995, 1930.

Dziewiatkowski, D. D., Benesch, R. E., and Benesch, R.: On the possible utilization of sulfate sulfur by the suckling rat for the synthesis of chondroitin sulfate as indicated by the use of radioactive sulfur, J. Biol. Chem. 178:931, 1949.

Ely, L. W., and Mensor, M. C.: Studies on the immobilization of the normal joints, Surg. Gynecol. Obstet. 57:212, 1933.

Evans, E. B., Eggers, G. W. N., Butler, J. K., and Blumel, J.: Experimental immobilization and remobilization of rat knee joints, J. Bone Joint Surg. 42A:737, 1960.

Frankshteyn, S.I.: Experimental studies on mechanism of development of contractures due to immobilization in casts, Khirurgiia 8:44, 1944.

Frugone, J. E., Thomsen, P., and Luco, J. V.: Changes in weight of muscles of arthritic and immobilized arthritic joints, Proc. Soc. Exp. Biol. Med. 61:31, 1946.

Gasser, H. S.: Contractures of skeletal muscle, Physiol. Rev. 10:35, 1930.

Hall, M. C.: Cartilage changes after experimental immobilization of the knee joint of the young rat, J. Bone Joint Surg. 45A:36, 1963.

Harrison, M. H. M., Schajowicz, F., and Trueta, J.: Osteoarthritis of the hip: a study of the nature and evolution of the disease, J. Bone Joint Surg. 35B:598, 1953.

Lucas-Championniére, J.: Précis du traitement des fractures par le massage et la mobilisation, Paris, 1910, G. Steinheil.

McLean, F. C., and Urist, M. R.: Bone: An introduction to the physiology of skeletal tissue, Chicago, 1955, University of Chicago Press.

Menzel, A.: Ueber die Erkrankung der Gelenke bei dauernder Ruhe derselben: eine experimentelle Studie, Arch. Klin. Chir. 12:990, 1871.

Müller, W.: Experimentelle Untersuchungen über die Wirkung langdauernder Immobilisierung auf die Gelenke, Z. Orthop. Chir. 44:478, 1924.

Peacock, E. E., Jr.: Some biochemical and biophysical aspects of joint stiffnes: role of collagen synthesis as opposed to altered molecular bonding, Ann. Surg. 164:1, 1966.

Ranson, S. W., and Sams, C. F.: A study of muscle in contracture: the permanent shortening of muscles caused by tenotomy and tetanus toxin, J. Neurol. Psychopathol. 8:304, 1923.

Salter, R. B., and Field, P.: The effects of continuous compression on living articular cartilage: an experimental investigation, J. Bone Joint Surg. 42A:31, 1960.

Scaglietti, O., and Casuccio, C.: Studio sperimentale degli effetti della immobilizzazione su articolazioni normali, Chir. Organi Mov. 20:469, 1936.

Sokoloff, L., and Jay, G. E., Jr.: Natural history of degenerative joint disease in the small laboratory animals. 4. Degenerative joint disease in the laboratory rat, Arch. Pathol. 62:140, 1956.

Solandt, D. Y., and Magladery, J. W.: A comparison of

effects of upper and lower motor neurone lesions on skeletal muscle, J. Neurophysiol. **5**:373, 1942.

Thaxter, T. H., Mann, R. A., and Anderson C. E.: Degeneration of immobilized knee joints in rats: Histological and autoradiographic study, J. Bone Joint Surg. **47A**:567, 1965.

Trias, A.: Effect of persistent pressure on the articular cartilage, J. Bone Joint Surg. **43B**:376, 1961.

Thomsen, P., and Luco, J. V.: Changes of weight and neuromuscular transmission in muscles of immobilized joints, J. Neurophysiol. **7**:245, 1944.

Tschmarke, G.: Experimentelle Untersuchungen über die Rolle des Muskeltonus in der Gelenkchirurgie. 3. Mitteilung: Fixationskontrakturen und die Beeinflussung ihrer Entwicklung, Arch. Klin. Chir. **164**:785, 1931.

Fractures and fracture-dislocations of the ankle joint

Ashhurst, A. P. C., and Bromer, R. S.: Classification and mechanism of fractures of the leg bones involving the ankle. Based on a study of three hundred cases from the Episcopal Hospital, Arch. Surg. **4**:51, 1922.

Aufranc, O. E.: Trimalleolar fracture dislocation, J.A.M.A. **174**:2221, 1960.

Bonnin, J. G.: Injuries to the ankle, ed. 1, New York, 1950, Grune & Stratton, Inc.

Bosworth, D. M.: Fracture-dislocation of the ankle with fixed displacement of the fibula behind the tibia, J. Bone Joint Surg. **29**:130, 1947.

Burwell, H. N., and Charnley, A. D.: The treatment of displaced fractures at the ankle by rigid internal fixation and early joint movement, J. Bone Joint Surg. **47B**:634, 1965.

Chapman, M. W., and Mahoney, M: The place of immediate internal fixation in the management of open fracture, Abbott Soc. Bull. **8**:85, May, 1976.

Charnley, J. The closed treatment of common fractures, Baltimore, 1963, The Williams & Wilkins Co.

Childress, H. M.: Vertical transarticular-pin fixation for unstable ankle fractures, J. Bone Joint Surg. **47A**:1323, 1965.

Coonrad, R. W., and Bugg, E. I.: Trapping of the posterior tibial tendon and interposition of soft tissue in severe fractures about the ankle joint, J. Bone Joint Surg. **36A**:744, 1954.

Dieterlé, J.: The use of Kirschner wire in maintaining reduction of fracture-dislocations of the ankle joint: a report of two cases, J. Bone Joint Surg. **17**:990, 1935.

Fleming, J. L., and Smith H. O.: Fracture-dislocation of the ankle with the fibula fixed behind the tibia, J. Bone Joint Surg. **36A**:556, 1954.

Glick, B. W.: The ankle fracture with inferior tibiofibular joint disruption, Surg. Gynecol. Obstet. **118**:549, 1964.

Gustilo, R. B., and Anderson, J. T.: Prevention of infection in the treatment of one thousand and twenty-five open fractures of long bones, J. Bone Joint Surg. **58A**:453, 1976.

Jergesen, F.: Open reduction of fractures and dislocations of the ankle, Am. J. Surg. **98**:136, 1959.

Kleiger, B.: The mechanism of ankle injuries, J. Bone Joint Surg. **38A**:59, 1956.

Lauge-Hansen, N: Fractures of the ankle: analytic historic survey as the basis of new experimental, roentgenologic and clinical investigations, Arch. Surg **56**:259, 1948.

Lauge-Hansen, N.: Fractures of the ankle. II. Combined experimental-surgical and experimental-roentgenologic investigations, Arch. Surg. **60**:957, 1950.

Lauge-Hansen, N.: Fractures of the ankle. IV. Clinical use of genetic roentgen diagnosis and genetic reduction, Arch. Surg. **64**:488, 1952.

Lauge-Hansen, N.: Fractures of the ankle. III. Genetic roentgenologic diagnosis of fracture of the ankle, Am. J. Roentgenol. Radium Ther. Nucl. Med. **71**:456, 1954.

Maisonneuve, J. G.: Recherches sur la fracture du perone, Arch. Gen. Med. **7**:165, 433, 1840.

Mayer, V., and Pohlidal, S.: Ankle mortise injuries, Surg. Gynecol. Obstet. **96**:99, 1953.

McDade, W. C.: Treatment of ankle fractures. In Instructional Course Lectures, American Academy of Orthopaedic Surgeons, vol. 24, St. Louis, 1975. The C. V. Mosby Co.

McDaniel, W. J., and Wilson, F.C.: Trimalleolar fractures of the ankle. And end result study, Clin. Orthop. **122**:37, 1977.

McMaster, J.H., and Scranton, P.E.: Tibiofibular synostosis: a cause of ankle disability, Clin. Orthop. **111**:172, 1975.

Meyers, M. H.: Fracture about the ankle joint with fixed displacement of the proximal fragment of the fibula behind the tibia, J. Bone Joint Surg. **39A**:441, 1957.

Müller, M. E., Allgower, M., and Willenegger, H.: Manual of external fixation, New York, 1970, Springer-Verlag New York, Inc.

Portis, R. B., and Mendelsohn, H. A.: Conservative management of fractures of the ankle involving the medial malleolus, J.A.M.A. **151**:102, 1953.

Scranton, P.E., McMaster, J.H., and Kelly, E.: Dynamic fibular function, a new concept, Clin. Orthop. **118**:76, 1976.

Wiggins, H. E.: Pronation-dorsiflexion fractures with involvement of distal tibial metaphysis—case studies. In Instructional Course Lectures, American Academy of Orthopaedic Surgeons, vol. 24, St. Louis, 1975, The C.V. Mosby Co.

Yablon, I.G., Heller, F.G., and Shouse, L.: The key role of the lateral malleolus in displaced fractures of the ankle, J Bone Joint Surg. **59A**:169, 1977.

Zuelzer, W.A.: Use of hookplate for fixation of ununited medial tibial malleolus, J.A.M.A. **167**:828, 1958.

Fractures and fracture-dislocations of the talus

Anderson, H.G.: The medical and surgical aspects of aviation, London, 1919, Hodder & Co.

Berndt, A.L., and Harty, M.: Transchondral fractures

(osteochondritis dissecans) of the talus, J. Bone Joint Surg. **41A**:988, 1959.

Blair, H.C.: Comminuted fracture and fracture-dislocations of the body of the astragalus; operative treatment, Am. J. Surg. **59**:37, 1943.

Boyd, H.B., and Knight, R.A.: Fractures of the astragalus, South. Med. J. **35**:160, 1942.

Coltart, W.D.: Aviator's astragalus, J. Bone Joint Surg. **34B**:545, 1952.

Davidson, A.M., Steele, H.D., MacKenzie, D.A., and Penny, J.A.: A review of twenty-one cases of transchondral fracture of the talus, J. Trauma **7**:378, 1967.

Davis, M.W.: Bilateral talus osteochondritis dissecans, J. Bone Joint Surg. **52A**:168, 1970.

Dunn, A.R., Jacobs, B., and Campbell, R.D.: Fractures of the talus, J. Trauma **6**:443, 1966.

Fjeldborg, O.: Fracture of the lateral process of the talus, Acta Orthop. Scand. **39**:407, 1968.

Gustilo, R.B., and Gordon S.S.: Osteochondral fractures of the talus, Minn. Med. **51**:237, 1968.

Haliburton, R.A., Sullivan, C.R., Kelly P.J., and Peterson, L.F.A.: The extra-osseous and intra-osseus blood supply of the talus, J. Bone Joint Surg. **40A**:1115, 1958.

Hawkins, L.G.: Fracture of the lateral process of the talus, J. Bone Joint Surg. **47A**:1170, 1965.

Hawkins: L.G.: Fractures of the neck of the talus, J. Bone Joint Surg. **52B**:991, 1970.

Kelly, P.J., and Sullivan, C.R.: Blood supply of the talus, Clin. Orthop. **30**:37, 1964.

Kenwright, J., and Taylor, M.A.: Major injuries of the talus, J. Bone Joint Surg. **52B**:36, 1970.

Marks, K.L.: Flake fracture of the talus progressing to osteochondritis dissecans, J. Bone Joint Surg. **34B**:90, 1952.

McKeever, F.M.: Treatment of complications of fractures and dislocations of the talus, Clin. Orthop. **30**:45, 1963.

Mindell, E.R., Cisek, E.E., Kartalian, G., and Dziob, J.M.: Late results of injuries to the talus: analysis of forty cases, J. Bone Joint Surg. **45A**:221, 1963.

Mukherjee, S.K., Pringle, R.M., and Baxter, A.D.: Fracture of the lateral process of the talus, J. Bone Joint Surg. **56B**:263, 1974.

Mukherjee, S.K., and Young, A.B.: Dome fracture of the talus, J. Bone Joint Surg. **55B**:319, 1973.

Mulfinger, G.L., and Trueta, J.: The blood supply of the talus, J. Bone Joint Surg. **52B**:160, 1970.

Pantazopoulos, T., Galenos, P., Vayanos, E., Mitsow, A., and Hartofilakidis-Garofalidis, G.: Fractures of the neck of the talus, Acta Orthop. Scand. **45**:296, 1974.

Pennal, G.F.: Fractures of the talus, Clin. Orthop. **30**:53, 1963.

Ray, A.: Fractures de l'astragale (à propos de 34 observations), Rev. Chir. Orthop. **53**:279, 1967.

Rendu, A.: Fracture intra-acticulaire parcellaire de la poulie astragalienne, Lyon Med. **150**:220, 1932.

Rosenberg, N.J.: Fractures of talar dome, J. Bone Joint Surg. **47A**:1279, 1965.

Sneed, W.L.: The astragalus: a case of dislocation, excision and replacement. An attempt to demonstrate the circulation in this bone, J. Bone Joint Surg. **7**:384, 1925.

Taylor, R.G.: Immobilization of unstable fracture dislocations by the use of Kirschner wires, Proc. R. Soc. Med. **55**:449, 1962.

Watson-Jones, R.: Fractures and joint injuries, ed. 4, vol. 2, Baltimore, 1955, The Williams & Wilkins Co.

Wildenauer, E. Die Blutversorgung des Talus, Z. Anat. Entwicklungsgesch. **115**:32, 1950.

Yvars, M.F.: Osteochondral fractures of the dome of the talus, Clin. Orthop. **114**:185, 1976.

Fractures of the calcaneus

Bankart, A. S. B.: Fractures of the os calcis, Lancet **2**:175, 1942.

Barnard, L., and Odegard, J.K.: Conservative approach in the treatment of fractures of the calcaneus, J. Bone Joint Surg. **52A**:1689, 1970.

Bertelsen, A., and Hasner, E.: Primary results of treatment of fracture of the os calcis by "foot-free walking bandage" and early movement, Acta Orthop. Scand. **21**:140, 1951.

Böhler, L.: The treatment of fractures, ed. 5, vol. 3, New York, 1958, Grune & Stratton, Inc.

Brattström, H.: Primary arthrodesis in severe fractures of the calcaneum, Nord. Med. **50**:1510, 1953.

Carothers, R.G., and Lyons, J.F.: Early mobilization in treatment of os calcis fractures, Am. J. Surg. **83**:279, 1952.

Conwell, H.E., and Reynolds, F.C.: Key and Conwell's management of fractures, dislocations, and sprains, ed. 7, St. Louis, 1961, The C.V. Mosby Co.

Cotton, F.J., and Henderson, F.F.: Results of fracture of the os calcis, Am. J. Orthop. Surg. **14**:290, 1916.

Cotton, F. J., and Wilson, L. T.: Fractures of the os calcis, Boston Med. Surg. J. **159**:559, 1908.

Dautry, P.: Sur le traitement des fractures du calcanéum, Acad. Chir. Mem. **87**:249, 1961.

Deyerle, W.M.: Long term follow-up of fractures of the os calcis, Orthop. Clin. North Am. **4**:213, 1973.

Dragonetti, L.: A proposito del trattamento incruento delle fratture di calcagno, Arch. Ortop. **82**:381, 1969.

Essex-Lopresti, P.: The mechanism, reduction technique and results in fractures of the os calcis, Br. J. Surg. **39**:395, 1952.

Gallie, W.E.: Subastragalar arthrodesis in fractures of the os calcis, J. Bone Joint Surg. **25**:731, 1943.

Gellman, M.: Fractures of the anterior process of the calcaneus, J. Bone Joint Surg. **33A**:382, 1951.

Goff, C.W.: Fresh fracture of the os calcis, Arch. Surg. **36**:744, 1938.

Gossett, J.: In Nosny, P., et al., editors: Mobilisation précoce après réduction et contention par broches des fractures du tarse postérieur, Acad. Chir. Mem. **95**:370, 1969.

Hall, M.C., and Pennal, G.F.: Primary subtalar arthrodesis in the treatment of severe fractures of the calcaneum, J. Bone Joint Surg. **42**:336, 1960.

Harris, R.I.: Fractures of the os calcis: treatment by early subtalar arthrodesis, Chin. Orthop. **30:**100, 1963.

Hazlett: J.W.: Open reduction of fractures of the calcaneum, Can. J. Surg. **12:**310, 1969.

Hunt, D.D.: Compression fracture of the anterior articular surface of the calcaneus, J. Bone Joint Surg. **52A:**1637, 1970.

Kiaer, S. and Anthonsen, W.: Fracture of the calcaneus treated with arthrodesis, Acta Chir. Scand. **87**(supp. 76):191, 1942.

Lance, E.M., Carey, E.J., and Wade, P.A.: Fractures of the os calcis: treatment by early mobilization, Clin. Orthop. **30:**76, 1963.

Leonard, M.H.: Treatment of fractures of the os calcis, Arch. Surg. **75:**990, 1957.

Leriche, R.: Ostéosynthèse primitive pour fracture par écrasement du calcanéum à sept fragments, Lyon Chir. **19:**559, 1922.

Lindsay, W.R.N., and Dewar, F.D.: Fractures of the os calcis, Am. J. Surg. **95:**555, 1958.

Maxfield, J.E.: Treatment of calcaneal fractures by open reduction, J. Bone Joint Surg. **45A:**868, 1963.

Maxfield, J.E., and McDermott, F.J.: Experiences with the Palmer open reduction of fractures of the calcaneus, J. Bone Surg. **37A:**99, 1955.

Moberg, E., and Erfors, C.G.: Primär terapi vid grava intraartikulära Kalcaneusfrakturer, Nord. Med. **49:**150, 1953.

Mooney, V.: Avulsion of the epiphysis of the os calcis, J. Bone Joint Surg. **17:**1056, 1935.

Morretti, O., and Piovani, C.: Trattamento ed esiti in 90 osservazioni di fratture del calcagno, Chir. Organi Mov. **56:**441, 1967.

Nosny, P., Bourrel, P., and Caron, J.-J.: Mobilisation précoce après réduction et contention par broches des fractures du tarse postérieur, Acad. Chir. Mem. **95:**365, 1969.

O'Connell, F., Mital, M.A., and Rowe, C.R.: Evaluation of modern management of fractures of the os calcis, Clin. Orthop. **83:**214, 1972.

Palmer, I.: The mechanism and treatment of fractures of the calcaneus. Open reduction with the use of cancellous grafts, J. Bone Joint Surg. **30A:**2, 1948.

Piatt, A.D.: Fracture of the promontory of the calcaneus, Radiology **67:**386, 1956.

Rotheberg, A.S.: Avulsion fracture of the os calcis, J. Bone Joint Surg. **21:**218, 1939.

Rowe, C.R., Sakellarides, H.T., Freeman, P.A., and Sorbie, C.: Fractures of the os calcis; a long-term follow-up study of 146 patients, J.A.M.A. **184:**920, 1963.

Thompson K.R., and Friesen, C.M.: Treatment of comminuted fractures of the calcaneus by primary triple arthrodesis, J. Bone Joint Surg. **41A:**1423, 1959.

Vestad, E.: Fractures of the calcaneum: open reduction and bone grafting, Acta Chir. Scand. **134:**617, 1968.

Warrick, C.K., and Bremner, A.E.: Fractures of the calcaneum: with an atlas illustrating the various types of fracture, J. Bone Joint Surg. **35B:**33, 1953.

Watson-Jones, R.: Fractures and joint injuries, ed. 4,

vol. 2, Baltimore, 1955, The Williams & Wilkins Co.

Widén, A.: Fractures of the calcaneus: a clinical study with special reference to the technique and results of open reduction, Acta Chir. Scand. (supp. 108), 1954.

Wilson, P.D.: Treatment of fractures of the os calcis by arthrodesis of the subastragalar joint, J.A.M.A. **89:**1676, 1927.

Zagra, A., and Bellistri, D.: L'artrodesi sottoastragalica immediata nelle fratture talamiche del calcagno, Minerva Ortop. **21:**574, 1970.

Fractures of the cuboid

Böhler, L.: The treatment of fractures, ed. 5, vol. 3, New York, 1958, Grune & Stratton, Inc.

Conwell, H.E., and Reynolds, F.C.: Key and Conwell's management of fractures, dislocations, and sprains, ed. 7, St. Louis, 1961, The C.V. Mosby Co.

Hermel, M.B., and Gershon-Cohen, J.: The nutcracker fracture of the cuboid by indirect violence, Radiology **60:**850, 1953.

Jackson, W.S.T., and Dickson, D.D.: Fractures and dislocations. In Du Vries, H.L.: Surgery of the foot, ed. 2, St. Louis, 1965, The C.V. Mosby Co.

Watson-Jones, R.: Fractures and joint injuries, ed. 4, vol. 2, Baltimore, 1955, The Williams & Wilkins Co.

Wilson, P.D.: Fractures and dislocations of the tarsal bones, South. Med. J. **26:**833, 1933.

Fractures of the navicular

Böhler, L.: The treatment of fractures, ed 5, vol, 3, New York, 1958, Grune & Stratton, Inc.

Conwell, H.E., and Reynolds, F.C.: Key and Conwell's management of fractures, dislocations, and sprains, ed. 7, St. Louis, 1961, The C.V. Mosby Co.

Crossan, E.T.: Fractures of the tarsal scaphoid and of the os calcis, Surg. Clin. North Am. **10:**1477, 1930.

Day, A.J.: The treatment of injuries to the tarsal navicular, J. Bone Joint Surg. **29:**359, 1947.

De Palma, A.F.: The management of fractures and dislocations: an atlas, Philadelphia, 1959, W.B. Saunders Co.

Dick, I.L.: Impacted fracture-dislocation of the tarsal navicular, Proc. R. Soc. Med. **35:**760, 1942.

Eftekhar, N.M., Lyddon, D.W., and Stevens, J.: An unusual fracture-dislocation of the tarsal navicular, J. Bone Joint Surg. **51A:**577, 1969.

Eichenholtz, S.N., and Levine, D.B.: Fractures of the tarsal navicular bone, Clin. Orthop. **34:**142, 1964.

Finsterer, H.: Ueber Verletzungen im Bereiche de Fusswurzelknochen mit besonderer Berücksichtigung des Os naviculare, Beitr. Klin. Chir. **59:**99, 1908.

Heck, C.V.: Fractures of the bones of the foot (except the talus), Surg. Clin. North Am. **45:**103, 1965.

Henderson, M.S.: Fractures of the bones of the foot—except the os calcis, Surg. Gynecol. Obstet. **64:**454, 1937.

Hoffman, A.: Ueber die isolierte Fraktur des Os naviculare tarsi, Beitr. Klin. Chir. **59:**217, 1908.

Joplin, R.J.: Injuries of the foot. In Cave, E.F., editor:

Fractures and other injuries, Chicago, 1958, Year Book Medical Publishers, Inc.

Lehman, E.P., and Eskeles, I.H.: Fractures of tarsal scaphoid: with notes on the mechanism, J. Bone Joint Surg. **10**:108, 1928.

Morrison, G.M.: Fractures of the bones of the feet, Am. J. Surg. **38**:721, 1937.

Penhallow, D.P.: An unusual fracture-dislocation of the tarsal scaphoid wih dislocation of the cuboid, J. Bone Joint Surg. **19**:517, 1937.

Perriard, M., Dieterlé, J., and Jeannet, E.: Les lésions traumatiques récentes comprises entre les articulations de Chopart et de Lisfranc, incluses, Z. Unfallmed. Berufskr. **63**:318, 1970.

Speed, K.: A text-book of fractures and dislocations covering their pathology, diagnosis and treatment, ed. 4, Philadelphia, 1942, Lea & Febiger.

Waters, C.H., Jr.: Midtarsal fractures and dislocations. In Instructional Course Lectures, American Acadamy of Orthopaedic Surgeons, vol. 9, Ann Arbor, 1952, J.W. Edwards.

Watson-Jones, R.: Fractures and joint injuries, ed. 4, vol. 2, Baltimore, 1955, The Williams & Wilkins Co.

Wilson, P.D.: Fractures and dislocations of the tarsal bones, South. Med. J. **26**:833, 1933.

Fatigue (march, stress) fractures

Morris, J.M., and Blickenstaff, L.D.: Fatigue fractures: a clinical study, Springfield, Ill., 1967, Charles C Thomas, Publisher.

Dislocations of the subtalar joint

Böhler, L.: The treatment of fractures, ed. 5, vol. 3, New York, 1958, Grune & Stratton, Inc.

Leitner, B: Behandlung und Behandlungsergebnisse von 42 frischen Fällen von Luxatio pedis sub talo im Unfallkrankenhaus Wien in den Jahren 1925-1950, Ergeb. Chir. Orthop. **37**:501, 1952.

Leitner, B.: Obstacles to reduction in subtalar dislocations, J. Bone Joint Surg. **36A**:299, 1954.

Soustelle, J., Meyer, P., and Sauvage, Y.: Luxation sous-astragalienne fermée, Lyon Chir. **60**:119, 1964.

von Vogt, H.: Drei seltene Verrenkungsformen im Talusbereich, Schweiz. Med. Wochenschr. **89**:1005, 1959.

Dislocations of the midtarsal (Chopart's) joint

Böhler, L.: The treatment of fractures, ed. 5, vol. 3, New York, 1958, Grune & Stratton.

Boidard, C.A.L.: Contribution à l'étude des luxations astragalo-scaphoidiennes. Thesis, University of Bordeaux, 1939.

Conwell, H.E., and Reynolds, F.C.: Key and Conwell's management of fractures, dislocations, and sprains, ed. 7, St. Louis, 1961, The C.V. Mosby Co.

Dewar, F.P., and Evans, D.C: Occult fracture-subluxation of the midtarsal joint, J. Bone Joint Surg. **50B**:386, 1968.

Gilland, F. A. E.: Les luxations isolées du scaphoide tarsien. Thesis, University of Nancy, 1936.

Watson-Jones, R.: Fractures and joint injuries, ed. 4, vol. 2, Baltimore, 1955, The Williams & Wilkins Co.

Weh, R.: Ueber die isolierte Luxation im Talonaviculargelenk. Thesis, University of Munich, 1939.

Willigens, J. E. F.: Contribution à l'étude de la luxation du scaphoide tarsien. Thesis, University of Nancy, 1936.

Dislocations of the cuboid

Drummond, D.S., and Hastings, D.E.: Total dislocation of the cuboid bone: report of a case, J. Bone Joint Surg. **51B**:716, 1969.

Dislocations of the tarsometatarsal (Lisfranc's) joint

Aitken, A.P., and Poulson, D.: Dislocations of the tarsometatarsal joint, J. Bone Joint Surg. **45A**:246, 1963.

Arenberg, A.A.: Vyvikhi v sustave lisfranka [Dislocation of Lisfanc's joint], Vestn. Khir. **102**:126, 1969.

Ballerio, A.: Un caso raro di lussazione tarso metatarsale isolata, Chir. Organi Mov. **38**:286, 1953.

Cherkes-Zade, D.I.: Pepelomy-vyvikhi v sustave lisfranka [Fracture-dislocation of Lisfranc's joint], Vestn. Khir. **103**:102, 1969.

Collett, H.S., Hood, T.K., and Andrews, R.E.: Tarsometatarsal fracture dislocations, Surg. Gynecol. Obstet. **106**:623, 1958.

del Sel, J.M.: The surgical treatment of tarsometatarsal fracture-dislocations, J. Bone Joint Surg. **37B**:203, 1955.

Detlefsen, M.: Die Luxation im Lisfrancschen Gelenk als typische Verletzung des Montorradfahrers, Beitr. Orthop. Traumatol. **15**:242, 1968.

Fitte, M., and Garacotche, I.: Luxation-fracture de l'articulation de Lisfranc, J. Chir. **56**:367, 1940.

Geckeler, E.O.: Dislocations and fracture-dislocations of the foot: transfixion with Kirschner wires, Surgery **25**:730, 1949.

Gissane, W.: A dangerous type of fracture of the foot, J. Bone Joint Surg. **33B**:535, 1951.

Groulier, P., and Pinaud, J.-C.: Les luxations tarsométatarsiennes (à propos de dix observations), Rev. Chir. Orthop. **56**:303, 1970.

Huet, P., and Lecoeur, P.: Sur 4 cas de luxation tarso-métatarsienne, Acad. Chir. Mem. **72**:124, 1946.

Perriard, M., Deterlé, J., and Jeannet, E.: Les lésions traumatiques récentes comprises entre les articulations de Chopart et de Lisfranc, incluses, Z. Unfallmed. Berufskr. **63**:318, 1970.

Quénu, E., and Küss, G.: Etude sur les luxations du métatarse, Rev. Chir. **39**:1, 1909.

Taussig, G., Hautier, S., and Maschas, A.: Les fractures-luxations de l'articulation de Lisfranc, Ann. Chir. **23**:1131, 1969.

Schiller, M.G., and Ray, R.D.: Isolated dislocation of the medical cuneiform bone—a rare injury of the tarsus, J. Bone Joint Surg. **52A**:1632, 1970.

Tondeur, G.: Un cas de luxation-fracture tarsométatarsienne, Acta Orthop. Belg. **27**:286, 1961.

7

TRAUMATIC INJURIES TO THE SOFT TISSUES OF THE FOOT AND ANKLE

James M. Glick

BURNS, FREEZING, AND FOREIGN BODIES

A comprehensive discussion of burns and freezing is not within the scope of this text; however, because of the high incidence of frostbite of the foot and because burns of the foot from irradiation are not uncommon, at least brief recognition of theses injuries is in order.

Burns

Burns are caused by exposure to intense heat, by contact with strong chemicals or live electricity, or by overexposure to roentgen rays or radium. Burns of the soles of the feet can occur from walking on hot objects without wearing shoes, but today this causation is unlikely. In industries that require the handling of molten materials the danger of burning a foot through a shoe is always present (Fig. 7-1).

London (1953), reporting on 301 burns of the feet, found that more burns occurred as a result of domestic accidents (e.g., during cooking or washing) than as a result of work accidents.

Classification. Artz and Reiss (1957) classified the depth of burns into first, second, and third degrees. This classification is oversim-

plified, but the changes are directly related to the amount of tissue destroyed. First-degree burns may be caused by the sun or by a minor flash and are characterized by erythema and dryness of the skin, usually without blistering. Second-degree burns are caused by flash or hot liquid; mottled redness of the skin occurs, with blistering, moistness, or edema. Third-degree burns, caused by contact with flame or chemicals, may be identified by the charred or pearly-white appearance and dryness of the skin. Unfortunately, it is difficult to determine the depth of a burn on first examination; but this description of the appearance may be helpful.

The first-degree burn involves the outer layer of the epidermis, while in the second-degree burn, generally the whole epidermal layer is affected. London (1953) suggested the use of a sterile safety pin to test for pain sensation in the burned area. Although both first and second-degree burns are painful, the first-degree burn is hyperesthetic to pinprick whereas the second-degree burn is hypesthetic. The third-degree burn acts upon the subcutaneous fat and, in its most severe form, the underlying structures such as neurovascular bundles and bone. The burned part is relatively insensitive to pain and is anesthetic to pinprick.

205

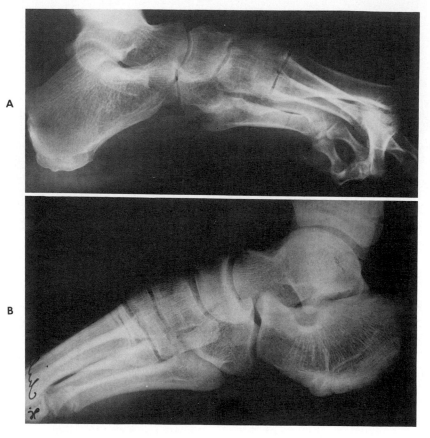

Fig. 7-1. A, Severe plantar contracture of the toes resulting from a third-degree burn. **B,** Destruction of the calcaneal tuberosity by a third-degree burn.

Other agents used to help determine the depth or degree of the burn, which make it possible for the practitioner to devise a more complete treatment plan, are radioactive isotopes (Bennett and Dingman, 1957), fluorescein dye injection (Meyers, 1962) and tetracycline injection, and thermography (Randolph et al., 1964).

Treatment. According to London (1953) adherence to the following principles is important in ensuring the greatest opportunity for recovery: (1) Lost skin must be replaced as soon as possible. Partly destroyed skin that may possibly regenerate must be given the best opportunity to do so, and totally destroyed skin must be replaced as soon as possible by grafting. (2) To facilitate the functional recovery of moving parts, measures should be taken to avoid infection, limit edema, and reduce pain as much as possible. (3) If neces-

sary, reconstructive procedures may be carried out at a later time.

Artz and Reiss (1957) contend that in order to save as much of the foot as possible, it is probably better to wait to debride the eschar on the foot until sequestration has begun. This recommendation contrasts with the advice given for burns of other parts of the body. Artz and Reiss suggest treatment by the exposure method and emphasize that the foot should be immobilized in proper position (i.e., dorsiflexion to prevent possible tendo Achillis contracture).

For chemical burns, Artz and Reiss (1957) recommend washing (not soaking) with water initially. If the burn is from dry lime, however the lime should only be brushed off since lime and water cause a chemical reaction. Attempts to neutralize the chemical agent which caused the burn are not recommended because some neutralizing methods have adverse effects. Baking soda for acid burns and vinegar for alkali burns are two household products that may be used without harm. Areas of the foot having been burned by phosphorus must be protected from the air; after the burn has been washed with water, moist dressings should be applied.

Radiation burns are manifested from 6 months to a year after excessive exposure. They are common on the plantar surface of the foot because of the extensive use of radiotherapy for verrucae plantares. Radiation burns are resistant to all forms of therapy; however, the area should be kept clean and free of all pressures so as to stimulate healing and growth of skin. In many cases grafting of new skin is necessary.

Freezing

Response to cold is individual and variable and therefore unpredictable. Duration and severity of exposure alter the clinical appearance. In general, the area first becomes blanched or white in response to the cold. As exposure continues, the area may become stiff and brittle. Freezing produces local sequelae similar to those of burns. Freezing injuries may be grouped as cryopathies and are classified by two principal environmental factors, wet and cold (Hermann et al., 1963). They are also divided into two categories: frostbite, caused by freezing cold, and immersion foot, caused by a combination of wet and cold. Like burns, freezing injuries have been classified by degree of severity; unlike burns, however, the value of this classification for assessing prognosis and planning care is limited.

Frost injuries are of essentially two types: those resulting from vasomotor disturbance caused by *exposure to cold* and those resulting from pathologic change caused by *actual freezing* of blood vessel walls or of blood. If the skin has been frozen, the following effects are invariably detected: (1) local and active dilatation of the minute vessels, (2) surrounding flush caused by an arteriolar dilatation, and (3) local whealing and blistering of the skin when freezing has been extreme.

Frostbite. Frostbite represents a borderline condition between actual freezing and immersion foot (Bigelow, 1942; Brownrigg, 1943). Frostbite implies superficial freezing; however, Vinson and Schatzki (1954) observed radiographic changes in the bone resulting from frostbite. Edwards and Leeper (1952) analyzed seventy-one cases of frostbite of the extremities. All showed necrosis, the extent of which was in direct relation to the duration of freezing after onset of symptoms. Chronic vasospasm or hyperhidrosis, cold injury, wounds, and possibly smoking were thought to be personal contributing factors.

The residual of severe freezing may be the formidable problem of necrosis and its consequences (Lewis, 1941). Blair et al. (1957) reported studying 100 cases of freezing in which the persistent symptoms were cold feet, numbness, pain, hyperhidrosis, deformed nails, scarring, and mutilation of the terminal phalanges.

Treatment. Lack of understanding of the pathophysiology of frostbite makes it difficult to recommend definitive principles of care. However, two kinds of treatment are necessary: (1) the foot should be rewarmed, and (2) local care should be maintained.

Contrary to the old belief that thawing should be gradual, it is now generally held that rapid warming of the injured part is advisable. The major benefit of rapid warming is a reduction in the total time of cold exposure. The condition of treatment is explicit: the frozen part should be placed in a water bath at a temperature of between 40° C. and 42° C. (104° F. to 107° F.). Harmful effects will occur if the temperature is higher than 42° C., and maximum benefits will not be obtained if the temperature is any lower. Heavy sedation may be necessary during the rewarming period.

In the local care of the frozen foot, strict cleanliness and asepsis must be observed for the first 7 to 10 days. Either the dressing method or the exposure method may be used. The foot should be immobilized in a functional position during the acute phase, but mobilization should be started as early as possible even if the area is gangrenous. Amputation should not be rushed into; as long as there is motion, there is still a chance for revitalization of the part.

Another area of treatment includes measures designed to diminish secondary vascular damage. The effectiveness of these methods, however, has been challenged. Hermann et al. (1963) believe that sympathectomy probably is of no value, at least in the early stages of treatment. Intra-arterial vasodilatation, sympathetic blocking agents (priscoline), and anticoagulants generally have not increased the good results of treatment. These measures may control pain, but most patients require no more than the usual analgesic agents to control the pain of frostbite.

Chilblain (pernio). Repeated mild frostbite produces vasomotor instability resulting in chilblain or pernio. The condition is characterized by recurrent attacks of hyperemia, burning, and tenderness. When the foot is affected, the symptoms generally are manifested over a bony prominence, especially the lateral side of the head of the fifth metatarsal.

Treatment is essentially mechanical and negative—the avoidance of pressure over the part by padding or shoe appliances and the avoidance of further chilling.

Immersion foot. Not until World War II was immersion foot given serious attention (Fausel and Hemphill, 1945). Webster (1942) studied 142 cases of long submersion of the feet in cold water. The limbs had been immobile and constricted by boots. The result was comparable to so-called trench foot and shelter foot and to ordinary frostbite.

The symptoms were increased on removal of the feet from the water. With the rapid swelling that occurred, the feet became red and hyperemic, and the temperature of the parts became extremely elevated, although there was no sweating. The pulses in the vessesls of the feet were strong. There were livid cyanosis, blebs, and extravasation of blood with ecchymosis, vasodilatation, and vascular wall impairment, especially over the medial aspects of the first metatarsophalangeal joint and the longitudinal arch. There were various degrees and patterns of anesthesia, hyperesthesia, and paresthesia.

Treatment. Treatment was by dry cooling and refrigeration, effected by the application of icebags, exposure to a fan, and then slow dry cooling at room temperature while the feet were elevated. Patients were comfortable within a few hours, blebs resorbed without breaking, and the average hospitalization was about a month, although minor symptoms often persisted for up to two years.

Ungley (1943) suggested that massage is contraindicated and that active movements aid circulation, although walking or positions restricting circulation are dangerous. He pointed out that although body warmth is necessary the extremities must be exposed to the air under dry coolness and the feet should be elevated on pillows. Bed rest and nutritional support assist the local condition. Amputation is rarely necessary.

The effects of any form of freezing are poorly understood. Experimental studies such as those of Hermann et al. (1963) show that a profound reduction of blood flow occurs as a result of freezing and that ischemia occurs even though frozen tissues require less oxygen. It has also been shown that in the process of freezing the tissues become opaque; then upon thawing, small blood vessels rupture and edema occurs. Also there is immediate intense vasoconstriction at the junction of the involved with the uninvolved tissues.

The best treatment, of course, is prophylaxis. Subsequent therapy is generally supportive. If one's feet are going to be exposed to cold, one should wear wool socks underneath a snugly fitting windproof and waterproof shoe, which will make use of the insulating properties of still air. Knize et al. (1969), in a study of 163 cases of frostbite, found that some tissue was lost in victims who, while in contact with metal or moisture, were exposed to temperatures of less than $-6.7°$ C for 1 hour or more and that a relationship existed between the duration of exposure and the amount of tissue loss.

Foreign bodies

Foreign bodies may produce acute symptoms or may remain asymptomatic, notwithstanding their presence in the tissues for a long time. Radiographs should be taken to help locate foreign bodies before any surgical attempt is made to remove them. Location of these pieces is usually difficult. In the case of a metallic foreign body, sometimes a rust spot can be observed in the fatty tissue near the foreign body and is helpful in localizing the position of the object.

Brown (1958) described a method to localize a foreign body accurately (Fig. 7-2). In this procedure two needles are inserted at right angles to each other into the area; vertical and horizontal radiographs are then taken. The needles may have to be replaced until their points are located in the exact region of the foreign body. With this method, tissue damage and the effects of surgery are reduced to a minimum.

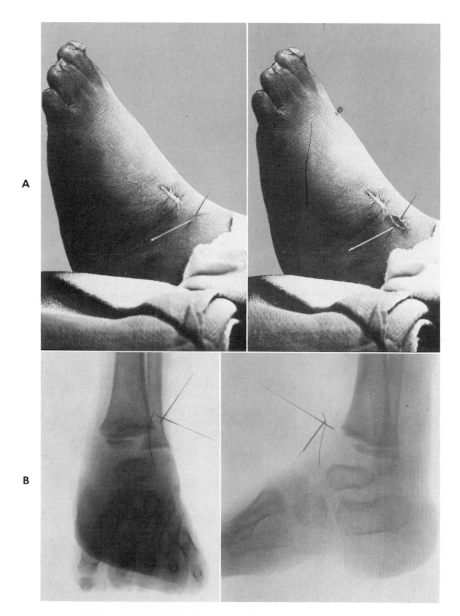

Fig. 7-2. Localization of a foreign body. **A,** Two needles at right angles to each other in the region of the foreign body. Incision made between the two needles. **B,** Biplane radiographs show needles localizing the foreign body.

Needles. Needles are the most common type of foreign body to penetrate the deep structures of the foot (Fig. 7-3). Most patients are seen soon after the accident because of disabling pain; however, asymptomatic cases are often disclosed when patients are being examined for another purpose (Fig. 7-4, A).

The presence of a needle in the tissues sometimes becomes symptomatic after being dormant for years, especially if the needle is embedded in the plantar surface (Fig. 7-4, B). A needle that has been embedded a long time and has not caused symptoms does not call for removal, but a needle that causes pain should be excised. Radiographic location of the needle in the foot should precede operation. A metal detector is helpful in locating the foreign body at operation (Moorhead, 1958). Unless the needle is close to the surface, its removal may be difficult.

Glass. Small pieces of glass occasionally penetrate below the skin and become encapsulated (Fig. 7-5); they remain relatively superficial and are readily excised. Larger fragments may become wedged in an intermetatarsal space; when they are not removed, necrosis may result (Fig. 7-6).

There are two main types of glass (Jennett and Watson, 1958). One is ordinary glass, composed of a soda lime silicate compound, from which windows, mirrors, and bottles are made. The other is lead or barium glass, found in the base of light bulbs, in fluoroscopic screens, and in expensive crystal glass. The former is of relatively low density and is not easily seen on radiographs. The latter is high-density glass and can readily be seen on radiographs. According to Roberts (1958), however, it should be possible to see all glass that is lodged around the foot if proper radiographs are taken.

Exogenous hair. Exogenous hair in the sole of the foot may become painful. While walking barefooted a person may pick up a hair which becomes embedded in the epidermis of the sole of the foot, where it remains invisible and inert. At a later date the hair may set up an acute inflammatory process. Sometimes the area must be probed under magnification until the hair is found. When the area suppurates, the hair may be exuded with the suppurative material.

Gunshot particles. Remaining particles of gunshot (Fig. 7-7) often produce delayed

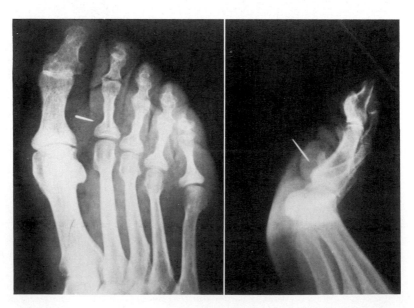

Fig. 7-3. Part of a needle in the foot. Acute symptoms occurred immediately after entrance.

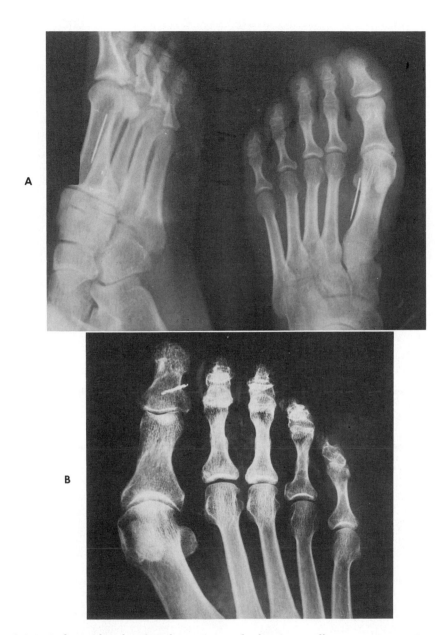

Fig. 7-4. A, Radiographs taken for other purposes disclosing a needle; asymptomatic. **B,** Part of a needle in the great toe. This foreign body, dormant for a long time, suddenly became symptomatic.

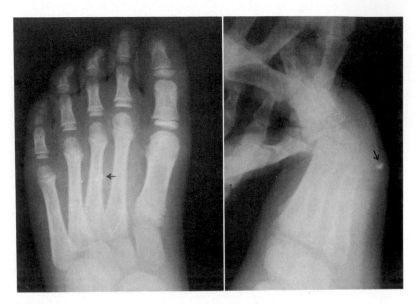

Fig. 7-5. Small piece of glass embedded in the subcutaneous tissue of the plantar surface; painful.

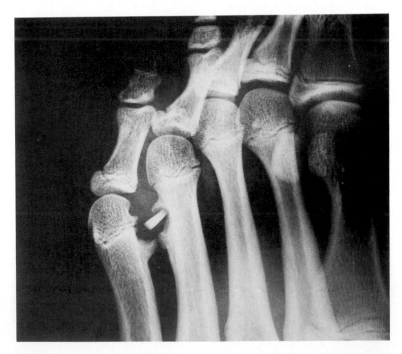

Fig. 7-6. Sharp piece of glass embedded between the fourth and fifth metatarsal heads; extensive osseous proliferation.

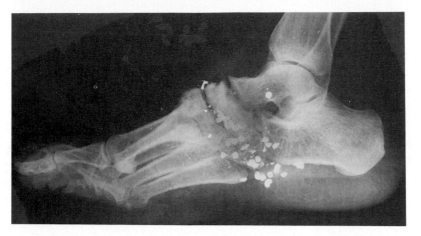

Fig. 7-7. Fragments of gunshot; constant pain in the tarsal joints.

symptoms of varying extensiveness. Only particles that produce pain require excision. Pinpointing the site of the particles in the foot by radiography is always necessary preparatory to excision.

SPRAINS, CONTUSIONS, AND ABRASIONS

A sprain is a wrenched or twisted joint. A strain is a condition of muscles, tendons, or ligaments induced by overuse or stretching in which there is no significant tear.

Sudden injuries of the foot may be grouped as those that occur during violent accidents and those that occur during the normal use of the foot. Sudden injury as the result of an accident includes any degree of crushing, tearing, or breaking of one structure or of a group of structural components of the foot and ankle. Sudden injuries that take place during normal use involve, for the most part, the ligaments. Frequently ligaments are torn from their attachments along with a small fragment of bone. These injuries are termed sprains or chip fractures.

The foot and ankle are more subject to sprains than is any other part of the body. Injuries vary from mild to severe, depending on the force involved, and may best be classified in degrees, as found in the *Standard Nomenclature of Athletic Injuries* (1966). A first-degree sprain is considered a mild injury, a second-degree a moderate one, and a third-

degree a severe injury. The third-degree injury therefore is a complete rupture of the involved ligaments, tendons, or muscles. A sprain of the lateral aspect of the foot and ankle is, by far, the most common.

Anatomy

The distal ends of the tibia and fibula form a mortise which maintains the trochlear surface of the talus and allows for a hinge motion in this joint. The lateral malleolus lies posterior to the medial malleolus, thereby placing the foot in slight external rotation with relation to the tibia. The articular surface of the talus is wider anteriorly. Inman (1976) has shown that the malleolar surfaces of the tibia closely approximate the sides of the talus in all positions from full plantar flexion to full dorsiflexion. Contrary to previous beliefs, there is no appreciable instability when the ankle is in full plantar flexion.

The ligaments about the ankle joint maintain the anatomic mortise. There are three groups of ligaments: (1) medial collateral (deltoid), (2) lateral collateral, and (3) inferior tibiofibular (syndesmosis) (Fig. 7-8).

The medial collateral (deltoid) ligament originates from the medial malleolus and extends anteriorly to attach to most of the medial aspect of the talus and the sustentaculum tali, with some filaments inserting into the navicular.

The lateral collateral ligament is composed

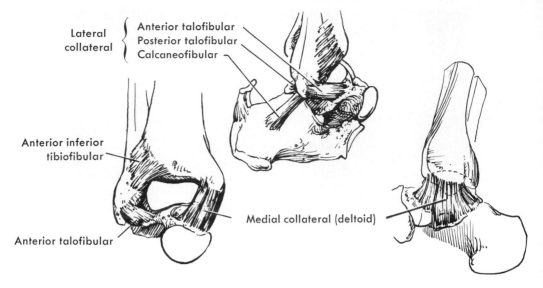

Lateral collateral { Anterior talofibular / Posterior talofibular / Calcaneofibular

Anterior inferior tibiofibular

Anterior talofibular

Medial collateral (deltoid)

Fig. 7-8. Ligaments of the foot: medial collateral (deltoid), lateral collateral, and inferior tibiofibular.

of three separate and distinct fascial bands: the posterior talofibular ligament, the anterior talofibular ligament, and the calcaneofibular ligament.

These are the collateral ligaments commonly affected in an ankle sprain.

According to Broström (1964) the ligament most frequently injured is the anterior talofibular; to be exact, in two thirds of the cases. Next in order of frequency of injury is the combined anterior talofibular and calcaneofibular ligaments, occurring in one fifth of the cases. Other lesions are rare.

Mechanism

Although the foot may assume varying positions of plantar flexion or dorsiflexion at the time a sprain injury is incurred, either inversion or eversion is the principal mechanism initiating the ligamentous injury. Normally the thrust of the body weight in motion is transmitted through the leg to the talus and then through the foot to the supporting surface. When the foot is turned suddenly in extreme inversion or eversion, which may happen during walking or running, the line of force goes through the ankle laterally or medially to the body of the talus. At that moment weight is not transferred through the foot; the line of force escapes through the side of the ankle, thus spraining or lacerating the ligament not capable of absorbing the force.

Kelly (1952) is of the opinion that common ankle injuries are caused by an exaggeration of one basic foot motion, either inversion or eversion. Inversion injuries are the more common ones, however, and can generally be separated into those with only partial disruption of the lateral collateral ligament system and those with complete disruption and associated instability.

The frequent observation that a severe ankle sprain is worse than a fractured ankle may, on occasion, be true if treatment is inadequate. A fracture is readily recognized; therefore appropriate treatment is instituted at once. Sprains are often regarded lightly, except in rare cases with evident ankle dislocation. Collateral ligaments may be ruptured completely in ankle sprains, and there may be an associated separation of the ankle mortise. Such sprains often reduce spontaneously and are often neglected and not treated by complete immobilization or repair of the ligaments. The resulting unstable ankle may require major surgical repair at a later date.

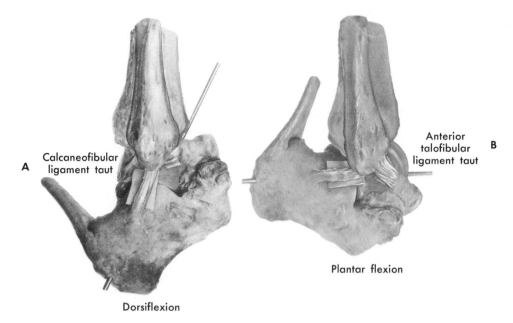

Fig. 7-9. Ligaments on the lateral side of the ankle joint. **A,** Stability of the ankle is maintained by the calcaneofibular ligament. **B,** Stability of the ankle is maintained by the anterior talofibular ligament.

Injuries to the lateral malleolar ligaments

Classification. There are three types of injury to the lateral malleolar ligaments: (1) sprains of the lateral collateral ligaments, (2) avulsion and momentary dislocation of the ankle joint, and (3) recurrent dislocations.

Recovery from simple, or first-degree, sprains is complete in a few weeks; nevertheless, every sprained ankle should be investigated to make certain that the sprain is actually simple. Most ankle injuries are second-degree sprains (moderate) or third-degree sprains (severe). Injury to the ligaments varies from extreme stretching of the collateral ligaments to tearing of the ligaments without complete avulsion. D'Anca (1970) has reported a case of simple rotatory dislocation of the ankle without fracture—a rare injury because of the mechanical efficiency of the mortise and the strength of the ligaments.

Symptoms. Swelling and local tenderness over the tarsal sinus, painful weight bearing, and increased discomfort on forced inversion of the foot comprise the symptoms. Edema and ecchymosis are accompanying manifestations of subdermal bleeding.

Diagnosis. First, the specific injured ligamentous structure must be sought. Usually it can be determined by palpating the three segments of the lateral collateral ligament. The anterior talofibular ligament is the one most commonly injured. Whether the distal tibiofibular ligaments have been injured should also be determined, but this is more difficult because the anterior and posterior talofibular ligaments overlie the tibiofibular ligaments. The area of swelling and discomfort helps indicate which structures are injured; also the amount of swelling and discomfort provides a clue as to the severity of the injury.

In order to make some decision about the stability of the injured ankle as compared with the ankle of the opposite side, the examiner can stress the ankle under radiographic control by inverting the foot while holding it first in equinus and then in dorsiflexion. When the foot is held in dorsiflexion, the calcaneofibular portion maintains the stability of the ankle (Fig. 7-9, A); when it is held in plantar flexion, the anterior talofibular portion of the lateral collateral ligament becomes the stabilizer

(Fig. 7-9, *B*). Some 25% of normal ankles which show no talar tilt in dorsiflexion will show varying degrees (6° to 28°) of talar tilt when stressed in equinus. This is apparently caused by the individual variations in the axis of the subtalar joint (the calcaneofibular ligament must be parallel with this axis in the sagittal plane) and not by the integrity of the ligaments. (See Chapter 1.)

Radiographs are helpful diagnostic tools. (See Chapter 3.) Lateral and AP views as well as views of the ankle internally rotated 30° should be taken. From these radiographs it is possible to see the tibiofibular syndesmosis. On occasion, one can see in the diastasis of the joint a suggestion of complete rupture of the distal tibiofibular ligaments (Fig. 7-10). Radiographs will not distinguish between the stable and the unstable sprain injury unless stress films are taken, which may not be

conclusive unless they are taken while the patient is under anesthesia (Fig. 7-11). The angle made between the dome of the talus and the articular surface of the tibia on these stress films will give the degree of the sprain (Fig. 7-12).

Anderson et al. (1952) stated that a 6° tilt of the talus as seen in a direct AP view (with the ankle in forced inversion) indicates that the anterior talofibular ligament alone is ruptured. Anderson and Lecocq (1954) showed that a 12° to 30° tilt means a combined tear of the anterior talofibular and calcaneofibular ligaments.

It must be kept in mind, however, that stress radiographs should be taken of both ankles, because of the normal variations in the axis of rotation. As stated previously, some normal ankles will demonstrate a significant talar tilt when stressed into inversion. Ber-

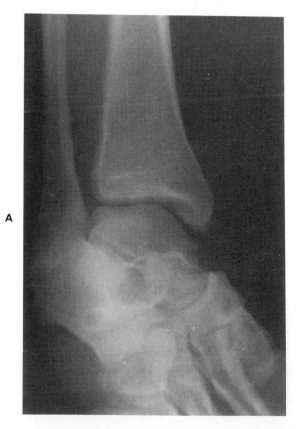

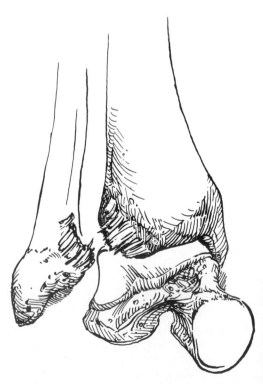

Fig. 7-10. Diastasis of the tibiofibular syndesmosis. **A,** Ankle internally rotated 30°. **B,** Tear of the distal tibiofibular ligaments.

ridge and Bonnin (1944) found that 4% to 5% of uninjured ankles they tested showed laxity of the lateral ligaments; the laxity was usually bilateral and occurred with talar tilt of from 5° to 25°.

From 1969 to 1974 (six seasons) inversion stress radiographs were taken of 396 ankles in 198 intercollegiate football players before they played. Sixty-two of the 396 ankles (16%) showed a significant talar tilt. Ankles which had a preexisting history of injury were included with those which did not, making the percentages significantly higher than the percentages in Berridge and Bonnin's (1944) study. It is interesting to note that the highest percentage of ankle injuries during these six

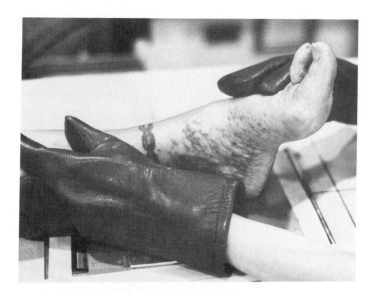

Fig. 7-11. Inversion stress of a tattooed ankle on a cassette for radiography.

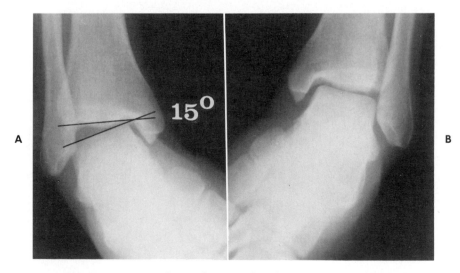

Fig. 7-12. Stress radiographs. **A,** Talar tilt of 15°; **B,** no talar tilt.

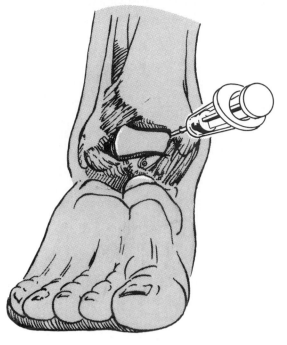

Fig. 7-13. Arthrography of the ankle. Dye is injected on the medial side for an injury to the lateral ligaments.

seasons occurred in the group manifesting a talar tilt of 5° or more (Glick et al., 1976).

Arthrographic studies of the ankle joint may also be made to aid diagnosis (Figs. 7-13 to 7-16). Leakage of the dye through a particular ligament or through the distal tibiofibular syndesmosis will pinpoint the structure torn. Probably the greatest benefit of this procedure is to demonstrate tears of the distal tibiofibular ligaments (Fig. 7-15). Arthrography also aids in determining whether the problem is fresh or old, especially in patients with developmental laxity of the ligaments. Berridge and Bonin (1944), and more recently Percy et al. (1969) and Gordon (1970), have described their methods of arthrography and their findings.

Fordyce and Horn (1972), in a series of patients with recent ligamentous injuries of the ankle, correlated the findings of stress radiographic and arthrographic studies with those of surgical exploration and found that, although arthrography may have been useful to demonstrate injury of the inferior tibiofibu-

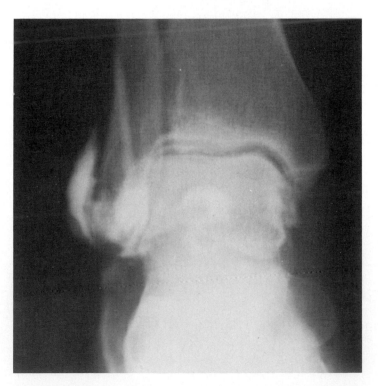

Fig. 7-14. Arthrogram showing a tear of the lateral collateral ligaments.

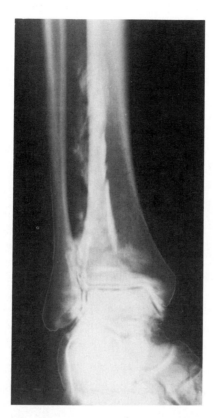

Fig. 7-15. Arthrogram showing a tear of the distal tibiofibular ligament. Note the seepage of dye through the ligament up into the interosseous membrane.

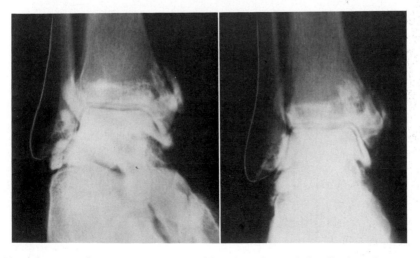

Fig. 7-16. Arthrogram showing extravasation of dye along the medial malleolus. There is a tear in the deltoid ligament.

lar ligaments and of the medial ligament, both radiography and arthrography were unreliable in the diagnosis of injuries to the "lateral ligament" of the ankle.

Broström et al. (1965), however, found arthrography helpful in diagnosing recent lesions of the ankle ligaments and in deciding which of these structures had been torn. The authors observed that escape of contrast media around the tip of and anterior to the lateral malleolus was associated with recent complete ruptures of the anterior talofibular ligament and that leakage into the peroneal tendon sheath was caused by a tear of the calcaneofibular ligament.

Arthrography can be performed as an office procedure. Gordon (1970) offered the following technique: The needle is inserted into the side of the ankle joint opposite the side of the suspected lesion. A 1½-inch needle (22 gauge) is used. Hypaque-50 diluted with an equal amount of sterile saline to make a 25% solution is injected. Five to 10 ml of this diluted

dye is then injected, depending on the amount of resistance the joint gives.

Treatment. The treatment for contusions, sprains, and strains is as follows: (1) cold applications to constrict the arterial beds and reduce subdermal bleeding, (2) compression to arrest active subdermal bleeding, (3) elevation of the injured part to decrease edema, and (4) rest.

Obviously, excessive manipulation of the foot aggravates a recent injury and consequently lengthens the period of disability. Cold applications begin to lose their value after 24 to 48 hours, whereas compression and elevation may be helpful for several days. Cold applications and compression are used guardedly for aged patients or patients with peripheral vascular disease.

Upon removing the compression dressing after 24 to 48 hours, assess the extent of the injury. By palpation and gentle manipulation, ascertain whether there has been a simple stretching or complete avulsion of the liga-

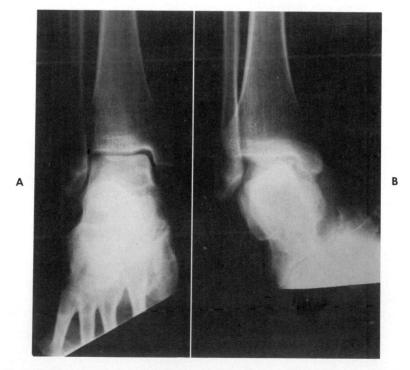

Fig. 7-17. Complete ruptures of the lateral collateral and deltoid ligaments. **A,** No stress applied. **B,** Inversion stress applied showing rupture of the lateral collateral ligaments. **C,** Eversion stress applied showing rupture of the deltoid ligaments.

ments. When the degree of injury is uncertain, radiographs should be taken with the ankle stressed in eversion and inversion to rule out complete rupture of the ligaments (Fig. 7-17). It may be necessary to place the patient under anesthesia to obtain these radiographs. Arthrography, as described, may be of value.

In about 36 hours, if edema is minimal, apply heat rather than cold to dilate peripheral vessels, thus speeding absorption at the site of injury.

In general, when swelling is moderate and complete rupture of the collateral ligament has been ruled out, partial immobilization with adhesive strapping or a firm ankle support, with or without the injection of procaine hydrochloride, permits healing while the patient is ambulatory. The Gibney basket-weave strapping, often used in athletic injuries, is a common method of taping the ankle. It is sometimes fortified with a heel lock. If more swelling is anticipated, the same type of ankle strapping, which leaves the ankle exposed in front, can be applied (Fig. 7-18).

Another excellent support is the Unna boot type of wrap. The Gelocast bandage (Fig. 7-19) is a modification of the Unna wrap and allows for faster drying. Gelocast bandages

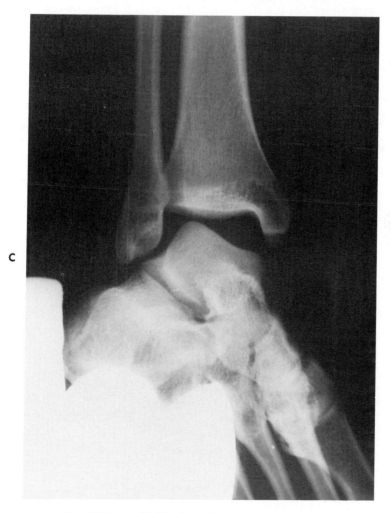

Fig. 7-17, cont'd. For legend see opposite page.

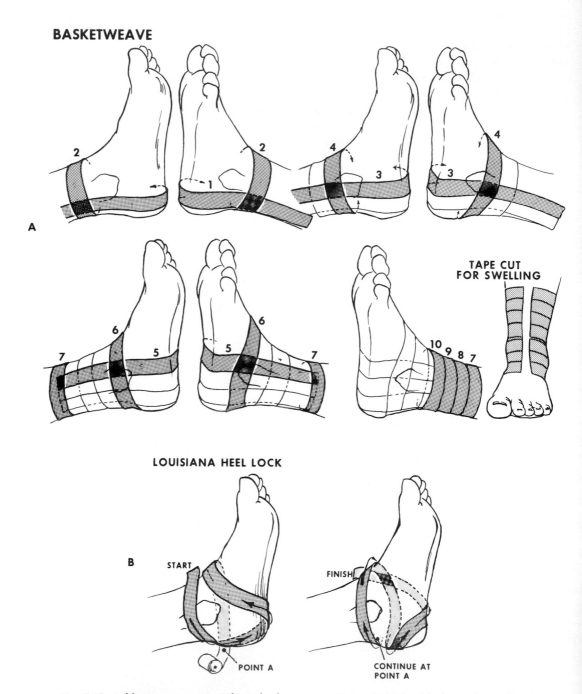

Fig. 7-18. Ankle strappings. **A,** Gibney basket-weave. **B,** Louisiana heel lock; can be applied in conjunction with the basket weave.

give better support than Ace bandages. To ensure even compression and optimal support, they should be applied from the toes to the tibial tubercle (Fig. 7-19, *A*); a few figure-eight turns are made around the ankle (Fig. 7-19, *B*). The bandages can usually be left on for 5 to 7 days, maintaining the same supportive quality throughout. For participants in athletic events, however, better support is given by tape.

The sprain type of injury without complete ligamentous disruption requires only protection from additional injury and seldom requires plaster immobilization. That significant ankle instability rarely follows such common injuries as ankles sprains tends to support the concept that operative repair is seldom necessary.

A plaster cast will assure maximal immobilization and may be used for patients in whom the severity of injury is undetermined or who cannot get along with other forms of immobilization. Some physicians advocate immobilization in a short leg cast for 3 to 6 weeks for inversion injuries with demonstrable tilting of the talus of ± 15° as compared to the opposite side. The use of plaster cast immobilization, however, has met with mixed feelings among physicians who continually treat and follow soft tissue injuries of the ankle.

Infiltration of 5 to 10 ml of 1% procaine hydrochloride has been advocated by many for sprained ankle without avulsion of the ligaments. McMaster (1943) reported 400 cases of sprained ankle in which 200 were treated by injection of procaine hydrochloride alone and 200 were treated by immobilization with adhesive strapping. Treatment by injection of procaine hydrochloride alone uniformly gave better results.

Avulsion of the collateral ligaments

Avulsion of the collateral ligaments is the most severe of all injuries to the lateral side of the ankle. In most instances the collateral ligaments are so completely torn that total lateral instability of the ankle results.

Leonard (1949) experimented with seven cadaver ankles and studied fifty-one sprained ankles. He concluded that the most important component of the collateral group in avulsion is the anterior talofibular ligament. In all

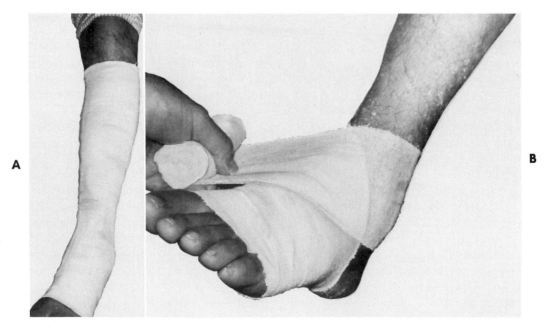

Fig. 7-19. Gelocast bandage. **A,** Completed application from the toes to the tibial tubercle. **B,** Figure-eight wrap around the ankle.

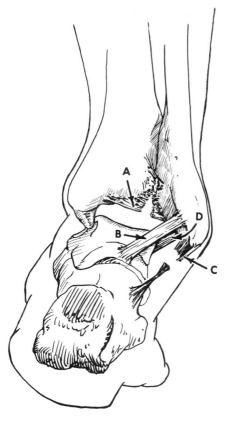

Fig. 7-20. Collateral ligaments. *A*, Torn posterior tibiofibular; *B*, posterior talofibular; *C*, torn calcaneofibular; *D*, anterior talofibular.

probability, the calcaneofibular ligament is equally important (Fig. 7-20).

Treatment. Anderson and Lecocq (1954) showed that ankle instability is greatest when either the calcaneofibular or the posterior tibiofibular ligament is torn with the anterior talofibular ligament. They stated that although a tear of the anterior tibiofibular ligament is a severe injury it may be treated conservatively; but combined tears should be treated surgically. Percy et al. (1969) believed that stress radiographs are unreliable and that an arthrogram is of more value in determining the extent of the injury.

Certainly there is a great deal of controversy—both about which methods provide the earliest and most accurate assessment of the injury and about which methods are proper for treatment. So much divergent thought on the treatment of this injury indicates that results of any form of therapy have been imperfect. Initial therapy as previously described has proved sound; further treatment, however, seems to vary with the whim of the physician.

Freeman (1965a) divided patients with lateral ligament avulsions into groups of three—each group receiving a different type of treatment. The first group were walking as soon as they were comfortable to do so. The second group had their injured ligaments immobilized in plaster casts for 6 weeks. The third group had operative repair with subsequent immobilization of the injured ankle for 6 weeks. The findings showed that maximum ankle stability was gained only by the patients in the third group, who had been treated operatively. Just 25% of these patients had symptom-free ankles after one year, however, whereas in the first group 58% were symptom-free after one year and in the second group, whose injured ligaments were only immobilized, 53% had symptom-free ankles after one year. Further evaluation of this study revealed that patients who were treated without surgery showed no more than 8° of instability on stress radiographs. Patients who were walking early were disabled an average of 12 weeks; those whose injured ligaments were immobilized for 6 weeks were disabled for 22 weeks; and those who had an operative repair followed by plaster casts were disabled for 26 weeks.

In another study Freeman (1965b) noted that the pathologic process which is usually responsible for functional instability of the ankle after a ligament injury is unknown. He and his co-workers postulated, however, that this functional instability, commonly known as giving-way, is caused by a proprioceptive deficit. Freeman therefore suggested a course of coordination exercises, for all types of ankle sprain, designed to control swelling and facilitate recovery of a full range of motion and muscle strength. In the group of patients treated thus, only 7% complained of giving-way whereas 40% reported complaints of giving-way after other forms of treatment. In

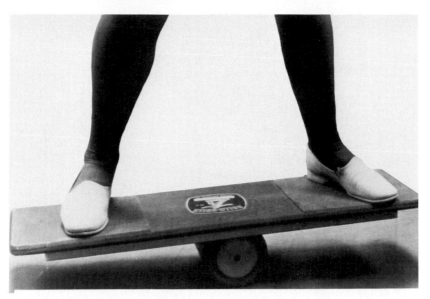

Fig. 7-21. Tilt board.

conclusion, Freeman suggested that the patient perform controlled tilting exercises of the ankle as soon as he is able to stand. At first the patient stands on a board balanced (like a seesaw) on a stable object and tilts the board from side to side. After mastering this exercise, he performs another series of tilting exercises on the board, which is now placed across a spherical object (Fig. 7-21).

Despite Freeman's (1965a,b) most interesting studies, many authors still claim that primary operative repair of ligaments yields the best result with the least disability. Anderson and Lecocq (1954), reporting on twenty-seven cases of repair of the fibular collateral ligaments, observed that many so-called minor ankle sprains are actually complete ruptures of these ligaments and that early surgical repair is paramount. Percy et al. (1969) believed that minor sprain should be treated by early mobilization, partial tear by immobilization, and complete tear by surgical repair. They also suggested that the degree of sprain can be diagnosed properly only with the aid of an arthrogram. Gillespie and Boucher (1971), in a study utilizing the Watson-Jones technique to repair lateral instability of the ankle in twenty patients, showed 80% excellent or good and 20% fair or poor

results. They also stated that the presence of arthritic changes in the ankle preoperatively may contraindicate this procedure.

Isolated posttraumatic lesions of the anterior tibiofibular ligament and of the anterior talofibular portion of the lateral collateral ligament are rare and difficult to diagnose. Disruption of the anterior talofibular ligament as described by Anderson et al. (1952) and by Landeros et al. (1968) may be more common than is generally recognized. This disruption can be demonstrated by the response of anterior subluxation of the talus to passive manipulation of the foot, the same kind of manipulation being used as when attempting to produce the anterior drawer sign at the knee (Fig. 7-22).

Injuries to the medial malleolar ligaments

The discussion thus far has been entirely about lateral collateral ligament sprain, which is indeed appropriate since it is the most common type of ankle sprain. Injuries to the medial collateral (or deltoid) ligament do not occur often; but when they do, they are generally caused by sudden eversion of the foot, subjecting the medial collateral ligament to an extreme abduction stress. Rupture of the medial collateral ligament is a rare entity as an

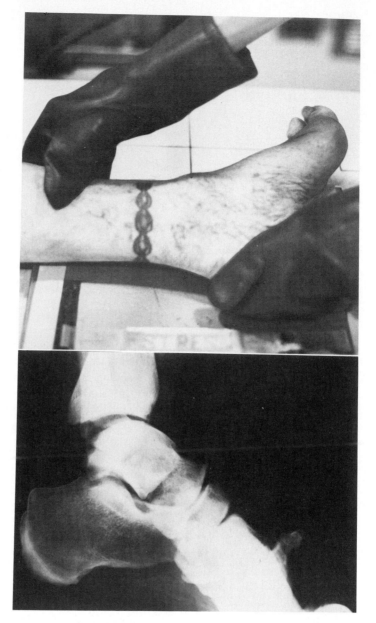

Fig. 7-22. Disruption of the anterior talofibular ligament. **A,** Anterior stress on a tattooed ankle. **B,** Anterior instability of the ankle. Note the anterior subluxation of the talus.

isolated lesion but frequently accompanies the bimalleolar type of fracture-dislocation of the ankle.

When rupture of the deltoid ligament occurs without a fracture of the lateral side of the ankle, a tear of the distal tibiofibular liga-ment complex must be suspected. This is not an unusual combination (Fig. 7-23).

Conservative treatment. Most sprains of the medial collateral ligament, even if the distal tibiofibular ligaments are torn, can be treated by adhesive or Unna boot wraps as in

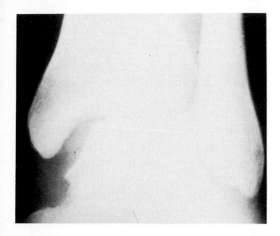

Fig. 7-23. An eversion stress radiograph shows spreading of the medial side of the ankle mortise and the distal tibiofibular syndesmosis, suggesting tears of the respective ligaments.

injuries to the lateral collateral ligaments. Similarly, plaster immobilization is debatable but is used mainly for patients who cannot tolerate the various wraps and require support.

The shape and form of the deltoid ligament allow for maintenance of apposition of the torn ends; therefore operative repair is seldom necessary. Dziob (1956) suggested that in the treatment of medial avulsion of the ankle, when the tilt of the talus in inversion under stress radiography is less than 15°, plaster immobilization of the foot and leg for 6 to 8 weeks is adequate; however, when greater then 15°, the torn ligaments must be sutured. (For surgical treatment, see Chapter 19.) Bonnin (1965), in an editorial, stated that rupture of the deltoid ligament "can safely be left to itself in most cases."

My criteria for surgery are when injuries involving the deltoid ligament are irreducible due to interposition or combined ruptures of the deltoid and distal tibiofibular ligaments.

Recurrent sprained ankles

"Recurrent dislocation of the ankle," "weak ankles," and "chronic sprains" are terms loosely applied to injured ankle ligaments. Recurrent episodes of overstretching and spraining of ankle ligaments ultimately leave the ligaments completely stretched or torn. The condition may be caused by sudden avulsion of the collateral ligaments with spontaneous reduction of the talus dislocation, which, if not properly treated, results in an unstable ankle. A sprained ankle may and often does lead to permanent disability (Bonnin, 1944).

In a report of fifty-seven cases of injury to the ankle without bony changes, Hughes (1942) recorded some lateral tilting of the ankle in about half the cases when radiographs were made with the ankle held in forced inversion. Bosien et al. (1955) followed 133 cases of ankle sprain for an average of 27 months. Among their patients 36% had had previous injury to the same ankle and 33% had had continuous residual ankle symptoms. Broström (1966a,b) related significant residual symptoms in 20% of 186 patients treated by nonsurgical methods and in only 3% of ninety-five patients treated by primary surgical repair.

Repeated twisting or giving-way of the ankle is typical, especially when the patient walks on irregular ground or wears heels worn down on the outer posterior surface. Among women, recurrent ankle sprain often results from previous injuries to the ankle coupled with the wearing of high-heeled shoes.

Supportive treatment. A good supportive shoe in addition to an elastic ankle support in some cases stabilizes the ankle sufficiently to prevent further sprains. Some patients are helped by a short leg brace with a lateral T-strap to prevent inversion. If this supportive treatment does not alleviate the problem, a reconstruction procedure may be necessary. (For surgical treatment, see Chapter 19.)

Forefoot sprain or sprain of the calcaneocuboid joint

This injury is a type of inversion sprain that involves a portion of the ligaments overlying the calcaneocuboid joint (Fig. 7-24). It causes immediate severe disability with pain, swelling, and tenderness localized to the region of the calcaneocuboid joint. Restriction of weight bearing for 48 hours usually brings enough relief to the injured patient so he can

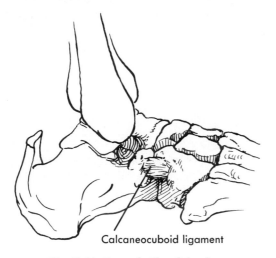

Calcaneocuboid ligament

Fig. 7-24. Lateral side of the foot.

begin to walk; thereafter, progressive healing continues to occur. On resumption of weight bearing, an Ace bandage wrap, tape strapping, or Gelocast should be worn. Any of these will provide sufficient support to the injured part and can probably be removed within a week.

Sprains of the first metatarsophalangeal joint and plantar fascia

First metatarsophalangeal joint. The first metatarsophalangeal joint is sometimes sprained by stubbing the toe or by extreme dorsiflexion. Swelling over the joint and pain on motion are symptomatic. Such sprains are, for the most part, simple sprains and respond to partial immobilization with adhesive tape and the wearing of a rigid-soled shoe.

Plantar fascia. The plantar fascia may be sprained by jumping, especially from heights. The sprain may be anywhere along the length of the fascia but is seen most often at its origin. Sprains of the plantar fascia respond to strapping and the wearing of a shoe with a rigid shank and a longitudinal arch support.

Contusions and abrasions

Treatment. These injuries are best treated by ice, local compression, elevation, and protective padding when the patient begins to ambulate.

ATHLETIC INJURIES
Differentiation

Athletic injuries in many respects are different from the usual injuries seen in clinical practice; thus their treatment deserves special consideration.

The patient is young and active, and the purpose of medical attention is not only to treat the injury so it heals properly but also to treat it in such a way that the patient can return to competition as quickly as possible.

The majority of athletic injuries are relatively minor ones such as mild sprains, strains, or contusions. Although people of other occupations with mild sprains, strains, or contusions probably can discharge their work and social responsibilities while they limp about, athletes cannot. For example, a mild ankle strain prevents a football player from cutting effectively but may be essentially asymptomatic while he is walking. Thus, even though these injuries are less serious than fractures and dislocations, they tax the acumen and judgment of the physician associated with athletic medicine.

Sites of injury. The foot and ankle are commonly traumatized during athletics; a sprained ankle is always a threat in sports such as baseball, football, and hockey. Thorndike (1962), in an analysis of athletic injuries on the Harvard football team for fifteen years, found 585 ankle sprains and 15 fractured ankles. Glick and Katch (1970), in a study in which 120 joggers were observed over an 11-week period, reported that of the 241 injuries occurring, twenty were ankle sprains and forty-three were other problems of the foot consisting of blisters, arch strains, sore heels, heel bursitides, toenail injuries, bruises, metatarsalgias, and corns.

Preventive treatment is essential. Athletes who are exposed to violent twisting of the ankle should have their ankles strapped with adhesive tape to limit inversion and eversion. A nonelastic ankle support may also be worn during games. This applies especially to athletes who have had recurrent ankle sprains. For protection of the forefoot, shoes should have rigid or metal toe boxing and firm soles.

Treatment. Treatment for specific injuries

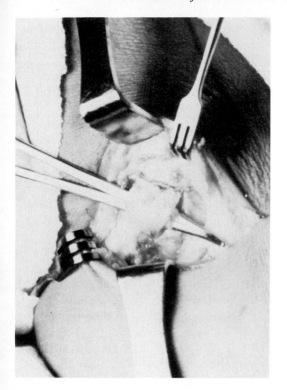

Fig. 7-25. Torn intact anterior talofibular ligament one year after injury. This was easily reattached to the lateral malleolus with sutures through drill holes. No other reinforcement procedure was used. The final result was a stable ankle.

is discussed under appropriate headings elsewhere in this book.

Most soft tissue injuries of the foot and ankle should initially be treated by the application of ice and a compression bandage; the foot should be elevated and weight bearing should be restricted. Following this treatment, graduated rehabilitative measures should be commenced under close supervision of the physician. Jogging can usually be started as soon as the athlete is comfortable enough to walk without a limp. Jogging usually should then progress to running and then to running in circles or in tight figure-eights before the athlete is allowed to participate in a particular sport. If in the progression of these activities swelling of the part or increased pain occurs, progress should be terminated and the athlete should return to one of the earlier activities mentioned.

Hirata (1968) stressed the advantages of performing these rehabilitative measures right on the playing field during practice session. He also emphasized the importance of frequent examination for signs of increased swelling and pain.

My contention is that if the ankle sprain treated conservatively in athletes does not improve in a week or two serious consideration of a surgical repair in the manner of Broström (1966a,b) should be made. I have been able to confirm Broström's findings that a good repairable ligament remains many months and even years after a complete rupture (Fig. 7-25).

Raising or lowering the heel counters of the shoe is effective in treating heel bursitis. Achilles tendinitis is best treated by elevating the heel with a ¼-to-½-inch pad. Either wearing thicker socks or placing petroleum jelly on top of and between toes seems to yield the best results for the athlete with toe blisters. Dancers frequently wrap tape around their blistered toes and do not remove the tape until it falls off by itself. For the athlete who has a contused foot, taping the protective pad over the outside of the shoe is the easiest method of application. Sprains of the first metatarsophalangeal joint will probably incapacitate the athlete for 3 weeks. He may be able to walk without pain in 1 week; but when he starts to run, more stress will be placed on this joint and the condition will be reactivated. Therefore, if the athlete with a sprain of the first metatarsophalangeal joint is allowed to return to competition too early a longer period of disability will probably ensue.

TRAUMATIC INJURIES TO THE TENDONS OF THE FOOT AND ANKLE

In general, traumatic rupture of the tendons about the foot and ankle is rare except for rupture of the tendo Achillis. Traumatic tenosynovitis and peritendinitis occur more often but are usually more difficult to treat. Tenosynovitis is inflammation of a tendon sheath; peritendinitis is inflammation of a tendon that possesses no sheath. All the tendons across the foot and ankle, except the tendo Achillis, have sheaths.

Traumatic tenosynovitis or peritendinitis

Process, symptoms, and treatment. Lipscomb (1950) stated that the tendons of human beings will not tolerate over 1,500 to 2,000 manipulations per hour. Acceleration of the speed of physical work, prolonged exertion, or extraordinary activity (e.g., the sudden playing of three sets of tennis by a person who is usually sedentary) may cause the trauma which initiates this condition. Lipscomb (1950) also showed that the pathologic process of tenosynovitis and peritendinitis is one of either acute inflammation or chronic fibrosis. The symptom is predominantly neuritic pain; the signs are localized heat, redness, and tenderness or pain when the specific tendon is moved.

These conditions may be acute or chronic. If the patient is seen early enough, treatment should include the application of ice, elevation of the foot, and rest. After the first 24 to 48 hours, diathermic or infrared heat may be applied. Rest, frequently best accomplished by plaster immobilization, is the most effective form of treatment. In mild cases adhesive strappings or Gelocast wraps suffice. Local steroid injections will frequently relieve acute symptoms in a short period of time but should not be expected to heal the lesion more quickly. Repeated steroid injections, in fact, should be performed cautiously, for they may weaken the tendon and produce spontaneous rupture.

Severe cases and cases of repeated traumatic tenosynovitis or peritendinitis may produce a great deal of scarification and may freeze the tendon so it requires extensive repair, including the formation of a new gliding mechanism. Therefore, in the more severe cases of tenosynovitis, surgical excision of the inflamed tissues in which the tendon glides may be the most conservative form of treatment.

Injuries caused by improper footwear generally involve the extensor hallucis longus tendon or the tendo Achillis. The extensor hallucis longus is most prominent over the dorsum of the forefoot. This is why it is often impinged upon by the margins of the vamps of pumps. Sometimes a protective fibroma of the skin and subcutaneous tissue forms just behind the first metatarsal head and may cause recurrent infection and formation of a draining sinus in its center. The entire mass of scar must be excised, and at times the gliding mechanism must be repaired.

A comparable condition is observed just above the insertion of the tendo Achillis, a condition that also results from friction and pressure—in this instance of the shoe counter. The condition is commonly known as "pump bump" because it is frequently seen in women who wear high-heeled shoes (Fig. 7-26). Moreover, the fad of laceless shoes and loafers (shoes which must fit closely in the area of the long axis of the foot) has caused an alarming increase of pump bumps. Although it is anatomically related to the apophysis of the calcaneus, a pump bump is reactive membranous bone formation that becomes an exostosis. (See Fig. 8-50.) A common anatomic variation of the calcaneus is a tuberous prominence; perhaps this variation of the normal heel predisposes to the formation of such exostoses.

A locally inflamed heel at the posterosuperior surface of the calcaneus lateral or medial to the tendo Achillis is a symptom of pump bump. The presence of the disorder, which occurs predominantly in adolescent and young adult females, is confirmed radiographically. It is best treated conservatively. The wearing of sandals or larger, laced, shoes has been effective in promoting quiescence. At times an adventitial bursa will develop over the exostosis and will respond to local antiinflammatory treatment. In very select cases, excision may be considered if symptoms persist. Brahms (1967) pointed out that if the mass occurs in the midline it is apt to be a rheumatoid nodule instead of a pump bump, which usually occurs laterally.

Keck and Kelly (1965) reported on a series of eighteen patients operated upon for symptomatic bursitis of the posterior part of the heel. They found that the posterosuperior border of the calcaneus was prominent in patients with this condition. Two surgical procedures were used. The first involved resection of the superior prominence of the

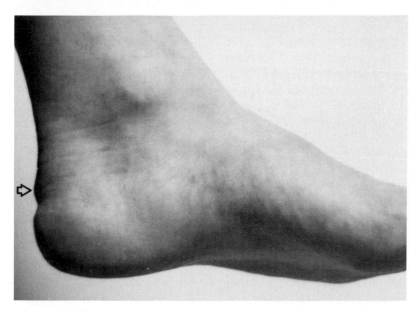

Fig. 7-26. "Pump bump."

calcaneal tuberosity with removal of the bursa, and the second consisted of a wedge osteotomy of the calcaneus with removal of a dorsally based wedge. Better results were achieved from the first operation, but a true statistical analysis could not be made because too few of the second operation were performed. Dickinson et al. (1966) reported good results from excision of the posterosuperior prominence of the calcaneus in twenty-one patients. They stressed, however, that only a small number of patients with this condition required surgical treatment; most had few or no symptoms, and those with symptoms were relieved by conservative measures.

Hemorrhagic tenosynovitis. Hemorrhagic tenosynovitis is an infrequent complication of an injury to a tendon. A direct blow to the tendon or an excessive strain of the tendon may break the endothelial lining of the tendon sheath, causing hemorrhage into the sheath, from which the blood cannnot escape and therefore clots. The blood clots assume the character of a foreign body, thereby becoming an irritant and often producing muscle spasm. This accounts for the continuous pain, even when the limb is at rest. The irritation tends to induce an increase in the production of syno-

vial fluid in the sheath, causing fluctuation over the area.

Acute pain and swelling over the injured tendon begin from 24 to 48 hours after trauma. Pain becomes worse and cannot be relieved; rest or change in position of the limb does not modify the symptoms. The area over the tendon is swollen, fluctuant, and tender to touch. The condition is differentiated from a pyogenic tenosynovitis by its rapid onset of symptoms after injury, the absence of signs of infection, and persistent acute pain over the injured tendon. These symptoms are incompatible with simple injuries to a tendon.

Exquisite pain and fluctuation pinpoint the site of the hematoma, which must be excised through an incision in the tendon sheath. Only rarely is the clot absorbed without excision.

Injuries to specific tendons

Lapidus and Seidenstein (1950) reported three cases of chronic nonspecific tenosynovitis. Two involved the tibialis posterior, and one the flexor hallucis longus, tendon. In all cases pain was intermittent. In the case involving the flexor hallucis longus, the condition had remained unrecognized for several months. In the cases involving the tibialis posterior, recognition did not occur until after one and three years, respectively. Treatment consisted of opening the tendon sheath to evacuate excess fluid and excising the thickened portion of the sheath.

In a study of tendon problems of the foot done at the Mayo Clinic, Lipscomb (1950) found tenosynovitis of the anterior tibial tendon in 24%, peritendinitis of the tendo Achillis in 20%, and tenosynovitis of the posterior tibial and peroneal tendons in 16% of cases. Tenosynovitis of the anterior tibial tendon was often associated with involvement of the extensor digitorum communis and was frequently caused by irritation from shoes or boots. Although in some cases the synovial sheath in front of the ankle had to be excised, for the most part tenosynovitis of these tendons responded to conservative treatment. Peritendinitis of the tendo Achillis was more difficult to treat. Because this condition was usually caused by irritation of the shoe counter or by unusually prolonged ambulation, the most successful treatment consisted of removal of the shoe counter, followed by heel elevation and rest. Tenosynovitis of the posterior tibial tendon and tenosynovitis of the peroneal tendon were often associated with static deformities of the foot. One case was reported in which the posterior tibial and flexor digitorum communis occupied the same tendon sheath. For the treatment of this condition Lipscomb (1950) suggested shoe correction, contrast baths, foot exercise, and radiotherapy.

Ghormley and Spear (1953) reviewed twenty-one cases of tenosynovitis of the tibialis posterior diagnosed and treated at the Mayo Clinic between 1935 and 1951. Eleven of these cases were the result of anomalies of the tibialis posterior with accessory tendons, which were excised at the time of operation. The remaining ten patients were treated conservatively with radiotherapy and strapping.

Williams (1963) reported on fifty-two patients with chronic tenosynovitis of the tibialis posterior tendon. The changes were regarded as nonspecific, with the exception of one case that showed associated manifestations of rheumatoid arthritis. Twelve patients in whom conservative treatment had failed were treated by surgical release of the tendon sheath, with complete relief resulting in eleven patients.

Cohen and Reid (1935) reported seven cases of tenosynovitis crepitans associated with oxaluria. Parvin and Ford (1956) reported two cases of stenosing tenosynovitis of the common peroneal tendon sheath, and Gunn (1959) reported a similar case. Pain in the area behind the lateral malleolus was produced by forced inversion as well as eversion of the foot. Tenderness and swelling overlying the peroneal tendons were relieved by surgical release of the thickened inferior retinaculum below the edge of the lateral malleolus (Fig. 7-27).

Compression of the posterior tibial nerve at the level of the medial malleolus (tarsal tunnel syndrome) should be considered in painful conditions of the foot. This problem is discussed in Chapter 15.

Traumatic subcutaneous rupture of tendons

In a review of twenty patients with traumatic subcutaneous ruptures of tendons, Griffiths (1965) found most of the ruptures to be associated with open wounds. In his experience the extensor hallucis longus repaired itself spontaneously. In one adult patient who had late repair of the posterior tibial tendon and in one who had late repair of the anterior tibial tendon, Griffiths found no functional impairment. He observed that after successful and early repair, complete functional recovery can generally be expected in adults. However, because of the plastic nature of the foot during childhood, late repair of these tendons causes deformity in children.

The two most commonly reported tendon ruptures of the foot are of the tibialis anterior and the tendo Achillis.

Rupture of anterior tibial tendon. Els (1910) was one of the first to report a rupture of the tibialis anterior tendon. Burman (1934) was first to report such a case in America. Lapidus (1941) reported two cases. Menso

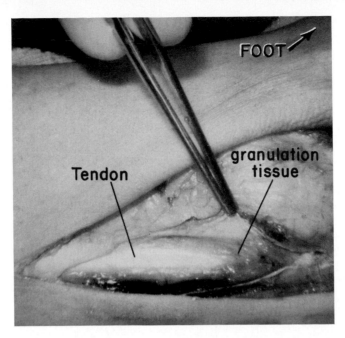

Fig. 7-27. Tenosynovitis of the peroneal tendon below the edge of the lateral malleolus. Note the granulation tissue overlying the tendon. The retinaculum has already been cut.

and Ordway (1953) reported two cases and reviewed the published reports, of which only ten had appeared up to that time. Lipscomb and Kelly (1955) reported twelve cases of injuries to the extensor tendons of the foot treated at the Mayo Clinic between 1938 and 1952; in nine of the cases the tibialis anterior tendon was involved.

Trauma causing avulsion may be powerful or mild. Usually it is a fall or twisting of the ankle, especailly when extreme plantar flexion is exerted. Sometimes the same area has been previously injured, probably with residual fraying of the terminal end of the tendon, predisposing to complete rupture.

Symptoms of a ruptured tibialis anterior tendon are sudden sharp pain and swelling over the first cuneiform, accompanied by an inability to coordinate normal foot motion. Dorsiflexion of the foot may be difficult and there may be a tendency to stub the toes. A few days after injury, extensive ecchymosis may occur over the insertion of the tendon. On palpation, a rupture defect is observed in the tendon channel at the terminal end of the tibialis anterior. When edema subsides, the defect may become visible. The terminal end of the ruptured tendon feels like a bulbous mass.

Recommended treatment. To repair a ruptured tibialis anterior, perform the following steps:

1. Make an incision over the tibialis anterior just above the transverse crural ligament.

2. Make a second incision over the insertion of the tibialis anterior.

3. Pull out the tibialis anterior through the first incision and thread a stainless steel wire through the tendon from above downward. At the proximal end of the wire, loop a pullout wire.

4. Replace the wired tendon in its original tunnel.

5. Suture the frayed ends of the tendon to each other and to the periosteum and cortex of the first cuneiform.

6. Pass the stainless steel wires through the plantar skin surface by means of Keith needles and tie them over a button (Fig. 7-28). Bunnell (1964) may be credited with being the first to use the button innovation. Apply a

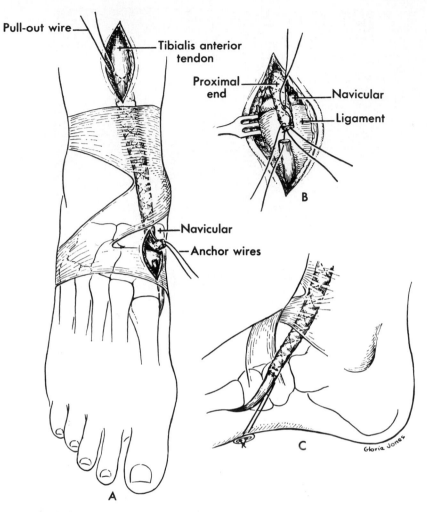

Fig. 7-28. Repair of a ruptured anterior tibial tendon. **A,** Incision over the tendon just above the transverse crural ligament. Second incision over the insertion of the tibialis anterior. The tendon is pulled out through the first incision. Stainless steel wire is threaded through the tendon from above downward. At the proximal end a pullout wire is looped under the wire and the tendon is guided through its original channel. **B,** Fragmented ends sutured to each other. **C,** Both ends of the stainless steel wire are passed through the plantar surface by a Keith needle and tied over a button.

boot cast for 6 weeks. After its removal, cut the wire at the bottom; the pullout wire permits extraction of the wire.

Rupture of tendo Achillis. Fresh rupture of the calcaneal tendon is most often seen in men in their fifth decade.

In a review of fifty-six cases Hooker (1963) noted the incidence of this entity in men with sedentary occupations who indulged occasionally in strenuous sports. The acute tendon rupture occurred significantly more often in the left leg than in the right leg. Histologic degeneration was evident in only some cases. Hooker's suggestion was that there were three main causes of rupture: (1) sudden extra strain on a taut tendon, (2) sudden passive stretching of a relaxed tendon into dorsiflexion, and (3) a direct blow over a taut tendon. Since pain is not always a constant factor, rupture is often unnoticed. There may or may

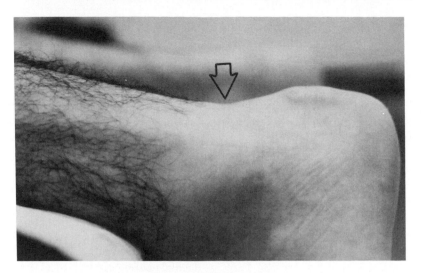

Fig. 7-29. Rupture of the tendo Achillis. Note the palpable gap.

not be a palpable gap and obvious impairment of plantar flexion in acute tendon rupture (Fig. 7-29).

Avulsion of the tendo Achillis is seen frequently, even in the young. This is because of the unfavorable leverage of a long forefoot and a short posterior lever (Milgram, 1953). Rupture of the tendo Achillis at its musculotendinous junction is seen more often in young persons, with the tendon fibers usually torn into irregular longitudinal strips near this junction.

Lea and Smith (1968) reported satisfactory results in eight patients treated nonsurgically. Their method consisted of a walking boot cast with the foot in gravity equinus position (without plantar flexion force) for 8 weeks, then crutches and a 2.5 cm elevated heel for 4 weeks.

Treatment. Many surgical methods have been recorded for repair of the tendo Achillis. None have given perfect results; even after solid repair, residual weakness remains and adhesions often occur.

There is still debate regarding operative and nonoperative methods of treating the ruptured tendo Achillis. Ingles et al. (1976) have compared the two methods of treatment in healthy athletic individuals and found a better return of power and endurance in patients treated surgically than in those treated by the equinus cast technique. The surgical patients were also more satisfied with the results. Nine reruptures occurred in the thirty-one nonoperated patients and none in the forty-eight who were treated operatively. Lea and Smith (1972) reported seven reruptures in sixty-six patients treated nonoperatively. They believed that these seven reruptures occurred because immobilization was not long enough. It appears that young athletic people gain a more satisfactory result from an operative repair.

Rupture of posterior tibial tendon. Spontaneous disruption of the posterior tibial tendon is an uncommon occurrence. Only a few cases have been recorded in the literature. Kettelkamp and Alexander (1969) reported four cases, three which were preceded by tenosynovitis.

The posterior tibial tendon courses behind the medial malleolus and inserts on the plantar surface of the tarsal navicular bone. It helps maintain the arch. When it ruptures or stretches, progressive loss of the longitudinal arch may occur. A flatfoot deformity with pain and tenderness along the course of the posterior tibial tendon should alert the examiner that the tendon is inefficient and probably torn.

Operative treatment is indicated for a ruptured posterior tibial tendon. Goldner et al. (1974) have described the transference of the flexor hallucis longus for ruptures that cannot be repaired primarily.

Rupture of peroneus longus tendon. Traumatic subcutaneous rupture of the peroneus longus is a rare condition caused by a sharp inversion force to the foot and ankle while the muscle is contracted. It may mimic an injury to the lateral collateral ligament; the tenderness and swelling are at the same location, in the area of the lateral malleolus.

Griffiths (1965) reported four cases of nonspontaneous rupture of the peroneal tendon, all caused by lacerations. Three of the four ruptures occurred in children, and only one of these was repaired immediately. The two that were repaired late yielded unsatisfactory results consisting of supination deformities of the foot and failure of the first metatarsal to reach the ground during standing. The rupture in the adult was repaired immediately, with satisfactory results. In the same article Griffiths reported a case of spontaneous rupture of the tibialis posterior tendon in an adult which healed satisfactorily although never repaired.

There are few reports on the results of these ruptures in adults. The implication is that the condition should be repaired reasonably soon after the diagnosis is made. If the tendon is not repaired in an adult, the patient may be left with an unbalanced foot and may be unable to place the first metatarsal firmly on the ground prior to lift-off, which would increase the pressure on the lateral border of the foot and lead to plantar callosities along the lateral metatarsals and to metatarsalgia.

To avoid a deformed foot in children with rupture of the peroneus longus tendon, it is mandatory that immediate repair be performed.

Tendon subluxations

Tendon subluxations are a slipping of a tendon from its natural groove. They are usually associated with congenital malformations and deformities; however, they may result from injury, arthritis, or malunited fractures. The most symptomatic tendon subluxations of the foot are of the peroneus longus.

Subluxations of the peroneus longus, characterized by recurrent episodes of sudden slipping of the tendon during walking, are caused by a poorly formed groove on the posterior surface of the lateral malleolus which permits the tendon to slip over it. This slipping often makes the patient fall because the peroneus longus goes immediately into spasm, thereby abducting and plantar flexing the foot. The condition can usually be reduced manually, but the attacks tend to recur with increasing frequency because the lateral fibulocalcaneal ligament is stretched further with each episode.

Treatment. At first occurrence the deformity is reduced and the foot immobilized for 5 to 8 weeks in a plaster cast. There are often no more recurrences. If there are recurrences, surgical intervention may be indicated (p. 540).

MISCELLANEOUS SOFT TISSUE INJURIES OF THE FOOT

The purpose of this section of the chapter is to discuss soft tissue injuries of the foot that have not been classified under previous headings and to investigate conditions which are not a direct response to trauma but may be associated with or be a sequela of trauma.

Crush injuries to the foot

A patient may complain of foot pain following an accident in which a heavy object landed on his foot although there is no outward evidence of injury and radiographs show no fracture. In this case a soft compression bandage should be applied and the foot should be elevated. Skin sloughing is to be expected (Fig. 7-30).

Late sequelae of crush injuries include pain and stiffness, which in turn may be a result of sympathetic dystrophy and soft tissue contractures. Curtiss (1966) described hematoma formation in the subfascial space on the dorsum of the foot obstructing venous flow from the distal forefoot. This may lead to the necessity of splitting cruciate and transverse

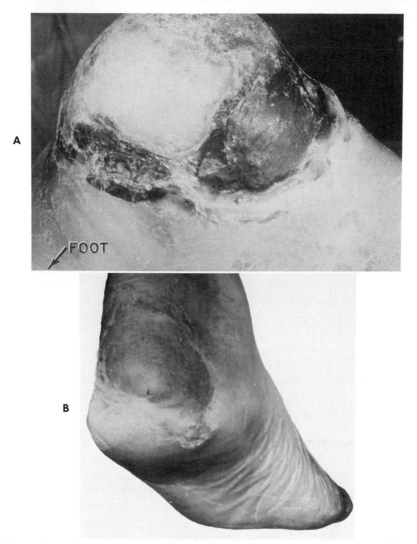

Fig. 7-30. A, Crush injury of the heel showing full-thickness skin loss. **B,** After a full-thickness cross-leg pedicle skin graft.

ligaments over the dorsum of the foot and ankle in order to restore circulation.

The treatment for sympathetic dystrophy and related conditions is a prompt return to as normal weight bearing as possible. Cast immobilization with a walking heel may be necessary to afford this weight bearing in the face of pain (p. 468).

Traumatic ulcers

Traumatic ulcers can occur as a result of various types of sudden injury such as chemical, thermal, or mechanical injury. In the early stages they may be treated conservatively however, for those that are accompanied by extensive skin damage and those that become intractable, grafting of skin on the area usually probides acceptable results.

Murray and Goldwyn (1966) treated fifteen patients with intractable plantar ulcers by means of split grafts and pedicle flaps. In thirteen of the patients the procedures were completely successful.

Traumatic ulcers are usually caused by excessive pressure on a weight-bearing area (see p. 419).

Volkmann's ischemic contracture

Contracture of one muscle or a group of muscles as a result of the replacement of the muscle cells by connective tissue is caused by an interference with the blood supply to the muscle involved. The condition is known as Volkmann's ischemic contracture (Fig. 7-31). A tourniquet or cast, especially over the arm, may cause the contracture by injury to a major artery. Trauma may be directly to the artery supplying the muscle or to a distal portion of the vessel, resulting in reflex vasospasm along its course through the leg. The foot is affected only indirectly.

Seddon (1966) found this condition to be more common in adults than in children. Monk (1966) reported a case of Volkmann's ischemic contracture of the lower extremity that resulted from a contusion to the calf muscles. He postulated that the contusion led to edema and decreased venous return, which ultimately resulted in a lack of blood supply to the muscles of the leg. The peripheral pulses in the foot remained, which demonstrated that the presence of these pulses does not contraindicate appropriate treatment.

In the early stage the loss of blood supply produces necrosis (muscle sequestrum) in the body of the muscle. With the passage of time, fibrous connective tissue replaces dead muscle fibers. The fibrous connective tissue contracts and shortens, thereby producing a deformity of the limb.

This serious condition occurs frequently enough after injuries to the lower extremity to warrant a more determined effort to prevent it. Early signs of tenseness of the thigh or more commonly of the calf and anterior compartment, along with equinus of the foot and pain on attempted dorsiflexion of the foot, should alert the examiner to the possibility of impending ischemia. All pressure should be released. Excision of the deep fascia and possibly evacuation of a hematoma beneath the muscles may save the threatened underlying structures. If the femoral or popliteal artery is injured, exploration and repair should be performed immediately.

Treatment for an already contracted lower extremity is simple because there is so little that can be done. It is primarily directed toward overcoming the deformity, for the muscle fibers cannot be revived. Treatment consists of prolonged stretching, tendon lengthening, or sectioning of the contracted muscle. Amputation may be necessary.

Compartment syndromes. A compartment syndrome results from increased tissue pressure within the various osteofascial compartment of the tibia (Fig. 7-32). If it is not treated effectively within 12 hours, a Volkmann contracture may occur. The syndrome follows trauma (e.g., a crush injury or a fractured tibia), surgical procedures (e.g., tibial osteotomies), burns, and exercise. Since increased compartment pressure is the underlying pa-

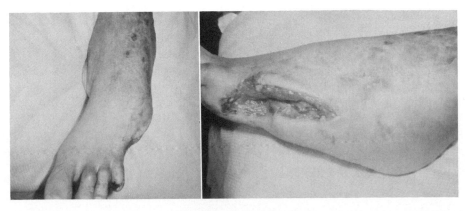

Fig. 7-31. Volkmann's ischemic contracture of the foot resulting from an injury to the knee. The blood supply to the foot was compromised. Removal of a toe was necessary because of gangrene.

thognomonic factor, prompt fascial decompression is the treatment of choice.

Pain, pallor, and paralysis of the foot are the signs and symptoms of a compartment syndrome. The peripheral pulses may still be present and should not confuse the issue. When these signs and symptoms occur, the physician should be alerted to this dangerous condition. The promptness of fascial decompression will determine the amount of functional loss that may result. The duration of the time period during which functional losses are reversible is unknown. Sheridan and Matsen (1976) showed that early fasciotomy, within 12 hours of the onset of symptoms, resulted in significantly better results than did later fasciotomies. Therefore it is best to perform the procedure as soon as the diagnosis is expected.

Prevention of a compartment syndrome is the most important defense against its disabling sequelae. Tight unyielding dressings or wraps should not be applied over the lower extremity initially following trauma or surgery. Casts should be windowed or split; and the extremity should be elevated, iced, and

checked frequently. Any hint of the syndrome warrants complete removal of all circular wraps. Pain in front of the shin during exercise is a warning sign to stop immediately. If peculiar sensations are experienced in the foot, hospitalization for elevation, ice application, and observation should be considered.

The factors that cause functional loss no matter how early fasciotomy is performed are unclear. Murbarak et al. (1976) have devised a technique of monitoring tissue pressure continuously in order to establish a criterion for fascial decompression. Their method is useful in patients who have experienced trauma or have had surgery associated with the risk of a compartment syndrome. A significant rise over the normal values plus increasing discomfort helps to make an early diagnosis.

When a single compartment is involved, a fasciotomy of that compartment is performed. It may be done by the open method (through a large skin incision extending the length of the fascia) or by the closed method (through several small incisions).

When all four compartments are affected, the procedure becomes more complicated.

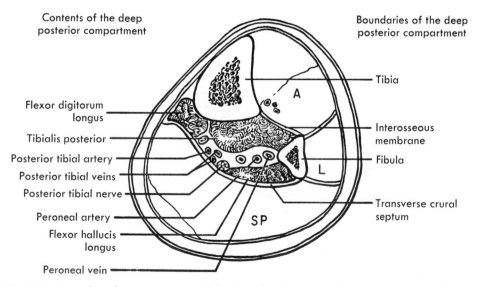

Fig. 7-32. Osteofascial compartments of the leg. The deep posterior compartment is shown in detail; the superficial compartments are represented by letters: *A* (anterior), *L* (lateral), and *SP* (superficial posterior). (From Matsen, F. A., III, and Clawson, D. K.: J. Bone Joint Surg. **57A:** 34, 1975.)

Kelley and Whitesides (1967) suggested a partial fibulectomy through a single incision as a means of releasing the fascia of all four compartments. Murbarak and Owen (1977) believe the double incision technique is easier, faster, and safer in obtaining a four-compartment fasciotomy. The incisions are placed anterolaterally and posteromedially. No matter what procedure is used early fasciotomy is the key to the best results.

REFERENCES

Anderson, K. J., and Lecocq, J. F.: Operative treatment of injury to the fibular collateral ligament of the ankle, J. Bone Joint Surg. 36A:825, 1954.

Anderson, K. J., Lecocq, J. F., and Lecocq, E. A.: Recurrent anterior subluxation of the ankle joint: a report of two cases and an experimental study, J. Bone Joint Surg. 34A:853, 1952.

Artz, C. P., and Reiss, E.: The treatment of burns, Philadelphia, 1957, W. B. Saunders Co.

Bennett, J. E., and Dingman, R. O.: Evaluation of burn depth by the use of radioactive isotopes—an experimental study, Plast. Reconstr. Surg. 20:261, 1957.

Berridge, F. R., and Bonnin, J. G.: The radiographic examination of the ankle joint including arthrography, Surg. Gynecol. Obstet. 79:383, 1944.

Bigelow, W. G.: The modern conception and treatment of frostbite, Can. Med. Assoc. J. 47:529, 1942.

Blair, J. R., Schatzki, R., and Orr, K. D.: Sequelae to cold injury in one hundred patients, J.A.M.A. 163:1203, 1957.

Bonnin, J.: The hypermobile ankle, Proc. R. Soc. Med. 37:282, 1944.

Bonnin, J. G.: Injury to the ligaments of the ankle, J. Bone Joint Surg. 47B:609, 1965.

Bosien, W. R., Staples, O. S., and Russell, S. W.: Residual disability following acute ankle sprains, J. Bone Joint Surg. 37A:1237, 1955.

Brahms, M. A.: Common foot problems, J. Bone Joint Surg. 49A:1653, 1967.

Broström, L.: Sprained ankles. I. Anatomic lesions in recent sprains, Acta Chir. Scand. 128:483, 1964.

Broström, L.: Sprained ankles. V. Treatment and prognosis in recent ligament ruptures, Acta Chir. Scand. 132:537, 1966a.

Broström, L. : Sprained ankles. VI. Surgical treatment of chronic ligament ruptures, Acta Chir. Scand. 132:551, 1966b.

Broström, L., Liljedahl, S. O., and Lindvall, N.: Sprained ankles. II. Arthrographic diagnoses of recent ligament ruptures, Acta Chir. Scand. 129:485, 1965.

Brown, J. R.: Localization of foreign bodies, Ohio Med. J. 54:908, 1958.

Brownrigg, G. M.: Frostbite in shipwrecked mariners, Am. J. Surg. 59:232, 1943.

Bunnell's surgery of the hand, ed. 4 (revised by Joseph H. Boyes), Philadelphia, 1964, J. B. Lippincott Co.

Burman, M. S.: Subcutaneous rupture of the tendon of the tibialis anticus, Ann. Surg. 100:368, 1934.

Cohen, H., and Reid, J. B.: Tenosynovitis crepitans associated with oxaluria, Liverpool Med. Chir. J. 43:193, 1935.

Curtiss, P. H.: Vascular problems in trauma of the foot, J. Bone Joint Surg. 48B:389, 1966.

D'Anca, A. F.: Lateral rotatory dislocation of the ankle without fracture, J. Bone Joint Surg. 52A:1643, 1970.

Dickinson, P. H., Coutts, M. B., Woodward, E. P., and Handler, D.: Tendo achillis bursitis, J. Bone Joint Surg. 48A:77, 1966.

Dziob, J. M.: Ligamentous injuries about the ankle joint, Am. J. Surg. 91:692, 1956.

Edwards, E. A., and Leeper, R. W.: Frostbite: an analysis of seventy-one cases, J.A.M.A. 149:1199, 1952.

Els, H.: Ueber eine Abrissfraktur des Tibialisanticus-Ansatzes, Dtsch. Z. Chir. 106:610, 1910.

Fausel, E. G., and Hemphill, J. A.: Study of the late symptoms of cases of immersion foot, Surg. Gynecol. Obstet. 81:500, 1945.

Fordyce, A. J. W., and Horn, C. V.: Arthrography in recent injuries of the ligaments of the ankle, J. Bone Joint Surg. 54B:116, 1972.

Freeman, M. A. R.: Instability of the foot after injuries to the lateral ligament of the ankle, J. Bone Joint Surg. 47B:669, 1965a.

Freeman, M. A. R.: Treatment of ruptures of the lateral ligament of the ankle, J. Bone Joint Surg. 47B:661, 1965b.

Ghormley, R. K., and Spear, I. M.: Anomalies of the posterior tibial tendon: a cause of persistent pain about ankle, Arch. Surg. 66:512, 1953.

Gillespie, H., and Boucher, P.: Watson-Jones repair of lateral instability of the ankle, J. Bone Joint Surg. 53A:920, 1971.

Glick, J. M. Gordon, R. B., and Nishimoto, D.: The prevention and treatment of ankle injuries, Am. J. Sports Med. 4:136, 1976.

Glick, J. M., and Katch, L.: Musculoskeletal injuries in jogging, Arch. Phys. Med. 51:123, 1970.

Goldner, J. L., Keats, P. K., Bassett, F. H., and Clippinger, F. W.: Progressive talipes equinovalgus due to trauma or degeneration of the posterior tibial tendon and medial plantar ligament, Orthop. Clin. North Am. 5:39, 1974.

Gordon, R. B.: Arthrography of the ankle joint, J. Bone Joint Surg. 52A:1623, 1970.

Griffiths, J. C.: Tendon injuries around the ankle, J. Bone Joint Surg. 47B:686, 1965.

Gunn, D. R.: Stenosing tenosynovitis of the common peroneal tendon sheath, Br. Med. J. 1:691, 1959.

Hermann, G., Schechter, D. C., Owens, J. C., and Starzl, T. E.: The problem of frostbite in civilian medical practice, Surg. Clin. North Am. 43:519, 1963.

Hirata, I.: The doctor and the athlete, Philadelphia, 1968, J. B. Lippincott Co.

Hooker, C. H.: Rupture of the tendo calcaneus, J. Bone Joint Surg. 45B:360, 1963.

Hughes, J. R.: Sprains and subluxations of ankle-joint, Proc. R. Soc. Med. **35**:765, 1942.

Inglis, A. E., Scott, W. N., Sculco, T. P., and Patterson, A. H.: Ruptures of the tendo Achillis: an objective assessment of surgical and nonsurgical treatment, J. Bone Joint Surg. **58A**:990, 1976.

Inman, V. T.: The joints of the ankle, Baltimore, 1976, The Williams & Wilkins Co.

Jennett, W. B., and Watson, J. A.: The radio-opacity of glass foreign bodies, with report of a case of injury of the cauda equina by fragments of glass, Br. J. Surg. **46**:244, 1958.

Keck, S. W., and Kelly, P. J.: Bursitis of the posterior part of the heel, J. Bone Joint Surg. **47A**:267, 1965.

Kelley, R. P., and Whitesides, R. E., Jr.: Transfibular route for fasciotomy of the leg, J. Bone Joint Surg. **49A**:1022, 1967.

Kelly, R. P.: Ankle injuries, Kentucky Med. J. **50**:281, 1952.

Kettelkamp, D. B., and Alexander, H. H.: Spontaneous rupture of the posterior tibial tendon, J. Bone Joint Surg. **51A**:759, 1969.

Knize, D. M., Weatherley-White, R. C. A., Paton, B. C., and Owens, J. C.: Prognostic factors in the management of frostbite, J. Trauma **9**:749, 1969.

Landeros, O., Frost, H. M., and Higgins, C. C.: Post-traumatic anterior ankle instability, Clin. Orthop. **56**:169, 1968.

Lapidus, P. W.: Indirect subcutaneous rupture of the anterior tibial tendon: report of two cases, Bull. N. Y. Hosp. Joint Dis. **2**:119, 1941.

Lapidus, P. W., and Seidenstein, H.: Chronic nonspecific tenosynovitis with effusion about the ankle, J. Bone Joint Surg. **32A**:175, 1950.

Lea, R. B., and Smith, L.: Ruptures of the Achilles tendon: nonsurgical treatment, Clin. Orthop. **60**:115, 1968.

Lea, R. B. and Smith, L.: Non-surgical treatment of tendo Achillis rupture J. Bone Joint Surg. **54A**:1398, 1972.

Leonard, M. H.: Injuries of the lateral ligaments of the ankle: a clinical and experimental study, J. Bone Joint Surg. **31A**:373, 1949.

Lewis, T.: Observations on some normal and injurious effects of cold upon the skin and underlying tissues: frostbite, Br. Med. J. **2**:869, 1941.

Lipscomb, P. R.: Nonsuppurative tenosynovitis and para-tendinitis. In American Academy of Orthopaedic Surgeons, Instructional Course Lectures, vol. 7, Ann Arbor, 1950, J. W. Edwards.

Lipscomb, P. R., and Kelley, P. J.: Injuries of the extensor tendons in the distal part of the leg and in the ankle, J. Bone Joint Surg. **37A**:1206, 1955.

London, P. S.: The burnt foot, Br. J. Surg. **40**:293, 1953.

Matsen, F. A., III, and Clawson, D. K.: The deep posterior compartmental syndrome of the leg, J. Bone Joint Surg. **57A**:34, 1975.

McMaster, P. E.: Treatment of ankle sprain: observations

in more than five hundred cases, J.A.M.A. **122**:659, 1943.

Mensor, M. C., and Ordway, G. L.: Traumatic subcutaneous rupture of the tibialis anterior tendon, J. Bone Joint Surg. **35A**:675, 1953.

Meyers, M. B.: Prediction of skin sloughs at the time of operation with the use of fluorescein dye, Surgery **51**:158, 1962.

Milgram, J. E.: Muscles ruptures and avulsions, with particular reference to the lower extremities. In American Academy of Orthopaedic Surgeons, Instructional Course Lectures, vol. 10, Ann Arbor, 1953, J. W. Edwards.

Monk, C. J. E.: Traumatic ischaemia of the calf, J. Bone Joint Surg. **48B**:150, 1966.

Moorhead, J. J.: Locating and removing foreign bodies, Am. J. Surg. **95**:108, 1958.

Murbarak, S. J., Hargens, A. R., Owen, C. A., Garretto, B. A., and Akeson, W. H.: The wick catheter technique for measurement of intramuscular pressure, J. Bone Joint Surg. **58A**:1016, 1976.

Murbarak, S. J., and Owen, C. A.: Double incision fasciotomy of the ligament for recompression in compartment syndromes, J. Bone Joint Surg. **59A**:184, 1977.

Murray, J. E., and Goldwyn, R. M.: Definitive treatment of intractable plantar ulcers, J.A.M.A. **196**:311, 1966.

Parvin, R. W., and Ford, L. T.: Stenosing tenosynovitis of the common peroneal tendon sheath, J. Bone Joint Surg. **38A**:1352, 1956.

Percy, E. C., Hill, R. O., and Callaghan, J. E.: The "sprained" ankle, J. Trauma, **9**:972, 1969.

Randolph, J. G., Leape, L. L., and Gross, R. E.: The early surgical treatment of burns. I. Experimental studies utilizing intravenous vital dye for determining the degree of injury, Surgery **56**:193, 1964.

Roberts, W. C.: Radiographic characteristics of glass, Arch. Ind. Health **18**:470, 1958.

Seddon, H. J.: Volkmann's ischaemia in the lower limb, J. Bone Joint Surg. **48B**:627, 1966.

Sheridan, G. W., and Matsen, F. A., 3rd: Fasciotomy in the treatment of the acute compartment syndrome, J. Bone Joint Surg. **58A**:112, 1976.

Standard nomenclature of athletic injuries. Prepared by the Subcommittee on Classification of Sports Injuries, American Medical Association, Committee on the Medical Aspects of Sports, Chicago, 1966, American Medical Association.

Thorndike, A.: Athletic injuries: prevention, diagnosis and treatment, Philadelphia, 1962, Lea & Febiger.

Ungley, C. C.: Treatment of immersion foot by dry cooling, Lancet **1**:681, 1943.

Vinson, H. A., and Schatzki, R.: Roentgenologic bone changes encountered in frostbite, Korea 1950-51, Radiology **63**:685, 1954.

Webster, D. R., Woolhouse, F. M., and Johnston, J. L.: Immersion foot, J. Bone Joint Surg. **24**:785, 1942.

Williams, R.: Chronic non-specific tendovaginitis of tibialis posterior, J. Bone Joint Surg. **45B**:542, 1963.

8

ACQUIRED NONTRAUMATIC DEFORMITIES OF THE FOOT

Roger A. Mann and Henri L. DuVries

The foot, more than any other skeletal unit, is subject to static deformities. Its weight-transmitting and propulsive functions are restricted daily by a relatively nonyielding foot covering. Anatomic variation in the shape and stability of the joint surfaces may predispose, resist, or modify the deforming force of such footwear.

Modern civilization disregards the physiology of the foot. Fashion and eye appeal rather than function determine shoe design, especially the forepart of the foot, where most disabilities and deformities occur. It is probably because the styles of women's footwear are more extreme than those of men that 80% of all forefoot problems occur in women. Men also are guilty of wearing ill-fitting shoes (Fig. 8-1), but to a lesser degree.

The restrictive force of poorly fitting shoes produces little deformity on the tarsus, because the tarsus is made up of short heavy bones and normal movement in the tarsal joints is limited inasmuch as the articular surfaces of the tarsal joints are comparatively flat. However, the phalanges and metatarsals are long thin bones with a normally wide range of joint motion. Restrictive force on these bones can produce static deformities of the forefoot—e.g., most first metatarsophalangeal joint deformities, including hammertoe, tailor's bunion, overlapping toes, and many other conditions that are deviations from the normal.

The human foot is uniquely specialized. The metatarsals and toes allow man to stand erect. The versatility of the forefoot permits him to retain his upright stance and gives him grace in walking, dancing, and athletics.

A well-developed and strong foot withstands surprising abuse; morbid changes take place only when maltreatment becomes excessive. An underdeveloped and frail foot may fail under ordinary stress and strain.

INCIDENCE AND CAUSE OF FOOT DISORDERS

Between 40% and 50% of civilized society has, or will have, some foot disorder. Of all disorders of the foot, 90% occur in the forefoot and many are essentially induced by ill-fitting shoes.

The forefoot is a modified square (Fig. 8-2, A). We have been endeavoring to educate people to this fact for many years. The forepart of a shoe, however, is generally triangular instead of conforming to the shape of the foot (Fig. 8-2, B). Obviously a square cannot be forced into a triangle, yet history tells us that for many thousands of years man has been forcing his foot into triangular-shaped coverings. Ordinarily shoes are without elasticity. Living tissue, however, yields to unrelenting

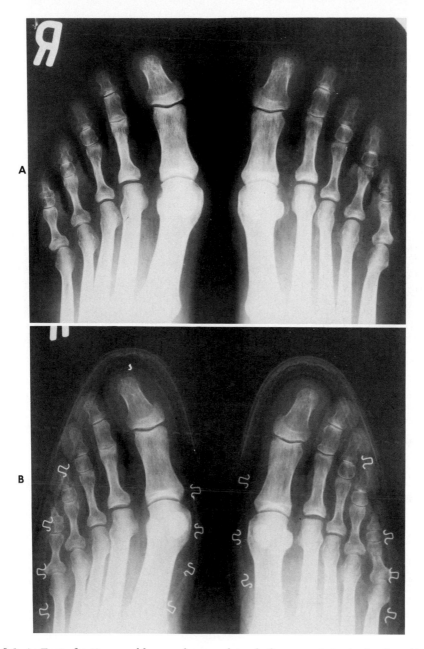

Fig. 8-1. **A,** Feet of a 42-year-old man who complained of vague pain in the forefoot. (As a rule the forefeet are modified squares; these are more oblique than usual.) **B,** In shoes.

restriction and pressure, even though mild. The foot accommodates itself gradually to the shape of the shoe; and deformities result in accordance with Wolff's law, which maintains that "primary changes in form and function are followed by determinable changes in the outer shape and the inner architecture of the involved bone."*

*Weinmann, J. P., and Sicher, H.: Bone and bones: fundamentals of bone biology, ed. 2, St. Louis, 1955, The C. V. Mosby Co., p. 174.

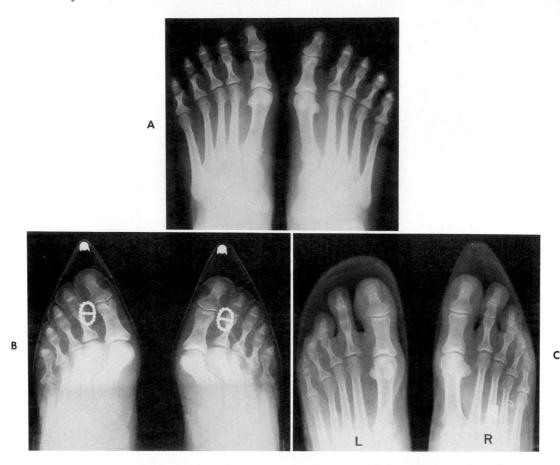

Fig. 8-2. A, Average normal feet of a young woman during weight bearing. **B,** In shoes during weight bearing. Note that she is developing hallux valgus. **C,** Effects of different types of shoes. The left shoe permits freedom of forefoot function; the right shoe restricts function of the four lesser toes.

DEFORMITIES OF THE FIRST METATARSOPHALANGEAL JOINT

The most frequent severely disabling affliction of the forefoot involves the first metatarsophalangeal joint. Anatomically this joint is the most complex part of the forefoot (Fig. 8-3); it is composed of relatively large bones with powerful intrinsic muscles inserted into the base of the proximal phalanx. It also is influenced in its function by the extensor and flexor hallucis longis, the tibialis anterior, and the peroneus longus. It plays a major role in the transmission of body weight in locomotion. General diseases, such as gout, rheumatoid arthritis, and neuropathies of the foot, have a predilection for this joint.

Bunions

The term "bunion," derived from the Latin *bunio* meaning "turnip," has been confusingly misapplied to disorders of the first metatarsophalangeal joint. It is often loosely used to connote any enlargement or deformity of this joint and has included such diverse conditions as ganglion, a congenitally wide head of the first metatarsal, hallux valgus, hallux rigidus, proliferation of the dorsum of the first metatarsophalangeal joint (dorsal bunion), and proliferative change secondary to arthritides.

Hallux valgus, actually a symptom complex, is the most common and disabling group of deformities included under the heading "bunion." When applied to the fifth metatar-

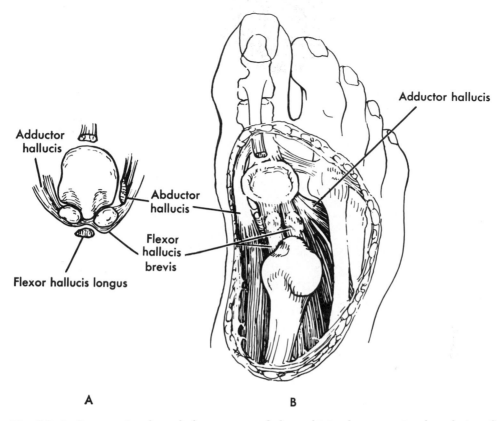

Fig. 8-3. **A,** Cross section through the metatarsophalangeal joint demonstrating the relation of the sesamoids and tendons to the first metatarsal head. **B,** Dorsal view of the first metatarso-phalangeal joint with the toe in plantar flexion.

sal head (bunionette or tailor's bunion), bun-ion has been mistakenly assumed to connote lateral bending of the head, a congenitally wide head, and chronic thickening of soft tissue structures over the head. As a corollary, "bunionectomy" is an equally unscientific term.

The numerous disorders in this category will be considered separately.

Congenitally wide first metatarsal head

A congenitally wide first metatarsal head (Fig. 8-4) often becomes a pressure area on the medial side of the great toe joint. Whether or not it is associated with hallux valgus, it may become a problem. The medial side becomes the most prominent point on the inner surface of the foot, creating an area for pressure by footwear and resulting in a chronic inflammatory process of the capsular structures over

the area. The inflammation produces addi-tional thickening of the capsule and enlarge-ment of the prominence.

Symptoms. The symptoms of a congenitally wide first metatarsal head are chronic pain and welling over the medial side. A shoe cut out over this area gives relief but treatment requires excision of the tibial condylar process of the first metatarsal head (Fig. 8-5).

Technique for reduction. The technique for reduction is as follows:

1. Make a semilunar incision with its apex extending dorsally from the middle of the tib-ial side of the first proximal phalanx to a point about 3 cm proximal to the head on the tibial side of the first metatarsal.

2. Dissect the skin flap to expose the tibial side of the great toe joint. Carefully expose and retract the dorsal medial cutaneous nerve to the hallux.

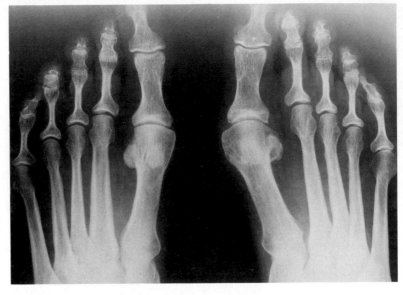

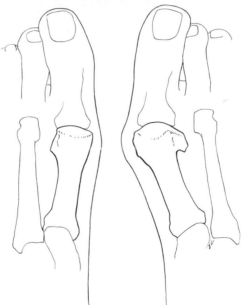

Fig. 8-4. Left. Normally shaped metatarsal head; right, congenitally wide metatarsal head.

3. Excise all excess hypertrophied or adventitious bursal tissue.

4. Make a longitudinal incision in the dorsal medial aspect of the joint capsule, dissecting it from the head of the first metatarsal.

5. Retract the capsule with the skin flap, exposing the tibial condyle of the first metatarsal head.

6. Incise the metatarsophalangeal interarticular ligament and deliver the metatarsal head from the wound with a periosteal or Chandler elevator.

7. The condylar (sagittal) ridge on the artic-

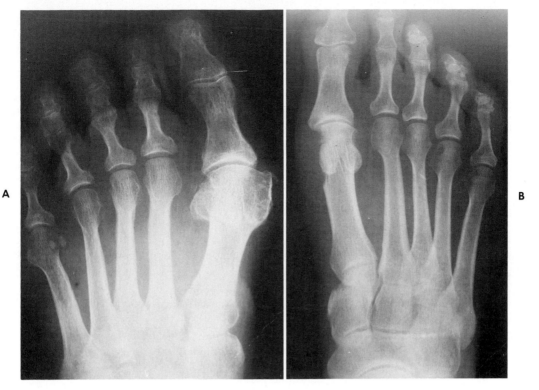

Fig. 8-5. Congenitally wide first metatarsal head. **A,** There is some osteophytic change as a result of pressure. **B,** Postoperative following a condylectomy.

ular surface of the metatarsal head is an ideal landmark for removal of the tibial condylar process. After excising the condylar process with an osteotome, round the sharp margins with a rasp or rongeur.

8. Make certain that the insertion of the abductor hallucis is intact. If it is not, repair it; otherwise, the patient will develop a postoperative hallux valgus.

9. Suture the capsule and skin in layers, and apply a compression bandage.

Ambulation may begin in 24 hours. Full use of the joint is usually possible in 3 to 4 weeks. Complications and disability are minimal.

Hallux valgus

Lateral deviation of the great toe with medial deviation of the head of the first metatarsal is technically classified as hallux valgus. The deformity is a static partial dislocation or subluxation of the first metatarsophalangeal joint that occurs with or without an accom-

panying painful soft tissue reaction over the medial prominence (bunion). In addition to the obvious lateralward deviation of the great toe, there is a varus or medial deviation of the first metatarsal shaft. The hallux valgus deformity is often accompanied by rotation of the great toe around its longitudinal axis. A variable degree of periosteal reaction on the medial side of the head of the first metatarsal is usually present.

With increasing angulation of the metatarsophalangeal joint, two displacements of the sesamoids occur. These displacements can be better comprehended if the sesamoids are considered to be related anatomically and functionally more to the proximal phalanx than to the head of the first metatarsal. With increasing valgus, the head of the first metatarsal progressively moves medially off the sesamoids, which retain their anatomic relationship to the proximal phalanx. With increasing valgus deformity of the proximal phalanx, proximal displacement of the fibular sesamoid and distal displacement of the tibial sesamoid, which are often seen in the weight-bearing AP projection of the foot, can be easily understood.

Etiology. Since hallux valgus occurs almost exclusively in people who wear shoes, investigators agree that the shoe must be an important etiologic factor. It is interesting to note, however, that even among unshod people, hallux valgus, although infrequent, has been reported to occur.*

Whereas the shoe appears to have been an essential element in the causation of hallux valgus, the fact remains that many individuals who wear modern footwear do not develop this deformity. There must be predisposing factors which make some feet more vulnerable to the effects of footwear and cause some unshod feet to exhibit a tendency toward the development of hallux valgus. Rare cases of hallux valgus seen in children (juvenile type) may also be explained by these predisposing factors.

Although there is no doubt that the skeletal abnormalities just mentioned are all present in the full-blown case of hallux valgus, yet var-

*Engle and Morton, 1931; Wells, 1931; Barnicot and Hardy, 1955; Lam Sim-Fook and Hodgson, 1958; Shine, 1965; Maclennan, 1966.

ious authors have seized upon single aspects of the deformity as major etiologic factors. These may be summarized under separate headings.

Shoes. That modern footwear is the principal contributor to the development of hallux valgus appears to be a certainty. A study of shoe-wearing and non–shoe-wearing persons of the same genetic background by Lam Sim-Fook and Hodgson (1958) revealed that 33% of the shod individuals had some degree of hallux valgus as compared with 1.9% among the unshod.

All studies which provide statistical data on the frequency of hallux valgus among shoe-wearing populations report that the condition is more frequent in females than in males. Wilkins (1941), in a study of feet with reference to schoolchildren, reported a proportion of 2 to 1 in the general population. Investigators reporting from surveys made among male and female recruits (Marwil and Brantingham, 1943; Hewitt et al., 1953) place the proportion at approximately 3 to 1, whereas authors whose statistics were obtained from clinical practice report the proportion to be 15 to 1 (Creer, 1938; Hardy and Clapham, 1951). Certainly the shoes worn by females are less physiologic than those worn by males, and shoes of any type are prone to lead to hallux

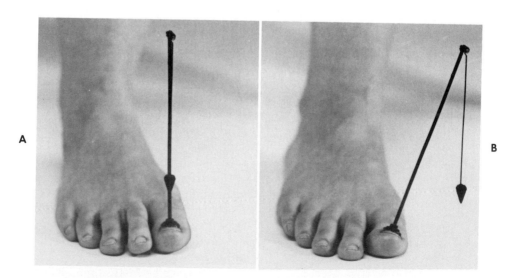

A   B

Fig. 8-6. Longitudinal rotation of the first ray with supination, **A,** and pronation, **B.** A pendulum is glued to the nail of the great toe.

valgus in susceptible individuals (Figs. 8-1 and 8-2).

Pes planus. The tendency for the pronated foot to develop a hallux valgus has been noted by many authors.* Hohmann (1925) was the most definite, asserting that hallux valgus is always combined with pes valgus and that pes

---

*Ewald, 1912; Mayo, 1920; Stein, 1938; Galland and Jordan, 1938; Joplin, 1950; Craigmile, 1953.

valgus is always the causative factor in hallux valgus.

The role played by pronation of the foot in the life history of hallux valgus generally has received little attention in the world literature, yet the effect of pronation as a possible initiating factor is readily demonstrated in any normal foot, as depicted in Figs. 8-6 to 8-10.

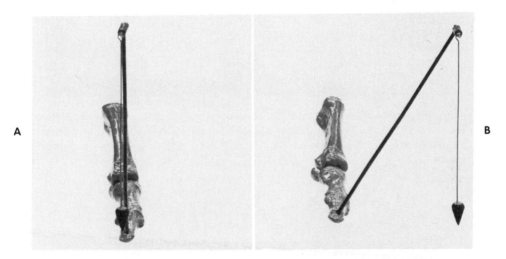

Fig. 8-7. Skeletal model of the demonstration in Fig. 8-6. **A,** Supination; **B,** pronation.

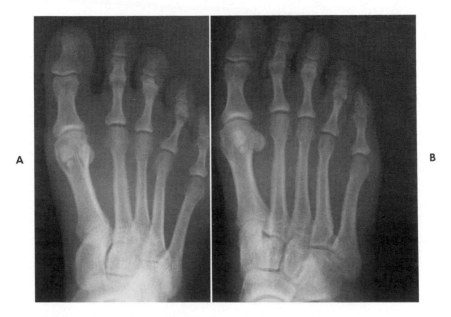

Fig. 8-8. Foot in Fig. 8-6 during weight bearing. **A,** Supination. **B,** Pronation. Note the apparent lateral displacement of the sesamoids.

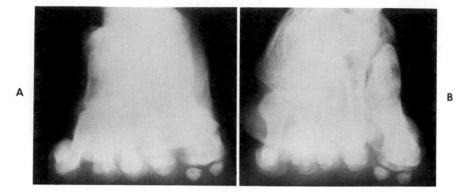

Fig. 8-9. Tangential views of the sesamoids during weight bearing. **A,** Supination. **B,** Pronation. The degree of longitudinal rotation of the metatarsal is clearly demonstrated by the position of the sesamoids, which still retain a normal relationship to their facets on the underside of the metatarsal head.

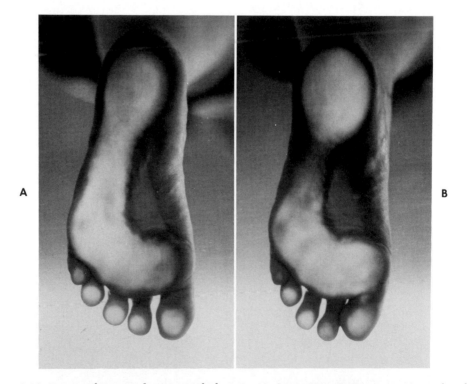

Fig. 8-10. Barographic view during weight bearing. **A,** Supination. **B,** Pronation. Note that the pressure area of the great toe has moved medially and has produced a mild hallux valgus.

In Fig. 8-6 a pendulum has been glued to the nail of the great toe. As the foot is pronated, the rotation of the first ray around its longitudinal axis is clearly shown. In Fig. 8-7 a skeletal model has been photographed. Note that with longitudinal rotation of the first metatarsal the fibular sesamoid becomes visible on the lateral side of the first metatarsal head. In Fig. 8-8 a dorsoventral weight-bearing radiograph is shown of the same foot as in Fig. 8-6. Note that in the pronated position the sesamoids appear to have been displaced laterally. The fibular sesamoid is now visible in the interval between the first and second metatarsals, as would be anticipated from the skeletal model in Fig. 8-7. That this appearance is due solely to the longitudinal rotation of the first metatarsal and not to an actual lateral displacement is revealed in tangential radiographs of the foot, in which the sesamoids can be seen to remain in a normal relationship to their facets located on the plantar surface of the metatarsal head (Fig. 8-9). In Fig. 8-10 the distribution of weight bearing through the sole of the foot is demonstrated by the barograph. Note that in the pronated foot the area of weight bearing transmitted through the great toe has been displaced medially and a degree of hallux valgus has been created.

Pronation of the foot imposes a longitudinal rotation of the first ray (metatarsal and phalanges) which places the axis of the metatarsophalangeal joint in an oblique plane relative to the floor. In this position it appears to be less able to withstand the deforming pressures exerted on it either by the shoes or by weight bearing. Unfortunately there are no data available on the relationship between the degree of pes planus and the degree of hallux valgus in the small percentage of unshod individuals who develop the condition. Furthermore, authors who have noted a relationship between pes planus and hallux valgus in shod individuals have presented no quantitative data.

In children who have severe pes planus secondary to a neuromuscular disorder such as poliomyelitis or cerebral palsy, there is a much higher incidence of hallux valgus deformity because these children exert pressure along the medial border of their foot during the stance and lift-off phase of walking, thereby forcing the great toe laterally or into valgus. This, in effect, stretches the medial capsular structures and produces a severe rapidly occurring hallux valgus deformity.

Metatarsus varus. The concomitant occurrence of hallux valgus and metatarsus varus has been noted by almost all clinicians.

In a careful statistical study of patients with hallux valgus, Hardy and Clapham (1951) found that, of all the possible correlations between various measurements on the foot, the correlation between the degree of hallux valgus and the size of the intermetatarsal angle was the "most striking" (coefficient, 0.71). This study confirmed that hallux valgus and metatarsus varus go together. The question is still unanswered as to which is the cause and which the result.

Ewald (1912), while emphasizing the relationship of hallux valgus and metatarsus varus, stated categorically that the "primary source" of hallux valgus was metatarsus varus of the first metatarsal. Truslow (1925) claimed to have presented a new name, "metatarsus primus varus," for a congenital abnormality which, if present, inevitably results in hallux valgus when the individual is forced to wear shoes. The studies of Hardy and Clapham (1951) and Craigmile (1953) on schoolchildren, however, seem to indicate that the metatarsus varus is secondary to the hallux valgus. In either case, any surgeon who is considering an operative correction of this deformity should be aware of the close relationship between the degree of metatarsus varus and hallux valgus.

Length of first metatarsal. Based upon minimal anthropometric data and unsubstantiated by mathematical analysis, both a short first metatarsal (Morton, 1935) and a long first metatarsal (Mayo, 1908, 1920) have been proposed as essential factors in the development of the hallux valgus (Fig. 8-11). It appears to us that the relationship between metatarsal length and the development of hallux valgus is fortuitous and not a direct etiologic factor.

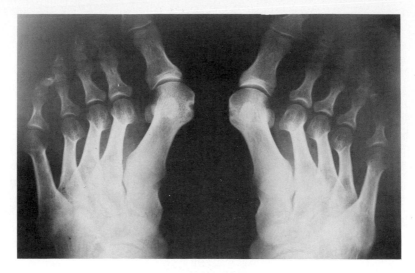

Fig. 8-11. First metatarsal longer than the second.

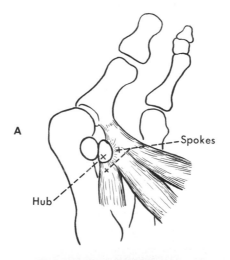

A

Spokes

Hub

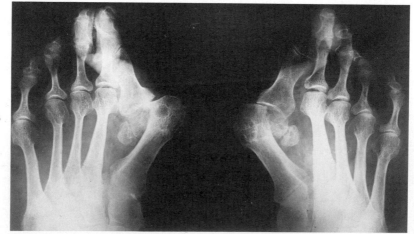

B

Fig. 8-12. A, The proximal phalanx and sesamoids are anchored by the conjoint tendon consisting of the adductor hallucis and fibular portion of the flexor hallucis brevis. B, As the first metatarsal head drifts medialward, it slides off the sesamoids, which become displaced into the first interspace, and the proximal phalanx is pulled into valgus.

Anatomic and physiologic variations in muscles. There appears to be no question that in the presence of the typical skeletal deformities seen in a case of marked hallux valgus, an alteration in the action of the intrinsic and extrinsic muscles is acting on the components of the first ray. It seems reasonable to believe that these alterations in muscular action may expedite an increasing deformity.

Whether anatomic variations in the muscles or abnormalities in their function are basic etiologic factors in hallux valgus remains unproved. Only Kaplan (1955) has described a constant anatomic variation occurring in routinely dissected cadaver feet. In laboratory specimens which demonstrated a definite hallux valgus, he reported that the tendon of the tibialis posterior was "thicker" than in normal feet and possessed an extension of its insertion into the lateral head of the flexor hallucis brevis. This condition was not present in feet without hallux valgus.

The evidence to date is too meager to evaluate the role of the muscles alone in the production of hallux valgus. One has the intuitive feeling that the muscular variations are but a single component among several which make some feet more prone than others to develop hallux valgus. Once the deformity begins, however, the relationship of the conjoined tendon to the fibular sesamoid becomes an important element producing the deformity (Fig. 8-12).

Contracture of the tendo Achillis so as not to permit normal active dorsiflexion causes the patient to externally rotate the foot and roll off the medial border of the hallux. This condition is most evident in cerebral palsy but also occurs in people without demonstrable neuromuscular disease.

Anatomic variations of the first metatarsal. There are several anatomic variations of the first metatarsal noted on AP weight-bearing projections that either help to resist or predispose a person to develop the hallux valgus deformity. Since these variations of the metatarsophalangeal joint and metatarsocuneiform joint are noted on radiographs, the examiner should keep in mind that they may or may not be real because rotation of the first ray can produce apparent anatomic variations due to the projection of the joint in a single AP plane. Some of the variations of the first metatarsal head are seen in Figs. 8-13 and 8-14, and the

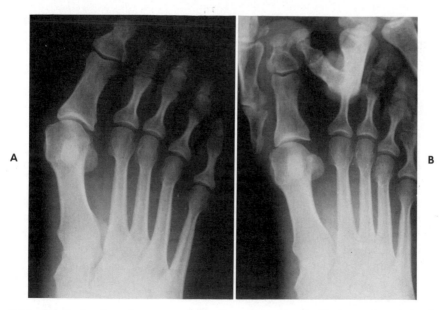

Fig. 8-13. Peculiarly shaped metatarsal head. It slopes on its fibular aspect to produce a congential hallux valgus. **A,** Normal articulation. **B,** Held in a straight line by an assistant. Note the gap in the articular surface at the fibular side of this joint.

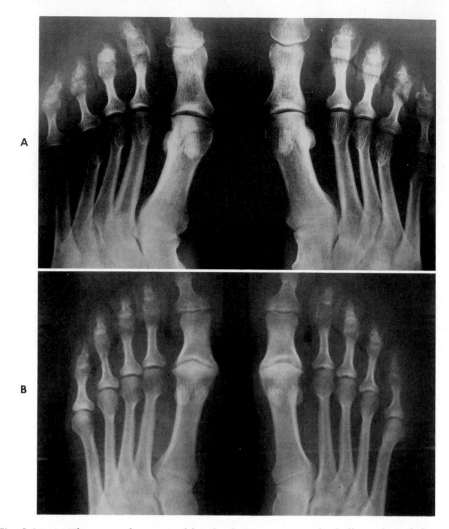

Fig. 8-14. **A,** Flat type of metatarsal head. This type resists the hallux valgus deformity. **B,** Peculiarly shaped metatarsal heads. This type resists movement of the great toe into valgus.

variations of the metatarsocuneiform joint are seen in Figs. 8-15 to 8-17.

Miscellaneous factors. Amputation of the second toe will usually result in a hallux valgus deformity (Fig. 8-18). This is probably due to loss of the support afforded by the second toe. A milder form of hallux valgus can be seen after resection of the second metatarsal head. Ganglionic cysts involving the medial capsule of the first metatarsophalangeal joint can sufficiently attenuate the capsule to permit development of a hallux valgus deformity in a foot

which might have only a slight predisposition toward it (Fig. 8-19).

Pathologic anatomy of hallux valgus. The precise factors which initiate the hallux valgus deformity are certainly conjecture at the present time.

From a clinical standpoint, most patients with a hallux valgus deformity have a mild flatfoot associated with a somewhat broad forefoot. The forcing of this anatomic configuration into a shoe is probably the most common etiologic factor in the production of a

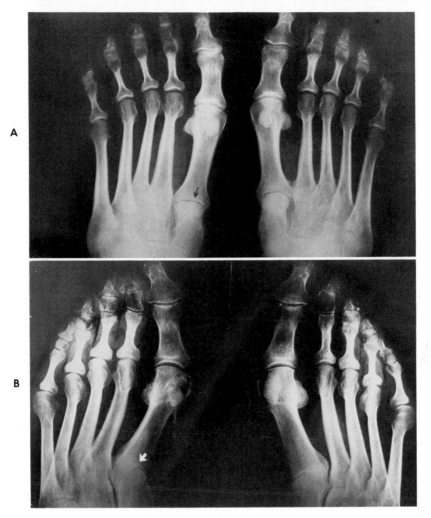

Fig. 8-15. A, Articulation of the base of the metatarsal with the first cuneiform at a right angle, resisting hallux valgus. **B,** Articulation of the base of the first metatarsal with the first cuneiform at an obtuse angle predisposing to hallux valgus.

hallux valgus. Such a foot within a shoe has pressure applied along the medial side of the great toe which, over a period of years, produces a certain degree of laxity of the medial capsular structures of the metatarsophalangeal joint and leads to the initial imbalance of the joint that evolves gradually into a hallux valgus deformity of varying degree. Other predisposing factors have been mentioned.

There are several factors to account for the other anatomic changes seen in hallux valgus.

The adductor hallucis tendon is a fixed structure which, besides blending with the lateral head of the flexor hallucis brevis to insert into the base of the proximal phalanx, anchors the sesamoids so they cannot drift medially. The lateral collateral ligament of the metatarsophalangeal joint, also a very dense structure, blends with the lateral joint capsule and adductor hallucis tendon to insert into the base of the proximal phalanx. As the hallux valgus deformity progresses, the great toe is forced lateralward by the shoe and by the

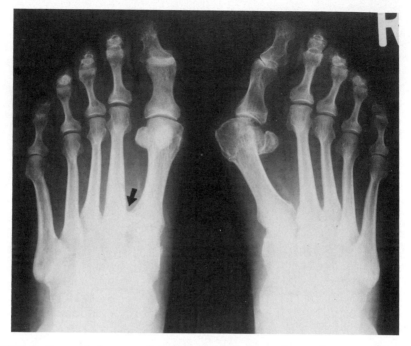

Fig. 8-16. Left, Congenital synostosis at the bases of the first and second metatarsals, preventing hallux valgus. Right, Absence of the anomaly, predisposing to hallux valgus deformity.

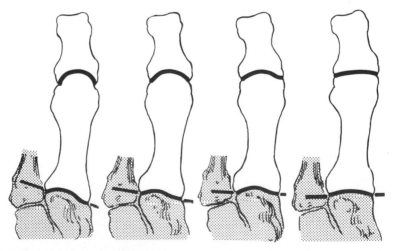

Fig. 8-17. Variations in the shape of the first metatarsal head and the angle of the articulation of the first metatarsal–medial cuneiform joint of the right foot. These may contribute to or resist deformity of the first metatarsophalangeal joint. A round metatarsal head predisposes to a hallux valgus, as does an obtuse first metatarsocuneiform joint.

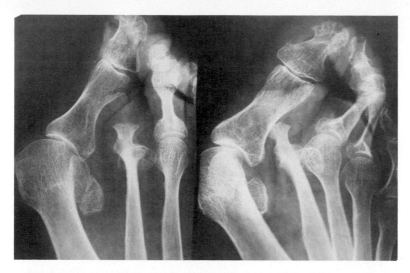

Fig. 8-18. Severe hallux valgus following amputation of the second toe.

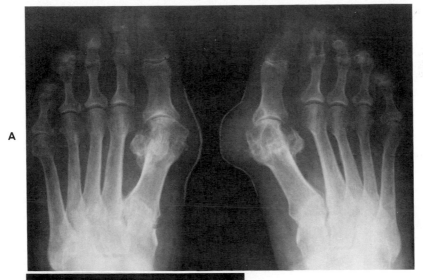

A

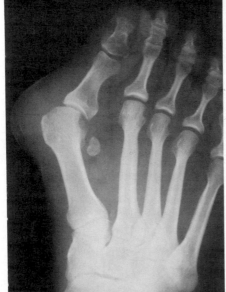

B

Fig. 8-19. A, Moderately advanced hallux valgus with a large associated ganglionic cyst on the right. **B,** Advanced hallux valgus.

pressure exerted along the medial side of the hallux during weight bearing. The base of the proximal phalanx, in effect, pushes the metatarsal head medialward. As the metatarsal head is pushed medialward, it attenuates the medial capsule and literally slides off the sesamoids, which are firmly anchored by the adductor hallucis.

Sesamoid views (Fig. 8-20) confirm the progressive displacement of the first metatarsal head off the sesamoid bones. As the metatarsal head is pushed off the sesamoids, the medial joint capsule is further attenuated; and the abductor hallucis tendon, forced medially, is pulled by the medial sesamoid under the metatarsal head. The base of the proximal phalanx meanwhile remains firmly anchored to the adductor hallucis and the lateral sesamoid; thus, as the metatarsal head drifts medially, the base of the proximal phalanx is not only held laterally but also forced to rotate on its long axis with the pivot point being the area where the lateral collateral ligament and

the adductor hallucis tendon blend (Fig. 8-21).

The first metatarsal shaft does not, we believe, rotate significantly along its longitudinal axis to contribute to the formation of a hallux valgus deformity. In a pronated foot there is some rotation of the entire first ray. (Figs. 8-6 to 8-10). If the medial drift of the metatarsal head continues unabated, in time there will be subluxation and then frank dislocation of the metatarsophalangeal joint with the result that the fibular, and sometimes the tibial, sesamoid becomes displaced between the first and second metarsal heads (Fig. 8-12). The flexor hallucis longus tendon travels with the sesamoid but the extensor hallucis longus tendon tends to drift laterally with the hallux. These tendons may become secondarily contracted in long-standing severe deformities.

Other secondary changes include callus formation along the plantar medial aspect of the hallux resulting from the pressure applied

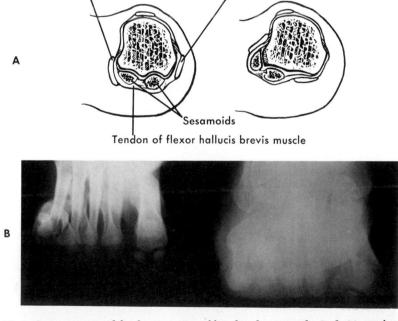

Tendon of Adductor hallucis muscle   Tendon of Abductor hallucis muscle

A

Sesamoids

Tendon of flexor hallucis brevis muscle

B

Fig. 8-20. A, Cross section of the first metatarsal head and sesamoids. Left, Normal relationship between the metatarsal head, the sesamoids, and the tendons crossing the area. Right, Hallux valgus. Note the distortion of structures around the metatarsal head. **B,** Sesamoids. Left, Normal position. Right, Hallux valgus. Note that the fibular sesamoid is in the metatarsal interspace.

to it by its abnormal rotation. A plantar callosity may be observed underneath the second metatarsal head due to the increased weight bearing caused by loss of stability of the first metatarsophalangeal joint. Enlargement of the adventitious bursa over the first metatarsal head can be severe and at times even break down to form a chronic draining sinus. The lesser toes are pushed laterally by the hallux, and at times the hallux will underlap the second toe.

Treatment. Over 100 surgical procedures for the treatment of hallux valgus have been described in the world literature. These vary from simple bunionectomies with capsular plication to more extensive operations such as tendon sectioning or transfers, resections of bony components, arthodeses of joints (particularly the first metatarsocuneiform joint), and osteotomies of the first metatarsal.

Before the surgeon chooses a definitive surgical procedure, he should examine the entire foot carefully, paying particular attention to its weight bearing. The aforementioned predisposing factors of hallux valgus must be carefully sought and evaluated along with the neurocirculatory status of the foot. If the surgeon neglects to evaluate the entire patient and foot properly, both he and the patient may be disappointed in the results of the surgical procedures.

For a complete discussion of treatment procedures, see Chapter 20.

Hallux varus

When the great toe deviates tibialward, the deformity is called hallux varus. The condition can either be congenital or acquired. The congenital type is rare. (See Chapter 4.) The acquired type results from a surgical procedure—usually a McBride bunionectomy—on the metatarsophalangeal joint of the great toe (Fig. 8-22) or from trauma such as avulsion of the adductor hallucis insertion. Besides deviating tibialward, the postoperative hallux varus deformity may also demonstrate extension of the metatarsophalangeal joint and flexion of the interphalangeal joint.

Etiology. The postoperative hallux varus can result from one or more of the following:

1. Overplication of the medial capsular structures
2. Medial displacement of the tibial sesamoid
3. Overpull of the abductor hallucis secondary to transposition of the muscle
4. Failure to properly repair the adductor

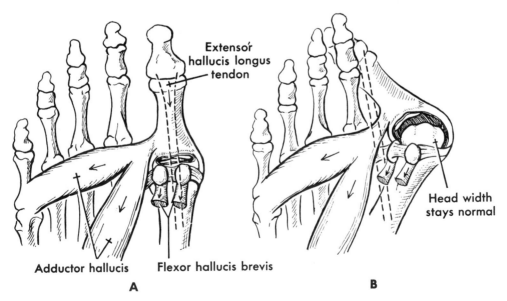

Fig. 8-21. Pathologic anatomy of hallux valgus. **A,** Normal anatomic configuration of the first metatarsophalangeal joint. **B,** Hallux valgus with distortion of anatomic structures around the first metatarsophalangeal joint.

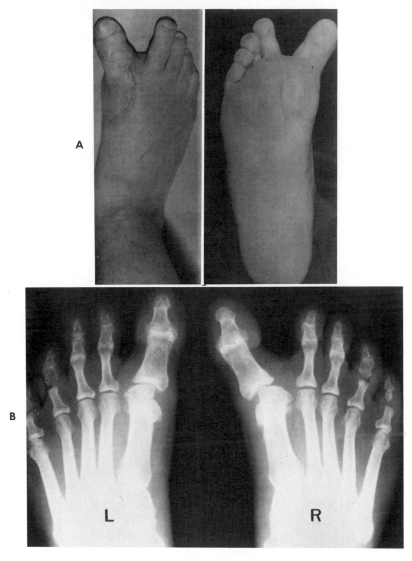

Fig. 8-22. A, Postoperative hallux varus caused by excessive shortening of the abductor hallucis tendon. **B,** Bilateral postoperative hallux varus following a McBride procedure.

tendon after its release from the fibular sesamoid and base of the proximal phalanx

5. Excessive resection of the exostosis from the medial aspect of the metatarsal head

6. Improper postoperative dressing or casts holding the metatarsophalangeal joint in a varus position.

Since no standardized procedure exists to correct all deformities, it is most important in each case of hallux varus that the surgeon carefully evaluate the pathomechanics producing the deformity to determine which corrective procedure to employ. Our experience has been that in some cases a correction of the deformity by a soft tissue procedure is not possible and that arthrodesis of the metatarsophalangeal joint will be necessary to obtain a satisfactory end result. As just mentioned, postoperative hallux varus is usually a complication of a McBride procedure but

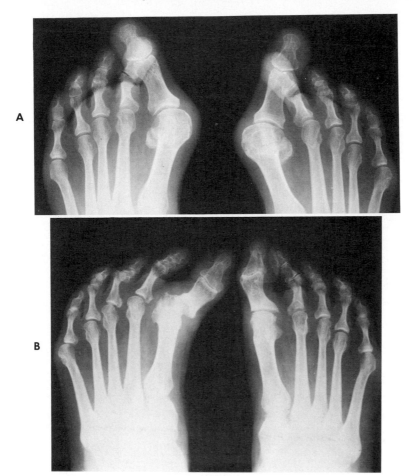

Fig. 8-23. A, Preoperative. Hallux valgus and overlapping second toes. **B,** Two years after a Keller procedure.

hallux varus may ensue after bunion procedures as well (Fig. 8-23).

Treatment

1. If the hallux varus is caused by overplication of the tibial capsular structures, some type of a release of the capsular structures is indicated. Carry this out through an incision on the medial side of the metatarsophalangeal joint, being extremely cautious so as not to interrupt the dorsal and plantar digital nerves; these may be involved in scar tissue. The medial capsule can be released by creating a flap which will slide so the toe can be brought back into a neutral or slight valgus position. Postoperatively it is important to support the great toe in satisfactory alignment for 6 weeks to prevent varus or valgus migration.

2. When the tibial sesamoid has been displaced medialward, replace it if possible under the first metatarsal head. Be extremely careful, however, because excision of the sesamoid, particularly when the fibular sesamoid has been excised, may result in a hallux extensus deformity. Repair of a postoperative hallux varus secondary to medial deviation of the tibial sesamoid can be achieved as follows:

   a. Drill a horizontal hole through the body of the sesamoid.
   b. Free all adhesions holding the sesamoid in its abnormal position.

c. Loop a wire through the hole and around the plantar aspect of the sesamoid.
d. Thread both ends of the wire into a ligature carrier.
e. Pass the ligature carrier under the first and second metatarsal heads and bring it out onto the dorsal aspect of the second interspace.

f. Retrieve both ends of the wire and remove the needle.
g. Fasten wires over a button on the dorsum of the second and third metatarsal heads, using moderate tension (Fig. 8-24, *B*).
h. In about 8 weeks, remove the terminal ends of the wire and the button. The

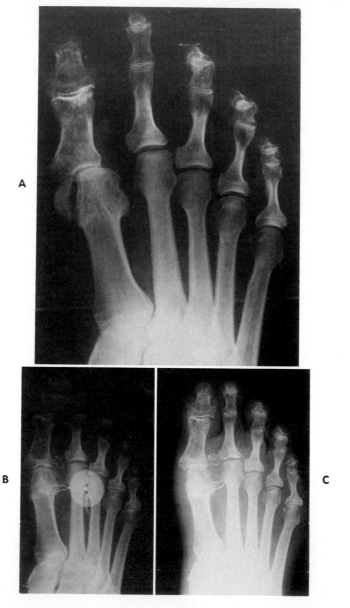

Fig. 8-24. A, Postoperative hallux varus (weight-bearing radiograph). Note the tibial sesamoid lying vertically on the tibial side of the first metatarsal head. **B,** Sesamoid held in normal position by a wire threaded through the body and anchored to a button on the dorsum of the foot. **C,** Two years postoperative. The sesamoid is in position and the hallux varus is corrected.

sesamoid will usually remain in its normal position (Fig. 8-24, *C*).

3. Overpull of the abductor hallucis is usually correctable by lengthening the tendon of the abductor hallucis or removing it from its transplanted position and moving it back onto the proximal phalanx whence it originated. Postoperatively the toe should be supported in proper alignment for 8 weeks.

4. If the hallux varus is secondary to failure to adequately repair the adductor tendon, the repair can be difficult due to the scarring which occurs in the web space between the first and second metatarsals. Remember, in carrying out a McBride procedure, that when the fibular sesamoid is removed and the capsule on the fibular side is released the end of the adductor hallucis is laid across the area of the defect so it will postoperatively help reestablish the continuity of the lateral capsular structures. If the adductor tendon is either cut off or allowed to remain plantarward, adequate scarring of the tissues will not occur and there will not be a competent lateral capsular structure. If the problem is too severe or the hallux varus has recurred,

consider arthrodesing the metatarsophalangeal joint of the great toe.

5. If too much of the metatarsal head has been resected, an arthrodesis of the metatarsophalangeal joint must be done because the stability of the joint has been lost. In the future it may be possible to carry out some type of hinged arthroplasty on the metatarsophalangeal joint; but at the present time we believe an arthrodesis gives the most consistent result.

6. If the varus is due to the position in which the hallux was held by a cast or soft dressing, usually a release of the medial capsular structures will correct the situation.

Hallux rigidus (hallux limitus)

Hallux rigidus, or hallux limitus, is second to hallux valgus in prevalence among disabling deformities of the great toe joint. Indeed, it may be more disabling than hallux valgus because in hallux valgus the patient is distressed mainly by the inability to obtain shoes to accommodate the deformity. In hallux rigidus the patient cannot obtain relief

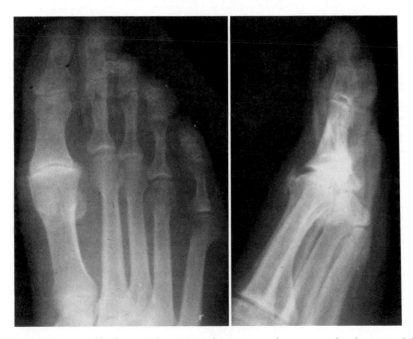

Fig. 8-25. Classic case of hallux rigidus. Note the osseous changes on the dorsum of the first metatarsal head which block dorsiflexion. (See Fig. 8-32, *A*.)

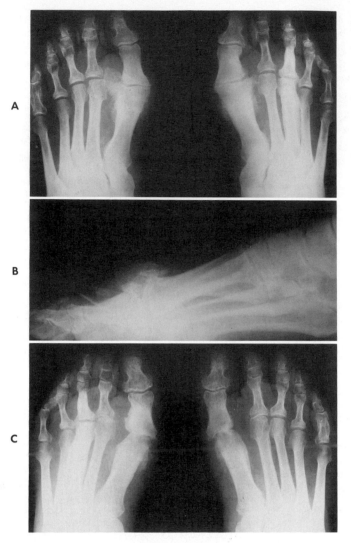

Fig. 8-26. A, Severe case of hallus rigidus secondary to degenerative arthritis. The third metatarsophalangeal joint on the right side also shows degenerative changes. **B,** Note the extensive new growth of bone on the dorsum of the first metatarsophalangeal joint. **C,** After correction by cheilectomy.

even when not wearing shoes because dorsiflexion of the metatarsophalangeal joint of the great toe is severely limited and painful. The main complaint is the pain in the metatarsophalangeal joint of the great toe, which is well localized to the dorsal aspect of the joint. The degree of disability is directly related to the extent of the deformity and the limitation of dorsiflexion.

The pathologic anatomy of hallux rigidus demonstrates degenerative arthritis of the metatarsophalangeal joint of the great toe. As a result the great toe is either fixed in plantar flexion or limited in dorsiflexion because of proliferation of bone around the articular surface of the head of the first metatarsal, particularly on the dorsal aspect. The bony proliferation usually does not involve the plantar surface of the metatarsal head. Not infrequently concomitant degenerative changes are noted about the base of the proximal phalanx (Figs. 8-25 and 8-26). In advanced cases

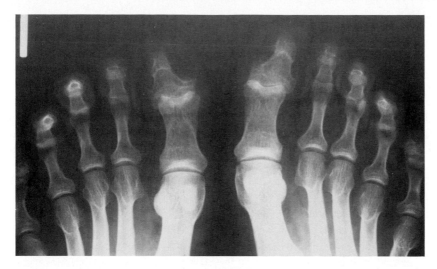

Fig. 8-27. Congenitally flat metatarsal heads of both feet.

the entire hallux is fixed in a plantar attitude, which forces the patient to walk on the outer border of the foot, thereby inverting the ankle and frequently producing secondary changes in the soft tissues and bones of the whole foot.

Etiology. For convenience, hallux rigidus may be divided into three types: (1) congenital (Chapter 4), (2) acquired as a result of traumatic arthritis, and (3) acquired secondary to one of the general arthritides.

Acquired. The acquired type of hallux rigidus is more common than the congenital type. It is essentially a traumatic osteoarthritis resulting from a combination of any of the following factors: (1) intra-articular fracture, (2) osteochondritis dissecans of the first metatarsal head, (3) repeated use of the great toe as a striking or anchor point, (4) extraordinary occupational weight bearing on the great toe joint, (5) a congenitally flat head of the first metatarsal (Figs. 8-27 and 8-28, *B*).

The metatarsophalangeal joint of the hallux has a moderate ball-and-socket articulation, and the periarticular structures have normal resistance to external pressure. If abnormal stress is applied to the hallux by a short and/or a pointed-toe shoe, excessive pressure can be brought against the articular surface of the joint. If the joint has a ball-and-socket type of relationship (Fig. 8-28, *A*), a hallux valgus may result. Conversely, the flatter the articular

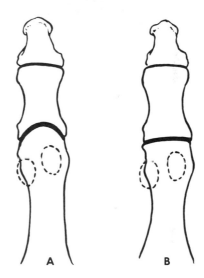

Fig. 8-28. Extreme variations in the shape of the first metatarsal head. **A,** Oval. The medial side of the shoe will force the hallux into a valgus position, producing a hallux valgus. **B,** Flat. The pressure of the side of the shoe cannot push the hallux into valgus but will cause constant trauma to the articular surface of the base of the proximal phalanx and to the head of the first metatarsal. Ultimately a traumatic osteoarthritis will occur, resulting in hallux rigidus.

surface of this joint (Fig. 8-28, *B*) and the more resistant the periarticular structures, the greater will be the pressure applied in an irregular manner; and this pressure may, over a period of time, lead to traumatic osteoarthritis and to a hallux rigidus.

Acquired secondary to one of the general arthritides. Gout and psoriatic or rheumatoid arthritis are likely causes of hallux rigidus. In gout the great toe joint is often the only joint of the foot involved, whereas in rheumatoid and psoriatic arthritis other joints of the foot are also affected. Complete ankylosis of the joint may be consequent to infection after surgical correction for hallux valgus.

From a historical standpoint, other theories have been advanced as to the etiology of hallux rigidus. Mau (1928) believed that an inefficient foot such as a pes valgus or a pes valgoplanus is the forerunner of hallux rigidus. Miller and Arendt (1940) expressed the opinion that hallux rigidus is related to a congenital proximal displacement of the sesamoid. Bingold and Collins (1950) stated it is due to a gait abnormality.

Treatment. Conservative treatment for hallux rigidus is directed toward alleviating the pain at the metatarsophalangeal joint of the great toe and can be accomplished by obtaining a shoe large enough to prevent excessive pressure against the enlarged joint. A stiff-soled shoe will help decrease motion at the metatarsophalangeal joint, thereby alleviating some discomfort. (See Fig. 17-3.) Alleviation can also be accomplished, particularly in adolescence, by placing the patient in a short leg cast, which extends out over the toes, to immobilize the joint for a 4-to-6-week period. Occasionally intraarticular injection of steroid will be of benefit. If conservative methods fail, surgical intervention may be indicated.

Treatment for congenital cases differs because the deformity varies. The faulty articular surface of the joint must be carefully evaluated in each case and an arthroplasty performed so a nearly normal ball-and-socket articular relation will be reestablished between the base of the proximal phalanx and the head of the first metatarsal.

Surgical treatment of hallux rigidus in adults is directed toward establishing a pain-free metatarsophalangeal joint and can be accomplished by arthrodesis of the first metatarsophalangeal joint, which eliminates the motion and hence the pain. Such a procedure has been advocated by Harrison and Harvey

(1963) and by Moynihan (1967). To permit more dorsiflexion of the metatarsophalangeal joint, Kessel and Bonney (1958) recommended a wedge osteotomy on the dorsum of the base of the proximal phalanx to bring the great toe out of its plantar-flexed position and into some dorsiflexion, thereby reducing the pressure against the joint during walking. Procedures to reestablish motion at the metatarsophalangeal joint usually do so at the expense of stability of the joint. The arthroplasty using a Silastic implant in the base of the proximal phalanx has been advocated for this condition. In our experience there have been as many poor results secondary to soft tissue reaction, joint stiffness, and loosening of the prosthesis as there have been satisfactory results with establishment of some dorsiflexion.

DuVries (1965) advocated a cheilectomy for the treatment of hallux rigidus. The procedure is applicable in essentially all acquired types of hallux rigidus and involves removal of the proliferative bone around the metatarsal head, thus allowing dorsiflexion to recur at the joint. With the return of dorsiflexion, the joint pain is effectively eliminated. The procedure has the advantage that if it happens to fail (which occurs in less than 10% of the patients) an arthrodesis can still be easily effected at the metatarsophalangeal joint.

Over a thirty-year period DuVries (1965) performed more than 400 cheilectomies for acquired hallux rigidus. The procedure has given satisfactory results in about 90% of the cases.

The surgical technique of cheilectomy is as follows:

1. Make a longitudinal incision immediately over the first metatarsophalangeal joint on either side of the extensor hallucis longus, extending it from the middle of the proximal phalanx to a point about the middle of the shaft of the first metatarsal.

2. Retract the skin and extensor hallucis longus.

3. Incise the joint capsule longitudinally and free it from the proliferative bone to which it is usually attached; retract the margins.

4. Deliver the head of the first metatarsal

dorsally. Plantar flexion of the great toe at this stage aids delivery (Fig. 8-29, *A*).

5. Observation of the articular surface of the first metatarsal head will demonstrate the outline of the original articular cartilage. Using this as the starting point, remove proliferative bone on the dorsum and sides of the metatarsal head. The bone is often granitelike in consistency. Include some of the normal bone of the head to form an accentuated rounded dorsal surface but never a pointed surface (Fig. 8-29, *B*).

6. Smooth the surface with a rasp. Be sure 45° of extension has been achieved. If the base of the proximal phalanx is also exostotic, remove excess bone and smooth (Fig.8-29, *C* and *D*).

7. Instill 1 ml of steroid into the joint space to help inhibit formation of extensive scar tissue in the capsule.

8. Suture the capsule if possible with fine chromic; close the skin as usual. Apply a compression bandage for 24 hours.

9. Institute gentle motion of the great toe joint on the third or fourth postoperative day, to be increased in vigor and extent daily for 3 months, to prevent formation of adhesions in the periarticular structures. The patient can usually be ambulatory by the second or third postoperative day in a wooden shoe worn for 2 weeks.

In most cases the patient will experience no pain and have satisfactory motion of the great toe joint in about 2 months (Figs. 8-30 to 8-32). Sometimes adhesions form and there is residual limitation of motion after complete

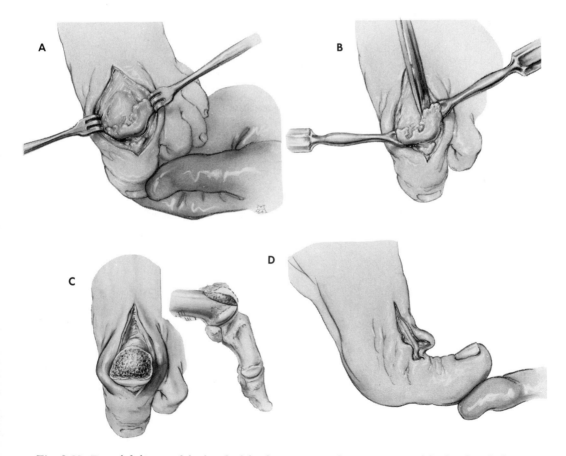

Fig. 8-29. Dorsal delivery of the head of the first metatarsal. **A,** Exposure of the head with the hallux plantar flexed, showing the proliferated bony change. **B,** Removal of excess bone with an osteotome. **C,** Smoothing and rounding the raw bone surface. **D,** Dorsiflexion of the hallux in normal excursion.

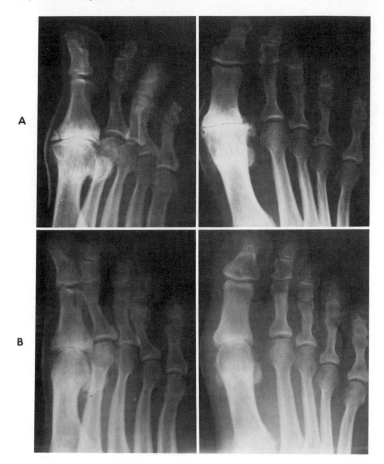

Fig. 8-30. A, Preoperative. Right foot of a 52-year-old man with hallux rigidus. **B,** Postoperative following a cheilectomy.

healing. Although some limitation of motion may be encountered, adequate dorsiflexion is present and will allow the patient to ambulate essentially pain free.

Hallux flexus (dorsal bunion)

Most cases of hallux flexus are the result of hallux rigidus because the bony proliferation on the dorsum of the head of the first metatarsal is so extensive it holds the hallux in a constant plantar-flexed position (Fig. 8-33). Only rarely (because the action of each step normally causes dorsiflexion of the great toe) is the plantar flexion of the great toe maintained by the unopposed pull of the flexor muscles (Fig. 8-34).

Lapidus (1940) classified the different types of hallux flexus or dosal bunion into four groups: (1) cases secondary to hallux rigidus, (2) cases caused by a paralytic deformity of the foot, both flaccid and spastic, (3) cases associated with congenital clubfeet, and (4) cases associated with severe congenital talipes planovalgus (Lapidus attributed this to compensation for a short tendo Achillis).

Hallux flexus has been observed by us in several cases in which there was severe trauma to the foot and ankle region that caused scarring about the flexor hallucis longus and led to its being so bound down as to hold the hallux in a plantar-flexed position. These patients often develop a callus or ulcer on the tip of the great toe due to excessive pressure in this area.

Surgical approach to treatment should be based on an evaluation of the pathologic anat-

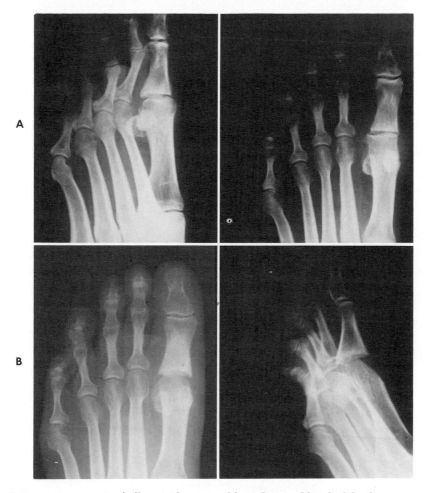

Fig. 8-31. A, Preoperative hallux rigidus caused by a flattened head of the first metatarsal. **B,** Two years after cheilectomy of the first metatarsal head.

omy in each case. When the periarticular structures, including the tendons, are involved, it is sufficient to lengthen tendons that are shortened and shorten tendons that are lengthened. When bony proliferation (hallux rigidus) limits dorsiflexion of the great toe, a cheilectomy of the first metatarsophalangeal joint may be performed.

Hallux extensus

Normally the metatarsophalangeal joint of the great toe is balanced by the pull of the extensor muscles, namely the extensor hallucis longus and extensor digitorum brevis (on the dorsum of the foot) and the flexor hallucis longus and flexor hallucis brevis (on the plantar aspect of the foot). When this balance is disturbed on the plantar aspect, a hallux extensus deformity may result. The etiology of the loss of flexor function can be divided into two groups: (1) following some type of trauma and (2) following surgery about the great toe.

The traumatic type is caused by stepping on a sharp object which lacerates the flexor hallucis longus tendon. Occasionally the flexor hallucis brevis will be completely lacerated, but this is unusual because of its greater breadth. After a foreign body laceration an infection may result in the plantar aspect of

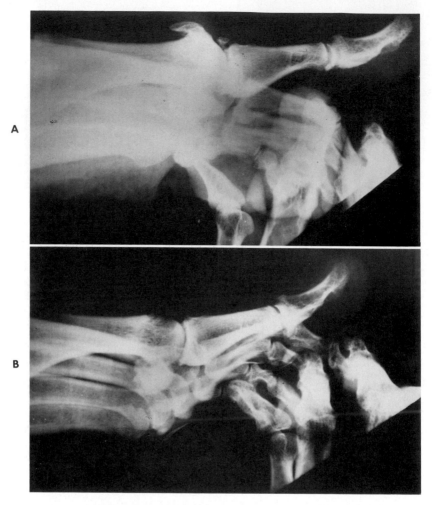

Fig. 8-32. Hallux rigidus; severe dorsal proliferation and joint mouse. **A,** Preoperative; **B,** 8 months postoperative.

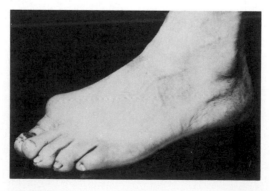

Fig. 8-33. Hallux flexus resulting from a severe hallux rigidus.

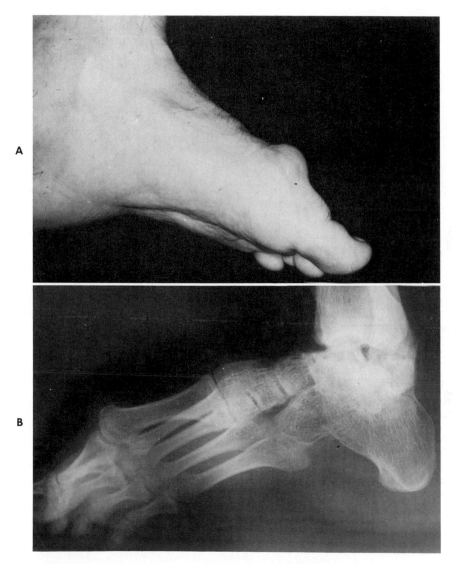

Fig. 8-34. A, Hallux flexus caused by paralysis of the extensors as a result of poliomyelitis. **B,** After a triple arthrodesis.

the foot in the area of the metatarsophalangeal joint and this too can cause the loss of flexor function.

When the hallux extensus follows surgery, it is because the flexor hallucis longus tendon was inadvertently cut while a sesamoid was being excised. If the laceration of the flexor hallucis longus goes unnoticed, a hallux extensus will result. Occasionally if both sesamoid bones are removed during a bunion procedure, the insertion of the flexor hallucis brevis is destroyed and a hallux extensus will result (Fig. 8-35). If the base of the proximal phalanx is removed, as is done in a Keller procedure, again the insertion of the flexor hallucis brevis is destroyed and a hallux extensus may result. The hallux extensus resulting from a loss of function of the flexor hallucis longus tendon is that of dorsiflexion or extension of the metatarsophalangeal joint; if flexor hallucis brevis function is lost, flexion of the interphalangeal joint will occur along with the extension of the metatarsophalangeal joint.

The treatment of an acute hallux extensus—e.g., if the flexor hallucis longus tendon were cut at the time of surgery or as a result of stepping on a sharp object—would be to repair the tendon. This assumes that the tendon is cut in the distal portion of the forefoot. Once the deformity has become established, reattaching the flexor hallucis longus or flexor hallucis brevis tendons is rarely feasible. In these cases a reconstructive procedure must be carried out, depending in part on the etiology of the condition.

If the etiology is loss of the flexor hallucis longus tendon function so the flexor hallucis brevis is still functioning, then a first toe Jones procedure (p. 589), in which the extensor hallucis longus is transposed to the distal head of the first metatarsal, would probably correct the deformity. The interphalangeal joint of the great toe would have to be arthrodesed in this case since there would no longer be any functioning muscle present across the joint. When the metarsophalangeal joint of the great toe has been completely dislocated or severely subluxated or there has been damage due to infection of the metatarsophalangeal joint, one is better off to arthrodese the metatarsophalangeal joint than to attempt a reconstructive procedure.

When the base of the proximal phalanx has been lost and the great toe becomes subluxated dorsally, again an arthrodesis is the procedure of choice; but then possibly a bone graft would have to be added if too much of the

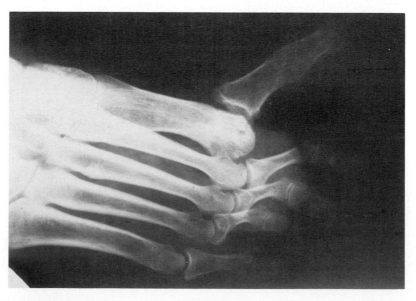

Fig. 8-35. Hallux extensus after excision of both sesamoids with arthrodesis of the interphalangeal joint of the hallux. A Jones tendon transfer reduced the deformity.

proximal phalanx had been surgically removed. At times following the surgical removal of the base of the proximal phalanx as is done in the Keller procedure and when a cock-up or hallux extensus deformity develops, lengthening of the extensor hallucis longus tendon will help bring the great toe down to satisfactory alignment. Occasionally this will have to be accompanied by a capsulotomy to correct the problem.

Tailor's bunion (bunionette)

The term "tailor's bunion" is applied to any enlargement of the fibular side of the fifth metatarsophalangeal joint. In times past, tailors would sit with their legs crossed as they sewed clothes by hand, thereby placing abnormal pressure on the fifth metatarsal head and often causing painful symptoms. Hence the name "tailor's bunion."

The enlargement may be the result of one or a combination of three conditions: (1) hypertrophy of the soft tissue overlying the fifth metatarsophalangeal joint, (2) a congenitally wide dumbbell-shaped fifth metatarsal head (Fig. 8-36, A), or (3) lateral deviation of the fifth metatarsal shaft and head (Fig. 8-36, B).

Etiology. As a result of the prominence of the metatarsal head, regardless of the etiology, increased pressure results over the fifth metatarsophalangeal joint due to the wearing of tight shoes. In response to the pressure over a period of time, a thickened bursa results which becomes progressively more symptomatic. Once this bursa becomes too large, even placing the patient in broad-toed shoes will not adequately correct the problem.

Occasionally, besides lateral deviation of the metatarsal head, some plantar deviation is present. In these cases, along with a developing bursa over the fibular side of the joint, there is an intractable plantar keratosis beneath the metatarsal head.

Symptoms. The overlying bursa becomes painful, swollen, and tender. The symptoms are usually aggravated by wearing any shoe that places pressure on the area and alleviated by going barefoot or cutting out this area of the shoe.

In patients with plantar flexion of the metatarsal shaft and head, an intractable plantar keratosis develops accompanied by subsequent pain and disability.

Treatment. In mild and moderate cases treatment with a broad-toed shoe and sometimes padding will help alleviate the symptoms. In protracted cases, however, operative correction is indicated. In the patient who has a congenitally wide fifth metatarsal head, the recommended surgical procedure is as follows:

1. Make a longitudinal incision over the dorsolateral aspect of the fifth metatarsophalangeal joint, extending it proximally from the middle of the proximal phalanx to the juncture of the middle and distal thirds of the fifth metatarsal. The dorsal cutaneous nerve to the fifth toe should then be identified (Fig. 8-37, A).

2. Retract the skin, subcutaneous tissue, and dorsal cutaneous nerve to expose the joint capsule.

3. Incise the joint capsule longitudinally just dorsal to the insertion of the abductor digiti minimi tendon.

4. Denude the fibular border of its capsule. At this point the dorsal capsular flap may be retracted dorsally and the abductor digiti minimi retracted plantarward to expose the fibular condyle of the metatarsal head.

5. Excise the fibular condylar process longitudinally by means of an osteotome. The sharp edges should be rounded off with a rasp or rongeur (Fig. 8-37, B). Do not excise the adventitious bursa unless excessively thickened. If the bursa is greatly enlarged and needs to be excised, be sure to identify the dorsal cutaneous nerve to the small toe to prevent cutting it when the bursa is removed.

6. Repair the capsule by suturing the dorsal capsule to the abductor digiti minimi (Fig. 8-37, C and D). Failure to do this may result in dislocation of the fifth metatarsophalangeal joint. Figs. 8-38 and 8-39 show the end result of the operation.

When there is a mild intractable plantar keratosis, excision of the plantar condyle is indicated at the time the fibular condyle is

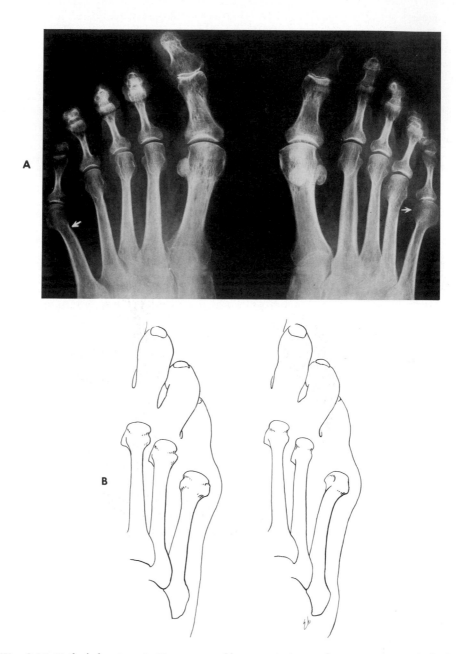

Fig. 8-36. Tailor's bunion. **A,** Two types of bone variation in the same person: Left, Lateral bending at the neck of the fifth metatarsal. Right, wide fifth metatarsal head. **B,** Schematic drawing: left, wide head; right, lateral deviation of the head.

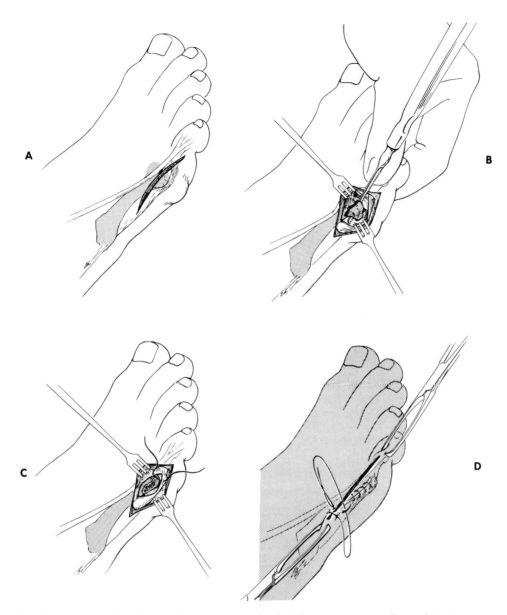

Fig. 8-37. DuVries' technique for correction of tailor's bunion. **A,** Semielliptical incision over the dorsum of the fifth metatarsophalangeal joint. **B,** Skin, capsule, and tendon of the abductor digiti minimi retracted. The fibular condyle of the fifth metatarsal head is excised with a nasal saw or osteotome. **C,** Capsule and tendon of the abductor digiti minimi sutured. **D,** Skin closed.

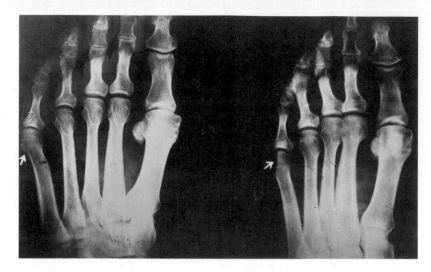

Fig. 8-38. Tailor's bunion. Left, Preoperative lateral deviation of the fifth metatarsal head. Right, Postoperatively.

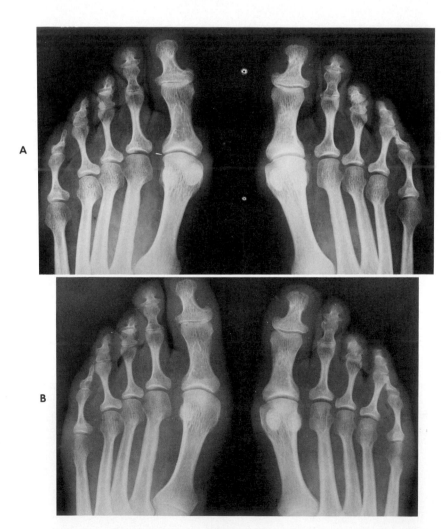

Fig. 8-39. Tailor's bunion caused by a wide fifth metatarsal head. **A,** Preoperative; **B,** postoperative.

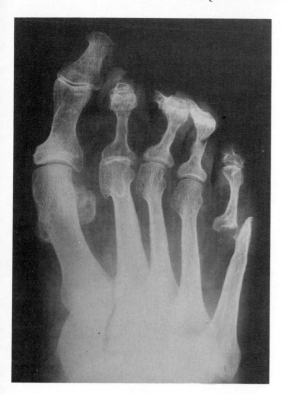

Fig. 8-40. Result of failure to suture the capsule and tendon of the abductor digiti minimi and excessive removal of the head of the fifth metatarsal.

removed. With marked lateral and plantar deviation of the fifth metatarsal shaft, the treatment of choice is osteotomy on an oblique plane to allow the metatarsal head to rise dorsally and at the same time move medialward to narrow the foot.

Occasionally a complication develops because of failure to suture the capsule and tendon of the abductor digiti minimi or because an excess amount of the fifth metatarsal head is removed, or both. This results in an imbalance of the head and a dislocation of the joint (Fig. 8-40). Correction can be accomplished by remodeling the fifth metatarsal head and repairing the capsule and tendon of the abductor digiti minimi tendon on the fibular side of the fifth metatarsophalangeal joint.

DISLOCATIONS OF THE SECOND METATARSOPHALANGEAL JOINT

Dorsal dislocation of the base of the second proximal phalanx (Fig. 8-41, *A*) is common

(Branch, 1937). It is the most frequent static complete dislocation in the forefoot (DuVries, 1956). Isolated dislocations of the other metatarsophalangeal joints are rare (Fig. 8-41, *B*). Partial or complete dislocation of all the lesser metatarsophalangeal joints is sometimes associated with cavus, clawfoot, or a generalized arthritic condition (e.g., rheumatoid arthritis).

Etiology. The etiology of an isolated dislocation of a second metatarsophalangeal joint is in part related to the fact that the second ray (consisting of the second metatarsal and the phalanges) is the longest in the foot. Due to the backward pressure of the shoe against the second toe, which causes the toe to buckle, the proximal phalanx has a tendency to gradually ride up onto the dorsum of the head of the second metatarsal. This results partially from the fact that the base of the proximal phalanx normally sits in slight dorsiflexion relative to the metatarsal head.

Over a period of time with intermittent pressure, a dorsal imbalance of the joint evolves and is accentuated by the two dorsal interossei which insert into each side of the base of the proximal phalanx. Once the joint is imbalanced, the proximal phalanx drifts dorsally and a contracture of the dorsal structures (capsular and extensor tendons) ensues. Occasionally a flattened area develops on the dorsal aspect of the metatarsal head that not infrequently is associated with an advanced hallux valgus deformity (Fig. 8-42, *A*). In these cases the deformity occurs rapidly because the second toe is lifted up by the lateral deviation of the great toe.

Symptoms. The symptoms result because the proximal phalanx sits on top of the head of the metatarsal, causing the toe to strike the top of the shoe and to produce a painful lesion over the proximal interphalangeal joint. The shoe, in turn, forces the dislocated proximal phalanx down against the metatarsal head and into the skin on the plantar aspect of the foot—which then develops a large diffuse intractable plantar keratosis that often becomes extremely symptomatic.

Treatment. If the dislocation is an isolated entity, an open reduction will correct most cases and significantly improve the remainder

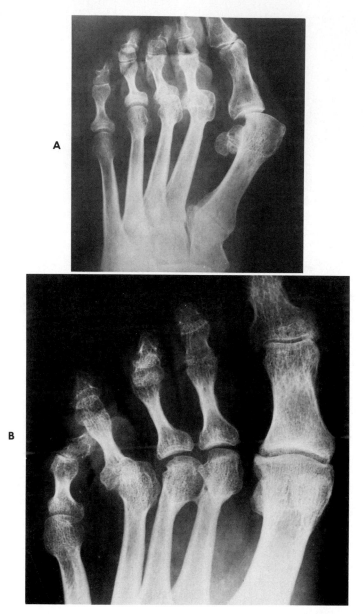

Fig. 8-41. A, Complete static dislocation of the second metatarsophalangeal joint and partial dislocation of the third metatarsophalangeal joint. **B,** Complete static dislocation of the fourth metatarsophalangeal joint.

(Fig. 8-42, *B*). If the dislocation is associated with a hallux valgus deformity, however, unless the hallux valgus is corrected any attempt to correct the dislocated metatarsophalangeal joint will be fruitless.

For the isolated dislocation of the metatarsophalangeal joint the recommended surgical technique is as follows:

1. Make a longitudinal incision starting in the web space and proceeding proximally, extending the incision over the affected metatarsal head and shaft. (A straight incision should not be used over the dorsal aspect of the metatarsophalangeal joint because contracture of the scar could redislocate the joint after correction had been achieved or the toe

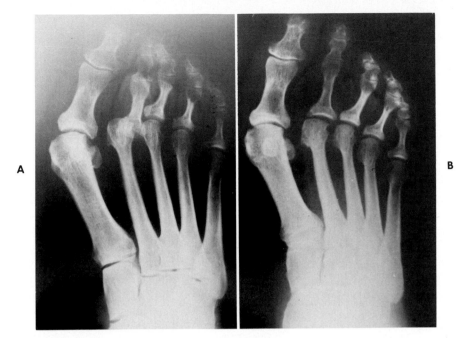

Fig. 8-42. Complete static dislocation of the second metatarsophalangeal joint. **A,** Preoperative; **B,** two years postoperative.

could be elevated dorsally by the contracting scar.)

2. Retract the skin and extensor tendon. In some cases extensor tendons have to be severed or extensively lengthened.

3. Open the capsule longitudinally if possible; however, if there are marked thickening of the capsule and adhesions, the capsule must be sectioned transversely along with the lateral ligaments in order to reduce the dislocation. At times some of the thickened capsule is excised.

4. Reduce the dislocation so that when the ankle joint is brought to neutral position the metatarsophalangeal joint will stay in place without force. If this does not occur, the dorsal contracture has not been sufficiently released to permit complete relocation of the joint. Occasionally a smooth Kirschner wire is needed to hold the joint in place; but there are problems attendant to this, namely breakage of the wire within the joint and possible migration of the wire.

5. Suture the dorsal capsule if feasible and close the skin.

6. Occasionally the dorsal surface of the metatarsal head demonstrates flattening, which precludes maintaining the reduction; then an arthroplasty of the metatarsal head is indicated.

7. The dressing should be applied in such a manner as to hold the metatarsophalangeal joint in proper alignment for a period of 6 weeks.

When this condition is present during repair of a hallux valgus deformity, the surgical procedure should be done through the incision in the first web space.

If a hammertoe is present and associated with the dislocation, no attempt should be made to correct it at the time the dislocation is reduced because the neurovascular structures may have been compromised during the reduction and, if more surgery is done on the toe distal to this, the blood supply to the tip of the toe could be impaired. We tend to wait approximately 8 weeks following reduction of the metatarsophalangeal joint before repairing a hammertoe.

Mallet toe, hammertoe, and clawtoe deformities

Because they are used interchangeably by various authors in describing deformities of the toes, the definitions of mallet toe, hammertoe, and clawtoe deformities have been confused. The nomenclature adopted for this book, we believe, is simple and to a certain extent follows the nomenclature that is used to describe deformities of the fingers. A mallet toe involves the distal interphalangeal joint; i.e., the distal phalanx is flexed on the middle phalanx. A hammertoe involves the proximal interphalangeal joint; the middle and distal phalanges are flexed on the proximal phalanx. In a clawtoe there is dorsiflexion (extension) deformity at the metatarsophalangeal joint associated with a hammertoe deformity.

With regard to the great toe, a hammertoe deformity involves the interphalangeal joint but no mallet toe deformity exists in the hallux (Fig. 8-43). A clawtoe deformity, which is essentially synonomous with a cock-up deformity of the great toe, occurs when there is hyperextension of the metatarsophalangeal joint. All these deformities may be mild and passively correctable at one extreme or rigidly contracted at the other extreme.

Both the mallet toe and the hammertoe deformities are acquired and may occur in one or several toes of the same foot but rarely involve all the toes. The clawtoe deformity is also acquired but usually involves all the toes of the foot, including the great toe (clawfoot).

These deformities occur with varying frequency among different populations but are much more common in shoe-wearing people. Reports dealing with deformities of the forefoot in natives who wear no shoes rarely mention mallet toe, hammertoe, and clawtoe (Engle and Morton, 1931; Wells, 1931; James, 1939; Barnicot and Hardy, 1955).

In various surveys regarding the incidence of these deformities among industrial workers (Creer, 1938), women reserves (Marwil and Brantingham, 1943), and wartime male recruits (Hewitt et al., 1953), the incidence of hammertoe and clawtoe deformities varies from 2% to 20%. All the studies seem to indicate, however, that these deformities develop slowly and insidiously, their incidence in-

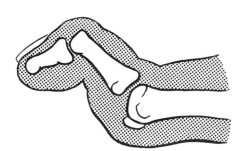

Fig. 8-43. Hammered great toe. Note the articulation of the distal phalanx with the plantar surface of the head of the proximal phalanx.

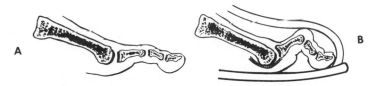

Fig. 8-44. A, Phalanx extended to its normal length. **B,** Buckling of the phalanx caused by restriction of the end of the shoe. Interphalangeal joints and metatarsophalangeal joints become partially dislocated; over time, the dislocation may become fixed.

creasing almost linearly with age. The hammertoe deformity rarely is seen in infants (Higgs, 1931).

Etiology. Shoes generally play the most important role in the direct cause of hammertoe, mallet toe, and clawtoe deformities. As has been stated, for centuries man has usually chosen to cover the forepart of his foot (a modified square) with a shoe whose forepart was in varying degrees triangular or too short. Thus toes have had to conform to a small space and, in order to do so, have buckled dorsally (Figs. 8-44 and 8-45). This fact unquestionably explains why acquired mallet toe and hammertoe are among the most common deformities of the forefoot in shoe-wearing societies. Shoes restrict the normal movements of the joints and impede the actions of the intrinsic muscles of the foot. It must be kept in mind, however, that anatomic predisposing factors vary extensively so a large number of shod people do escape these and other deformities of the forefoot.

The specific etiology of *mallet toe* is unknown, but this deformity is probably secondary to pressure of the toe against the shoe. A

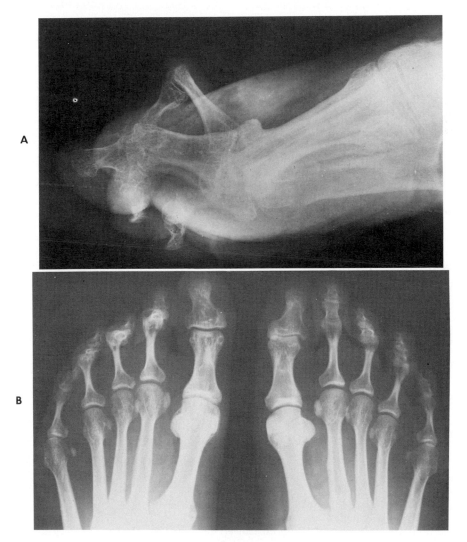

Fig. 8-45. A, Hammered second toe. Note the articulation of the middle phalanx with the plantar surface of the head of the proximal phalanx. **B,** Right foot: hammered third and fourth toes. The second toe is normal. Left foot: hammered second, third, and fourth toes.

mallet toe usually occurs in the second toe and the second ray (which is most often the longest in the foot). Due to pressure against the tip of the shoe, the toe becomes plantar flexed at the distal interphalangeal joint. We have also seen tightness of the flexor digitorum longus tendon in patients who developed a mallet toe deformity, but whether this tightness was a primary or a secondary change in these patients we do not know.

The specific etiology of *hammertoe* is difficult to state with any assuredness. There seem to be several factors.

1. Most commonly the hammertoe is brought about by the prolonged wearing of shoes which are too small and cause the toes to be buckled for a long period of time. High-heeled shoes serve to further aggravate the deformity.

2. At times the hammertoe is due to tightness of the flexor digitorum longus tendon; we believe that when not associated with a joint contracture this condition represents a *dynamic* hammertoe as opposed to the *fixed* hammertoe seen following the continual pressure against the toe by a small shoe. In a dynamic hammertoe, when the ankle joint is brought up into neutral position or slight dorsiflexion, hammering of the toes is produced. If the foot is allowed to drop into plantar flexion, the toes straighten out and there is no deformity present. An argument can be made that this condition is due to tightness of the flexor digitorum brevis tendon, but the fact that it seems to be dependent on the position of the ankle makes the flexor digitorum brevis unlikely to be the basic cause.

3. Hammertoe deformity is associated with

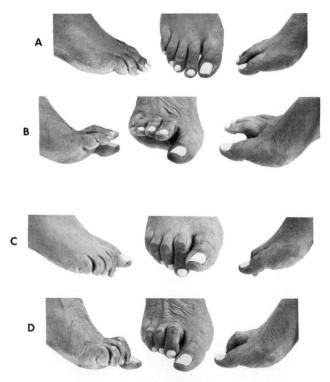

Fig. 8-46. Action of the muscles in clawtoe deformity. Fresh cadaver foot. **A,** At rest. **B,** Tension on the extensor digitorum longus alone. Note the extension of the metatarsophalangeal joints and the minimal extension of the interphalangeal joints. **C,** Tension on the flexor digitorum longus alone. Note that maximal flexion occurs in the interphalangeal joints. **D,** Tension simultaneously on the extensor digitorum longus and flexor digitorum longus. Note the resulting deformities in all but the great toe.

neuromuscular diseases such as cerebral palsy, polio, myelodysplasia, Charcot-Marie-Tooth, and multiple sclerosis; and in these cases it is probably secondary to muscle imbalance.

4. Patients with rheumatoid arthritis may also develop hammertoes, and the deformity is sometimes seen in patients with psoriatic arthritis.

5. Occasionally, following fractures of the tibia, progressive hammering of the toes is observed probably secondary to a compartment syndrome that resulted in ischemia of some of the calf and/or intrinsic muscles of the foot.

The precise etiology of *clawtoe* is as much in doubt as is the etiology of mallet toe and hammertoe. There is no question that simultaneous contracture of the long flexors and extensors of the toes without the modifying action of the intrinsic muscles of the foot causes the typical deformity seen in this condition (as was pointed out by Duchenne in 1867) (Figs. 8-46 and 8-47). Quite obviously the clawtoe deformity is a result of muscle imbalance between the intrinsic and extrinsic musculature. Taylor (1951), however, found no abnormality of the intrinsic muscles in a series of sixty-eight patients with clawtoes when he studied the muscles by gross inspection, stimulation, and microscopic examination of biopsy material.

The clawtoe deformity usually involves multiple toes and frequently both feet. It often occurs with a cavus foot. It can be associated with the same neuromuscular diseases as hammertoes and may be associated with rheumatoid and psoriatic arthritis as well as

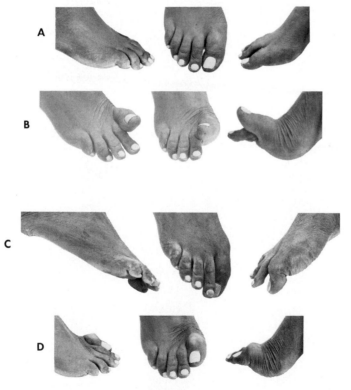

Fig. 8-47. Action of the muscles in clawtoe deformity. Cadaver foot. **A,** At rest. **B,** Tension on the extensor hallucis longus alone. Note the extension of the metatarsophalangeal and interphalangeal joints. **C,** Tension on the flexor hallucis longus alone. Note the maximal flexion in the interphalangeal joint. **D,** Simultaneous tension on the extensor hallucis longus and flexor hallucis longus, with resulting hammertoe deformity.

diabetes. Occasionally the deformity is seen with a mild heel cord contracture. It can itself be either flexible or rigid. The overall condition of clawtoes is often made worse by the fact that the person cannot find an adequate shoe and, as a result, develops a painful bursa over the proximal interphalangeal joint which at times ulcerates (Fig. 8-48).

As the claw deformity becomes more rigid and the toes strike the top of the shoe, the metatarsal heads are forced into the plantar aspect of the foot. As the toes are drawn up onto the metatarsal heads, the fat pad is pulled distally and the metatarsal heads become more prominent on the plantar aspect of the foot. These can result in painful plantar callosities which may ulcerate in severe cases, particularly if sensation to the foot is impaired.

Treatment. In the treatment of the aforementioned toe deformities, many factors must be taken into consideration. The young patient whose deformity is not fixed should be treated by conservative measures. The most important conservative measure is to get the patient into a broad-toed shoe, preferably with a crepe sole. This avoids pressure on the toes and the development of painful callosities. The shoe itself may be modified by using

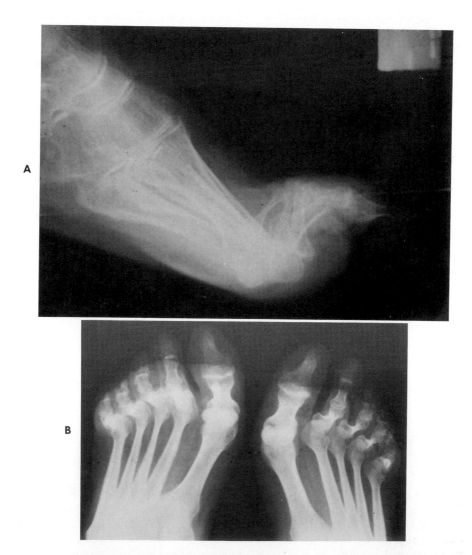

Fig. 8-48. **A,** Dorsal dislocation of all interphalangeal and metatarsophalangeal joints in clawtoe deformity. **B,** Clawing of all toes.

a metatarsal bar to relieve metatarsal head pressure. The use of an extra-depth shoe (with a Plastizote insole), to distribute pressure equally on the plantar aspect of the foot is helpful. The patient should also be started on a program of daily manipulation of the toes to help keep them flexible.

Unfortunately, with time, and even with good conservative management, most of these deformities become fixed and often require surgical correction. We believe it most important that if surgery is required the procedure be carefully selected depending on the specific etiology of the deformity.

Additional discussions of treatment for these conditions, including presentations of surgical technique for correction of hammered toes, can be found on pp. 588 to 596.

MORTON'S SYNDROME

A short first metatarsal, a hypermobile first metatarsal segment, and posterior displacement of the sesamoids comprise the syndrome described by Morton (1935). Not to be confused with Morton's neuralgia, this syndrome causes hypertrophy of the second metatarsal, tenderness at the base of the second metatarsal, and callosities under the heads of the second and third metatarsals. Morton observed that a high percentage of weak feet and feet with metatarsalgia are directly related to the syndrome. He thought that the hypermobility of the first metatarsal bones was caused by their shortness, which permits abnormally free motion in the joint between the first cuneiform and the navicular and between the first and middle cuneiforms. The resulting instability is reflected in malfunction of the metatarsal and of the longitudinal arch of the foot.

Statistical studies by Hawkes (1914), among others, regarding the relative length of the metatarsals had demonstrated that in about 80% of human feet the first metatarsal is shorter than the second. This is in agreement with Jones (1944), who stated: "The only alternative is to assume that there is such a thing as ideal foot function and that this function could presumably be carried out by an ideal but not by the normal foot."

Harris and Beath (1949) took issue with Morton's interpretation; nevertheless, in 1952 Morton again supported and enlarged his theory.

ACQUIRED NONTRAUMATIC DISORDERS OF THE CALCANEUS
Haglund's disease (prominent posterosuperior tuberosity of the calcaneus) and related conditions

Haglund (1928) appears to have been the first to call attention to the possible relationship between the shape of the calcaneus and the appearance of pump bumps, tendo Achillis bursitis, retrocalcaneal bursitis, and small spurs at the attachment of the tendo Achillis. Saxl (1929) emphasized that if the upper surface of the tuberosity of the calcaneus was too prominent the soft tissues were compressed between the counter of the shoe and the underlying bone, thus producing the variety of conditions just mentioned. Both surgeons recommended that the upper posterior lip of the calcaneus be surgically removed if chronic irritation persisted in spite of shoe modifications (Fig. 8-49).

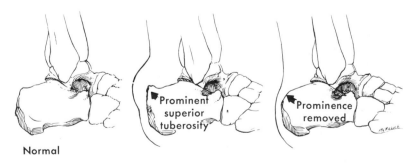

Normal

Fig. 8-49. Normally shaped calcaneus; prominent superior tuberosity (Haglund's disease) removal of the posterior lip of the calcaneus in Haglund's disease.

Anatomically the posterosuperior tuberosity of the calcaneus may be variously shaped (Fig. 8-50). Occasionally it is markedly prominent (Figs. 8-50, A, and 13-20); and when it is, it usually results in constant pain when the patient wears shoes. Hohmann (1948) referred to such a prominence as Haglund's disease.

A congenital anomaly of the posterior tuberosity of the calcaneus (Fig. 8-51) can lead to painful symptoms from the pressure of shoes. At times a tendo Achillis bursitis is produced, which may result in a subdermal enlargement immediately above the tendo Achillis insertion. The condition is caused by prolonged pressure from the upper margin of the shoe counter. Any extraordinary shape or a prominent posterosuperior border of the calcaneus (see Fig. 13-20) is usually the predisposing cause.

Fowler and Philip (1945) called attention to the association of such a prominence with bursitis above the tendo Achillis. They not only related the shape of the tuberosity to the development of these painful lesions but also considered the significance of the angle made between the posterior surface and the plantar surface of the calcaneus (Fig. 8-52) as seen on the lateral radiograph. The normal range of the angle is between 44° and 69°. If the angle

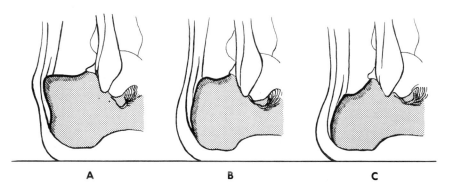

Fig. 8-50. Variations in shape of the superior tuberosity of the calcaneus. **A,** Hyperconvex (so-called Haglund's disease); **B,** normal; **C,** hypoconvex.

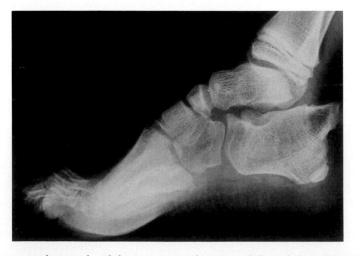

Fig. 8-51. Congenital anomaly of the posterior tuberosity of the calcaneus; painful from the pressure of shoes.

is too great (above 75°), abnormal pressures are likely to occur.

Although Keck and Kelly (1965) expressed concern as to the possibility of measuring this angle accurately, they stated that their cases demonstrated angles between 70° and 80°. From their series of twenty-six heels which were symptomatic just above the tendo Achillis insertion, they concluded that an abnormally large protuberance of the posterosuperior tuberosity of the calcaneus was a basic cause in these cases of tendo Achillis and retrocalcaneal bursitis. The vertical contour of the shoe counter is almost always semielliptical; therefore, when the posterosuperior margin of the heel bone is prominent, the upper margin of the counter constantly irritates the soft tissues over the prominence, producing hypertrophic changes. The condition usually becomes symptomatic in adolescence, before massive hypertrophy of the soft tissues develops.

For surgical treatment of these conditions, see Chapter 19.

Calcaneal spurs of the plantar tuberosity

A heel spur is an osteophytic outgrowth just anterior to the plantar tuberosity of the calcaneus, extending along its entire width for about 2 to 2.5 cm. The apex of the spur is embedded in the plantar fascia, directly anterior to its origin. The condition may exist without symptoms, or it may become painful, even disabling.

Calcaneal spurs are of three types:

1. Large but symptomless because the angle of growth is such that the spur does not become a weight-bearing point; or large but with inflammatory changes that have been arrested so the condition is disclosed only incidentally during radiographic examination of the foot for some other purpose.

2. Large and painful on weight bearing because the pitch of the calcaneus has been altered by a depression of the longitudinal arch, the spur thus becoming a weight-bearing point.

3. Having only a rudimentary proliferation and an irregular jagged outline accompanied by an area of decreased density around the origin of the plantar fascia, indicating a subacute inflammatory process (Fig. 8-53).

All calcaneal spurs undoubtedly begin as the third type; but only a few become symptomatic at that stage, because only in them are the etiologic factors acute.

Etiology. Before the availability of radiography, reports of painful heels had appeared sporadically in the medical literature but it was difficult to determine the cause of the pain until radiographs demonstrated an exostosis located at the calcaneal attachment of the plantar fascia.

Why at that time clinicians assumed an infectious agent rather than a mechanical factor to be the cause is not clear but, in any

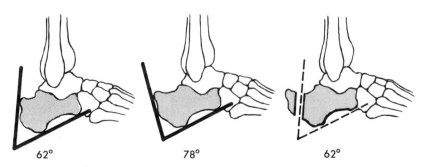

62°   78°   62°

Fig. 8-52. Variation in angles of the posterosuperior tuberosity of the calcaneus (observations of Fowler and Philip). Left, Normal. Center, Prominence predisposing to tendo Achillis bursitis. Right, Prominence excised. (Modified from Keck, S. W., and Kelly, P. J.: J. Bone Joint Surg. **47A**:267, 1965.)

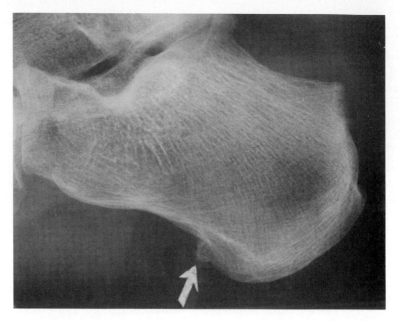

Fig. 8-53. Heel spur undergoing subacute inflammation.

event, Baer (1906) declared that "it seems fairly certain that we must consider the gonococcus to be the etiological factor in a great number of cases." He based this statement on his experience with six patients who had painful calcaneal spurs, all of whom had a history of gonorrhea. In one, a positive culture of gonococcus was obtained, and in two others cocci were demonstrated in the microscopic sections of the excised bone.

Baer's statement was accepted as truth for the next quarter of a century. As late as 1932 Liberson wrote: "The painful heel of gonorrhea is due to both bony exostosis and the soft tissue infiltration over it." Later writers suggested infectious diseases and trauma as causes of spur formation. Blokhin and Vinogradova (1937) reported thirty-three cases in which arteriosclerosis, gonorrhea, and syphilis were not at all causative. The spur resulted from functional overuse and/or an abnormality of the bones of the foot. The hereditary factor was suggested by Gould (1942), who reported exostosis of the heel in the father of six children; the third child, a son, had a spur. That son had four children, of whom the second child, a boy, had a heel spur. Gould suggested that the abnormality passed down

through the male side. Davis and Blair (1950) reported fifteen cases of calcaneal spurs associated with Strümpell-Marie disease.

In considering the differential diagnosis of symptomatic calcaneal spurs, the examiner should bear in mind the following conditions: rheumatoid arthritis, Reiter's syndrome, and gout.

Anatomically the plantar aponeurosis arises from the tuberosity of the calcaneus, passes forward, divides into five bands, and inserts into the base of the proximal phalanx; here it is continuous with the periosteum. During normal gait, as the body passes forward onto the toes the toes are forced into dorsiflexion pulling the plantar aponeurosis over the metatarsal heads (Hicks, 1954). This action of winding the plantar aponeurosis over the metatarsal head has been likened to a windlass mechanism (Fig. 8-54) and produces a greal deal of stress on the origin of the plantar aponeurosis. Over a long period of time, proliferative bony changes at the origin of the fascia may lead to formation of a spur.

Diagnosis. The principal symptom is pain of varying degree which is aggravated by weight bearing. It is usually well localized and does not involve the entire plantar surface of

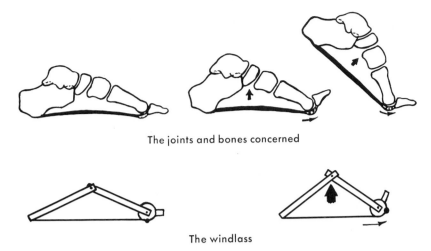

The joints and bones concerned

The windlass

Fig. 8-54. Windlass mechanism of the aponeurosis and the metatarsal head.

the heel. Rarely does it radiate from the heel area.

Physical examination demonstrates that on palpation the entire plantar surface of the heel may be tender but the point of maximum tenderness is usually just anterior and medial to the calcaneal tuberosity. This tender region may be pinpointed radiographically immediately beneath the spur.

In the early stages, fibrositis of low chronicity with or without pain anterior to the calcaneal tuberosity represents the pathologic change. Continuation of the process leads to osteophytic changes and bone deposits on the sulcus just anterior to the tuberosity. The accumulation of new bone is self-limiting; the final spur varies greatly in size and shape but mostly has a triangular bar shape. Occasionally an unusually shaped and painful spur is encountered (Fig. 8-55) which requires special evaluation.

In rare instances symptoms are caused by osteolytic changes in the plantar tuberosity itself (Fig. 8-56). These symptoms can become very disabling, and each case must be given careful study. Conservative measures, such as mechanical appliances for weight distribution, are used in the treatment of this disorder. Intractable cases require that the entire plantar tuberosity be excised surgically.

The usual mediolateral radiographic appearance of the spur is pointed like a tack but extending over the entire width of the tuberosity.

Treatment. Most calcaneal spurs are asymptomatic and do not require treatment. The major etiology of symptomatic spurs is believed to be mechanical, and many spurs do indeed respond to measures that reduce the forces acting on the plantar aponeurosis. Proper footwear which will decrease the impact at initial floor contact, such as a crepe sole, may be useful. A thick rubber sponge heel appliance with a sulcus to accommodate the heel spur is often helpful.

Reduction of the forces can further be accomplished by taping the foot into adduction and inversion to decrease the tension on the plantar aponeurosis. Similar reduction of stress can be achieved with shoe wedges, UCBL inserts, and other appliances that help invert the heel within the shoe.

If conservative measures fail to provide sufficient relief, anti-inflammatory medications such as phenylbutazone, indomethacin, and salicylates are often helpful. If medication fails to bring adequate relief, local injection of steroid with or without procaine from a plantar approach may be beneficial. Occasionally ultrasound has been successful in resistant cases. Some cases are very resistant to treat-

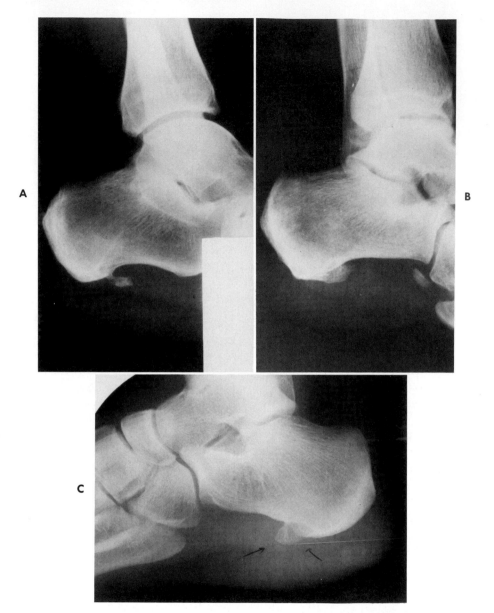

Fig. 8-55. Unusually shaped spurs requiring special evaluation. **A** and **B,** Painful spurs. **C,** Osseous cyst at the origin of the plantar fascia.

ment, whereas others respond well but have periodic recurrences.

Surgical excision of the spur has been performed in patients who have intractable pain that is unrelieved by conservative treatment. In our experience not more than 50% of these patients get prompt and permanent relief from the surgical procedure.

For a more complete discussion of treatment procedures, see Chapter 19.

Calcaneal spurs and osteosclerosis of the posterior tuberosity

Occasionally the surgeon encounters an abnormal insertion of the tendo Achillis that is probably caused by an inward angulation of

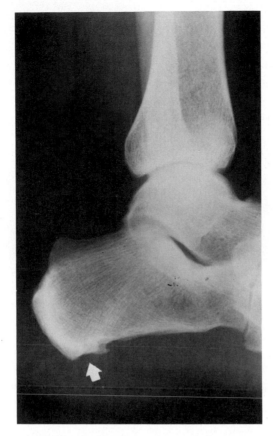

Fig. 8-56. Painful heel caused by osteolytic changes of unknown etiology in the plantar tuberosity of the calcaneus; asymptomatic.

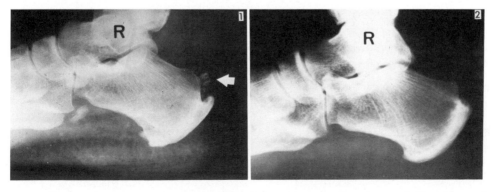

Fig. 8-57. Calcaneal spurs and osteosclerosis of the posterior tuberosity caused by abnormal insertion of the tendo Achillis. Note the presence of osteophytes in the retrocalcaneal bursa in *1*.

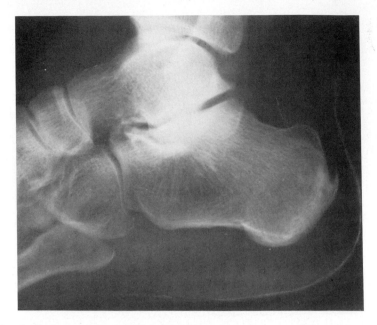

Fig. 8-58. Spur in the middle of the posterior tuberosity of the calcaneus.

the lower half of the posterior tuberosity. This angulation causes the tendo Achillis to begin its insertion at an abnormally low point; it creates an unusually deep retrocalcaneal bursa as well. Abnormal traction on the lower half of the posterior tuberosity produces a reactive osteosclerosis and the formation of a spur (Fig. 8-57). The hard leather counters of shoes undoubtedly aggravate these conditions and cause them to become painful. A sharp spur may form in the middle of the posterior tuberosity of the calcaneus (Fig. 8-58).

Only in rare instances are surgical procedures indicated. Usually if the patient avoids wearing shoes with hard and rigid counters (the part of the shoe that covers the posterior tuberosity must be made of soft leather), the symptoms will dissipate.

FLATFOOT (PES PLANUS) IN ADULTS

Flatfoot, weak foot, or fallen arches, as the disorder is variously called, is difficult to classify. There is no known standard by which the longitudinal arch may be considered flat, normal, or high. Some primitive peoples in Africa and Australia are all flatfooted; when they have painful feet, it is only as a result of injuries. In our modern society, however, many people with so-called normal arches experience pain on weight bearing.

Many people with flatfoot can walk as comfortably and as easily as others who have so-called normal arches, yet for some reason a myth exists that people with flatfoot will have difficulty with their feet. During World War II, thousands of men were rejected from the U.S. Army because they had asymptomatic flatfoot. Athletes with flatfoot (some long-distance runners, particularly) are not impeded by the condition. With few exceptions, black people have flatfoot at an early age but later usually develop strong "normal" arches. Perhaps one out of a thousand people with flatfoot will have pain from the condition because of congenital or acquired abnormalities (DuVries, 1967).

A precise classification of flatfoot deformities is difficult, but the following may be useful generally:

1. Flatfoot—congenital type
   a. Asymptomatic flexible flatfoot
   b. Symptomatic flexible flatfoot
   c. Peroneal spastic flatfoot
   d. Flatfoot secondary to an accessory navicular (prehallux)

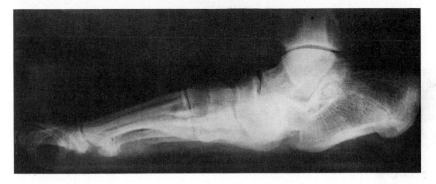

Fig. 8-59. Symptomatic severe flatfoot (rocker-bottom foot); required major stabilization.

e. Old congenital deformity (e.g., congenital vertical talus)

f. Associated with a generalized dysplasia (e.g., Marfan's syndrome)

2. Flatfoot—acquired type

a. Trauma

(1) Dysfunction of the subtalar joint secondary to a fracture

(2) Rupture of the posterior tibial tendon

b. Generalized arthritic condition (e.g., rheumatoid arthritis)

c. Neuromuscular imbalance (e.g., cerebral palsy, polio)

Flatfoot—congenital type

Asymptomatic flexible flatfoot

The asymptomatic flexible flatfoot does not require any treatment.

Symptomatic flexible flatfoot

It has always been somewhat puzzling to us why two feet which seem to be identical by both physical and x-ray examination can present two distinct clinical pictures. Why one flexible flatfoot is symptomatic and another is asymptomatic can be a perplexing and frustrating problem for the patient and the physician. This is particularly true if the patient has previously had an asymptomatic flatfoot. If, however, the patient gives a history of progressively recurring discomfort, it behooves the physician to make every effort to ascertain the etiology of the flatfoot condition.

Occasionally the patient will give a history of a radical change in work habits, such as increased standing for long periods of time on a hard floor or possibly having sustained an injury to the foot. As a result of some foot discomfort, the patient will often start to walk in an abnormal manner which will secondarily cause a strain on other areas of the foot. This type of problem can occur in a normal foot as well as in a flatfoot, although the flatfoot seems to be somewhat more prone to becoming symptomatic.

The history obtained from the patient is that the feet ache with weight bearing of greater than 2 or 3 hours. The pain is dull and poorly localized. The symptoms are usually aggravated by prolonged weight bearing and activities and relieved by getting off the feet.

The physical findings may demonstrate a normal-appearing arch when the patient is sitting on the examination table, but there is flattening of the longitudinal arch with weight bearing (Fig. 8-59). An associated valgus of the heel (Fig. 8-60) and abduction of the forefoot are noted. When the patient is asked to stand on his toes, the heel inverts normally. The range of motion of the subtalar joint may be somewhat increased, particularly in eversion; and the range of motion of the transverse tarsal joint is likewise increased, particularly into abduction (Fig. 8-61). There may be a decrease in ankle dorsiflexion due to tightness of the tendo Achillis. The motor function about the foot and ankle is normal.

Treatment of the symptomatic flexible flatfoot in adults should be conservative. It is most important to obtain an adequate shoe for the patient to wear. The use of a Thomas heel to support the talonavicular joint may be of

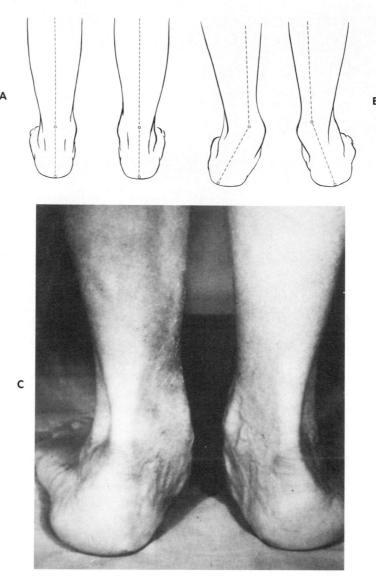

Fig. 8-60. A, Tendo Achillis in vertical line. **B,** Valgus heel. The tendo Achillis lies laterally behind the lateral malleolus. **C,** Patient with valgus heel. (**C** courtesy Dr. Milton Lewis.)

benefit. Various other shoe corrections, such as medial lift to help tilt the calcaneus into varus, may also be useful. Corrections within the shoes consist of felt, leather, metal, or plastic arch supports. Any shoe correction should be made gradually to allow the foot time to accommodate. It is ill-advised to start out hastily with an expensive plastic insert.

In the more acute cases adhesive strapping to hold the foot in an adducted and inverted position along with a felt arch support will often give satisfactory results. Occasionally the use of a short leg cast with a well-molded arch will benefit the patient.

If all methods of conservative treatment fail and the patient continues to be extremely symptomatic, consideration can be given to a double or triple arthrodesis. It should be kept in mind, however, that these procedures place increased stress on the ankle joint and

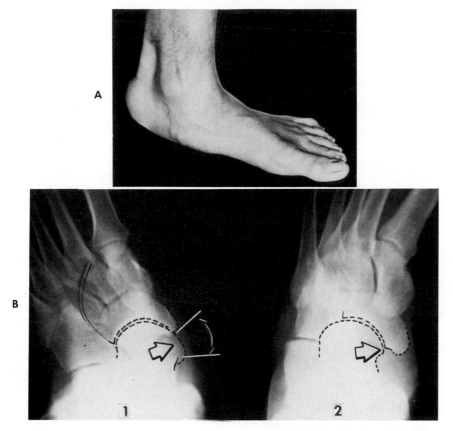

Fig. 8-61. A, Flatfoot with eversion and abduction of the forefoot in a 43-year-old man. **B,** Demonstration of, *1,* abduction and, *2,* extreme adduction in this man. Note the excursion of the navicular over the head of the talus.

this may become a source of further discomfort to the patient. (A brief discussion of treatment appears on p. 556.)

Peroneal spastic flatfoot

Etiology. The rigid type of peroneal spastic flatfoot in adults is often the end result of the flexible type.

Harris and Beath (1948) believed that the rigid type was always caused by an anomalous talocalcaneal bridge or by a calcaneonavicular bar (Figs. 8-62 to 8-64). Webster and Roberts (1951) supported this theory. A tarsal coalition can initially begin as a fibrous lesion and then in time progress to a cartilaginous, and finally to an osseous, lesion (Cowell, 1972). This is probably why some cases are initially flexible and then become rigid. There are also secondary bone changes in the subtalar and trans-

verse tarsal joints which also contribute to the progressive rigidity of the foot.

The etiology of the peroneal spasm per se is unknown except that it is probably a compensatory reflex spasm secondary to irritation of the subtalar joint mechanism.

We have seen several cases of acquired peroneal spastic flatfoot in adults in which no etiology could be found. In several of these patients, after failure of conservative treatment a subtalar arthrodesis was undertaken. At the time of surgery, early degenerative changes were noted in the posterior facet of the subtalar joint; however, the etiology for the onset of this problem could not be identified.

Symptoms. The patient with a peroneal spastic flatfoot will usually complain of pain in the hindfoot associated with a progressively

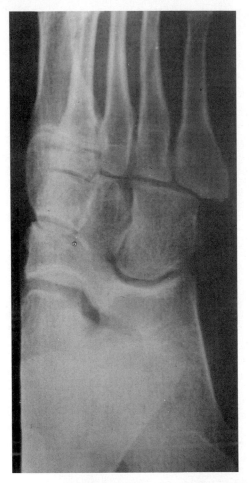

severe flatfoot deformity. He rarely can relate information that will aid in determining the etiology of the condition.

Physical examination. The physical findings demonstrate marked flattening of the longitudinal arch with eversion of the heel. When the patient is asked to stand on his toes, he is unable to invert the heel and it remains everted. The range of motion of the subtalar joint is either absent or considerably restricted. The calcaneus may be held rigidly in an everted position. Spasm of the peroneal tendon may be noted, and occasionally clonus can be elicited by strongly and sharply inverting the heel.

Treatment. The treatment in the adult patient whose foot can be brought back to neutral position or to slight varus is immobilization in a short-leg walking cast for a period of 6 weeks. Approximately 50% of patients will respond to this form of treatment, and in some cases it will have to be repeated. In patients whose foot cannot be brought to neutral, a general anesthetic is necessary for proper

Fig. 8-62. Calcaneonavicular bar completely ossified (synostosis).

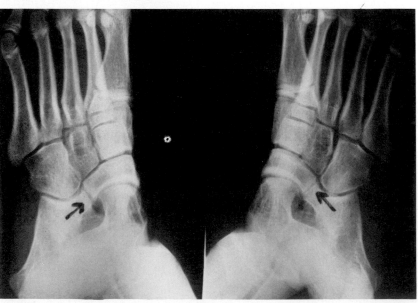

Fig. 8-63. Calcaneonavicular synchondrosis.

alignment and the application of a short-leg walking cast.

In the patient whose foot is very rigid with extensive secondary changes present in the subtalar and talonavicular joint, treatment by immobilization in a short-leg walking cast is much less successful. A molded leather ankle brace with medial and lateral metal stays to immobilize the foot and ankle may be of some benefit. If conservative measures fail to give adequate relief, a triple arthrodesis is indicated.

Flatfoot secondary to an accessory navicular (prehallux)

In some patients with a prehallux the normal support of the longitudinal arch by the posterior tibial tendon is inefficient. Kidner (1929) pointed out that this is because the posterior tibial tendon inserts into the prehallux, which is connected to the navicular by a fibrous union, and at other times the prehallux acts as an irritation to the posterior tibial tendon, causing it to reflexly lose function.

Symptoms. An accessory navicular becomes symptomatic much more frequently during adolescence than during adult life. In adults who have been previously asymptomatic, a history of trauma to the foot and ankle,

usually in the form of a twisting injury, is elicited. The patient will complain of pain which is fairly well localized over the prominence on the medial side of the foot. The pain is often caused by the rubbing of the shoe against the prominence, but at times the patient experiences discomfort in the longitudinal arch.

Physical examination. The physical findings demonstrate a prominence on the medial side of the tarsal navicular bone. There is often local irritation of the skin, and a bursa is noted over the prominence. Approximately half the patients with an accessory navicular have a normal arch, and half demonstrate some loss of height of the longitudinal arch. Palpation usually causes discomfort. The function of the posterior tibial tendon, secondary to pain, is somewhat weak. When the patient stands, there may be further flattening of the longitudinal arch. The range of motion of the ankle, subtalar, and transverse tarsal joints is normal.

Treatment. Treatment of the symptomatic accessory navicular is initially conservative and consists of immobilization in a short-leg walking cast, use of anti-inflammatory medications, and occasionally an injection of steroid into the area of maximum pain and

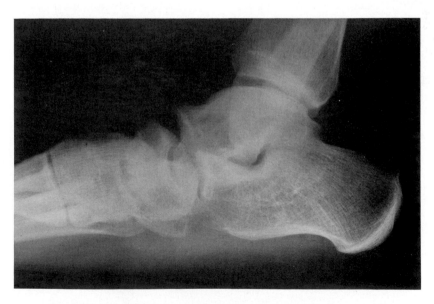

Fig.8-64. Planovalgus caused by congential talonavicular anomaly.

tenderness. If conservative measures fail, a Kidner procedure will usually give a satisfactory result (p. 107).

Miscellaneous types of congenital flatfoot

The flatfoot deformity associated with an old congenital or generalized dysplasia rarely becomes sufficiently symptomatic to cause the patient to seek orthopaedic attention. If help is sought, however, the conservative measures just enumerated are applicable. If the foot remains symptomatic, some type of stabilization procedure is indicated.

Flatfoot—acquired type
Trauma

Dysfunction of subtalar joint. Occasionally following a fracture that extends into the posterior facet of the subtalar joint, a progressive flatfoot deformity will develop. Again the conservative treatment outlined earlier in this section should be applied; but if this fails, stabilization of the subtalar joint is indicated.

Rupture of posterior tibial tendon. From whatever cause, this usually leads to the rapid development of a severe symptomatic flatfoot deformity. The etiology should be suspected whenever a unilateral pes planus rapidly appears. These ruptures usually occur in middle-aged persons and are usually spontaneous although they may follow minor trauma or possibly an injection of steroids into the sheath of the posterior tibial tendon.

The physical examination will demonstrate that there is weakness of inversion of the foot. When the patient is asked to rise on his toes, he will find it difficult to do so on the involved side and there will be little or no inversion of the heel.

Treatment. The methods of treatment are dependent on the age of the patient and the acuteness of the rupture. In a young active individual with an acute rupture, surgical correction consisting of repair or reconstruction of the posterior tibial tendon is indicated. (Goldner et al., 1974). In the older less active individual, surgical stabilization by a subtalar or triple arthrodesis may be indicated.

Generalized arthritic condition (e.g., rheumatoid arthritis)

Patients with rheumatoid arthritis can develop a progressively severe flatfoot deformity due to the loss of integrity of the ligamentous structures about the longitudinal arch as well as the joints of the hindfoot. This type of flatfoot occurs insidiously over a period of years and is rarely symptomatic until a severe deformity is present.

Conservative treatment for the problem consists of using a UCBL insert to control the hindfoot. A short leg brace with a medial T strap can also be useful.

Unfortunately the generalized arthritides are most resistant to conservative measures, and a subtalar or triple arthrodesis is indicated if the patient is sufficiently symptomatic.

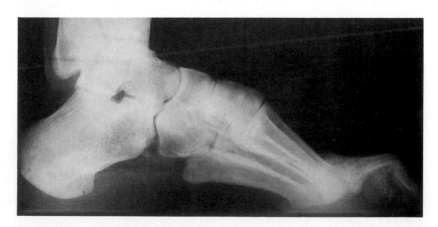

Fig. 8-65. Clawfoot. Note the high longitudinal arch and the contracture of all the toes.

Neuromuscular imbalance (e.g., cerebral palsy, polio)

A slow progressive type of flatfoot deformity can result from a neuromuscular imbalance of the foot, such as that associated with cerebral palsy and polio. Although quite deformed, the foot is rarely symptomatic. The imbalance is usually associated with tightness of the heel cord, a mild rocker-bottom type of foot, and often a hallux valgus. This deformity has been acquired over a period of many years secondary to tightness of the tendo Achillis as well as to spasticity of the calf muscles concomitant with cerebral palsy and secondary to muscle imbalance and ligamentous laxity following poliomyelitis.

The foot is usually not symptomatic; but if it is symptomatic, conservative measures will produce a satisfied patient. Surgery in this type of flatfoot is reserved only for symptomatic cases.

Treatment would include a triple arthrodesis and possible lengthening of the tendo Achillis in the patient with cerebral palsy and a triple arthrodesis and possible tendon transfer in the patient with poliomyelitis. It must be kept in mind, however, that any hindfoot stabilization procedure results in increased stress on the ankle joint.

CLAWFOOT

Clawfoot, also known as hollow foot, pes cavus, or pes arcuatus, is a distinct deformity (Fig. 8-65) that begins after the age of 3 years and differs from congenital talipes equinus or calcaneus as well as from paralytic pes calcaneocavus ("posterior pes cavus"). Characteristics of the typical condition are (1) an exaggeration in the height of the longitudinal arch, (2) slight shortening of the foot, (3) prominence of the metatarsal heads in the sole, (4) distal migration of the plantar fat pad, (5) clawing of the toes, (6) loss of flexibility of the joints of the foot, (7) reduction of the weight-bearing surface, and (8) often limited dorsiflexion at the ankle joint. Dorsal contracture and dislocation of the metatarsophalangeal joints are typical. The apex of the deformity on the inner border of the foot is usually the naviculocuneiform joint. The degree of the cavus ranges from a simple high arch and dorsally elevated midfoot area to an extreme concavity of the longitudinal arch. Often the forefoot is in equinus, and the deformity may be accompanied by a true hindfoot equinus brought about by contracture of the calf muscles; it may also be combined with varying degrees of malposition of the calcaneus as a result of previous lengthening of the heel cord.

A varus component to the deformity of the hindfoot may also be present (hence the name pes cavovarus); then too much weight is thrown on the outer border, often causing the base of the fifth metatarsal to become a weight-bearing, pressured point. In clawfoot the base of the metatarsals is so high that the heads of the metatarsals strike the ground pointedly; consequently, most patients have heavy callosities and sometimes traumatic ulcers under one or more of the heads.

Etiology. The pathomechanics of clawfoot are poorly understood. The deformity has been ascribed to (1) imbalance of the instrinsic muscles, a theory first proposed by Duchenne in 1867, and (2) imbalance of various extrinsic muscles (Bentzon, 1933; Hallgrímsson, 1939).

Brewerton et al. (1963), in studying the causes of clawfoot, found that in 66% of their seventy-seven cases neurologic signs could be detected during clinical examination. The most commonly made diagnosis was peroneal muscular atrophy (Charcot-Marie-Tooth disease), which was found in one third of the patients. Myelodysplasia and poliomyelitis were next in frequency. Friedreich's ataxia, although much less common, must also be kept in mind with its absence of ankle jerks and progressive disturbance of balance. In the "idiopathic" group of Brewerton et al., eleven of twenty-six patients gave a family history of clawfoot. Seven of the twenty-six showed electromyographic and nerve conduction abnormalities, thus pointing up the importance of a thorough neurologic evaluation.

Clawfoot may be caused by any of a number of neurologic diseases, of both the central and the peripheral nervous systems; it may be the result of infectious and traumatic diseases as well. A certain percentage of cases undoubtedly represent formes frustes of hereditary conditions such as peroneal muscular atrophy and Friedreich's ataxia.

Symptoms. The degree of deformity is variable. Symptoms of the condition are inability to walk or stand for long periods, easily tiring feet, severe calluses (which may ulcerate) on the plantar aspect of the foot and on the tips of the toes, and often a heavy callosity under the base of the fifth metatarsal as a result of foot inversion.

Treatment. The aim of treatment should be to relieve symptoms, correct the deformity, and prevent recurrence. Every foot should be treated as an individual problem. Inasmuch as a method applicable to all cases cannot be offered, an outline of treatment based on the degree of deformity is herewith suggested.

Slight deformity. In mild cases (especially in early cases in which the feet remain flexible, with moderate cavus that disappears on weight bearing), permanent contracture of the plantar structures can sometimes be prevented. The cavus and clawing of the toes can be kept to a minimum by getting the patient into carefully fitted shoes with low heels. A metatarsal bar and wedging appliances should be employed if callosities are present. Exercises are recommended to increase flexibility of the foot and to stretch the toes and muscles of the calf.

Moderate to severe deformity. Suggested procedures for the operative correction of clawfoot include tendon transfers and lengthening, fasciotomy, plantar muscle denervation, anterior tarsal wedge osteotomy, and triple arthrodesis.

Tendon transfer for the moderate to severe deformity was advocated by Sherman (1905). He created a sling from the long extensor tendon about the neck of the metatarsal bones. (Taking a somewhat different approach, Taylor [1951] recommended transplanting the long flexor tendon into the extensor tendon of the lesser toes.) Steindler (1917) advocated stripping the plantar fascia from the plantar surface of the calcaneus to release its bowstring action on the longitudinal arch. In 1919, Hibbs suggested transferring the extensor hallucis longus and extensor digitorum

longus into the cuneiforms. In moderate cases Cole (1940) employed Steindler's fasciotomy, followed by the use of a Thomas wrench and the Hibbs relocation procedure. Alvik (1954) extended the wedge osteotomy forward to include a wedge resection of the first and second cuneiforms and the base of the first and second metatarsals.

Whether such soft tissue operations as Steindler's fasciotomy and/or tendon transfers completely correct a clawfoot deformity is questionable. Steindler himself recommended the procedure only in the mildest of cases. Brockway (1940), in discussing Steindler's operation, stated that it was surprising how little correction could be obtained and how frequently relapse occurred. The technique is of value, however, when combined with other procedures.

Garceau and Brahms (1956) and Garceau (1961), in the belief that clawfoot is the result of intrinsic muscle imbalance, recommended selective plantar neurectomy if (1) the foot is flail, except for functioning plantar muscles which cause the cavus, (2) there is dorsal bunion with cavus, (3) poorly opposed flexor muscles in calcaneocavus deformity are present, and (4) there is cavoadductus deformity due to cerebral palsy. Results are best when procedures are performed before the development of the foot is complete.

McElvenny and Caldwell (1958) described a procedure in which elevation and supination of the first metatarsal are performed along with fusion of the tarsometatarsal and, if necessary, the naviculocuneiform joints. This operation is employed when the deformity is primarily of the medial portion of the foot; however, they combine the operation with plantar fasciotomy, triple arthrodesis, and first metatarsocuneiform fusion to correct severe deformities.

Dwyer's (1959) calcaneal osteotomy is useful in children in whom a varus deformity of the hindfoot is present; it should be combined with plantar fasciotomy. He reported good results in forty-one children from 3 to 16 years of age. Dwyer's calcaneal osteotomy is probably the procedure of choice for children with deformities in which heel varus is prominent.

He believes this correction of the weight-bearing alignment of the foot will result in progressive improvement of the deformity.

When the hindfoot is not deformed, anterior tarsal wedge osteotomy (Cole, 1940; Japas, 1968) is indicated for severe deformity in the skeletally mature foot. For older patients Dwyer (1959) also used the calcaneal osteotomy, combined with removal of a dorsally based wedge from the tarsometatarsal region.

If the hindfoot is deformed, stabilization by the "beak" triple arthrodesis as described by Siffert et al. (1966) may be indicated for the mature severely deformed foot.

For a more complete discussion of treatment procedures, see Chapter 19.

REFERENCES

Alvik, I.: Operative treatment of pes cavus, Acta Orthop. Scand. **23**:137, 1954.

Baer, W. S.: Gonorrheal exostosis of the os calcis, Surg. Gynecol. Obstet. **2**:172, 1906.

Barnicot, N. A., and Hardy, R. H.: The position of the hallux in West Africans, J. Anat. **89**:355, 1955.

Bentzon, P. G. K.: Pes cavus and the M. peroneus longus, Acta Orthop. Scand. **4**:50, 1933.

Bingold, A. C., and Collins, D. H.: Hallux rigidus, J. Bone Joint Surg. **32B**:214, 1950.

Blokhin, V. N., and Vinogradova, T. P.: Shpory pyatochnykh kostey [Calcaneal spurs], Ortop. Travmatol. Protez. **11**:96, 1937.

Branch, H. E.: Pathological dislocation of the second toe, J. Bone Joint Surg. **19**:978, 1937.

Brewerton, D. A., Sandifer, P. H., and Sweetnam, D. R.: "Idiopathic" pes cavus: an investigation into its aetiology, Br. Med. J. **2**:659, 1963.

Brockway, A.: Surgical correction of talipes cavus deformities, J. Bone Joint Surg. **22**:81, 1940.

Cole, W. H.: The treatment of claw-foot, J. Bone Joint Surg. **22**:895, 1940.

Cowell, H. R.: Talocalcaneal coalition and new causes of peroneal spastic flatfoot, Clin. Orthop. **85**:16, 1972.

Craigmile, D. A.: Incidence, origin, and prevention of certain foot defects, Br. Med. J. **2**:749, 1953.

Creer, W. S.: The feet of the industrial worker. Clinical aspect: relation to footwear, Lancet **2**:1482, 1938.

Davis, J. B., and Blair, H. C.: Spurs of calcaneus in Strümpell-Marie disease: report of 15 cases, J. Bone Joint Surg. **32A**:838, 1950.

Duchenne, G. B.: Physiology of motion (translated and edited by E. B. Kaplan), Philadelphia, 1949, J. B. Lippincott Co. (Original French edition, 1867.)

DuVries, H. L.: Dislocation of toe, J.A.M.A. **160**:728, 1956.

DuVries, H. L.: Surgery of the foot, ed. 2, St. Louis, 1965, The C. V. Mosby Co.

DuVries, H. L.: Five myths about your feet, Today's Health **45**:49, August 1967.

Dwyer, F. C.: Osteotomy of the calcaneum for pes cavus, J. Bone Joint Surg. **41B**:80, 1959.

Engle, E. T., and Morton, D. J.: Notes on foot disorders among natives of the Belgian Congo, J. Bone Joint Surg. **13**:311, 1931.

Ewald, P.: Die Aetiologie des Hallux valgus, Dtsch. Z. Chir. **114**:90, 1912.

Fowler, A., and Philip, J. F.: Abnormality of the calcaneus as a cause of painful heel, Br. J. Surg. **32**:494, 1945.

Galland, W. I., and Jordan, H.: Hallux valgus, Surg. Gynecol. Obstet. **66**:95, 1938.

Garceau, G. J.: Pes cavus. In Instructional Course Lectures, American Academy of Orthopaedic Surgeons, vol. 18, St. Louis, 1961, The C. V. Mosby Co.

Garceau, G. J., and Brahms, M. A.: A preliminary study of selective plantar-muscle denervation for pes cavus, J. Bone Joint Surg. **38A**:553, 1956.

Goldner, J. L., Keats, P. K., Bassett, F. H., and Clippinger, F. W.: progressive talipes equinovalgus due to trauma or degeneration of the posterior tibial tendon and medial plantar ligaments, Orthop. Clin. North Am. **5**:1, 39, 1974.

Gould, E. A.: Three generations of exostoses of the heel: inherited from father to son, J. Hered. **33**:228, 1942.

Haglund, P.: Beitrag zur Klinik der Achillessehne, Z. Orthop. Chir. **49**:49, 1928.

Hallgrímsson, S.: Pes cavus, seine Behandlung und einige Bemerkungen über seine Aetiologie, Acta Orthop. Scand. **10**:73, 1939.

Hardy, R. H., and Clapham, J. C. R.: Observations on hallux valgus, J. Bone Joint Surg. **33B**:376, 1951.

Harris, R. I., and Beath, T.: Etiology of peroneal spastic flat foot, J. Bone Joint Surg. **30B**:624, 1948.

Harris, R. I., and Beath, T.: The short first metatarsal: its incidence and clinical significance, J. Bone Joint Surg. **31A**:553, 1949.

Harrison, M. H., and Harvey, F. J.: Arthrodesis of the first metatarsophalangeal joint for hallux valgus and rigidus, J. Bone Joint Surg. **45A**:471, 1963.

Hawkes, O. A. M.: On the relative lengths of the first and second toes of the human foot from the point of view of occurrence, anatomy and heredity, J. Genet. **3**:249, 1914.

Hewitt, D., Stewart, A. M., and Webb, J. W.: The prevalence of foot defects among wartime recruits, Br. Med. J. **2**:745, 1953.

Hibbs, R. A.: An operation for "claw foot," J.A.M.A. **73**:1583, 1919.

Hicks, J. H.: The mechanics of the foot. II. The plantar aponeurosis and the arch, J. Anat. **88**:25, 1954.

Higgs, S. L.: "Hammer-toe," Postgrad. Med. J. **6**:130, 1931.

Hohmann, K. G. G.: IV. Der Hallux valgus und die

übrigen Zehenverkrümmungen, Ergeb. Chir. Orthop. 18:308, 1925.

Hohmann, K. G. G.: Fuss and Bein, ihre Erkrankungen und deren Behandlung, ed. 4, Munich, 1948, J. F. Bergmann.

James, C. S.: Footprints and feet of natives of the Soloman Islands, Lancet 2:1390, 1939.

Japas, L. M.: Surgical treatment of pes cavus by tarsal V-osteotomy, J. Bone Joint Surg. 50A:927, 1968.

Jones, F. W.: Structure and function as seen in the foot, Baltimore, 1944, The Williams & Wilkins Co.

Joplin, R. J.: Sling procedure for correction of splay-foot, metatarsus primus varus, and hallux valgus, J. Bone Joint Surg. 32A:779, 1950.

Kaplan, E. B.: The tibialis posterior muscle in relation to hallux valgus, Bull. Hosp. Joint Dis. 16:88, 1955.

Keck, S. W., and Kelly, P. J.: Bursitis of the posterior part of the heel: evaluation of surgical treatment of eighteen patients, J. Bone Joint Surg. 47A:267, 1965.

Kessel, L., and Bonney, G.: Hallux rigidus in the adolescent, J. Bone Joint Surg. 40B:668, 1958.

Kidner, F. C.: The prehallux (accessory scaphoid) in its relation to flat-foot, J. Bone Joint Surg. 11:831, 1929.

Lam Sim-Fook and Hodgson, A. R.: A comparison of foot forms among the non-shoe and shoe-wearing Chinese population, J. Bone Joint Surg. 40A:1058, 1958.

Lapidus, P. W.: "Dorsal bunion": its mechanics and operative correction, J. Bone Joint Surg. 22:627, 1940.

Liberson, F.: Deep x ray therapy in the treatment of "painful heel," J. Urol. 28:115, 1932.

Maclennan, R.: Prevalence of hallux valgus in a neolithic New Guinea population, Lancet 1:1398, 1966.

McElvenny, R. T., and Caldwell, G. D.: A new operation for correction of cavus foot: fusion of first metatarso-cuneiformnavicular joints, Clin. Orthop. 11:85, 1958.

Marwil, T. B., and Brantingham, C. R.: Foot problems of women's reserve, Hosp. Corps Q. 16:98, 1943.

Mau, C.: Das Krankheitsbild des Hallux rigidus, Munch. Med. Wochenschr. 75:1193, 1928.

Mayo, C. H.: The surgical treatment of bunion, Ann. Surg. 48:300, 1908.

Mayo, C. H.: The surgical treatment of bunions, Minn. Med. 3:326, 1920.

Miller, L. F., and Arendt, J.: Deformity of first metatarsal head due to faulty foot mechanics, J. Bone Joint Surg. 22:349, 1940.

Morton, D. J.: The human foot, New York, 1935, Columbia University Press.

Morton, D. J.: Human locomotion and body form: a study of gravity and man, Baltimore, 1952, The Williams & Wilkins Co.

Moynihan, F. J.: Arthrodesis of the metatarsophalangeal joint of the great toe, J. Bone Joint Surg. 49B:544, 1967.

Saxl, A.: Die Schuhgeschwulst der Ferse, Z. Orthop. Chir. 51:312, 1929.

Sherman, H. M.: The operative treatment for pes cavus, Am. J. Orthop. Surg. 2:374, 1905.

Shine, I. B.: Incidence of hallux valgus in a partially shoe-wearing community, Br. Med. J. 1:1648, 1965.

Siffert, R. S., Forester, R. I., and Nachamle, B.: "Beak" triple arthrodesis for correction of severe cavus deformity, Clin. Orthop. 45:101, 1966.

Stein, H. C.: Clinical surgery: hallux valgus, Surg. Gynecol. Obstet. 66:889, 1938.

Steindler, A.: Operative treatment of pes cavus: stripping of the os calcis, Surg. Gynecol. Obstet. 24:612, 1917.

Taylor, R. G.: The treatment of claw toes by multiple transfers of flexor into extensor tendons, J. Bone Joint Surg. 33B:539, 1951.

Truslow, W.: Metatarsus primus varus or hallux valgus? J. Bone Joint Surg. 7:98, 1925.

Webster, F. S., and Roberts, W. M.: Tarsal anomalies and peroneal spastic flatfoot, J.A.M.A. 146:1099, 1951.

Weinmann, J. P., and Sicher, H.: Bone and bones: fundamentals of bone biology, ed. 2, St. Louis, 1955, The C. V. Mosby Co.

Wells, L. H.: The foot of the South African native, Am. J. Phys. Anthropol. 15:185, 1931.

Wilkins, E. H.: Feet with particular reference to school-children, Med. Officer 66:5, 13, 21, 29, 1941.

9

CONGENITAL NEUROLOGIC DISORDERS OF THE FOOT

The foot in myelodysplasia

EARL N. FEIWELL

Definition of myelodysplasia: A developmental defect of the spinal cord usually associated with spina bifida with or without meningocele or myelomeningocele, absence of vertebrae (particularly sacral agenesis with or without absent lumbar vertebrae), diastematomyelia, or lipoma

GENERAL CONSIDERATIONS

The resultant foot problems secondary to myelodysplasia may be present at birth or may become progressive because of the unbalanced musculature about the foot. Sometimes progression occurs as a result of progressive paralysis during childhood from undiagnosed diastematomyelia, tethered cords, or lipomas.

The goal of treatment is dependent on the functional ability of the patient. All feet do not have to be perfect. The greater the neurologic deficit, the less normal will be the foot requirement. A full range of motion is not necessary for patients who will be wearing orthoses. For them 5° of dorsiflexion and plantar flexion is sufficient. Patients who walk should have plantigrade feet that do not provide excessive pressure on any portion of the plantar surface and that are not difficult to fit with shoes and orthoses. Patients who do not walk should have feet that are shoeable and sufficiently plantigrade to avoid pressures on areas other than plantar skin.

Foot care

The insensitive foot must be protected at all times. This fact must be emphasized to the patient as well as the parent. We strongly recommend foot coverings whether the patient is in a wheelchair, in an automobile, or ambulatory.

Insensitive feet must have protection at all times. Tennis shoes should be worn on the beach or in the water. It is satisfactory to allow swimming in bare feet in swimming pools; but shoes must be worn right up to the pool edge, for hot decking can cause severe burns.

Principles of surgical evaluation

Preoperatively the patient should have a careful evaluation of the deformities as well as muscle function performed by the physician as well as by an experienced physical therapist. The physical therapist should have several periods of observation; we recommend the use of faradic stimulation as advised by Sharrard and Grosfeld (1968) to determine muscles that contract but are not under volitional control. This is not a good objective test for evaluating transfers, but it will indicate muscles which may cause deforming forces or indicate functioning muscles not demonstrated on muscle testing.

The principles of poliomyelitis surgery are not completely applicable to the myelodysplasia patient. Factors making this difference are multiple but primarily include lack of sensa-

303

tion, presence of spasticity, muscles that are functioning but not under volitional control, and the patient's overall brain abnormalities which limit balance, motor planning and overall gait abilities. In addition, there seems to be a tendency toward increased stiffness of joints following casting or surgical treatment.

Casts

Gentle casting may be carried out preoperatively to help reduce deformity and stretch contractures. Casts should be applied with satisfactory padding. The casting should be very gentle, and good molding is necessary to avoid slipping of the foot within the cast and development of pressure areas. Plaster should extend beyond the toes to protect them from ulceration. Postoperative casting should be utilized only for protection of the foot and not for the maintenance or correction of deformities. Corrections should be made at the time of the surgery, and pins used for fixation of the bones to hold the position.

We generally utilize a cast that is split down to the skin postoperatively rather than bivalve a cast. A bivalved cast holds position poorly. Significant fevers several days postoperative or longer which are not definitely caused by respiratory or urinary tract infections require inspection of the wound by removing the cast and reapplying a new one if there is no question of problem in the foot.

Postoperative splinting, that is, splinting after the casts have been removed and the patient is beginning to be braced and splinted at night, should be very carefully and sparingly used on the insensitive foot, for pressure sores are common. Frequent checking of the foot must be done and the splint should be well padded, particularly in the areas of pressure on the back of the heel. There is a great tendency for the foot to slip upward and change position in the splints.

Orthoses

Orthoses should be planned preoperatively and measured, if possible, so patients who require protection when coming out of a cast will have their orthoses ready. As a result of swelling in the postoperative period, there is a great tendency for pressure areas to occur. The foot should be checked frequently when the orthosis is first received and any red areas immediately relieved or the patient placed back in a cast and the orthosis discontinued until appropriate corrections are carried out.

Incisions

Transverse incisions should be avoided whenever possible to protect the venous and lymphatic drainage. Myelodysplasia children usually require multiple surgical procedures throughout their life, so it is possible that three or four procedures can create circumferential scarring about the foot or ankle. An example of this is a patient who had a posteromedial release which gave her a relatively high scar from the Achilles tendon around to the midfoot. Later in life, she had a metatarsal osteotomy with a transverse foot incision and finally at age 12 a triple arthrodesis with a transverse scar placed as usual at the sinus tarsi running posteriorly. The patient eventually underwent bilateral amputations because of persistent swelling of the toes and ulcerations.

Arthrodesis

In general, it is best to avoid the development of rigid feet secondary to multiple bony fusions. The rigid foot cannot compensate for slight differences or irregularities on the plantar surface, and tendency for breakdown over these areas readily occurs. Arthrodesis is difficult to obtain in any joint of the insensitive foot. Internal fixation of the joint to be fused and avoidance of weight bearing even in the cast until there is radiographic evidence of bony bridging are necessary.

Pantalar arthrodesis is to be condemned because of the difficulty in obtaining a satisfactory ankle fusion, the prolonged period of immobilization necessary for healing, and the possibility of developing Charcot joints in areas of nonunion or even breakdown of fusion sites (Hayes et al., 1964). In addition, the late complications of metatarsal ulcers exist. There is no definite advantage to this surgical procedure because light bracing is available for the ankle and no great advantage of gait or comfort to the patient is gained.

Triple arthrodesis is satisfactory in feet with some sensation, but we generally avoid it if possible for the reasons just noted. The triple arthrodesis patient must be carefully evaluated preoperatively because of the possible problem of a preexistent abnormality in the ankle joint such as a flat or irregular-shaped talus from prior casting or excessive pressures during ambulation. These can go on to Charcot-type joints. The greater the number of joints that are movable, the greater is the possible compensation in avoidance of pressure areas.

BASIC FOOT DEFORMITIES

The primary types of deformities seen in myelomeningocele feet are equinus, equinovarus or equinovalgus, calcaneus with valgus or varus, valgus foot, convex pes valgus, cavus foot, and toe deformities.

Equinus

Equinus is seen primarily in completely paralyzed feet and is an early deformity. It apparently develops as a contracture of the gastrocsoleus despite the muscle's lack of function. At times isolated function is present within the gastrocsoleus which leads to contracture.

Treatment varies with the age group as well as with function. In the nonfunctioning gastrocsoleus, tendon lengthening can be done by subcutaneous tenotomy at a very early age. Frequently there is no sensation in the area and the procedure can be carried out (as done by Menelaus, 1976) without anesthesia in infants during the first few weeks of life. Correction should not be carried beyond neutral, and postoperative casting should be in a well-padded cast which does not apply significant pressure to one area. After the foot has been in a cast for 4 weeks, dorsiflexion can then be maintained by gentle manual range of motion. In patients who have function in the gastrocsoleus group, even though nonvolitional function, the gastrocsoleus tendon can be split and the medial half placed anterior to the dorsum of the foot. This procedure allows

for stability of the ankle and for maintenance of the neutral position during growth (Caldwell, 1958; Sharrard, 1967; Jolson, 1977).

In older patients with rigid ankle joints, who would not be improved by tendon and posterior capsular releases, anterior-based wedge osteotomies of the distal tibia have been successful in providing a plantigrade foot. Extreme deformities have been overcome with this method. In children with growing distal tibial epiphyses and fixed equinus, Sharrard and Grosfeld (1968) described posterior soft tissue release followed by anterior tibiofibular ligament release to allow for widening of the mortise and bringing the talus back up into neutral from its plantar-flexed position.

Equinovarus

According to Sharrard and Grosfeld (1968) and Menelaus (1971), equinovarus is the most common deformity seen in myelomeningocele feet. It occurs most frequently in paralysis above the L4 level. Etiology is again related to many causes. Primarily one can consider muscle imbalance, that is, an overpowering posterior tibialis; but more frequently the deformity seems to be related to intrauterine position. Iatrogenic cause is related to sectioning of the tendons or transfer of muscles without recognition of active medial forces (Menelaus, 1971).

Early treatment consists of gentle casting for several months to decrease contractures. Our policy has been that if correction is poor after several months we may wait until approximately 6 months of age and then carry out the full soft tissue release. Menelaus (1976) most recently described success with early posterior release and progressive casting treatment. He found that firmly fixed equinovarus deformities require a complete posteromedial plantar release, including lengthening of the Achilles tendon; if the posterior tibialis is functional, the tendon is lengthened significantly rather than simply sectioned. We avoid lateral anterior tibial transfer since in the older child this may bring on marked valgus deformity in a corrected foot and have no effect on an uncorrected foot.

The basic procedure consists of sectioning all ligaments and capsules across the posterior, medial, and plantar aspects of the subtalar, talonavicular, and calcaneocuboid joints as well as across the plantar area of the calcaneonavicular and naviculocuboid ligaments. We believe it is absolutely necessary to free these contracted tissues to establish the appropriate alignment of the tarsal bones. Leaving one area intact will preclude obtaining proper alignment and allow greater tendency for recurrence.

Staging the procedure should be avoided if possible since normal alignment of the tarsal bones cannot be obtained if free motion of all the bones does not occur at one time. Turco's (1971) approach through a straight medial incision plus postoperative pinning of the talonavicular joint provides a satisfactory method. If the subtalar joint appears to be unstable and tends to slide back into its prior malposition, then pinning the joint is also of benefit. Careful casting as previously described is performed. Avoidance of an incision curved posterior to the medial malleolus decreases the possibliity of slough, for the greatest tension always occurs at this angle after correction.

In patients who have tensions of the skin on closure due to marked deformity correction, the flap repair as described by Walker (1971) has been very useful (Fig. 9-1). This allows the operator to swing a flap utilizing the dorsum of the foot and thus bring the loose lateral skin over the dorsum and onto the new area of prominence where the talar head now lies on the medial side of the foot. Careful subcutaneous dissection is necessary to leave the dorsal venous system. When the flap procedure is performed, a well-padded compres-

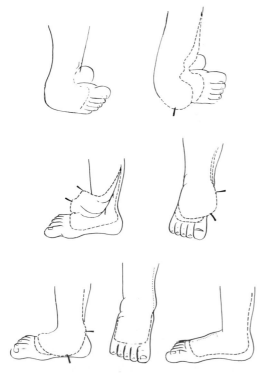

Fig. 9-1. Dorsal flap closure of a medial release. Top, Incision and raising the flap. Middle, Foot corrected. Bottom, Flap rotated and sutured in position with the foot corrected. (From Walker, G.: J. Bone Joint Surg. **53B**:462, 1971.)

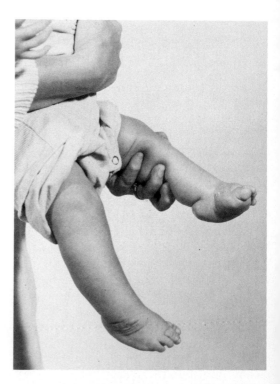

Fig. 9-2. Equinovarus feet; prominent head of the talus laterally in line with the tibia and patella. The medial midtarsal crease is where the tarsals and forefoot are medially displaced on the talus.

sion dressing is used and the plaster is merely placed around as a protective shell. The cast and compression dressing are changed in 3 days and removed at 2 weeks. Casting is maintained for approximately 4 months; then short orthoses and well-padded night splints are utilized for the next 4 to 8 months.

Satisfactory reduction of the hindfoot deformity in infants will correct the apparent forefoot adductus since this adductus is due to the medial displacement of the foot on the talus. The initial position of the talus is normal so the talar head is in line with the tibia; it is the rest of the foot which is swung around and malpositioned on the talus. Restoration of the proper relationship of foot to talus corrects what appears to be internal tibial torsion (Figs. 9-2 to 9-4). Our observations are that bony deformity of the talar neck into increased valgus (abduction) and bony forefoot

adductus are late deformities. Recurrent deformities undergo repeat releases. If satisfactory correction is not obtainable with additional releases in insensitive feet, then talectomy should be done at the same time.

It must be emphasized, however, that merely removing the talus does not correct the foot deformity. The relationships of the calcaneus, cuboid, and navicular are abnormal; therefore appropriate soft tissue releases in the same fashion as the posterior medial plantar release must be performed with the appropriate correction of the tarsal bones, thus bringing the foot out of forefoot supination and hind foot varus. The tibiofibular ligament release is frequently necessary to appropriately set the calcaneus posteriorly in the ankle mortise. Incomplete removal of the talus or subperiosteal dissection in the young child has allowed reformation of the talus.

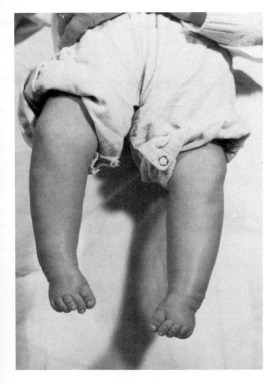

Fig. 9-3. The foot and leg appear to be internally rotated as compared with the knee.

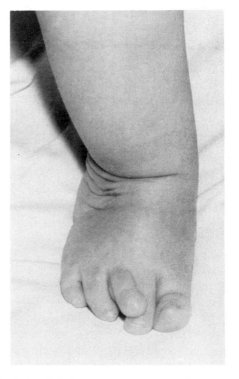

Fig. 9-4. All deformities are corrected by correcting the relationship of the calcaneus, navicular, and cuboid with the talus.

Talectomy has been of value in older patients who are not ambulatory but who have severe deformity to the extent that they are unable to wear shoes and cannot approximate the plantar surface of the foot to wheelchair footrests, thus causing pressure areas on the thin dorsal skin of the foot. The need for talectomy in well-treated feet should be rare (Menelaus, 1976).

Cuneiform-cuboid wedge osteotomy provides satisfactory correction in older children who ambulate but have a varus deformity causing bursal enlargement about the fifth metatarsal. This procedure can correct supination, adductus, and a mild degree of equinus. Its advantage is that it preserves all joints and allows maximum growth in a foot with lessened growth potential and greater plantar pressures than normal (Hay and Walker, 1975). We consider the procedure in children between the ages of 6 and 12, although it can be performed in older patients to avoid triple arthrodesis.

Surgery is carried out by two vertical incisions, one being between the first and second cuneiforms and the other around the junction of the third cuneiform and cuboid. The proximal and distal margins of the cuneiforms are located and the approximate wedges are planned; then the distal cut is made. The forefoot is rotated to correct the supination deformity. At this point, the proximal cut is made and the dorsal wedge removed in order to correct the equinus or cavus of the foot; adductus is corrected by a cuboid-based wedge with the apex at the first cuneiform. If cavus is being corrected, the surgeon must first cut the plantar fascia at the heel. Occasionally, if the bones are small and the deformity is great, the additional dorsal wedge must be removed from the navicular and the naviculocuneiform joint thus violated. We would rather violate the naviculocuneiform joint than the tarsometatarsal joints, since metatarsal pliability decreases the chance for plantar ulcers. We have not found residual heel varus to be a problem, and frequently it is partially balanced by a valgus ankle.

Triple arthrodesis is considered in patients over the age of 12 years. In addition to the multiple problems previously described, we have had difficulty completely correcting significantly deformed feet in the older child with a single-stage triple arthrodesis. Oftentimes, additional midfoot or forefoot surgery is required.

Calcaneus foot

The calcaneus foot has the tuber of the os calcis almost parallel with the tibia. The foot may be nearly aligned with the os calcis and point upward, or there may be some forefoot drop present with cavus. The deformity cannot be inhibited by bracing. Severe deformities defy the wearing of shoes because of lack of heel prominence. Gait is affected because there is no posterior stability. Placing the foot flat on the ground requires flexing the knee, thereby decreasing knee stability in stance. To keep up with their center of gravity, these patients walk in almost a running gait. Severe deformities cause pressure areas on the heel (Tachdjian, 1972).

Calcaneus deformity is due to a poor or absent gastrocsoleus and a strong dorsiflexor of the foot. The tibialis anterior comes in soonest of the muscles crossing the ankle, beginning at about the L4 area and being the strongest at approximately the L5 segment (Fig. 9-5). Thus a full-strength tibialis anterior is present before any gastrocsoleus strength. Additionally, dorsiflexors, particularly the peroneus tertius, are also present at this level.

Basic treatment consists of transferring the tibialis anterior through the interosseous membrane to the os calcis (Peabody procedure) (Peabody, 1949; Hayes et al., 1964; Turner and Cooper, 1971). The peroneus tertius, if functional, should also be transplanted. Fifteen degrees of plantar flexion is preferred preoperatively and obtained by casting in well-padded plaster. We do not attempt to achieve the full position if soft tissue tightness prevents it, for sectioning the tibialis anterior at surgery usually will allow a significant and adequate increase in plantar flexion. Lesser degrees of plantar flexion in the young child are accepted in order to avoid plastic skin lengthening anteriorly.

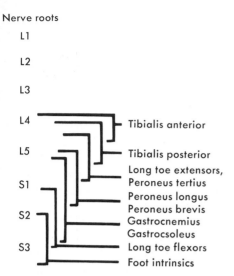

Nerve roots

L1

L2

L3

L4 — Tibialis anterior

L5 — Tibialis posterior

Long toe extensors, Peroneus tertius

S1 — Peroneus longus

Peroneus brevis

S2 — Gastrocnemius

Gastrocsoleus

S3 — Long toe flexors

Foot intrinsics

Fig. 9-5. Segmental innervation of the foot by musculature. (From Menelaus, M.: Orthopedic management of spina bifida cystica, Edinburgh, 1971, E. & S. Livingstone, Ltd.)

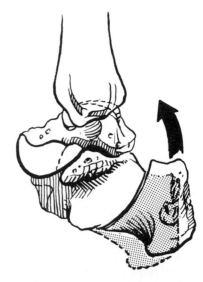

Fig. 9-6. The crescentic osteotomy of Samilson corrects a calcaneus deformity and improves the posterior lever arm of the calcaneus. Healing is as rapid as for a closing-wedge osteotomy. (From Samilson, R.: In Bateman, J. E., editor: Foot science, Philadelphia, 1976, W. B. Saunders Co.)

The basic procedure consists of obtaining the maximum length of tibialis anterior, bringing the tendon proximally to the junction of the proximal and middle thirds, and then passing the muscle belly through a completely resected interosseous membrane window. It is extremely important that the membrane not be in contact with the tendon. The tendon is fixed distally to the os calcis by varying techniques. Simple suture to the bone has been satisfactory. If we are unable to get satisfactory length of the anterior tibial tendon, we fix the anterior tibial to the calcaneal tendon as close to the bone as we can reach. After 6 weeks of casting, an adjustable double-upright ankle orthosis is utilized with the ankle being gradually brought up over the next 4 months to no greater than neutral position. Dorsiflexion is avoided.

These transfers are best performed at 6 months to 2 years of age in order to avoid excessive deformity and to provide maximum opportunity for growth correction. In addition, the distance between the posterior tip of the calcaneus and the ankle joint remains satisfactory and provides a better lever arm for effective muscle function. After 4 years of age, Samilson's (1976) crescentic osteotomy to

correct the deformity of the heel provides increased posterior length for an improved lever arm, restores the posterior prominence for better shoe fit, and increases the length of the plantar surface of the foot (Fig. 9-6). A tendon transfer can be accomplished then or at a secondary procedure later. Healing of the osteotomy is rapid because of the large cancellous surface. Some degree of valgus or varus of the heel can be corrected at the same time. If cavus of the foot is also present, it can be corrected by a tarsal osteotomy.

The primary purpose of this transfer is to provide some degree of posterior stability and to allow for a normal formation of the os calcis. Toe rises against gravity cannot be performed even with multiple tendon transfers. Calcaneal varus deformity may be present initially or may occur as a varus deformity after the transfer if unrecognized medial muscle is present (i.e., the tibialis posterior or long toe flexors) (Menelaus, 1971). If recognized initially or later, these muscles should be transferred to the os calcis. Calcaneal valgus is treated in the same manner by posterior transfer of the peronei to the medial side of the heel. The peroneus tertius can be transferred to the middorsum for some dorsiflexion balance, but usually it is transferred posteriorly with the tibialis anterior.

Continued foot valgus requires additional surgery, for this affects bracing, footwear, and stability. Valgus can be progressive despite removal of the active deformity forces. Achilles tenodesis will provide improved posterior stability and is useful when the anterior muscles are too weak for transfer. Under no circumstances should it be performed without a strong active muscle transfer when an active extensor muscle is present anteriorly. All eight feet in our series required reoperation when an attempt was made to tenodese the Achilles tendon, leaving the tibialis anterior in place. Most of our series of Achilles tenodeses have been to the tibia. However, tenodesis to the fibula as described by Westin (1975) is now done to improve fibular growth.

Valgus foot

Because the weight-bearing area lies medial to the subtalar joint, the valgus foot is an unstable foot for weight bearing. Pressure areas occur at the medial malleolus from orthoses (Fig. 9-7). If medial T-straps are used, the straps must continuously be loosened because of pain at the sensitive medial malleolus and ulcerations on the insensitive malleolus while the valgus deformity continues.

Problems appear to become most significant as the child gets heavier, about the age of 8 to 10 years.

The earliest and most severe deformities occur from muscle imbalance due to strong active lateral muscles, e.g., the peronei, and absent medial musculature. The posterior tibial muscle is commonly absent while the peroneals are intact. It has been our experience that the tibialis posterior does not function in as high a segmental level as Menelaus (1971) described. This function does not occur until after strong peronei are present.

In flaccid feet, valgus can occur progressively during growth—apparently due to several factors. As Makin (1965) pointed out, the fibula does not have adequate stimulation from muscle pull and becomes relatively short compared with the tibia. This then removes lateral containment of the talus and allows excessive lateral pressure on the distal tibial epiphysis with progressive valgus of the joint.

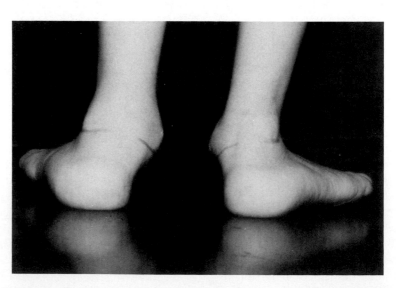

Fig. 9-7. Valgus feet place the weight-bearing line medial to the foot. The ankle is in valgus, as demonstrated by a more proximal tip of the lateral malleolus as compared with the medial. Pressure sores occur on the medial malleoli from bracing.

Weight bearing passes more medially, and the subtalar joint responds to its more valgus position accordingly by rocking further into valgus. If the subtalar joint was in valgus from the early postnatal period or from excessive correction of other deformities of the foot, then both the ankle and the subtalar deformities are accentuated with unprotected weight bearing.

External rotation deformities further accentuate the problem, particularly in patients with ankle-foot orthoses or no orthoses.

Early treatment consists of transferring the deforming tendons to a more medial position on the foot, or more medially on the calcaneus. Sectioning of tendons alone, particularly spastic tendons, may prevent immediate or active progression but does not change the deformity. As long as the valgus position persists in the weight-bearing patient, the deformity will progress. Tight-fitting plastic inserts holding the foot and ankle may help but are difficult to use in insensitive feet.

A Grice procedure after the age of 3 years reduces subtalar deformity and maintains a more stable and improved heel position. Tendon transfer or transection of deforming muscles must be done at the same time; however, a high rate of failure is present with the Grice fusion. The ankle must be immobilized for a more prolonged period and weight bearing not allowed, as it is in sensitive feet, during the healing period. Tibial grafts are not used because of fear of fracture in the normally weak bone structure of thin tibias in these children.

A recently described subtalar fusion by Alban et al. (1975) has shown promise. In this technique a single incision is used, extending from the sinus tarsi over the lateral heel, and a full thickness plug of bone is removed with a Cloward bone plug remover from the os calcis. This technique improves fusion and avoids complications of other types of grafts, and the bone is easy to obtain. The same device removes subtalar joint bone, and the donor plug is inserted across the joint.

Weight-bearing radiographs of the valgus ankle joint demonstrate the valgus position of the talus. The presence of a short fibula is usual in the paralytic foot and dorsiflexion of the ankle accentuates the valgus position. Achilles tenodesis to the fibula is satisfactory in young children because it decreases the dorsiflexion and stimulates the fibula to increase growth (Westin, 1975).

In a nonfunctioning gastrocsoleus muscle a short vertical incision 3 inches above the heel allows section of the tendon at the musculotendinous junction. With the ankle in 20° of plantar flexion, the tendon is pulled tightly to the fibula by a suture through the bone underneath a periosteal flap. The flap is then sutured to the tendon itself. Postoperative treatment is the same as described for the anterior tibial transfer.

The valgus ankle in patients 11 years of age or more is treated by a supramalleolar osteotomy. Our approach is medial as compared with Sharrard and Webb's (1974) anterior approach. From our more medial vantage the neurovascular bundle is visualized and protected and the widest portion of the osteotomy, a posteromedial wedge, is best performed. A closing wedge osteotomy is performed, and a step-cut staple utilized for stabilization. A slightly posteriorly based wedge is used because of the anterolateral deformity in the joint that is usually present. Open wedge osteotomies are avoided because of the poor healing and the probability of collapse of the graft. The fibula is not osteotomized. In most instances of late deformity, the subtalar joint is also deformed so the osteotomy as well as a subtalar fusion is necessary. In this situation the removed tibial wedge is used for the subtalar fusion.

Convex pes valgus (paralytic vertical talus)

Convex pes valgus is equinovalgus of the calcaneus with dorsal subluxation of the rest of the foot on the neck of the talus, the navicular lying on the neck of the talus, and the rest of the bones in line with the navicular. The cuboid is angulated and subluxated on the calcaneus. The talus assumes a vertical position. The overall deformity causes instability of the weight-bearing surface, a pressure area over the head of the talus, and in advanced states an impossibility to shoe (Fig. 9-8).

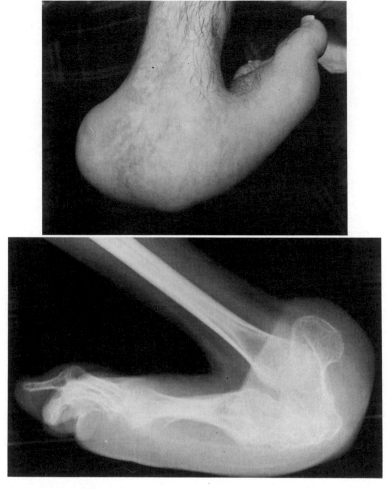

Fig. 9-8. Vertical talus deformity (equinovalgus) can cause pressure areas over the prominent head of the talus and is impossible to shoe when severe.

The etiology is related to the levels of paralysis that produce strong extension and eversion with weakness of balancing toe flexors, tibialis posterior, and intrinsics. A tight Achilles tendon is present but does not always demonstrate function. The functioning muscles may be involuntary.

Treatment is directed toward improving the balance of forces and correcting the bony deformities. This is an extremely difficult deformity to treat as it is in the congenital variety. Sharrad and Grosfeld (1968) had their highest rate of failure in treating this deformity. Multiple methods were utilized. Extensive surgery is necessary, regardless of the method, since the deforming tendons must be released and transferred, contracted ligaments released (as in a medial plantar release), and the navicular placed in the proper position to the talus, as with equinovarus. Differentiation must be made from those feet corrected by plantar flexion only.

Sharrard's present technique (1976) requires a medial and lateral release of the talus and lengthening of the Achilles tendon, toe extensors, peroneus tertius, and peroneus longus; transfers of the peroneus brevis posteriorly to the posterior tibial tendon and of the tibialis anterior to the talar neck are done. Pins are placed across the talonavicular joint and across the reduced subtalar joint through the heel.

In the older more rigid foot, talectomy and calcaneocuboid reduction is performed.

Cavus foot and clawtoes

The cavus foot has a prominent middorsal area with metatarsal heads protruding on the plantar surface and dorsally displaced toes with clawing. In similar sensitive feet painful callosities develop on the plantar surface and corns arise on the dorsal surface of the toes. In the insensitive foot these areas become intractable ulcers and special protective shoes must be worn to avoid ulceration. The deformities are usually seen in low-level lesions, notably the sacral level, in patients who have active long toe flexors and extensors but not intrinsics. Occasionally, spastic intrinsics are present in an otherwise paralyzed foot to give a cavus deformity.

Treatment is directed at balancing the forces of the foot, releasing spastic muscles, and correcting the bony deformity. These are generally the feet most successfully treated (Sharrard and Grosfeld, 1968).

The treatment is quite variable, depending on the deformity and its cause. In early childhood, before fixed bony deformities are present, the foot can be treated by release of the plantar fascia and short flexors at the heel and transfer of the long toe flexors to the extensor hood to provide metatarsophalangeal flexion and interphalangeal extension (the Girdlestone procedure of splitting the flexor tendons and bringing half up each side of the proximal phalanx) (Taylor, 1951).

Spastic intrinsics can be denervated by cutting the plantar nerves, if the foot is insensitive, or the Garceau (1956) technique of cutting only the motor branches, if sensory nerves are to be spared.

Bony deformities are corrected by cuneiform-cuboid osteotomies and, if calcaneus is present, the crescentic osteotomy of Samilson (1976). The latter must be done in conjunction with release of the plantar ligament.

Plantar ulcers will heal if the bony prominence is removed. This is accomplished by the appropriate correction of the deformities.

If chronic infection is present around the metatarsal heads, the cure is by excision of the offending metatarsal head and placement of a large metatarsal bar on the bottom of the shoe. The bar gives a rocker effect to the bottom of the shoe, distributing the weight on the sole and decreasing the metatarsophalangeal dorsiflexion on roll-off.

The foot in cerebral palsy
M. MARK HOFFER

A thorough understanding of orthopaedic surgery and cerebral palsy is required before making plans on a cerebral palsy patient's foot (Basset, 1971; Bank, 1975). It is important to ascertain whether the patient is a potential ambulator. Foot deformities rarely affect the child enough to prohibit ambulation. Neurologic balance is the key to ambulation. If the child has not achieved that balance by the first six years of life, he rarely will walk at a later date. Retention of perinatal reflexes in an obligatory fashion over the first few years of life also bodes poorly for the ambulatory or potentially ambulatory cerebral palsy child. Adults with cerebral palsy, especially those who walk very little, have poor tissue circulation in their feet. One should be very cautious about suggesting reconstructive surgery in these adults, for the complication rates far exceed the rates in children.

The child with motion disorders (athetosis, ataxia, dyskinesia) will have foot deformities that are difficult to analyze. This is because the deformities are inconsistent, are never fixed, and seem to depend to a large degree on writhing postures. Deformities due to spasticity are easier to analyze and the results of surgery are more predictable. It is important to differentiate fixed from flexible deformities in the spastic child. The increased tone in the muscles of spastic feet initially results in dynamic deformity, but eventually soft tissue and joint contracture occur.

In the diplegic child with bilateral involvement, the most frequent combination of deformities seems to be equinovalgus; in the hemiplegic spastic child, equinovarus is most often found.

EQUINUS DEFORMITIES

Equinus deformities should not be over-treated, for this may result in the more disabling calcaneus (Banks and Green, 1958). In these children we usually perform stretching exercises; we utilize progressive walking plasters and braces before resorting to surgical procedures.

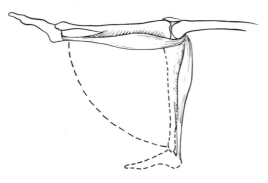

Fig. 9-9. Classic two-joint muscle test to differentiate gastrocnemius contracture from gastrocsoleus contracture.

Equinus deformities have often been analyzed by the two-joint muscle test (Fig. 9-9). This test utilizes the supposed difference in gastrocnemius contracture from gastrocsoleus contracture. We believe most children with cerebral palsy have a positive differential test clinically but not when tested by electromyography (Perry et al., 1974). Electromyograms in gait usually show increased activity of both gastrocnemius and soleus in the child with equinus deformities (Figs. 9-10 and 9-11). Therefore we usually advise an Achilles tendon lengthening rather than a gastrocnemius slide.

When performing an Achilles tendon lengthening procedure, we prefer the three-level cuts—distal and proximal on the medial side and central laterally (Fig. 9-12). We bring the ankle up to neutral only and do not overcorrect. We find this operative procedure works more consistently than the two-level operation, because of the variation in the spiraling of the Achilles tendon fibers from individual to individual. For fear of contract-

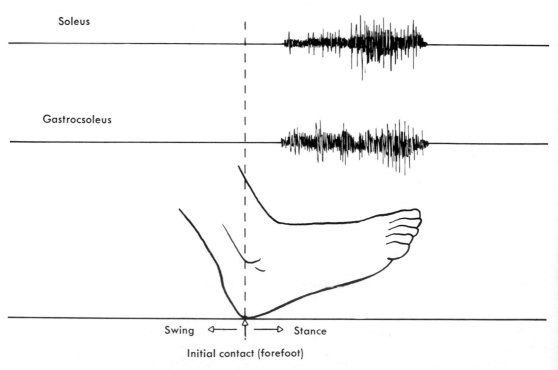

Fig. 9-10. EMG tracing of a normal triceps surae gait. Note the onset of activity well after heel strike.

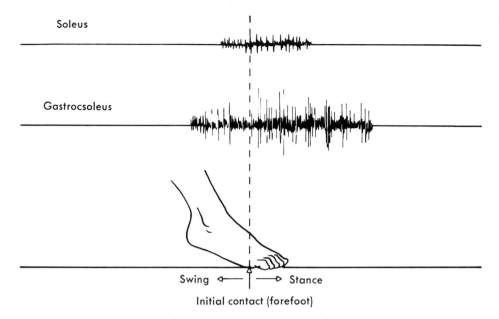

Fig. 9-11. EMG tracing of a cerebral palsy equinus gait. Note the onset of activity prior to initial floor contact.

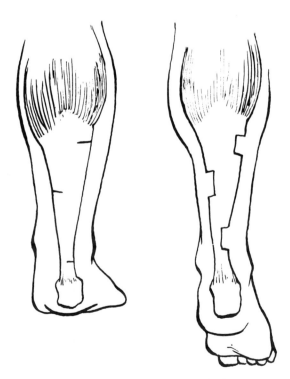

Fig. 9-12. Method of Achilles tendon lengthening through three short transverse skin and tendon incisions.

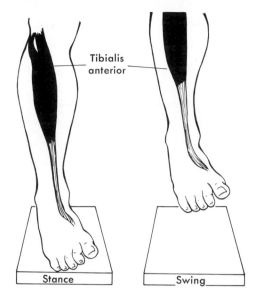

Fig. 9-13. Continuous anterior tibial activity in a varus cerebral palsy foot. Here split anterior tibial tendon transfer is performed.

ing scars, we do not ever use longitudinal posterior incisions. We generally utilize multiple transverse incisions. The patient is immobilized with a short-leg walking cast. The plaster is removed in 4 weeks and a brace is continued for at least a year.

VARUS DEFORMITIES

Varus deformities that are flexible may be due to overactivity of any of the muscles medial to the ankle joint. The triceps surae and the posterior tibial and anterior tibial muscles are most often implicated. These spastic deformities do not respond well to orthoses or inserts. Our general policy is to determine the dynamic deforming force by gait electromyography and perform either anterior tibial or posterior tibial surgery combined with Achilles tendon lengthening if necessary (Figs. 9-13 to 9-15).

The overactive anterior tibial muscle in stance and swing requires a split anterior

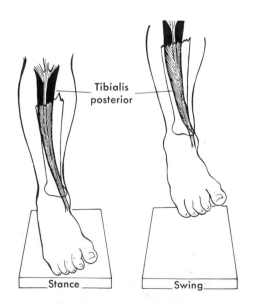

Fig. 9-14. Continous posterior tibial activity in a varus cerebral palsy foot. Here lengthening of the muscle is advised.

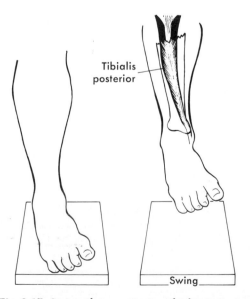

Fig. 9-15. Swing phase posterior tibial activity in a varus cerebral palsy foot. Here posterior tibial tendon transfer forward is advised.

tibial tendon transfer (Hoffer et al., 1974) (Fig. 9-16). The anterior tibial tendon is split longitudinally from its insertion to the ankle joint by two separate incisions. It is then transferred subcutaneously to the cuboid. Immediate ambulation in short leg plaster is permitted, and a brace is applied at 4 weeks to be worn for at least a year.

The overactive posterior tibial muscle in stance and swing requires lengthening at the musculotendinous junction (Root and Frost, 1971). In the rare situation when a posterior tibial muscle is active exclusively in swing, the muscle is transferred anteriorly (Root, 1951; Bisslar and Lewis, 1975). Here short leg plaster is utilized and removed in 4 weeks when therapy is begun. When good muscle function occurs (usually 6 to 8 weeks), weight bearing in a brace begins and is continued for at least a year.

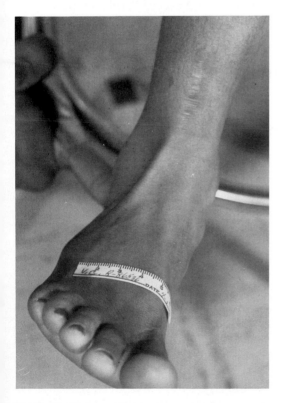

Fig. 9-16. Postoperative appearance of a properly performed split anterior tibial tendon transfer. (From Hoffer, M.M., et al.: Orthop. Clin. North. Am. **5**:31, 1974.)

When varus deformities have been allowed to become fixed, calcaneo-osteotomy in addition to the aforementioned procedures is advised (Silver et al., 1967).

VALGUS DEFORMITIES

Flexible valgus deformities may be due to hyperactivity of the triceps surae and/or peroneal muscles or to the position of the hips and knees. The adducted hip–valgus knee combination forces weight bearing on the medial aspect of the foot. The surgeon must be especially careful to get proper alignment and balance of these proximal joints before beginning treatment of the valgus of the foot.

Ankle-foot orthoses, especially polypropylene insert molded shells, can control minor flexible valgus of the hindfoot; but with increased tone these orthoses become ineffective. Heel cord lengthening and peroneal release-and-transfer have been suggested for the flexible hind part of the foot valgus (Sharrard, 1972). We have performed eight such peroneal tendon procedures. Six resulted in either overcorrection or undercorrection. We hope that dynamic electromyography will give more predictable results. At this point we advise that the hind part of foot valgus be treated with extra-articular subtalar arthrodesis. Currently we utilize iliac crest bone placed in the denuded sinus tarsi with talocalcaneal pin fixation. The smooth pin is removed at 8 weeks, when ambulation is allowed in a walking plaster. At 10 to 12 weeks, a molded polypropylene brace is applied below the knee and utilized for a year.

The procedure of extra-articular arthrodesis was first described using tibial bone (Grice, 1952); some surgeons utilize fibula. We do not use tibia or fibula, for fear of pathologic fracture in the first case and growth disturbances of the fibula in the second. A new, excellent, method has been described utilizing the calcaneus as a source of graft (Alban and Alban, 1975).

Triple arthrodesis is rarely indicated in cerebral palsy. For the mature foot with fixed valgus or varus deformity which interferes with function, however, triple arthrodesis is advised. Staples should be used for the joints in these spastic feet, and an attempt made to release deforming muscle forces to prevent recurrence.

FOREFOOT DEFORMITIES

The valgus hind part of the foot is often associated with a hallux valgus deformity of the first metatarsophalangeal joint (Fig. 9-17). Here we advise that, during correction of the valgus hindfoot, release of the adductor hallucis insertion and plication of the medial metatarsophalangeal joint capsule be performed. Pin fixation of the corrected metatarsophalangeal joint should be maintained for 6 weeks. Recurrence will happen if the hindfoot valgus is not corrected.

The long toe flexors are often spastic in cerebral palsy feet, but the contractures rarely become fixed. By contrast, a child with acquired brain damage will frequently develop severe toe flexor spasticity. Release of spastic toe flexors is easily accomplished by te-

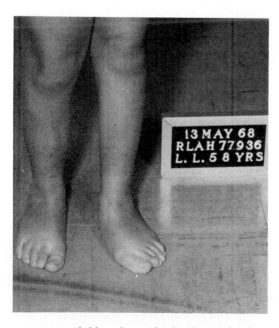

Fig. 9-17. Child with cerebral palsy and valgus hindfoot. He has also developed spastic hallux valgus. (From Proceedings of Foot Society, 1977.)

notomies in the proximal segment of the toes, a much more predictable procedure than lengthening these tendons at the ankle level. Prior to Achilles tendon lengthening in a spastic child, it is wise to study the activity of the toe flexors during barefoot gait. Even mild spasticity of these muscles can become significant after the lengthened Achilles tendon permits increased stretch. Therefore simultaneous Achilles tendon lengthening and toe flexor tenotomies may be necessary in appropriate cases.

Occasionally in cerebral palsy the great toe extensor will work selectively as a foot dorsiflexor more effectively than the anterior tibial muscle. Tohen et al. (1966) suggested that these muscles be transferred together to the dorsum of the foot.

It should be emphasized again that although the procedures are not difficult technically to perform they should be reserved for surgeons well indoctrinated in the care of the cerebral palsy child.

Foot surgery in motor unit disease
JOHN D. HSU

Motor unit disease consists of neuropathies and myopathies, diseases traditionally known as neuromuscular diseases. It defines the area better, although there are many instances in which neuromuscular diseases cross the motor unit barrier and become influenced by spinal cord or higher centers.

Neuropathies are generally stable conditions and involve the motor unit from the anterior horn cell to the neuromuscular junction. Nonprogressive examples include spinal muscular atrophy, Charcot-Marie-Tooth disease, and poliomyelitis. Landry-Guillain-Barré-Strohl disease represents a form of neuropathy in which progressive recovery of motor weaknesses is seen.

Myopathies, by contrast, are diseases that are directly attributable to degeneration of the muscle fiber. These conditions are generally progressive. Progression can be rapid as in Duchenne pseudohypertrophic muscular dystrophy, in which a victim succumbs to the disease in his early 20's, to slowly progressive as in the fascial-scapular-humeral type of muscular dystrophy or limb girdle type of dystrophy, a fairly stable condition. In certain congenital muscular dystrophies no progression of weakness can be seen.

It is not the scope of this section of the chapter to discuss generally identification or the clinical manifestations of these diseases; rather it is hoped that the foot changes can be described and current treatment methods summarized.

GOAL IN TREATMENT

The goal in treatment of the foot deformities in motor unit disease is to maintain function and comfort. The resultant position of the foot is the effect of a fine balance between agonist and antagonist muscle groups. Because of selective weaknesses, one group of muscles can become overpowering. Gravity, positioning, and adaptation to equipment may also help direct the foot into abnormal positions. Soft tissue contractures can occur resulting in the development of an abnormal position; and when this happens, additional factors may set up a vicious cycle of deformity production causing further loss of balance and function (Roy and Gibson, 1970).

DUCHENNE PSEUDOHYPERTROPHIC MUSCULAR DYSTROPHY (DMD)
Walking phase—early

The young child with DMD does not show any deformity. Early there is anterior tibial weakness. The gastrocnemius-soleus muscle remains strong. Coupled with gravitational forces in sitting and walking, there is a natural tendency for the ankle to be in equinus. Early management should include stretching, generally taught by the physician or the physical therapist to the family, and use of night splints to hold the ankle at a neutral position.

Walking phase—late

As the DMD child gets older (between 7 and 8 years of age), walking becomes more difficult. Weakness in the hip extensors and the quadriceps and anterior tibial muscles is significant, and the child rises and walks on his tiptoes. The posterior tibial muscle generally remains strong, turning the forefoot into varus and adductus (Fig. 9-18). Maintaining balance requires effort, and falling occurs frequently. To prolong ambulation, correction of the deformities followed by bracing is necessary.

Correction of equinus deformity. If equinus is the predominant deformity, lengthening the Achilles tendon percutaneously is the method of choice. Frequently this is used in conjunction with bracing and other procedures.

Correction of varus and adductus deformity. In the DMD patient the deformity of varus and adductus is generally caused by the pull of the relatively strong posterior tibial muscle. The posterior tibial tendon is transferred anteriorly through the interosseous membrane (Spencer, 1973; Hsu, 1976). A simplified method for the accomplishment of

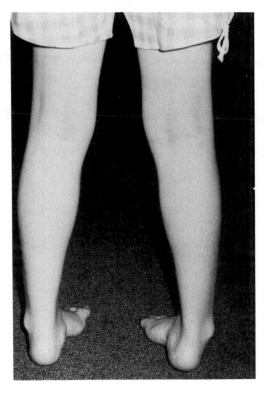

Fig. 9-18. DMD patient, age 10 years; varus and adductus deformity of the foot in the late walking phase.

this surgical procedure is illustrated in Fig. 9-19. We favor this method in DMD patients and in children because it minimizes surgical trauma and achieves a satisfactory result (Morris, 1971; Williams, 1976).

Postsurgical management. After surgical correction has been made, lightweight casts made of fiberglass (e.g., Lightcast) have been routinely used in our clinic. The patients are generally standing the day after surgery and walking in 3 to 4 days with training. Casts are

allowed to remain approximately 6 weeks and are then removed in favor of prefitted bilateral long leg braces.

Late stages—wheelchair patients

If preventive measures have not been instituted or corrections have not been made earlier, progressive foot deformity is frequently seen in the older DMD patient (Fig. 9-20, *C*). We believe this is attributable to previous deformity and to poor wheelchair adaptation and design; thus the feet do not reach the pedal, and gravitational forces pull the foot into further equinus. In the extreme varus position, pressure sores can occur on the dorsal and lateral aspects of the foot. In these cases, corrective measures need to be

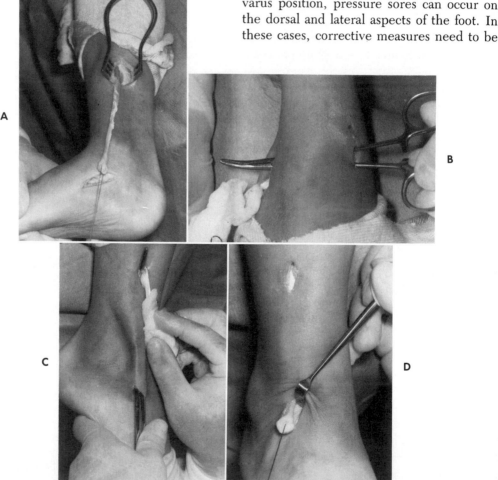

Fig. 9-19. Our procedure for a posterior tibial tendon transfer anteriorly through the interosseous membrane. **A,** Exposure of the posterior tibial tendon and removal from the medial side of the foot. **B,** Incisions used to bring the tendon anteriorly through the interosseous membrane. **C,** Tendon passer used to bring the tendon to the dorsum of the foot. **D,** Tendon ready for anchoring.

taken with tendon and contracture releases made. The following procedures can be used: (1) Achilles tendon lengthening, (2) release of the contracted medial structures, and (3) posterior tibial and anterior tibial release. Generally all these procedures can be done percutaneously followed by immobilization in the corrected position in short leg casts. After removal of the casts (3 to 4 weeks), short leg braces (e.g., a cosmetic-type AFO [ankle-foot orthosis]) can be used. Bracing is mandatory; otherwise the deformities will occur.

CHARCOT-MARIE-TOOTH DISEASE

Charcot-Marie-Tooth disease is an inherited condition involving peripheral motor neurons and showing progressive muscular atrophy of the feet and legs first (Dyck et al., 1975). Fig. 9-21 illustrates the foot deformities seen in an involved family. The general pattern of weakness occurs with wasting of the leg muscles, peroneal weakness, pes cavus, hammertoes, and clawing of the toes. This results in a steppage gait and shuffling of the feet. Foot drop and selective progressive muscle atrophy cause fixed deformities and

contractures to occur in the feet (Jacobs and Carr, 1950).

Initial treatment should be directed at support with splinting. When foot deformities persist, a careful assessment of the muscle strength by selective muscle testing is necessary. Frequently at an early age correction of the foot deformities can be made by appropriate tendon transfers to maintain balance. The anterior tibial tendon can be transferred to the lateral side, or the posterior tibial tendon can also be transferred through the interosseous membrane.

As the deformity increases, the foot develops into abnormal positions. With fixed bony deformities, wedge correction followed by triple arthrodesis is indicated and should be made at a time when bone growth has nearly ceased. (See also Chapter 10.)

SPINAL MUSCULAR ATROPHY

Spinal muscular atrophy represents a neuropathy due to selective degeneration of the anterior horn cells. It is a stable condition in most cases (Munsat et al., 1969). The primary feature is muscle atrophy; as the child grows,

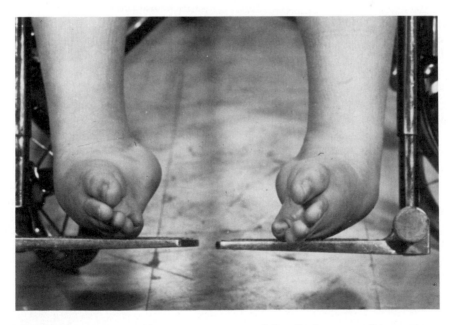

Fig. 9-20. DMD patient, age 13 years; equinovarus deformity in a nonwalking patient.

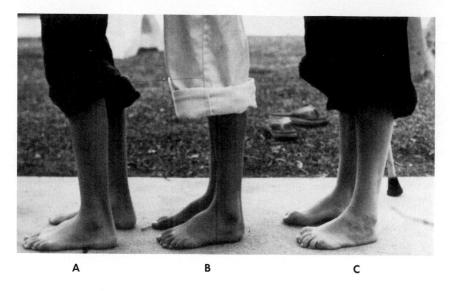

Fig. 9-21. Foot deformity in Charcot-Marie-Tooth disease. **A,** Daughter (age 12); **B,** daughter (age 14); **C,** mother (age 36); all show some degree of deformity.

the weakened muscles become unable to support the skeleton and collapse of the underlying bony architecture occurs. This is especially seen in the ankles and feet.

Initial treatment of foot deformities consists of cast correction of the contractures. Weakness in the distal extremity generally leads to a calcaneal valgus position of the feet. After muscle testing, if there is good function in the peroneal muscle, the procedure of choice is to transfer the peroneal tendons to pull in either dorsiflexion or plantar flexion in a balanced manner so the inversion and eversion deformities of the feet will be eliminated. With severe calcaneal valgus deformities in a young patient, a subtalar extra-articular bony stabilization procedure (Grice, 1955) is useful, followed later by triple arthrodesis if walking has been maintained.

LANDRY-GUILLAIN-BARRÉ-STROHL POLYNEURITIS

This syndrome, acute inflammatory polyradiculoneuropathy, causes paralysis of the respiratory muscles and extremities with gradual recovery. In a study of eighty-nine patients by Oryschak (1972) at Rancho Los Amigos Hospital, the foot deformities were classified as early or late. Full recovery is expected in the majority of cases within two years; thus treatment for the early phase should be directed toward protection of the weak muscles of the ankle and foot and passive correction of deformities. Splints and braces are generally quite adequate.

Residual weaknesses are seen in 15% of the patients and are manifested by lack of control of dorsiflexion of the foot and ankle. Residual dorsal bunion requires transfer of the extensor hallucis longus to the medial side of the foot and arthrodesis of the interphalangeal joint of the great toe (i.e., the modified Jones procedure). When there is difficulty supporting the ankle, appropriate tendon transfers should be made. If tendon transfers cannot satisfactorily correct the problem, fusion must be considered. In a recent study by Gordon (1977) certain patients with persistent deformities have required transfer of the peroneus longus to the second cuneiform to strengthen weakened or absent dorsiflexors with satisfactory results.

REFERENCES
The foot in myelodysplasia

Alban, S., Alban, H., and Fixler, R.: Subtalar arthrodesis utilizing autogenous calcaneal graft, J. Bone Joint Surg. 57A:133, 1975.

Caldwell, G. D.: Correction of paralytic footdrop by hemigastrocsoleus transplantation, Clin. Orthop. 11:81, 1958.

Garceau, G. J., and Brahms, M. A.: A preliminary study of selective plantar-muscle denervation for pes cavus, J. Bone Joint Surg. 38A:553, 1956.

Hay, M., and Walker, G.: Plantar pressures in healthy children and in children with myelomeningocele, J. Bone Joint Surg. 55B:828, 1975.

Hayes, J. T., Gross, H. P., and Dow, S.: Survey for paralytic defects in myelomeningocele, J. Bone Joint Surg. 46A:1577, 1964.

Jolson, R.: Split triceps transfer for recurrent equinus. In McLaurin, R., editor: Myelomeningocele, New York, 1977, Grune & Stratton, Inc.

Makin, M.: Tibio-fibular relationship in paralyzed limbs, J. Bone Joint Surg. 47B:500, 1965.

Menelaus, M.: Orthopaedic management of spina bifida cystica, Edinburgh, 1971, E. & S. Livingstone, Ltd.

Menelaus, M. B.: Talectomy for equinovarus deformity in arthrogryposis and spina bifida, J. Bone Joint Surg. 53B:468, 1971.

Menelaus, M. B.: Orthopaedic management of children with myelomeningocele: a plea for realistic goals, Dev. Med. Child Neurol. 18(supp. 37):3, 1976.

Peabody, C.: Tendon transplantation in the lower extremity. In Instructional Course Lectures, American Academy of Orthopaedic Surgeons, vol. 6, Ann Arbor, 1949, J. W. Edwards.

Samilson, R.: Crescentic osteotomy of the os calcis for calcaneocavus feet. In Bateman, J. E., editor: Foot science, Philadelphia, 1976, W. B. Saunders Co.

Sharrard, W. J. W.: Paralytic deformities in the lower limb, J. Bone Joint Surg. 49B:731, 1967.

Sharrard, W. J. W., and Grosfeld, I.: Management of foot deformities in myelomeningocele, J. Bone Joint Surg. 50B:456, 1968.

Sharrard W. J. W., and Webb, J.: Supramalleolar wedge osteotomy of the tibia in children with myelomeningocele, J. Bone Joint Surg. 56:458, 1974.

Sharrard, W. J. W.: Paralytic convex pes valgus. In McLauren, R., editor: Myelomeningocle, New York, 1977, Grune & Stratton, Inc.

Tachdjian, M.: Pediatric orthopaedics, Philadelphia, 1972, W. B. Saunders Co.

Taylor, R. G.: Treatment of claw toes by multiple transfer flexors to extensor tendon, J. Bone Joint Surg. 33B:539, 1951.

Turco, V. J.: Surgical correction of resistant club feet, J. Bone Joint Surg. 53A:477, 1971.

Turner, J., and Cooper, R.: Posterior transposition of tibialis anterior through the interosseus membrane, Clin. Orthop. 79:71, 1971.

Walker, G.: Early management of varus feet, J. Bone Joint Surg. 53B:462, 1971.

Westin, G. W.: Achilles tenodesis to fibula. Personal communication, 1975.

The foot in cerebral palsy

Alban, S., and Alban, H.: Subtalar extra-articular arthrodesis with calcaneal bone in children with cerebral palsy. Proceedings, American Academy of Cerebral Palsy, 1975.

Banks, H. H.: Orthopedic aspects of cerebral palsy. In Samilson, R. L., editor: Foot deformities in orthopedic aspects of cerebral palsy, Philadelphia, 1975, J. B. Lippincott Co.

Banks, H. H., and Green, W. T.: Correction of equinus deformity in cerebral palsy, J. Bone Joint Surg. 40A:13, 1958.

Basset, F. H.: Deformities of the foot in cerebral palsy. In Instructional Course Lectures, American Academy of Orthopaedic Surgeons, vol. 20, St. Louis, 1971, The C. V. Mosby Co.

Bisslar, R. S., and Lewis, H. L.: Transfer of the tibialis posterior tendon in cerebral palsy, J. Bone Joint Surg. 52A:137, 1975.

Grice, D. S.: Extra-articular arthrodesis of the subastragalar joint with paralytic flat foot of children, J. Bone Joint Surg. 9:927, 1952.

Hoffer, M., Rieswig, J., Garret, A. A., and Perry, J.: Split anterior tendon transfer in cerebral palsy, Orthop. Clin. North Am. 5:31, 1974.

Perry, J., Hoffer, M., Antonelli, D., Giovan, P., and Greenberg, R.: Electromyography of the triceps surae in cerebral palsy, J. Bone Joint Surg. 56A:511, 1974.

Root, L.: Transfer of posterior tibial tendon in cerebral palsy, Proceedings, American Academy of Cerebral Palsy, 1971.

Root, R., and Frost, H. M.: Spastic varus treated by inner muscular posterior tibial tendon lengthening, Clin. Orthop. 79:61, 1971.

Sharrard, W. J. W.: Personal communication, 1972.

Silver, C. M., Simon, S. D., Spindell, E., Litchman, H. M., and Scala, M.: Calcaneal osteotomy for valgus and varus deformities of the foot in cerebral palsy; a preliminary report on twenty-seven operations, J. Bone Joint Surg. 49A:232, 1967.

Tohen, A., Carmona, J., and Barrera, J.: The utilization of abnormal reflexes in the treatment of spastic foot deformities, Clin. Orthop. 47:77, 1966.

Foot surgery in motor unit disease

Dyck, P. J., Thomas, P. K., and Lambert, E. H., editors: Peripheral neuropathy, Philadelphia, 1975, W. B. Saunders Co.

Gordon, S. L., Morris, W. T., Stoner, M. A., and Greer, R. B., III: Residua of Guillain-Barré polyneuritis in children, J. Bone Joint Surg. 59A:193, 1977.

Grice, D. S.: Further experience with extra-articular arthrodesis of the subtalar joint, J. Bone Joint Surg. 37A:246, 1955.

Hsu, J. D.: Management of foot deformity in Duchenne's pseudohypertrophic muscular dystrophy, Orthop. Clin. North Am. 7:979, 1976.

Jacobs, J., and Carr, C. R.: Progressive muscular atrophy of the peroneal type (Charcot-Marie-Tooth disease), J. Bone Joint Surg. 32A:27, 1950.

Morris, H. D.: Personal communication, 1971.

Munsat, T. L., Woods, R., Fowler, W., and Pearson, C. M.: Neurogenic muscular atrophy of infancy with prolonged survival, Brain 92:9, 1969.

Oryschak, A. F.: The Guillain-Barré syndrome. A study of residual muscular weakness and disability, U.S.C. Orthop. Semin. **5**:341, 1972.

Roy, L., and Gibson, D. A.: Pseudohypertrophic muscular dystrophy and its surgical management. Review of 30 patients, Can. J. Surg. **13**:13, 1970.

Spencer, G. E., Jr.: Orthopaedic considerations in the management of muscular dystrophy, Curr. Pract. Orthop. Surg. **5**:279, 1973.

Williams, P. F.: Restoration of muscle balance of the foot by transfer of the tibialis posterior, J. Bone Joint Surg. **58B**:217, 1976.

10

ACQUIRED NEUROLOGIC DISORDERS OF THE ADULT FOOT

Robert L. Waters and Douglas E. Garland

In childhood, neurologic disorders of the lower extremity often bring about muscular imbalance of the foot and consequently may cause abnormalities of the bones and joints. The adult who acquires a neurologic illness after skeletal maturity usually has normal bone and joint structures. Correction of adult deformities can be obtained from proper orthotic management and appropriate tendon releases, tendon lengthenings, and tendon transfers to rebalance existing muscular forces.

Stroke and head trauma and spinal cord injury are the most common central neurologic disorders causing deformity about the foot and ankle. Peroneal nerve palsy is the most common disorder of the peripheral nerves requiring orthotic or surgical care. Charcot-Marie-Tooth disease, Friedreich's ataxia, and related posterior spinocerebellar degenerative diseases affect both upper and lower neurons and commonly require orthopaedic attention.

When muscle imbalance is due to a disorder of the peripheral nerves (poliomyelitis, peripheral nerve palsy), muscles may be presumed to demonstrate activity in the correct phase of the gait cycle. Variance of activity from the normal phase occurs only as a deliberate substitution to compensate for other gait abnormalities. By contrast, central nervous system diseases alter the normal inhibitory and facilitory responses on lower locomotor centers and spinal reflexes, and they may be completely or partially freed from regulation by higher centers. The result may be absence of muscle activity, no control of intensity of activity, loss of phasic activity, or variations of activity in relation to posture. Consequently, standard tests of voluntary muscle strength often have little relationship to the actual activity of the muscles during walking. Correct surgical and orthotic management depends on critical visual analysis of the subject during ambulation to determine which muscles are responsible for gait abnormalities. Gait electromyography gives more precise information about the phasic activity of those muscles.

STROKE

Equinus, varus, and toe curling acting alone or in various combinations are the most common disabilities in the lower extremity and most frequently require bracing and/or surgery. Often they occur in the same patient. Bracing is required initially since surgical correction is delayed until 6 months after the stroke. This waiting period allows time for completion of the majority of spontaneous neurologic recovery and for the patient to realize his gait disability is permanent.

We prefer the BICAAL (bi-channel adjustable ankle locking) orthosis for the initial treatment of most problems about the foot and ankle. Anterior and posterior stops allow precise adjustment of the ankle position for the patient. The BICAAL position is frequently adjusted several times in the first month after stroke. The BICAAL orthosis is oftentimes the permanent treatment of choice for patients with moderate equinus caused by spasticity or varus (Waters and Montgomery, 1974).

Plastic materials fabricated over a positive mold of the subject's leg have replaced the traditional spring-type orthoses. The amount of ankle flexibility can be decreased by extending the medial and lateral trim lines anteriorly or by incorporating ridges in the orthosis. These orthoses are lightweight and can be worn in any shoes the subject wears as long as they have the same heel height.

Equinus

Excessive plantar flexion is initially secondary to spasticity although later it may be due to a mixture of spasticity and myostatic contracture. It causes the patient to weight bear on the forefoot without heel contact (Fig. 10-1). In order to obtain heel contact, the tibia must be extended backward causing hyperextension of the knee.

When equinus is not satisfactorily corrected by an orthosis, surgical correction is indicated. The benefits of surgery are easily shown by performing an anesthetic block of the posterior tibial nerve at the popliteal fossa. In the absence of fixed contracture, paralysis of the triceps surae will relieve equinus and the heel will no longer piston out of an orthosis. This allows the patient to walk more easily and to appreciate the potential benefits of surgery.

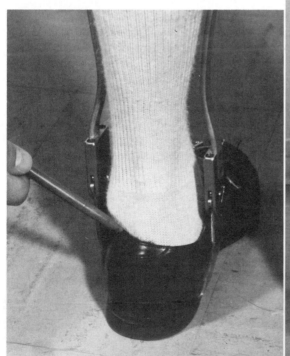
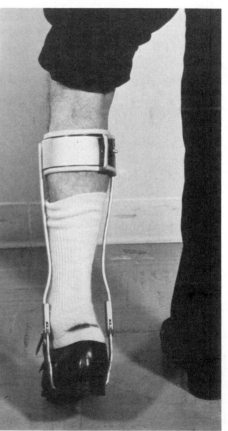

Fig. 10-1. **A,** A mark is placed on the sock with the heel firmly seated in the shoe. **B,** The patient is then asked to walk, and the heel is observed to see whether it pistons out of the shoe.

Achilles tendon lengthening may be an open or a percutaneous procedure. We prefer a modification of the Hoke triple hemisection tenotomy performed percutaneously. At surgery the knee is extended and the ankle dorsiflexed, placing tension on the Achilles tendon. This draws the tendon posteriorly away from the neurovascular structures. Tenotomy is performed and the ankle dorsiflexed to neutral but not beyond. A short-leg walking cast is applied with the ankle in approximately 5° of plantar flexion to prevent added stretch of the Achilles tendon while walking. Care should be taken to avoid overlengthening of the Achilles tendon since plantar flexion weakness can result. The cast is worn 6 weeks, and the ankle protected in an AFO during the day and a posterior splint at night for an additional 6 weeks. We have obtained serial x-ray examination of the Achilles tendon tagged on each end with metal clips, and they revealed that no further lengthening occurs despite immediate full weight bearing in a short leg cast.

Plantar flexion weakness is the most commonly overlooked gait abnormality in the hemiplegic patient, and the most frequently encountered complication of Achilles tendon lengthening. When present, the patient walks using one of two abnormal gait patterns. In the first and less common pattern the ankle assumes an excessively dorsiflexed position in stance with compensatory knee flexion; the knee is stabilized by the quadriceps. The substitution pattern is demanding and inefficient, however, and the patient soon learns the next pattern. In the second pattern he hyperextends his knee at heel strike, locking it in extension with the tibia directed backward from the vertical, and maintains posture during stance. This is purposely done to keep the center of gravity of the body behind the ankle joint and prevent excessive ankle dorsiflexion and knee flexion.

Forceful knee hyperextension will eventually lead to genu recurvatum and pain. The latter gait pattern, when observed at the knee, closely resembles the knee hyperextension thrust caused by excessive plantar flexion (equinus). The key to differentiating the two

patterns is observation of the foot. Patients with plantar flexion weakness weight bear primarily on the heel whereas patients with hyperactive triceps (equinus) weight bear initially on the forefoot. The "standing test" also aids differentiation.

If active toe flexion is present prior to surgery, long toe flexor release is performed at the time of Achilles tendon lengthening even if toe flexion is not painful. Correction of equinus causes relative shortening of the long toe flexors. Patients with asymptomatic toe curling prior to surgery may have increased toe curling and pain after surgery.

After Achilles tendon lengthening, the foot is positioned with an orthosis. Most patients require continued orthotic support after corrective surgery. Patients whose only deformity is equinus usually have a weak or absent contraction of the tibialis anterior, and an AFO is required to prevent foot drop. In patients with spasticity, it is difficult to lengthen the Achilles tendon "just the right amount." The stretch response is one of the major determinants of muscle activity in the spastic triceps surae. The amplitude of this response varies in each patient and is highly sensitive to the length and velocity of muscle extension. Correction of equinus by Achilles tendon lengthening alters the range and velocity of extension, particularly if heel contact is reestablished. Slight differences in the amount of lengthening can result in persistent equinus or plantar flexion weakness; both conditions benefit from continued orthotic support. It is best to err by underlengthening than by overlengthening the Achilles tendon. Patients can be brace free with slight flexion deformities, but a resultant weakened calf more often requires bracing.

Varus

Surgical correction of varus is indicated when, despite use of a well-fitted orthosis, the foot twists in the shoe causing the patient to weight bear on the lateral edge of the foot (Fig. 10-2).

Five muscles may contribute to varus: the soleus, flexor hallucis longus, flexor digitorum longus, tibialis posterior, and tibialis anterior.

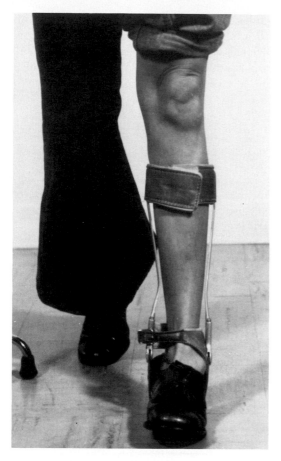

Fig. 10-2. Surgery is indicated when the varus persists despite application of an orthosis. The addition of a T-strap is usually insufficient to correct varus. If the strap is secured with sufficient force to improve the varus, excessive pressure is applied to the skin over the lateral malleolar area.

When the soleus significantly contributes to varus, equinus is also present. The contribution of the soleus to varus is diminished by heel cord lengthening. Similarly, when the long toe flexors significantly contribute to varus, toe curling is present; the contribution of the long toe flexors to varus is elminiated by their release.

It is not necessary to lengthen the tibialis posterior tendon unless the patient has marked hindfoot varus under anesthesia. Electromyographic studies performed on stroke patients reveal this muscle to be often inactive or, when active, usually displaying minimal activity. If the tibialis posterior is released or lengthened in association with the SPLATT procedure (split anterior tibial tendon transfer), there is a possibility that calcaneovalgus in conjunction with the excessive eversion of the forefoot will occur. This is particularly true in patients with pes planus associated with the collapse of the medial arch and pain prior to their stroke.

Observation and palpation of the tibialis anterior tendon reveal this muscle to be the key deforming force in forefoot varus. If forefoot varus is corrected, hindfoot varus is not a problem. The SPLATT procedure reliably corrects forefoot varus. The principle behind it is to transfer the lateral portion of the tibialis anterior tendon to the distal third cuneiform and cuboid and create an eversion force neutralizing the varus pull of the remaining proximal portion (Fig. 10-3).

The SPLATT is performed through a medial longitudinal incision in the arch of the foot. The distal one half to two thirds of the tendon is freed from its insertion in the base of the first metatarsal and a suture is placed around the free end. A second incision is made over the muscle-tendon junction of the tibialis anterior. The pretibial fascia and retinacular ligaments are divided by passing a scissors between the two incisions. The tendon suture is delivered to the proximal incision. When traction is applied on the suture, the tibialis anterior tendon splits lengthwise just beyond the muscle-tendon junction. A third transverse incision is placed over the cuneiform and cuboid bones. Drill holes are placed in each and interconnected. The tibialis anterior is passed subcutaneously on top of the retinacular ligaments, pulled lateral to medial through the holes in the cuboid and the third cuneiform, and sutured to itself. Failure of fixation with this method is uncommon. Passage of the transferred tendon subcutaneously rather than under the extensor retinaculum enables the tendon to "bowstring" anteriorly when the tibialis anterior contracts and thus increases the tendon's mechanical advantage.

Following surgery, a short-leg walking cast is applied. At 6 weeks the cast is removed.

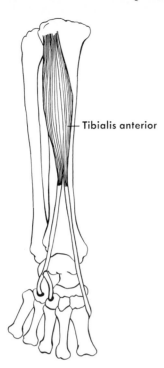

Tibialis anterior

Fig. 10-3. The split anterior tibial tendon transfer (SPLATT) is performed by passing the lateral two thirds of the tendon through two holes drilled in the cuboid and third cuneiform and sewing the tendon to itself.

The posterior half of the cast is worn at night, and an AFO is worn for activity an additional 4½ months to prevent plantar flexion and ensure satisfactory tendon healing. The SPLATT procedure has proved itself so reliable that when varus is the only significant deformity for which an AFO is worn one can predict the patient will walk orthosis-free after surgery.

Equinovarus

In most patients equinus, varus, and toe curling occur together. Achilles tendon lengthening, the SPLATT procedure, and long toe flexor release are performed simultaneously. Because the transferred portion of the tibialis anterior tendon is secured under tension, it serves as an active tenodesis to prevent drop foot in swing. After the transferred tendon has been protected 6 months, some patients are able to walk without an orthosis. There is a gradual tendency for the passive elements in the muscle to stretch, however, and foot drop or mild equinus to recur requiring orthotic support even if the tibialis anterior strongly contracts in swing. Electromyographic evaluation often reveals the triceps surae to be abnormally active in terminal swing and to have presumably created a greater opposing force than the tibialis anterior can withstand. Also, after surgery a plantar flexion force is now generated at the ankle at the time of heel strike due to the resultant forces of body weight and limb motion passing anterior to the point of heel contact.

If the Achilles tendon is consistently lengthened to such an extent that foot drop is not likely to recur, most patients will have evidence of plantar flexion in stance after surgery.

In an effort to prevent recurrent equinus without excessively lengthening the Achilles tendon, we are currently transferring the flexor hallucis longus or flexor digitorum longus through the interosseous membrane to the dorsum of the foot (Fig. 10-4). The procedure is performed on healthy young patients if the long toe flexors are active in swing. This can be determined visually or by gait electromyography. If the flexor hallucis longus and flexor digitorum longus are active, only the former is transferred. The tendon is passed through drill holes in the third cuneiform and cuboid along with the split portion of the tibialis anterior. The procedure is not performed on elderly patients or on patients with impaired circulation since it requires more surgical time and dissection.

Transfer of the toe flexor tendons is done by releasing the tendons in the foot (Fig. 10-5). Care should be taken to preserve as much of the tendon length as possible. A second incision is made along the posteromedial aspect of the tibia. The tendon transfers are pulled into the proximal incision. By the application of tension on the tendon and by blunt fingertip dissection, the muscle is stripped from its origin on the tibia, fibula, and interosseous membrane. A third incision is made anteriorly over the interval between the extensor hallucis longus and extensor digitorum communis.

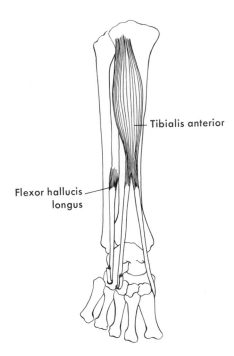

Tibialis anterior

Flexor hallucis longus

Fig. 10-4. The flexor hallucis longus is transferred through the interosseous membrane and inserted into the cuboid and third cuneiform to reinforce the SPLATT.

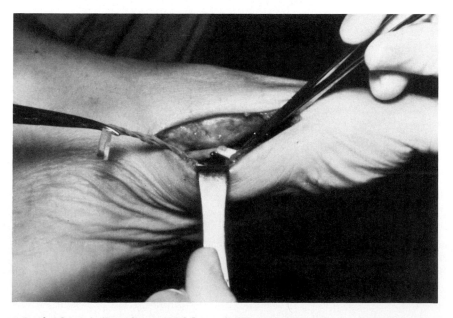

Fig. 10-5. The flexor hallucis longus and flexor digitorum communis are released by an incision along the medial arch of the foot. This same incision can be utilized to detach the distal portion of the tibialis anterior tendon when the SPLATT is performed.

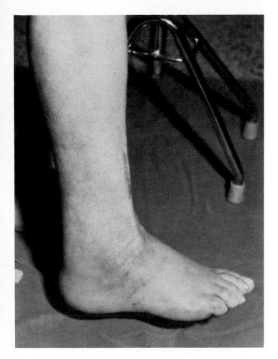

Fig. 10-6. Postoperative appearance of a foot following tendo Achillis lengthening, SPLATT, and reinforcement with the flexor hallucis longus tendon. The transferred tendons are on the anterior aspect of the foot. Balance of the foot is excellent, the foot is maintained in neutral during swing, and varus is corrected.

A window is created in the interosseous membrane and the handle of a small osteotome is passed through the window. The interosseous membrane is bluntly stripped proximally and distally from the tibia and fibula. The window is placed sufficiently proximal on the leg (8 to 10 cm above the ankle mortise) so there is sufficient distance between the tibia and fibula for the tendon and its attached fibers to pass freely (Fig. 10-6).

Inadequate dorsiflexion

Inadequate dorsiflexion in swing (foot drop) is due to inactivity or paresis of the anterior tibialis. It occasionally is seen in patients without equinus. Gait electromyography performed on stroke patients generally fails to demonstrate suitable muscles for tendon transfer to restore dorsiflexion because the muscles are inactive during swing. This type of foot drop is corrected by an AFO (Fig. 10-7).

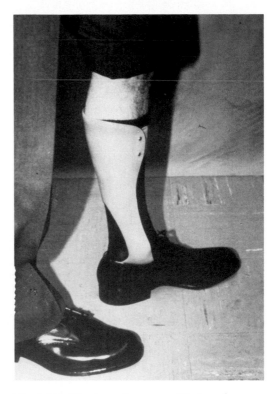

Fig. 10-7. Plastic orthoses are fabricated over a positive mold of the shank and foot. The foot plate of the orthosis is hidden inside the shoe.

Toe curling

Excessive toe flexion (toe curling) that causes pain in stroke patients is usually characterized by inactive toe extensors (Fig. 10-8). Correction is achieved by releasing the flexor hallucis longus and/or flexor digitorum communis tendons. If one or two toes are involved, tenotomy is performed at each toe. When all toes are involved, the tenotomy is more easily performed by sectioning the flexor hallucis longus and common tendon of the flexor digitorum longus in the sole of the foot, distal to the insertion of the quadratus plantae.

An incision is made in the medial aspect of the foot along the upper border of the abductor hallucis (Fig. 10-5). The abductor is reflected plantarward, and access to the flexor hallucis longus and flexor digitorum longus is obtained in the interval between the first and third layers of plantar muscles. This same incision is utilized to detach the distal portion of

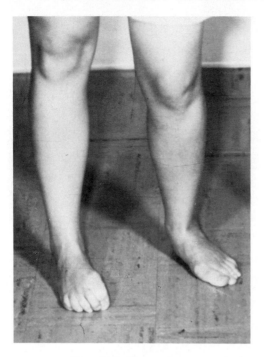

Fig. 10-8. Toe curling.

the tibialis anterior tendon when the SPLATT procedure is performed. Persistent flexion of the proximal interphalangeal joints is sometimes present after surgery due to spasticity of the short flexors, but it rarely causes discomfort in stroke patients.

Spasticity of the flexor hallucis longus, adductor hallucis, and lateral head of the flexor hallucis brevis will increase both valgus and varus deformities of the great toe if present prior to stroke. Correction of the dynamic component of these deformities is obtained by release of the flexor hallucis longus. We divide the conjoint tendon of the adductor hallucis and lateral head of the flexor digitorum brevis distal to the fibular sesamoid and leave the sesamoid in place. Additional bony procedures may be required to correct persistent structural deformity. Unless all tendons are released and the toe made flail, bony procedures to realign the toe will not prevent further deformities.

HEAD TRAUMA

Neurologic recovery in the head-injured patient occurs over a more prolonged period than does injury following stroke. Definitive surgical procedures should be delayed until at least 18 months have elapsed, at which time the majority of recovery has occurred. Surgery may be indicated in the subacute phase when equinus prevents ambulation or institution of a rehabilitation program.

The same surgical procedures described for the stroke patient may be applied to the head trauma patient for the management of deformities of the foot and ankle. Toe deformities in the head-injured patient are more difficult to treat than in the stroke patient, however, because of varying combinations of spasticity among the long toe flexors, short toe flexors, extensors, and intrinsic muscles.

Equinus and extensor rigidity

Following acute head trauma, equinus contractures are prevented by appropriate passive range of motion exercises and splinting. Casts may be applied to prevent deformity; serial casts may be required to correct established deformities. Patients who are initially decorticate or decerebrate develop extensor rigidity causing severe equinus. This is due to brain stem damage and does not occur in stroke patients, in whom the lesion is generally confined to the cerebral cortex. Anesthetic injection of the posterior tibial nerve will allow a decrease in the extensor tone and better positioning of the ankle prior to cast application.

Achilles tendon lengthening should not be performed during the first year. Electromyographic examination of patients with equinus due to extensor rigidity reveals excessive and continuous tibialis anterior activity while standing, despite equinus posture. This plus the fact that the extensor rigidity may later subside can cause excessive dorsiflexion, plantar flexion weakness, or calcaneal valgus if Achilles tendon lengthening is performed prior to neurologic stability.

When equinus (often associated with clonus) interferes with ambulation, phenol injection of the motor branches of the posterior tibial nerve can be safely performed in the first year to correct deformity or extensor rigidity that cannot be corrected by casting.

Initially, complete block is obtained and residual deformity due to myostatic contracture can be corrected by serial casting postoperatively. The majority of motor axons recover within 6 months. No additional surgical procedures are required if extensor rigidity clears.

Closed phenol injection to the posterior tibial nerve is not recommended since the loss of sensation is bothersome and injury to sensory fibers may precipitate causalgia. Closed motor point injection of phenol or alcohol is an acceptable alternative procedure.

Surgical exposure of the posterior tibial nerve is obtained through a short longitudinal midline incision. The incision begins at the popliteal crease and extends distally 10 cm. The posterior tibial nerve is identified between the heads of the gastrocnemius; the motor branches to the medial and lateral heads of the gastrocnemius are injected with phenol. Several branches may innervate each head. The posterior tibial nerve is traced to the border of the soleus. The motor branches to the soleus, tibialis posterior, and long toe flexors are identified with a nerve stimulator and injected with phenol by a 25-gauge needle. A solution of 3% phenol in glycerin is used for injection. This solution is bactericidal and should not be heat sterilized prior to injection.

Toe deformities

Toe deformities in the head-injured patient are more difficult to treat than in the stroke patient. Due to differing patterns of muscle imbalance, different types of deformities occur. The surgical procedure employed must be individualized. No single procedure can be applied to all deformities.

Unless fixed deformity is present, phalangectomy is contraindicated. The bony and ligamentous structures provide inherent lateral stability; without this support, lateral deviation of the toes may occur. The exception is when dorsal callosities are present in association with fixed contracture of the proximal interphalangeal joints. Proximal interphalangeal joint resection and arthrodesis are performed to maintain stability in association with tendon releases.

The objective of surgery is to release overactive muscles responsible for painful toe deformities and is most frequently accomplished by release of the long and short flexors with occasional lengthening of the extensors if markedly overactive. Loss of active toe flexion is not significant in this population. Excessive toe flexion at the proximal and distal interphalangeal joints in head trauma patients is usually due to both short and long toe flexor activity. If only the long toe flexors are released, flexion will persist at the proximal interphalangeal joint following surgery and still cause pain. Therefore tenotomy of both the long and the short flexors is performed via transverse incisions on the volar aspect of each toe.

In some patients excessive toe flexion is present only at the proximal interphalangeal joint and not the distal phalangeal joint (Fig. 10-9). This deformity is due to excessive short flexor activity and may be demonstrated by anesthetic block of the posterior tibial nerve at the ankle, paralyzing the short flexor muscles. If the deformity is corrected following block, only the short flexors are released.

Excessive dorsiflexion at the metatarsophalangeal joints is generally a passive response to excessive flexion at the interphalangeal joints rather than to excessive extensor activity. If the extensor tendons are markedly active, lengthening of the extensors is performed in association with toe flexor release. When extensor tenotomy is not performed, the patient is instructed that it may be necessary to release these tendons at a later date.

Transfer of the long flexor tendons to the extensors (Girdlestone-Taylor procedure) at times is useful in the spastic patient. Electromyographic studies reveal that the long toe flexor muscles remain active during terminal stance and during swing. If the long toe flexors are transferred to the extensors, this persistent activity may prevent dorsiflexion at the metatarsophalangeal joints in terminal stance.

Rarely the lateral four toes may assume an

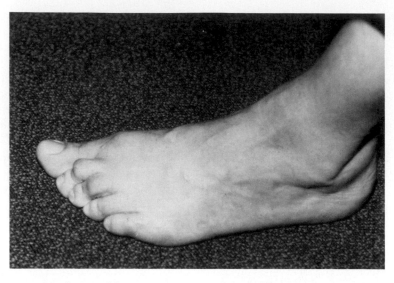

Fig. 10-9. Excessive flexion of the proximal interphalangeal joints of the lateral four toes is due to activity of the short toe flexors. The distal interphalangeal joints are extended, indicating that overactivity of the flexor digitorum communis is not present.

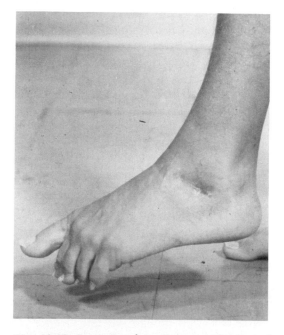

Fig. 10-10. Intrinsic plus posture, indicative of spasticity in the intrinsic muscles. The lateral four toes are flexed at the metatarsophalangeal joints and extended at the interphalangeal joints.

intrinsic plus posture with flexion at the metatarsophalangeal joints and extension at the interphalangeal joints (Fig. 10-10). The great toe may be hyperextended. This deformity is often caused by a positive tonic grasp or Babinski response that is triggered each time the sole of the foot contacts the ground. Surgical correction is obtained by release of the intrinsic tendons (short toe flexors, interossei, lumbricals).

CHARCOT-MARIE-TOOTH DISEASE

Charcot-Marie-Tooth or peroneal muscular atrophy was first described by H. H. Tooth of England and by J. M. Charcot and Pierre Marie of France in 1886. Although they considered it a myopathy, degenerative changes have been detected in the peripheral nerves, motor nerve roots, and spinal cord. It is both familial and hereditary.

Genetics

Allen (1939) demonstrated a triple pattern of inheritance: dominant, sex-linked recessive, and simple recessive. More important, and of great clinical significance, he believed that the pattern of inheritance determined the age of onset and the clinical pattern.

When the inheritance is dominant, the child receives a normal gene from one parent and a corresponding abnormal gene from the other parent. Symptoms become apparent around 30 years of age and may be mild to moderate. Pes cavus may be the only deformity.

When the inheritance is by a simple recessive gene, each parent contributes a defective gene. Since there is nothing to offset these genes, there is an early onset (before 8 years of age) with severe and progressive deformity. By the second decade the patient is usually disabled.

The sex-linked recessive pattern lies between the previous two in clinical severity. Boys receive a defective gene from their mother with no corresponding gene from their father. Since there is only one defective gene, onset is usually delayed until the second decade of life. Since there is no normal gene, however, the disease progresses and deformities become severe by the middle of the third decade. Offspring of these affected females will be normal; only males will be carriers. All patients and families should seek genetic counseling.

Clinical findings

The age of onset is between 5 and 20 years, although the dominant pattern may not have symptoms until after 30. After the initial symptoms the progression of involvement will continue and be symmetric. The peroneals are usually the first muscles involved. The intrinsics of the foot may be involved initially, but this involvement is subtle and difficult to define. There may be slight varus present, but early it can be controlled by footwear and the patient may not be seen until further progression has occurred.

The tibialis anterior is the next muscle involved. Progression of the disease may continue and involve the toe extensors and finally the gastrocnemius. Paresis of the peroneus brevis is generally more severe than of the peroneus longus. The peroneus longus is nearly always active in patients with progressive cavus and may be presumed to play an important role in the deformity. At this time cavovarus, equinovarus, cavus, and toe clawing may be evident. Equinus is often due to deformity of the forefoot rather than to gastrocnemius contracture. Gross muscle loss will be evident, and fibrillar twitching may be observed in the wasted muscles. Ankle jerk reflexes are decreased or absent, and knee jerks may eventually appear. Involvement is primarily motor, although areas of hypesthesia may be present.

Once gross muscle loss has become evident in the lower extremity, intrinsic weakness in the upper extremity may be detected followed by involvement of the forearm and clawing of the hands.

Surgery

Deformities in the young include cavus, equinovarus, and mild toe clawing. In adulthood cavus is the main deformity followed by toe clawing. In childhood the progression is so fast that some equinus develops secondarily to the other deformities and disuse and may become fixed. In the adult, due to slow progression and to both intrinsic and extrinsic involvement, cavus deformity develops with little equinus. Toe clawing is more common and may also be secondary to intrinsic and extrinsic muscle involvement. Toe clawing may also be secondary to a weakened tibialis anterior while the toe extensor remains strong and is used as the primary dorsiflexor of the foot (Fig. 10-11).

The basic surgery in the past was bone procedures, but deformities often recurred if there was not appropriate tendon transfer. In the child, even if the disease is progressing, soft tissue procedures may be performed and will minimize structural bony deformities. A plantar fasciotomy and Achilles tendon lengthening may be indicated early in the disease. The peroneus longus may be transferred to the peroneus brevis. If the patient has fixed equinovarus, he may already manifest bony changes. This gives the tibialis posterior an added mechanical advantage, and it may also become a deforming force. If varus of the heel is fixed or is detected with

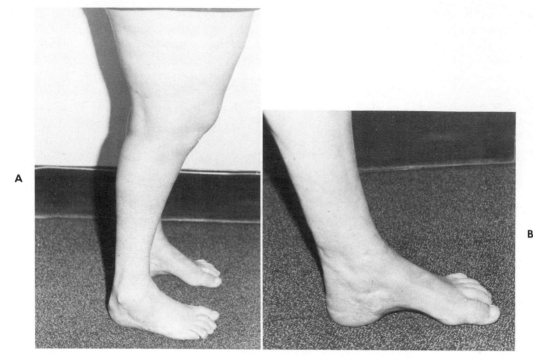

Fig. 10-11. A, Classic lower extremity picture of Charcot-Marie-Tooth deformity. Note the normal muscles proximally with marked wasting distally. **B,** Cavus deformity. A scar is present under the medial malleolus from transfer of the posterior tibial tendon.

standing, the posterior tibial tendon may need to be lengthened or sectioned. The tibialis posterior may be transferred anteriorly to the middle or lateral aspect of the forefoot, depending on the degree of varus. In the presence of fixed bone deformity subtalar or triple arthrodesis is performed. The SPLATT may rarely be employed to balance the forefoot. The tibialis anterior is usually involved and is therefore not always a strong enough muscle for transfer.

Once a stationary point in the progression of the disease is achieved, bone procedures can be undertaken with or without soft tissue procedures. The triple arthrodesis, frequently with an Achilles tendon lengthening and plantar fasciotomy, is the most frequent procedure to correct these deformities. A modification of the triple arthrodesis, such as the Lambrinudi, may be indicated when the anterior muscles are weakened and foot drop is present. If the foot is not balanced after the

triple arthrodesis, muscle transplantation should be employed to balance it or deformities will recur despite the triple arthrodesis.

In the adult foot, cavus and toe clawing are the most frequent deformities. The cavus may be corrected by a triple arthrodesis, a tarsal osteotomy, or osteotomies of the metatarsals depending on the severity of the deformity. A V-osteotomy of the tarsi rather than an anterior wedge osteotomy is recommended since the foot is not shortened by the former. Plantar fasciotomy is usually performed at the same time. If cavus is mild, sometimes its correction corrects the associated toe deformity. If toe clawing is present and not fixed, a Girdlestone-Taylor procedure is indicated. The ideal patient for a Gridlestone-Taylor does not have callosities under the metatarsal heads and weight bears on the ends of his toes. Metatarsalgia or callosities under the metatarsal heads usually are not corrected by the

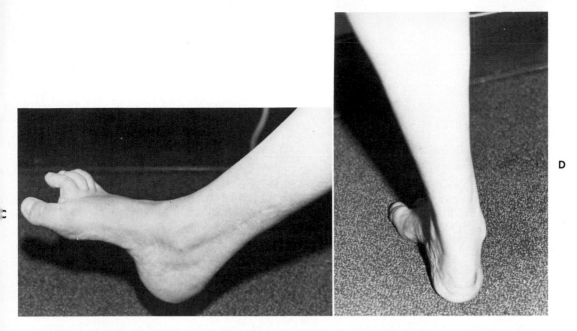

Fig. 10-11, cont'd. C, Attempted dorsiflexion. The only dorsiflexor present is the common toe extensors. The posterior tibial tendon was palpable but had only trace strength. **D,** Heel varus. Transfer of the posterior tibial tendon did not prevent further deformity. Subtalar arthrodesis can correct the varus deformity.

Girdlestone-Taylor operation alone. Tarsal osteotomies, transfer of extensor tendon with interphalangeal fusion, or partial phalangectomies will be required for this deformity. If the foot remains balanced but drops after the bone procedure, a polypropylene orthosis is indicated.

PERONEAL NERVE PALSY

The outlook for significant recovery of motor function following transection of the peroneal nerve in adults is poor after repair. Even when the nerve stroma remains following stretch injuries, the prognosis is variable unless recovery occurs in the early stages. After compression injuries full return may be anticipated if the compressive force is identified early and removed.

It is difficult to predict the chances for recovery based on results recorded in the literature. Outcome is often expressed as the time elapsed between injury and initial motor recovery. The return of some voluntary motion, however, does not always lead to sufficient recovery of strength to prevent foot drop. After a compression or stretch injury, if there is no advancing Tinel sign at 6 months or some voluntary contraction in 9 months, generally there will be minimal chance for functionally significant recovery.

Despite uncertainty regarding recovery of nerve function following acute injury, correction of foot drop can be initially obtained by a plastic shoe insert-type orthosis. Custom-fitted polypropylene orthoses fabricated over a positive mold of the patient's foot and ankle may be worn without discomfort. Shoes may be interchanged as long as they have approximately the same heel height. Objections to orthoses as a permanent method of correcting foot drop have been less frequent since the introduction of cosmetic plastic material that enables one to conceal the orthosis in socks, slacks, or trousers. These orthoses are superior to traditional orthoses with metal uprights. Consequently the cosmetic orthosis may also be the treatment of choice for many patients with a permanent foot drop.

Posterior tibial tendon transfer may be considered as a means of eliminating the need for an orthosis. The limitations of surgery, however, should be carefully considered. Despite favorable reports in the literature (Gunn and Molesworth), we have encountered the following problems after this tendon transfer: failure of automatic response of the tibialis posterior in the swing phase of gait, gradual passive stretching of the tibialis posterior, and planovalgus in patients with preexisting pes planus.

In our experience the posterior tibial tendon restores active voluntary dorsiflexion and fires in the swing phase only if the patient makes a conscious effort to contract this muscle with each step. Apparently good results occur initially when the tendon is transferred and tightly secured, acting mainly as a tenodesis. The patient may voluntarily dorsiflex the foot and not demonstrate a foot drop during ambulation because of the tenodesis effect. Careful questioning of the patient's family will reveal that during routine walking foot drop is usually present. The reason for this paradoxical response lies in the organization of the central nervous system. Direct corticospinal tracts enable the normal patient with an intact cerebral cortex to consciously fire the tibialis posterior in the swing phase. The basic locomotor mechanisms responsible for walking, however, are located subcortically. These mechanisms normally enable normal muscle activity to occur without conscious effort. Despite intensive therapy, it is not possible to reprogram the tibialis posterior to a swing-phase muscle in all patients.

Since the tibialis posterior is normally inactive at heel strike, however, it is subjective to tensile forces which stretch out passive elements of the muscle beyond their normal length. This is because the resultant body weight forces passes anterior to the point of heel contact. Consequently most patients examined several years after surgery have 20°

to 30° of foot drop unless they make a conscious effort to dorsiflex the foot. Dorsiflexion of the foot is preferable to complete foot drop; however greater correction can be usually obtained with an orthosis.

Patients with pes planus may not tolerate any loss of hindfoot varus support. If the tibialis posterior is transferred, calcaneal valgus may increase (associated with increased pronation) and collapse of the medial arch may occur and become symptomatic.

When tendon transfer is performed, we prefer to do a transfer of the flexor hallucis longus and flexor digitorum longus rather than of the tibialis posterior. This is based on the fact that the combined cross-sectional area of these two muscles and their combined strength are greater than those of the tibialis posterior alone. Also we are of the opinion that these muscles more easily convert to automatic swing phase activity although this has not occurred in all patients. The two tendons are passed through the interosseous membrane and inserted into the second cuneiform via the same surgical approaches as described for stroke patients.

SCIATIC NERVE PALSY

As with damage to the peroneal nerve, the outlook for recovery following complete sciatic palsy is poor unless early recovery occurs after a compression injury. Treatment consists of prescription of a rigid ankle-foot orthosis to provide ankle stability. Particular emphasis is placed on teaching the patient the importance of three-times-a-day foot inspection for signs of excessive pressure. Once pressure ulceration occurs and the normal protective covering of the foot pad is scarred, prevention of pressure sores becomes increasingly difficult.

Extreme care should be taken in the use of plastic orthoses. These devices rely on direct skin contact and must be fitted with extreme precision to avoid excessive skin pressure.

Pantalar arthrodesis is mentioned only to be condemned. The patient with complete sciatic palsy will have near-normal gait and walking tolerance with a well-fitted orthosis. Although the foot is held within the orthosis, some ankle and subtalar motion occurs. This motion is important and helps the foot adapt to the sole of the shoe and underlying terrain. Pantalar arthodesis robs the patient of this important adaptive mechanism and increases both pressure and shear stress on the insensitive skin.

HEREDITARY SPINOCEREBELLAR ATAXIA

Friedreich's ataxia is the most common of the spinocerebellar ataxias. Degeneration can be found in the Purkinje cells of the cerebellum, the spinocerebellar tracts, the posterior column, and the corticospinal tracts. The exact etiology is unknown, but the condition is transmitted by an autosomal recessive gene.

Clinical findings

The onset is during childhood and adolescence and may be insidious. Difficulty in ambulation (ataxia) is the major complaint. Foot problems and scoliosis are frequently present. As the disease progresses, ataxia is detected in the upper extremity and intensive tremor may be present. Speech abnormalities, nystagmus, and cardiac abnormalities can also become evident. With further progression a generalized hypotonia is noted, and death may occur in the fourth decade.

The most common foot deformity is a symmetric cavus with or without clawtoes. The great toe also demonstrates the clawtoe deformity. Equinus may be present, sometimes only the forefoot. Muscle imbalance, both intrinsic and extrinsic, must cause these deformities. Peroneal muscle weakness is the most common muscle abnormality. Weakness of the tibialis anterior is a less consistent finding. The knee and ankle jerks are usually absent, and a positive Babinski may be elicited. Two-point discrimination along with position and vibration sense may be diminished.

Surgery

Since cavus and toe clawing are the most common deformities, the majority of the surgical procedures are directed toward them. Surgery should be performed early in the milder cases to prevent further deformity, although not before skeletal maturity has been reached. Since some of the disease may be nonprogressive and the risks of surgery are no greater for cavus foot than for similar foot deformities of other etiologies, an aggressive surgical approach may be undertaken. A well-balanced stable foot will often aid in ambulation and lessen the effects of ataxia.

The most common operation is directed toward correcting the cavus deformity. Depending on the degree of the deformity and the surgeon's preference, a triple arthrodesis, a tarsal osteotomy, or metatarsal osteotomies may be performed. A plantar fasciotomy frequently is required at the same time.

Toe clawing is the second most common problem. For the great toe deformities, transfer of the long toe extensor to the first metatarsal and fusion of the interphalangeal joint (Jones procedure) is often indicated. If the deformities are not fixed, a Girdlestone-Taylor procedure can be employed on the other toes. For metatarsalgia or fixed clawtoe deformities, a Girdlestone-Taylor procedure is not indicated since it will not correct these deformities. Metatarsal osteotomies, transfer of the extensor tendons proximally, interphalangeal fusion, or resection are indicated for this problem.

The cavus and clawtoe deformities are secondary to intrinsic and extrinsic muscle imbalance. The toe clawing may be accentuated by a weakened tibialis anterior, and the common toe extensors aid in foot dorsiflexion.

A review by Makin (1953) stated that a frequently utilized procedure for this deformity was transfer of the extensor digitorum longus to the dorsum of the foot. Sixteen of the eighteen patients, however, subsequently developed hammertoes; and eight required interphalangeal arthrodesis. This is to be expected since the intrinsics are weak or the deformity would not develop. A Girdlestone-Taylor procedure would seem to be more logical. If foot drop were the problem, the extensor of the great toe could be transferred to the dorsum of the foot with interphalangeal fusion of the great toe.

A polypropylene orthosis should be employed for proprioceptive loss or weakened anterior muscles or to aid in stability.

REFERENCES

Allen, W.: Relation of hereditary pattern to clinical severity as illustrated by peroneal atrophy, Arch. Int. Med. **63:**1123. 1939.

Jacobs, J. E., and Carr, C. R.: Progressive muscular atrophy of the peroneal type, J. Bone Joint Surg. **32A:**27, 1950.

Makin, M.: The surgical management of Friedreich's ataxia, J. Bone Joint Surg. **35A:**425, 1953.

Tachdjian, M. O.: Pediatric orthopedics, Philadelphia, 1972, W. B. Saunders Co.

Waters, R., and Montgomery, J.: Lower extremity management of hemiparesis, Clin. Orthop. **102:**133, 1974.

11

THE DIABETIC FOOT AND AMPUTATIONS OF THE FOOT

F. William Wagner, Jr.

GENERAL CONSIDERATIONS

Gangrene occurring from trivial causes in persons presenting the appearance of usual health and in whom no evidences of atheromatous degeneration of the arteries can be detected should awaken the suspicion of the existence of diabetes, and no time should be lost in making a careful examination of the urine.*

This quote from Dr. Senn is just as true today as it was in 1890. Undiscovered diabetics are frequently "found" when an unhealing ulcer or patch of gangrene following a blister or trivial trauma brings them to the attention of the physician. Despite the discovery of insulin, antihyperglycemic agents, antibiotics, and other sophisticated diagnostic and treatment modalities, reports of difficulty in treating the diabetic foot arise from many centers and from individuals in private practice. Amputation statistics show diabetes mellitus to be one of the leading causes of limb loss of the lower extremity in the Western world (Goldner, 1960; Glattly, 1964; Sarmiento and Warren, 1969). The life expectancy for a person who is diabetic is nearly 70% that for a nondiabetic but appears to be increasing along with the life expectancies of the rest of

the population. Less than 30% of diabetic patients require insulin for the control of blood sugar, and very few die as a direct result of hyperglycemia or other carbohydrate abnormalities (Medical Staff Conference, 1974). All, however, may be afflicted with the long-term complications of vascular disease, retinopathy, nephropathy, and neuropathy. The duration and severity of the diabetes are not related directly to the severity of the complications. The vast majority of complications occur in patients with milder forms of the disease (Kramer and Perilstein, 1958).

There are an estimated 10,000,000 diabetic people in the United States: 2,000,000 known to have the disorder, 2,500,000 with carbohydrate intolerance, and 5,500,000 who are prediabetic. An infected foot is the most common septic problem leading to hospitalization of the diabetic patient (Pratt, 1975). With the numbers just mentioned, it can be seen that there is a large population at risk. The foot of the diabetic patient is especially susceptible to the complications from diabetic angiopathy and neuropathy. Blood vessel involvement can be at both macroscopic and microscopic levels.

The macrolesion (atherosclerotic) appears to be the same qualitatively in the diabetic as in the nondiabetic patient but appears at a

---

*Senn, N.: Principles of surgery, Philadelphia, 1890, F. A. Davis & Co., p. 193.

younger age and is more frequent, more severe, and of wider distribution. The microlesion (thickening of the capillary basement membrane) is also found as an aging phenomenon in nondiabetics and is more pronounced at distal levels of the lower extremity (Medical Staff Conference, 1974). In insulin-requiring diabetic patients there is an increase in the prevalence and magnitude of thickening with duration of the disease, appearing even when strict control of glucose levels is maintained. The inference can be made that the degenerative vascular changes occur through comparable mechanisms in the diabetic and the nondiabetic patient but are accelerated and exaggerated in the diabetic.

Unfortunately, specific treatment and a cure are not presently available for diabetes mellitus. Thus all treatment is aimed at the symptoms, laboratory findings, and complications. Atheromatous occlusion of large vessels produces symptoms and lesions ranging from cold feet through claudication to gangrene. Revascularization procedures such as endarterectomy, profundoplasty, and bypass grafts should be considered by the vascular surgeon before amputation. Long-term limb salvage is possible with femoral-tibial as well as other bypass procedures even when no significant popliteal segment runoff is present (Burgess and Marsden, 1974; Stabile and Wilson, 1977). Microangiopathy is less readily diagnosed. It comes as a shock to see a gangrenous toe in a foot with bounding dorsalis pedis and posterior tibial pulses. It is even a greater shock to have a simple toe amputation fail in such a foot. Evidently the interaction of angiopathy and neuropathy in the foot can produce a wide range of problems from simple nail hypertrophy and callus formation to severe involvement of soft tissues and bone. Breakdown of skin and subsequent infection can lead rapidly to gangrene, amputation, and even death.

The second foot

When breakdown has begun in one diabetic foot, it is not too long until problems start in the other (Greenbaum et al., 1964). Figures vary from clinic to clinic, but the same warning has been sounded that the "well" extremity must be protected with additional zeal once problems have started. It is predicted that when amputation has been performed for gangrene the other leg will begin to have problems within 18 to 36 months in 50% of patients (Goldner, 1960). Within five years about a third of patients will have died. Preventive and prophylactic measures are thus doubly important for the second foot.

Team approach

As in many areas of modern medicine, it is impossible for one person to know of and provide care in all aspects of treatment of the diabetic patient. At Rancho Los Amigos Hospital diabetic patients are cared for on a combined ortho-diabetic service. Orthopaedic and medical house staff as well as full-time senior staff are in daily attendance and hold joint conferences and bedside consultation

General surgery, vascular surgery, plastic surgery, urology, infectious disease service, and others are called as needed in consultation. At staff rounds necessary information is obtained from nursing service, social service, psychiatry and psychology, prosthetic and orthotic services, and physical and occupational therapy. Interns and medical students are assigned graded levels of care.

Surgical procedures are performed by the resident staff after demonstrations by attending surgeons. Toward the end of their rotation, residents are supervised by postgraduate fellows.

The overall mortality rate for all lower extremity surgical procedures has been 9%. The mortality rate for patients with foot and ankle procedures has been 1%. Close medical-surgical liaison on a service specializing in the care of these usually fragile patients with multisystem involvement results in decreased mortality (Kahn et al., 1974).

Ischemic index

Many tests do not have a high correlation with healing rate in the diabetic patient (Romano and Burgess, 1971; Holstein, 1973). There is no constant relationship between palpability of pulses and measured flow through the skin (Moore, 1973). Oscillometry, arteriography, plethysmography, ergometry, thermography, fluorescein, histamine wheal, and similar tests all have staunch advocates and vehement detractors. In recent years Doppler ultrasound has been used as a sensitive stethoscope to detect arterial flow and to measure systolic blood pressure in the lower extremity with peripheral arterial lesions (Mackereth and Lennihan, 1970; Yao, 1970; Carter, 1973; Barnes et al., 1976).

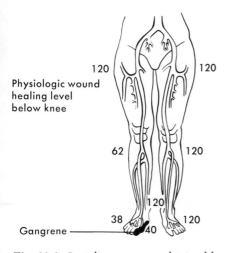

Fig. 11-1. Systolic pressures obtained by transcutaneous Doppler ultrasound. The ischemic index is determined by dividing the lower extremity systolic pressure by the brachial systolic pressure. Healing occurs when the index is above 0.45.

A study of limbs with diabetic ulcers led to conclusions that such lesions could heal if a certain minimum ratio existed between pressure in the brachial artery and pressure in arteries at the site of the lesion. At Rancho Los Amigos Hospital this work has been extended to surgical procedures in the diabetic foot. Level of amputation and prediction of healing of surgical procedures in the foot are determined by preoperative evaluation of brachial and lower extremity arterial blood flow velocity waves and systolic pressures by transcutaneous Doppler ultrasound (Fig. 11-1). Pressures are obtained in the involved lower extremity at various levels from hip to toe with blood pressure cuffs that are 120% the diameter of the extremity at the level being measured (Kirkendall et al., 1967). Digital waves and pressures are assessed by means of small toe cuffs (Gundersen, 1971). The ischemic index is derived by dividing the lower extremity pressure by the brachial pressure. Satisfactory healing can be predicted at a particular level if the flow is pulsatile and the ischemic index is over 0.45. We have found that with an index over 0.45, the systolic pressure has been near 70 mm Hg or higher and the flow has been pulsatile. The success rate for 134 consecutive procedures has been over 93% (Table 11-1).

Vascular reconstruction

Arterial reconstructive procedures should be considered in all patients with ulcers,

Table 11-1. Ischemic index of 0.45 or greater with pulsatile flow*

Level of amputation	No. of patients	Healed	Failures	Healing rates (%)	
Above knee	18	18	0		
Through knee	10	10	0		
Below knee	26	24	2	93.2	93.3
Syme's	37	34	3		
Ray and midtarsal	13	11	2		
Toes	13	12	1		
Midtarsal operation	17	16	1	94.1	

*Results are in 134 consecutive lower extremity surgical procedures for diabetic infection, gangrene, and/or deformity of the foot.

infection, and/or gangrene of the foot. The peripheral vascular service is an indispensible ally of the diabetic service. If the ischemic index is sufficient to indicate healing of the lesion or healing of a surgical procedure, local treatment is administered. If the index is below 0.45 and the patient is a rehabilitation candidate, arteriography is performed. If the patient is not a prosthetic candidate, amputation is done at the through-knee or above-knee level. Thromboendarterectomy, profundoplasty, and bypass grafts are carried out as indicated. Successful revascularization can lead to healing of an ulcer, success in a local surgical procedure, or lowering of the amputation by at least one level (Burgess and Marsden, 1974; Stabile and Wilson, 1977). Unsuccessful revascularization requires amputation, but below-knee levels can be achieved in a high percentage of cases (Burgess and Marsden, 1974).

CLASSIFICATION OF FOOT LESIONS AND METHODS OF TREATMENT

The usual consensus is that traditional treatment for ulcerations and infection has a poor prognosis. The admonition has been "don't whittle," but do a definitive one-time procedure which will heal. From this attitude came the 80% above-knee amputation rate of twenty years ago. With changing knowledge and better diagnostic procedures, 80% of amputations are now done below the knee and the level is being pushed even lower, into the ankle and foot (Rossini and Hare, 1976).

We believe that major arterial blockage is not the usual cause of breakdown in the typical diabetic foot lesions. Basement membrane thickening leads to a diffusion defect which interferes with normal tissue nutrition. The basement membrane of the Schwann cell is also thickened, and this, along with other metabolic changes, leads to diffuse and local neuropathy (Medical Staff Conference, 1974). Breakdown in the insensitive foot results from unappreciated local trauma, nutritional deficiencies, diminished microcirculation, loss of protective sensation, and lowered resistance to infection. There usually is an underlying bony deformity. Treatment is designed to improve tissue circulation, improve nutritional exchange, protect hypesthetic areas, and correct deformities (Goldner, 1960; Mooney and Wagner, 1977; Wagner, 1977).

Our classification of foot lesions has been designed on a service treating diabetics, but the basic principles are applicable to any insensitive or dysvascular foot (Mooney and Wagner, 1977). It was developed by studying the natural history from potential breakdown to total foot destruction and is divided into six grades:

Grade 0: Skin intact (may have bony deformities)
Grade 1: Localized superficial ulcer
Grade 2: Deep ulcer to tendon, bone, ligament, joint
Grade 3: Deep abscess, osteomyelitis
Grade 4: Gangrene of toes or forefoot
Grade 5: Gangrene of whole foot.

Treatment techniques and materials

1. Conventional orthopaedic operations for bony deformities such as bunionectomies and clawtoe and hammertoe revisions; relief of intrinsic bone pressure points by metatarsal osteotomies, proximal interphalangeal joint resections and fusion, and metatarsal head resections

2. Debriding and resection procedures such as toe and ray resections and transmetatarsal and Syme amputations

3. Use of tissue and potential dead space irrigation and lavage systems such as modified Shirley-type tube drain (Wagner, 1977), Kritter irrigation system through the suture line (Kritter, 1973), and direct injection of Collen's solution (Collens et al., 1962)

4. Biologic materials including wound dressings, such as porcine grafts, Epigard, and various enzymatic debriding agents

5. Iodine-containing materials such as organic complexes and the triple iodide solution of Collens (Collens et al., 1962)

6. Medical supportive treatment including intravenous antibiotics, close monitoring and control of blood glucose levels, electrolytes, and BUN, WBC, and hemoglobin levels (Kahn et al., 1974)

7. External supportive and pressure-re-

lieving devices such as total contact walking casts of plaster, fiberglass, and plastic (e.g., Hexcellite), polypropylene orthoses, and rocker bottom shoes; pressure-relief materials such as polyurethane foams, polyethylene foams, and microcellular rubber trimmed and fitted into shoes deep enough to accept the extra material (Mooney and Wagner, 1977)

Flow charts. Treatment techniques and healing requirements have been matched with the graded foot lesions and flow charts developed to aid in decision making (Kunin, 1975). The various parts of the flow chart are as follows:

Oval: A condition at the beginning of treatment or an end-result condition
Rectangle: A treatment or diagnostic procedure to be performed
Diamond: A question as to the result of a test or treatment; answered yes or no
Arrows: Progression of treatment and tests and direction depending on yes or no answer to the question in the diamond
Numbers: Explanations of the procedures and diagnostic tests to be performed (see "Treatment and Diagnostic Procedures")

Grading of foot lesions
Grade 0
Description. A grade 0 foot is one in which there are no open skin lesions. There may be multiple bony deformities, such as clawtoes, hallux valgus with bunions, neuropathic joints with bony prominences, depressed metatarsal heads with calluses, pressure points about the fifth metatarsal base, and navicular and calcaneal prominences (Figs. 11-2 to 11-4).

Treatment. The aim of treatment is to relieve pressures over the areas of potential breakdown (Fig. 11-5). Many times this can be done with shoes and pressure relief inserts (Mooney and Wagner, 1977). In addition, the patient must be taught about his disease and must be made a part of the treatment team. If the patient is older and has poor eyesight, a family member must be taught to assist in this daily care. Patient education is probably the single most important part of the whole treatment system. Without a cooperative patient or family member, most treatment fails and an amputation is the final outcome. The following list could well be posted in every diabetic clinic.

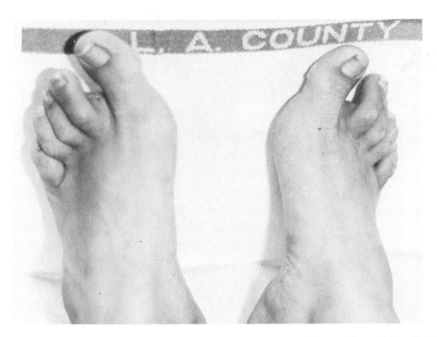

Fig. 11-2. Grade 0 foot, "at risk." Note the clawed toes, incurved toe nails, and dorsal calluses over the proximal interphalangeal joints.

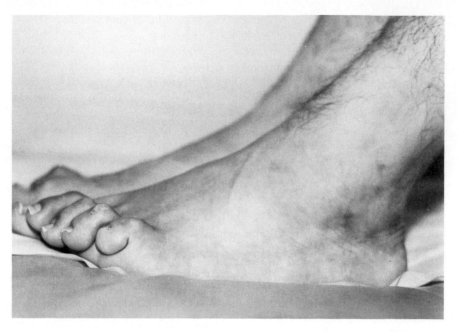

Fig. 11-3. Grade 0 foot: no open lesions. Clawtoes, depressed metatarsal heads, and dorsal calluses are present.

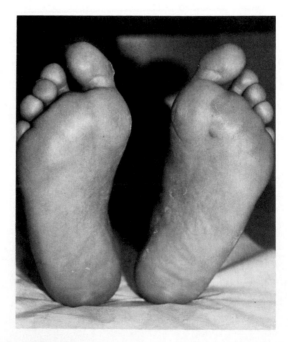

Fig. 11-4. Bottom of a grade 0 foot, no open lesions. Calluses under the depressed metatarsal heads are at risk of breakdown.

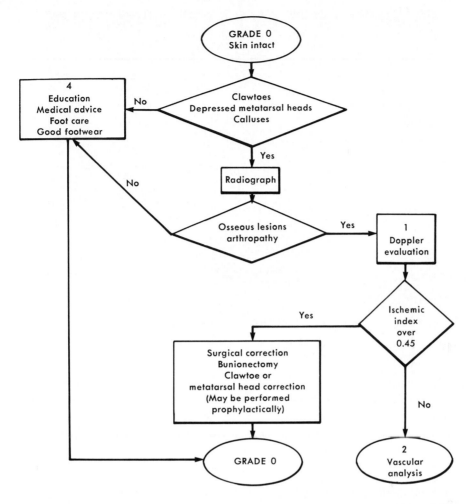

Fig. 11-5. Flow chart for a grade 0 foot, no open lesions. The foot is "at risk."

Patient and family instructions for care of diabetic foot

1. Inspect the feet daily for blisters, cuts and scratches and skin breakdown between the toes.
2. Wash the feet daily with mild soap. Dry carefully, especially between the toes. Use medicated foot powder as prescribed for fungal infections.
3. Avoid extremes of temperature. Test water before bathing. Use a part of the body other than the insensitive feet or hands to test. If the patient is unable, a member of the family should do this testing.
4. If the feet are cold at night, wear wool socks or down booties. Do not apply external sources of heat such as hot water bottle or heating pads. Do not place feet near the heater in an automobile.
5. Do not use chemical agents for the removal of corns and calluses, but have this performed by your doctor.
6. Inspect the insides of the shoes daily for foreign objects, protruding nails, torn linings, and bunching up of shoe construction material.
7. Wear properly fitted stockings. Do not wear mended stockings. Avoid stock-

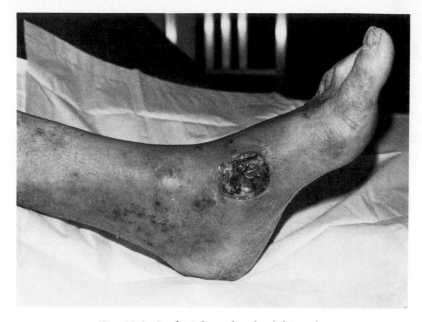

Fig. 11-6. Grade 1 foot: slough of skin only.

ings with seams. Change stockings daily. Be careful of pressure on the toes from the new stretch socks.

8. Do not wear garters that are circular. If garters are necessary, they should be attached to a garter belt.

9. Wear properly fitted shoes. Avoid pointed and open-toed shoes. Break in shoes gradually. If necessary have another member of the family inspect the feet after wearing new shoes for the first few times.

10. Never walk barefooted. This includes going to the bathroom at night.

11. Cut nails straight across. Do not cut into the corners.

12. Do not do "bathroom surgery" on corns and calluses. Follow special instructions from your doctor.

13. See your physician regularly and be sure that your feet are examined at each visit.

14. Be sure that anyone caring for your feet knows that you are a diabetic. This includes the shoe salesman. Recognize that as you get older your feet will tend to spread and require a wider and

longer shoe. Do not insist on the same size that you wore at age 19.

If the patient develops an ulcer which heals and then recurs when ambulation resumes, he is a candidate for some type of prophylactic surgical care to prevent further breakdown. When it is not possible to protect the foot completely from abnormal pressure by some type of external pressure relief, surgical intervention to relieve pressure is indicated. We have performed clawtoe procedures, bunionectomies, and resection of various bony prominences, with virtually 100% healing.

When surgery is contemplated or there appears to be a potential surgical lesion, Doppler evaluation is performed. If the ischemic index is under 0.45 in the foot, the patient is referred to the vascular service for further evaluation.

Grade 1. A grade 1 lesion presents with a superficial ulcer in the skin only. It may have a necrotic or a viable base (Fig. 11-6).

The treatment plan is to convert the ulcer to one with a viable base which will then heal either by epithelialization or with a skin graft (Fig. 11-7). Debriding can be performed with wet-to-dry dressings or various enzymatic

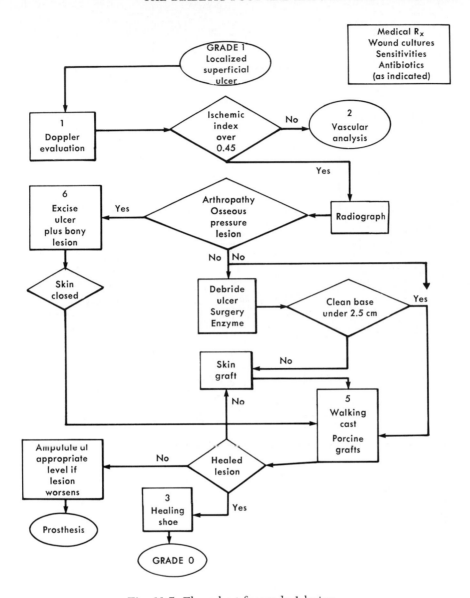

Fig. 11-7. Flow chart for grade 1 lesion.

agents or surgically. Porcine grafts, the patient's own skin, or Epigard can be used to seal the ulcer. We have found that this creates a virtually sterile wound. A walking cast is used to rest the wound and provide a rigid support; the cast controls edema and yet helps keep the patient mobile.

After the wound is healed primarily or by graft, a healing shoe of Plastizote may be used until the wound is mature enough to allow use of an ordinary shoe. If healing does not take place, resection of underlying bone must be performed. Very few treated grade 1 lesions progress to the point of requiring amputation.

Grade 2. A grade 2 lesion is deeper and the slough is to tendon, bone, ligament, or joint (Fig. 11-8). Such a lesion must usually be debrided. If it is on the plantar surface, the wound will frequently heal with rest, elevation, local debriding, and a walking cast. If it does not heal readily with these measures, removal of the bony prominence under the lesion is indicated.

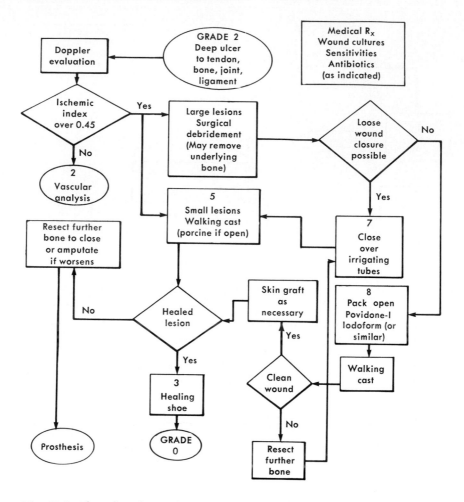

Fig. 11-8. Flow chart for grade 2 lesion: deep ulcer to tendon, bone, joint, ligament.

The ischemic index is obtained. If under 0.45, the patient is referred to the vascular service. If above 0.45, the patient is operated on and infected material removed. Excision of the metatarsal head results in rapid healing of the ulcer. Palpation of the adjoining heads at surgery will usually indicate whether these heads need resection or metatarsal osteotomy to prevent transfer of pressure. Most wounds are closed over irrigation tubes for 24 to 48 hours (Kritter, 1973). We have found that open surgical wounds heal less well than those closed. This is corroborated by Ecker and Jacobs (1970), who found that sixteen of thirty-six open wounds failed but only two of eighteen closed wounds failed.

Patients who return from revascularization procedures are treated as indicated from the grading of the wound. If the wound continues to heal and a grade 0 foot results, any remaining deformity can then be treated as necessary.

Grade 3. A grade 3 lesion represents further progression to a deep abscess or osteomyelitis (Fig. 11-9). Small incision and drainage openings are not sufficient unless performed very early. There must be complete removal of all infected and/or gangrenous tissues at the time of surgical treatment.

The exact timing of surgery is frequently difficult; however, we have found that with several days of bed rest, elevation, intrave-

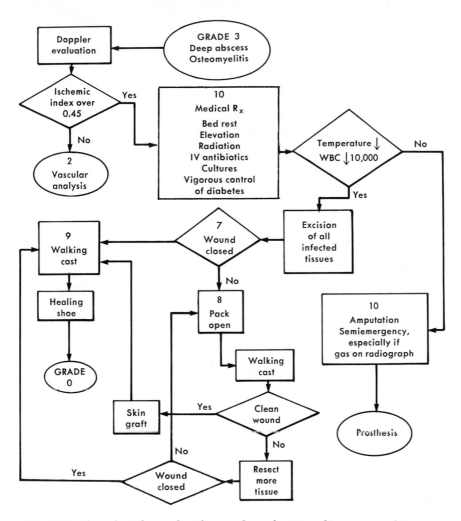

Fig. 11-9. Flow chart for grade 3 lesion: deep abscess and/or osteomyelitis.

nous antibiotics, and vigorous control of the diabetic problems, lesser procedures can be performed than if immediate surgery is done (Kahn et al., 1974). Surgical procedures can be performed when the temperature curve is decreasing and the WBC descends below 10,000. There must be complete removal of infected tissue, especially of osteomyelitic tissue. We have rarely seen osteomyelitis heal with antibiotics and rest if the ischemic index is much under 1.0. If there is gas on radiographs or by palpation, special care must be taken to rule out clostridial infection (Bessman and Wagner, 1975). We have found, however, that clostridial infection is relatively rare although gas appearing in the tissue is not

uncommon (Bessman and Wagner, 1975; Di Gioia et al., 1977). Palpable subcutaneous gas is usually associated with less severe cellulitis. Gas found by radiography in the muscle layer indicates myonecrosis. Amputation must be performed above this level (Bessman and Wagner, 1975; Di Gioia et al., 1977). Localized procedures can still be done in the presence of nonclostridial gas if all of the infected muscle is excised. On occasion, when dorsal wounds have been debrided to good tissue and there is not quite enough skin to close, we have used walking casts until a granulating base has resulted and a skin graft is then applied.

Again, the ultimate aim is to obtain a grade

0 foot with intact skin. Any residual deformity is then treated as necessary.

Grade 4. A grade 4 lesion includes gangrene of some portion of the forefoot (Figs. 11-10 and 11-11). If the gangrene is dry and limited to the distal portion of the toe, a toe amputation through the base will frequently suffice. More proximal involvement usually requires a metatarsal ray resection. Multiple toe involvement frequently requires a transmetatarsal or more proximal amputation.

The criteria of McKittrick et al. are as valid today as in 1949 and, along with the Doppler evaluation, help to determine the level of amputation. (See "Transmetatarsal Amputation," p. 366.)

If the gangrene is progressive and wet, immediate open or closed amputation may be necessary. Severe pain, increasing sedimentation rate, increasing WBC, increasing fever, and increasing need for insulin all indicate the necessity for immediate ablation. A first-stage Syme amputation is usually the lowest level

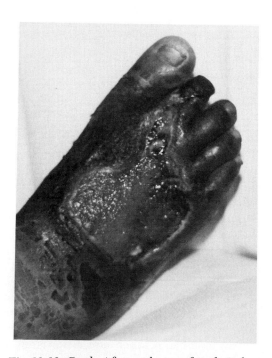

Fig. 11-10. Grade 4 foot with area of grade 2 ulceration.

indicated (Spittler et al., 1954) (Fig. 11-12). If the Doppler pressure and ischemic index are not sufficient at the Syme level, a below-knee, through-knee, or above-knee procedure must be performed as indicated by the vascular studies.

Grade 5. A grade 5 lesion represents complete foot involvement with no local procedures possible (Fig. 11-13). Below-knee, through-knee, or above-knee amputations are carried out depending on vascular analysis. Further assessment is made of the patient's suitability for prosthetic wear, state of the other limb, and social considerations. Through-knee levels are usually performed for patients who will not be prosthetic users.

Treatment and diagnostic procedures designated by numbers on flow charts

1. Doppler evaluation. Systolic blood pressures at hip, thigh, knee, calf, ankle, foot and toes are obtained by transcutaneous Doppler ultrasound acting as a hypersensitive stethoscope. The width of the blood pressure cuff must be 120% the diameter of the limb at the level being measured (Kirkendall, 1967). The pressure in the lower limb divided by the brachial artery pressure gives the ischemic index. If the ischemic index is over 0.45, there is a 93% + chance that a surgical procedure will heal (Table 11-1). Local lesions can heal with nonoperative treatment unless there is an abscess or osteomyelitis present. Flow patterns are also assessed; the flow should be pulsatile for healing to take place. We have found that if the index is over 0.45 virtually all the waves have been of a pulsatile nature and most of the local pressures have been over 70 mm Hg.

2. Vascular treatment. Foot lesions with an ischemic index below 0.45 are referred for possible revascularization procedures. Arteriography must usually be performed. There are some centers, however, that are using the Doppler ultrasound to map the blood flow and the consensus is that such a Doppler mapping can be almost as accurate as arteriography. Revascularization procedures such as profundoplasty, endarterectomy, and bypass grafts between various levels generally allow local

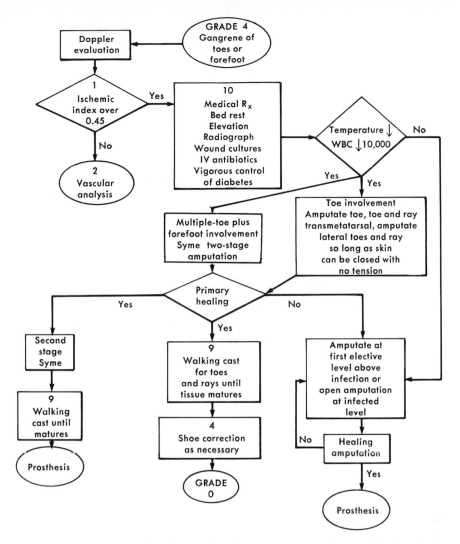

Fig. 11-11. Flow chart for grade 4 lesion: gangrene of toes and/or forefoot.

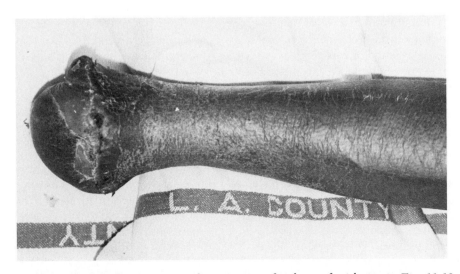

Fig. 11-12. Healing first-stage Syme's amputation for the grade 4 lesion in Fig. 11-10.

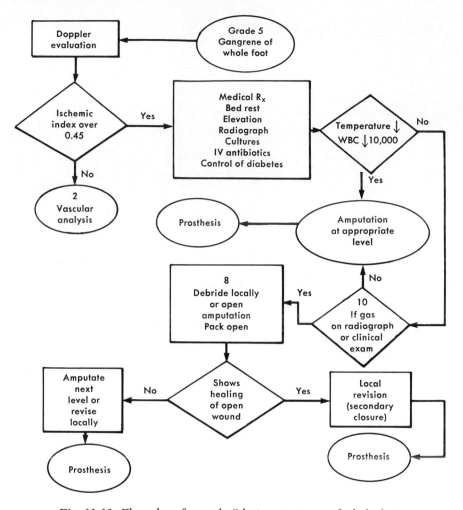

Fig. 11-13. Flow chart for grade 5 lesion: gangrene of whole foot.

healing, local surgical procedures, or lowering of the amputation by at least one level.

3. Walking cast. Total-contact walking casts have been found to rest tissues, reduce edema, prevent additional local trauma, keep the patient ambulatory, and after prolonged use even raise the ischemic index. The casts may be of fiberglass, Hexcellite, plaster, or combinations thereof. The ankle must be at neutral or slightly above neutral, or a rocker bottom must be applied to allow heel-to-toe progression in walking. If there is even slight plantar flexion of the forefoot, it is difficult or impossible for the average patient to walk without crutch assistance.

4. Healing shoe. Polyethylene foam is formed over an enlarged last to provide a soft forgiving shoe that allows ambulation as the lesion heals (Fig. 11-14). It is used frequently following a healing cast or is used at the onset of a relatively small lesion. The shoe is not permanent but lasts about 3 months. No dressings are used on open lesions. The patient wears white cotton stockings which are changed as necessary.

5. Education. The patient and the family are taught about diabetes mellitus, its control, and its complications. They are given repeated instruction in care of the foot. The patient is thus made a part of the treatment team, and much earlier care of incipient lesions is possible. Prevention is more reliable

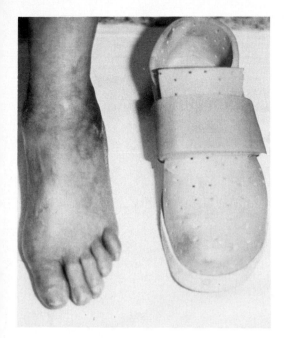

Fig. 11-14. Healing shoe. Formed of Plastizote over an enlarged last to allow room for toes, it provides excellent pressure relief.

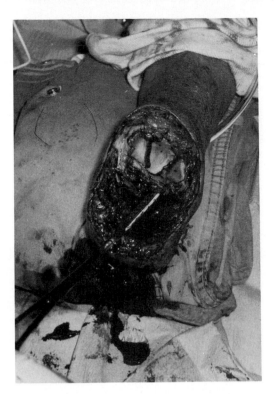

Fig. 11-15. Shirley drain drawn into the wound of a first-stage Syme amputation; white tubing for irrigating fluid, clear tubing for gravity drainage.

than treatment, and every diabetic patient should be taught the importance of foot hygiene and sensible foot wear.

6. Porcine graft. Open skin lesions are virtually 100% infected in diabetic patients. Sealing off the lesions with a split thickness graft, a porcine graft, or Epigard (a synthetic plastic skin) results in virtual sterilization of the wound. Lesions under 1.5 cm can epithelialize beneath porcine graft or Epigard and a walking cast for protection. Larger lesions must usually be grafted. After application of a split-thickness graft, a porcine graft or Epigard will act as an excellent surgical dressing.

7. Excision. A plantar ulcer is rarely excised unless there is a connection between it and the underlying bone, which is not usually the case. When bone is removed from a dorsal incision, virtually all ulcers heal with minimal local treatment.

8. Irrigating tubes. These are of two types depending on the size of the potential dead space.

After the first-stage Syme amputation a large potential space is formed at the ankle joint and must be drained. A Shirley sump drain is modified by removal of the air filter and introduction of an antibiotic solution through the tube (Wagner, 1977). No suction is used, but the fluid runs by gravity through the perforated exit tube (Fig. 11-15). This double-tube system is introduced through a separate stab incision and is removed at approximately 48 hours. The tip of the tube is cut off and cultured upon removal. If there has been evidence of cellulitis or synovitis, the tube is left in longer.

In small wounds an infant feeding tube or plastic intravenous needle is introduced through adjacent soft tissues into the depth of the wound (Figs. 11-16 and 11-17). Antibiotic fluid is run into the wound and acts to dilute the hematoma and remove minor bits of debris. Exit is between the sutures (Kritter, 1973).

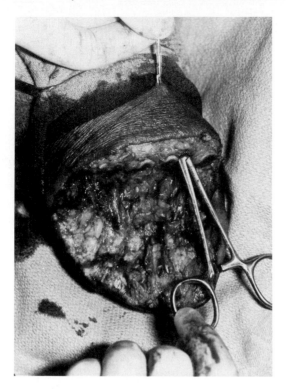

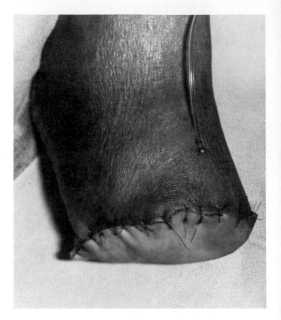

Fig. 11-17. Wound irrigation in a Kritter type of transmetatarsal amputation.

Fig. 11-16. Wound irrigation tubing brought through the small stab incision of a transmetatarsal amputation. Beveled metatarsal edges provide pressure relief.

9. Packing of open wounds. Opinions vary as to the efficacy of local antiseptic agents. We have found that iodine compounds such as povidone, iodoform, or Collen's solution aid in the local cleansing of such wounds. The pack must be so applied that infectious material is not sequestered. Packing is continued only until the wound is clean enough to skin graft or to close secondarily.

10. Medical treatment. Urgent surgical drainage of a fluctuant abscess may be required, but surgery should be delayed until maximal benefits have been derived from rest, elevation, antibiotics, and vigorous control of the diabetic state. Local foot procedures will frequently be possible when cellulitis has been controlled.

Neuropathy

The diabetic diathesis includes involvement of the nervous system (Lamontagne and Buchtal, 1970). The exact mechanisms are not known but appear to be part of the metabolic disorder and probably involve the sorbitol pathway (Chopra et al., 1969). Autopsy studies show loss of anterior horn cells, reduction in number of axone cylinders, and abnormalities of the Schwann cells (Greenbaum et al., 1964). The autonomic system is also involved and can affect the limbs.

Chronic sensory neuropathy is the most common form seen in our clinic. There is loss of ankle reflex, diminution or loss of vibratory sense, diminution in position sense, and diminution in pain appreciation. Symptoms of dysesthesia, hyperesthesia, and muscle and limb pains will be described variously as burning, aching, gnawing, ants crawling on the skin, or hot liquid flowing on the skin. These disappear as loss of sensation progresses.

Trophic and autonomic changes result in brittle hyperkeratotic skin, thickened deformed nails, atrophy of fat in the sole, and loss of function in the sebaceous and sweat glands.

The motor loss resembles an intrinsic muscle palsy. The metatarsophalangeal joints become extended and the proximal interphalan-

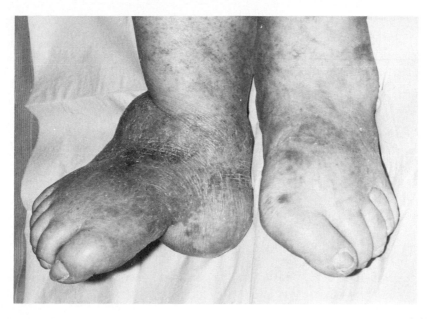

Fig. 11-18. Severe Charcot changes of the right foot with ulcer under the prominence of the talus following lateral dislocation of the tarsus. Grade 1 left foot "at risk" with bunion and hammered toes.

geal joints flexed, and typical clawed toes result. The plantar fat pad shifts distally, and the metatarsal head is covered with skin and subcutaneous tissue less able to withstand direct and shear pressures.

Bone changes are seen with diabetic neuropathy. Osteoporosis can occur as generalized demineralization of bone without a period of immobilization or other causative events. It seldom causes a clinical problem unless fracture occurs. Osteolysis is usually localized to the forefoot. In advanced cases the metatarsal shaft may narrow and shorten and lead to subluxation at the metatarsophalangeal joints. Local fracture may also lead to disruption of the joints.

Neuropathic joints are seen most frequently in the midfoot but can involve other joints (Figs. 11-18 and 11-19). The onset may be with minor trauma or with alteration of the mechanics of the foot. There may be pain at the onset, but usually the whole process is painless. Periarticular fractures occur, joint stability is lost, and complete destruction and disintegration may result. Repair processes lead to callus, periosteal new bone, and even spontaneous fusion of joints. Ulcers fre-

quently form under local protuberances formed as a result of bone healing.

Our treatment program for the neuropathic joint is based on complete rest at the onset, progressing to protected weight bearing in a cast or brace. Triple arthrodesis has been successfully performed in very early lesions before destruction is too severe. Prolonged casting has resulted in healing of adjacent fractures and spontaneous fusion of joints. Late cases show progressive deformity, ulcerate, become infected, and require a Syme two-stage amputation.

Treatment of the neuropathy itself is usually not successful. There is some indication that strict diabetic control and B-complex vitamins can give temporary relief in a case which has resulted from poor diabetic control. Cases with some regression of symptoms have been followed and have eventually shown progression of the neuropathy despite good control of the diabetic state. All patients who have had diabetes mellitus for twenty years manifest signs of diabetic neuropathy.

In our experience, ulcerative lesions occur mainly at bony prominences such as at the heel, under deformities, or at depressed

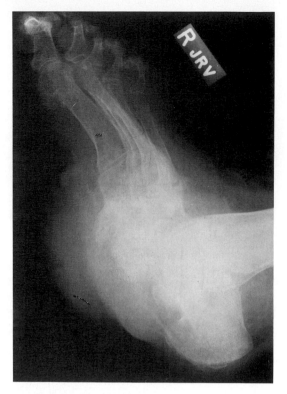

Fig. 11-19. Severe diabetic Charcot changes in right foot; virtual dissolution of the midtarsal structures.

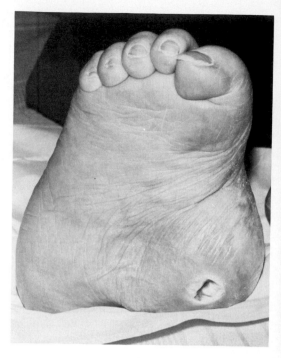

Fig. 11-20. Severe Charcot joint destruction; ulcer under the apex of the weight-bearing deformity.

metatarsal heads (Figs. 11-20 and 11-21). Ulcers can occur at other sites but usually only after some traumatic incident such as penetration of a foreign object. Many of these patients have no signs of vascular impairment. Prophylactic removal of bony prominences after healing of the ulcer can protect a patient from further breakdown. The usual onset of a plantar ulcer follows the formation of a thickened plantar callosity under a metatarsal head. The neuropathic foot is especially prone to the development of extra thick callosities. These callosities can act as foreign bodies and traumatize the tissues between the callus and the underlying bony prominence, with the ultimate production of an ulcer. Exudate from the ulcer breaks through, and the patient is first aware of the lesion when he notices moisture on his stocking. Trimming of the overlying callus can also reveal an undiscovered ulcer. Pressure relieving shoe inserts, rocker bottom shoes, and similar devices can help the

ulcer heal and prevent recurrence. However, if this is not successful, removal of the intrinsic bony pressure point by osteotomy or ostectomy is indicated.

If the ulcer progresses despite treatment, it may eventually reach deeper tissues and produce an abscess or osteomyelitis. Further treatment would be indicated as outlined in the treatment diagrams.

Bacteriologic studies in infected diabetic feet

Multiple organisms are usually cultured from infected diabetic gangrene and diabetic ulcers (Williams et al., 1974). Enteric gram-negative bacilli and enterococci have been incriminated in infection accompanied by subcutaneous gas (Bessman and Wagner, 1975; Di Gioia et al., 1977). In these studies the material for culture was obtained at the bedside from the draining lesion. With a mixed flora and varied bacterial sensitivities,

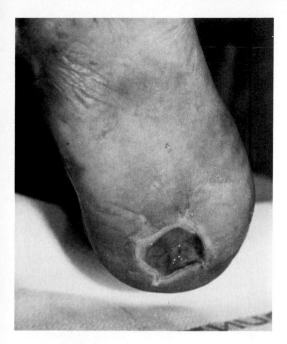

Fig. 11-21. Recurrent ulcer following partial calcanectomy. The patient walked without an ankle-foot orthosis for protection.

it is difficult to set up an antibiotic treatment program.

In an attempt to identify the pathogenic bacteria in the infected lesions, superficial wound exudates were contrasted with material dissected aseptically from the surgically excised specimen. Our study showed little agreement between cultures of the deep and superficial material. There was complete concordance in only ten patients (17%). In this group antibiotic therapy directed against all of the organisms failed to eradicate them.

In the majority of cases most but not all of the causative bacteria can be isolated at the bedside. The most common organisms are the Enterobacteriacae, enterococci, and staphylococci. Relatively few anaerobes are isolated, and no anaerobes have been isolated in pure culture. *Staphylococcus epidermidis* and *Corynebacterium* were cultured from both superficial and deep areas but were never isolated as the sole causative organisms.

Antibiotic treatment is selected not to eradicate the deep infection but to reduce and minimize the surrounding cellulitis. Gangrenous tissue, deep abscess, and osteomyelitis must be surgically drained or excised in the diabetic patient. A penicillin-type antibiotic plus an aminoglycoside appears to provide the best all-around results until cultures and sensitivities indicate a change. Since the aminoglycosides are ototoxic and nephrotoxic, close attention must be paid to hearing and kidney function.

Control of blood glucose in surgery

A high percentage of diabetic patients will undergo surgical procedures in their lifetimes. Most of these patients will be under the care of an internist, but occasionally a previously undiagnosed patient will be found to have the disease during his surgical course. It is not within the scope of this chapter to discuss the medical care of the diabetic patient, but the surgeon should be aware of problems in the perioperative period. A short time with a practical article should give him a good approach to blood glucose control in case of emergency. An especially good article is one by Rossini and Hare (1976).

Surgical techniques

Amputations. Ablative procedures are discussed more thoroughly in the section on amputations (p. 363).

Metatarsal osteotomies. Pressure from and pressure on the metatarsal heads can be relieved by a number of procedures that shorten the metatarsal and/or change the angle of the shaft.

Osteotomies close to the metatarsal head tend to develop hypertrophic callus in the diabetic patient. This callus can then become as much of a pressure point as the metatarsal head and lead to an ulcer. Osteotomies in the midshaft are more prone to nonunion and the development of Charcot-like changes in the nonunion which can lead to pressure points from the amount of bone formed.

Osteotomies in the cancellous bone at the metatarsal base appear to be superior. With relief of pressure on one head, transfer of pressure to the adjacent head is common. Palpation of the adjacent head at surgery will

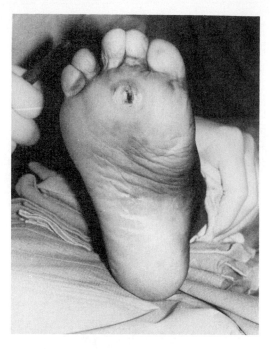

Fig. 11-22. Foot with severe ulcer under the second metatarsal head, disruption of the metatarsophalangeal joints, and previous resection of the metatarsal head for osteomyelitis.

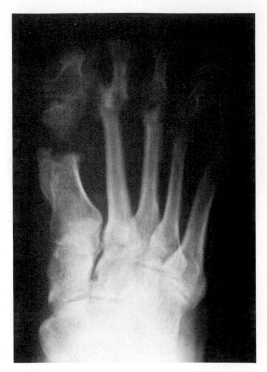

Fig. 11-23. Foot in Fig. 11-22; resection of previous osteomyelitis of the first metatarsal and breakdown of the metatarsophalangeal joints.

give an indication of its prominence and the probable necessity to osteotomize, shorten, or angulate the shaft to about 50% of the correction obtained with the first osteotomy.

If the protuberance of the fifth metatarsal head is especially large, it is best corrected by excision of the distal half of the metatarsal through an oblique osteotomy. Removal of the base of the proximal phalanx prevents a pressure point from the flare. Syndactylization of the fourth and fifth toes prevents proximal migration of the fifth. Partial fifth metatarsal head resection has frequently resulted in an unstable joint and further deformity and is no longer used.

Clawtoe and hammertoe repair. If clawtoes or hammertoes are not too severe, they can be corrected by dorsal capsulotomy, tendon lengthening, and proximal interphalangeal joint fusion. These procedures work in early cases with minimal deformities. Late cases

may show initial correction but almost all recur. The usual patient will not consider clawtoe surgery unless ulcers have recurred or the deformity is severe enough to interfere with the wearing of shoes. In older patients it is almost a truism that some bone must be removed and soft tissue procedures will not succeed.

Metatarsal head resection (Hoffman-Clayton procedure). Although this type of procedure was originally described for severe arthritic deformities with marked joint destruction, it is finding use in the diabetic patient with plantar callosities and ulceration (Figs. 11-22 to 11-27).

Single-head resection is performed for plantar ulceration. If the adjacent heads feel prominent at surgery, a dorsal wedge osteotomy of the adjacent shafts will prevent transfer lesions. To prevent hypertrophic callus near the head or distal shaft, the osteotomy is best performed at the base. The foot must be

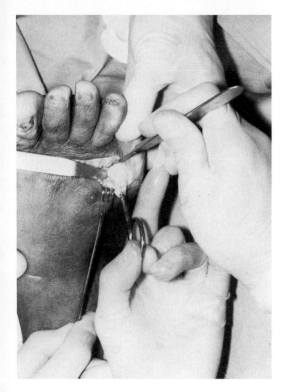

Fig. 11-24. Use of a screw to hold the metatarsal head during sharp dissection for removal of the head.

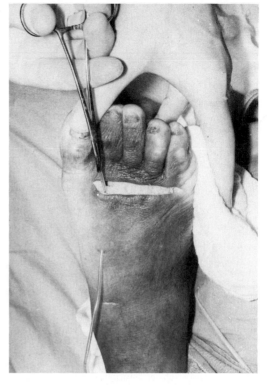

Fig. 11-25. Placing an irrigation tube through a separate stab incision.

protected in a walking cast for about 8 weeks to prevent neuropathic breakdown of the tarsometatarsal and midtarsal joints. We now advocate resection of the proximal portion of the proximal phalanx to further shorten the bony structures and thus provide relative lengthening of the soft tissue structures. This minimizes the tendency for the toes to be pulled dorsally as healing progresses. Pressure from the prominence of the flare is also avoided. Intramedullary Kirschner wires aid in toe and shaft alignment postoperatively and help prevent excessive toe retraction. If there has been recent infection, the wires are not used. Most of these patients have a flat-footed gait preoperatively and continue with the same gait in ordinary shoes. A rocker bottom stiff-soled shoe adds motion that converts the gait to an almost normal heel-toe progression.

Bunionectomy. The medial aspect of the first metatarsophalangeal joint is susceptible to pressure if hallux valgus is more than a few degrees. Once ulceration and scarring have occurred, the skin is especially prone to recurrent ulcers.

The Keller resection provides excellent relief of local pressure. Attachment of the flexor hallucis brevis to the base of the resected proximal phalanx aids in preventing hyperextension of the great toe.

Resection of bony prominences
Calcaneus. Enforced bed rest during an illness, following a cerebrovascular accident, or during convalescence from surgery such as open reduction and internal fixation of hip fracture frequently leads to pressure sores under the prominences around the heel.

If the ischemic index is over 0.45, the ulcer and underlying bone are removed to allow closure of the ulcer (Figs. 11-28 and 11-29). If the ischemic index is under 0.45, a below-

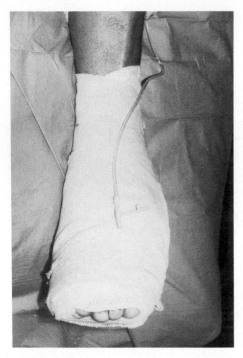

Fig. 11-26. Completed soft dressing with a Kritter-type irrigation system. Fluid exits through the incision.

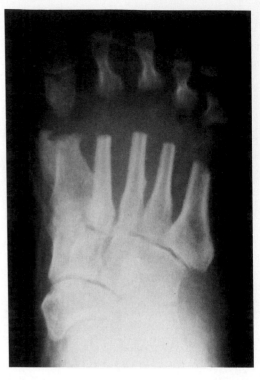

Fig. 11-27. Completed Hoffman procedure.

knee amputation usually must be performed. Postoperative drainage of the cavity is essential. After healing, a polypropylene ankle-foot orthosis allows almost normal gait. The patient must use the orthosis for all weight bearing.

Calcaneocuboid, cuboid–fifth metatarsal, and midtarsal joints. Charcot involvement of these joints can lead to disintegration with plantar angulation and subsequent bony protuberances, rapidly causing ulcers (Figs. 11-18 and 11-19).

Resection of the bone is accomplished through separate medial or lateral incisions approaching the protuberance subperiosteally. The prominence is resected flush with the surrounding bone. Wallking-cast treatment is started 10 to 12 days postoperatively and is continued until the surrounding bone is healed. This may take up to 6 months.

Summary

The number of diabetic patients is increasing. An infected foot is the most common septic problem requiring hospitalization of the diabetic patient. To aid in establishing treatment programs, diabetic foot lesions have been graded from 0 (intact skin) through 5 (gangrene of the whole foot). A flow chart has been constructed for each grade to indicate treatment at progressive stages.

An ischemic index has been developed to aid in assessment of vascular potential. Local healing, healing of operative procedures, and healing of amputations are all dependent on sufficient blood supply (Williams et al., 1974). The ischemic index represents the value obtained by dividing the various lower extremity systolic pressures by the brachial artery pressure. The leg pressures are obtained by transcutaneous Doppler ultrasound used as a sensitive stethoscope. If the ischemic index is over 0.45, 93%+ healing has occurred following surgical procedures.

Standard reconstructive procedures can be performed in the diabetic foot to relieve deformities and prevent breakdown of skin over bony protuberances. Partial-foot and

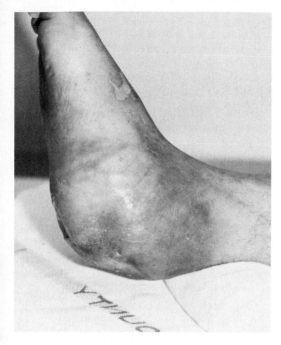

Fig. 11-28. One year after partial calcanectomy. The patient walked without an orthosis and caused a new ulcer.

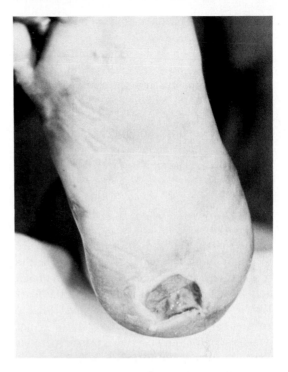

Fig. 11-29. Removal of the remainder of the calcaneus is necessary to heal the ulcer.

Syme's amputations have been performed in a large number of diabetic patients, with a high success rate.

Diabetic neuropathy is present to some degree in all patients with diabetes of twenty or more years' duration. Charcot arthropathy can be triggered by minor trauma or can be completely insidious in onset. Absolute rest followed by protection with walking casts may result in healing of juxta-articular fractures and even fusion of affected joints. Surgical fusion can be successful if performed early enough.

It is believed that the team approach with close cooperation between the medical and orthopaedic staffs has contributed to our low mortality rate and high healing rate.

FOOT AMPUTATIONS

Amputation is described as the process of cutting off (*ambi*, around; *putare*, to prune), especially by surgery of a portion of the body. In the lower extremity the causes, in descending order of frequency, are as follows:

1. Peripheral vascular disease (with diabetics forming the greater percentage of these patients)
2. Trauma (becoming more frequent in younger male patients)
3. Tumors
4. Chronic infection (e.g., osteomyelitis not responding to usual treatment)
5. Congenital and acquired deformities (e.g., fibular hemimelia)
6. Cosmesis (rare)

Level selection in foot amputations

In trauma, tumors, chronic infection, and congenital deformities, the level selection is usually dictated by the underlying pathologic process. All length is saved— as determined by skin viability in trauma, degree of malignancy of the tumor, or remaining function in the extremity with a congenital defect. Traumatic lesions that require prolonged casting can leave the patient with a stiff and painful partial foot. This is especially true at the Chopart and Lisfranc levels.

If a walkable partial foot is not possible by 6 months, serious consideration should be given to ablation as a reconstructive procedure. Longer delay raises false hope in the patient and frustration in the surgeon. Amputation should not be considered a procedure to hide failure of previous treatment; rather it is a further step in treatment of a badly injured foot. It should be done as a plastic procedure to provide a new interface between the patient and his new environment—the prosthesis.

In dysvascular patients new diagnostic procedures are aiding the assessment of healing at various levels. Noninvasive techniques are of major importance, for penetration of the diabetic or dysvascular foot can precipitate an acute infection or local thrombosis. Radioactive xenon has been reported to give reliable results (Moore, 1973) but frequently is not available in smaller hospitals. Transcutaneous Doppler ultrasound is being used as a sensitive stethoscope to assess blood flow in dysvascular limbs (Mackereth and Lennihan, 1970; Yao, 1970; Carter, 1973; Barnes et al.,

1976). The procedure is described at the beginning of the chapter. In the nondiabetic patient healing can occur with an ischemic index of 0.35.

Specific amputations

Toes. Loss of a part or all of the toe can usually be compensated by shoe correction, especially the rocker bottom shoe (Fig. 11-30). Partial amputation of a lesser toe may be necessary for gangrene of diabetes, arteriosclerosis, congenital deformity, tumor, or trauma.

Surgical techniques. Flaps may be of any shape, size, or description; they must only be long enough to close without tension. They may be long-dorsal, long-plantar, side-to-side, or fish-mouth; however, their length must not be over 50% greater than the width at the base. The flaps should be tested before suturing and the stump palpated to be sure that no bony prominence is present. Bone must be removed and angular areas rounded to relieve internal pressure and palpable external pressure. Flaps must close without

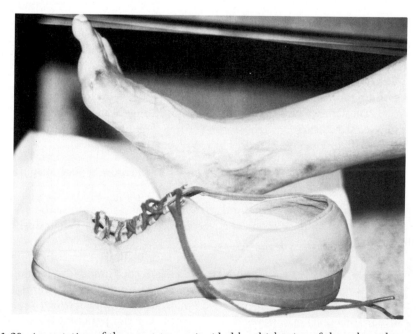

Fig. 11-30. Amputation of the great toe; gait aided by thickening of the sole and a moderate rocker of the sole.

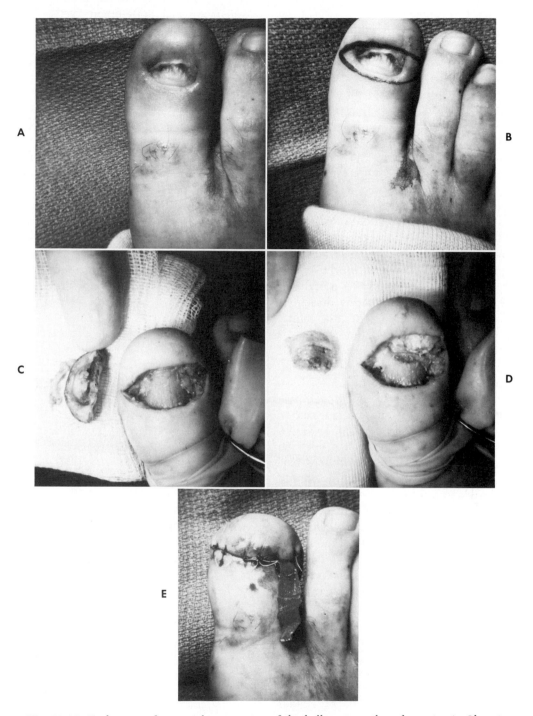

Fig. 11-31. Technique of terminal amputation of the hallux, toenail, and matrix. **A,** Chronic ingrown nail with fungal infection; has been debrided and treated with Collens solution. **B,** Elliptical incision to remove the nail and matrix. **C,** Nail and matrix removed. **D,** Distal 1 cm of bone removed to allow closure of the wound. **E,** Wound closed over iodoform wick to allow escape of the hematoma from raw bone.

tension. If such closure is not possible, more bone must be removed (Wagner, 1977).

Terminal amputation of hallux and toenail (terminal Syme). Deformity of the great toenail and recurrent severe infections may not respond to simple treatment. Partial phalangectomy and removal of the nail and matrix from the dorsum allow primary closure of the distal flap. If the closure is under tension, more bone must be removed (Fig. 11-31).

Amputation of great toe. The base of the proximal phalanx of the great toe is saved, if at all possible, to preserve the action of the flexor hallucis brevis. This appears to pull the fat pad and the proximal phalanx over the distal portion of the first metatarsal head to provide cushioning at roll-off. If disarticulation is necessary, plantar skin should be used over the metatarsal head. In the lesser toes no distinction is made between amputating through a phalanx and disarticulating at the joints. Again, flaps must close without tension. If there is a contracture of a joint that would leave a protruding stump, this must be corrected.

Amputation of toes and metatarsal rays. Any or all of the lateral toes and rays can be taken through an oblique incision, leaving a remarkably effective foot. The flap must be wide and long enough to close without tension. Antibiotic solution lavage is brought into the wound and exits between the sutures. This aids in the evacuation of hematoma and debris (Kritter, 1973). A Plastizote filler is used to compensate for the loss of the lateral toes (Fig. 11-32).

Resection of osteomyelitic bone without amputation. A satisfactory toe stub may result if osteomyelitic bone is excised leaving the soft tissue behind. This is usually indicated in the great toe and fifth toe. A medial or lateral incision is made along the extent of the infected bone. The bone is then dissected extraperiosteally. The wound either is packed open with povidone, iodoform, or similar packs or is closed over antibiotic irrigation tubes. The residual soft tissue shrinks as it heals and provides a pad for the metatarsal head.

Transmetatarsal amputation. McKittrick

et al. (1949) outlined the indications for a transmetatarsal amputation in the diabetic patient. Their criteria are as valid today as they were then:

1. Gangrene of all or part of one or more toes, provided the gangrene and accompanying infection have become stabilized and the gangrene has not involved the dorsal or plantar aspect of the foot
2. A stabilized infection or open wound involving the distal portion of the foot, when total excision of the infected area with primary or delayed closure can be accomplished
3. An open infected lesion in a neurogenic foot as a curative procedure when the entire area of anesthesia can be excised or as a delayed procedure when the area of infection can be excised but the line of incision is through the area of anesthesia

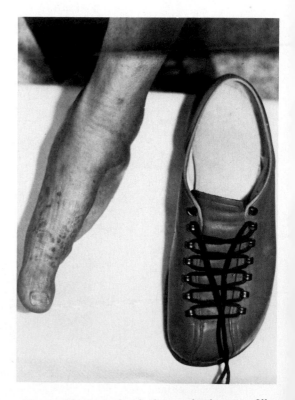

Fig. 11-32. Extra-depth shoe with Plastizote filler for resection of the lateral toes and rays.

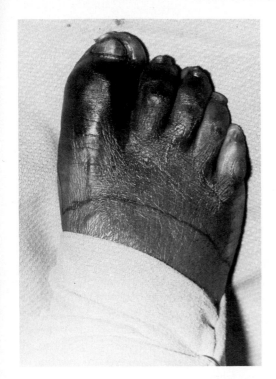

Fig. 11-33. Skin incision for transmetatarsal amputation; grade 4 foot with infected gangrene of the great toe.

In dysvascular patients the addition of the ischemic index obtained with the transcutaneous Doppler ultrasound has allowed selection of the level of amputation more easily than could be done by clinical means alone.

This amputation is also indicated after crushing injuries to the toes and metatarsal heads if sufficient plantar skin is available.

Surgical technique. Bone section is planned proximal to the metatarsal heads (Fig. 11-33). The skin incision on the dorsum passes from medial to lateral at the level of the bone section.

If skin is involved with gangrene or infection, the bone is shortened until sufficient good skin is available to close without tension. The incision goes distally at the midlevel of the metatarsal shafts and swings to the plantar surface (Fig. 11-34). The plantar incision parallels the flexion crease at the base of the toes about 1 cm more proximal.

The metatarsals are cut through with an oscillating saw; the first is beveled medially, and the fifth laterally as well as inferiorly so no sharp corners remain. The line of division of the metatarsals deviate about 15° from the

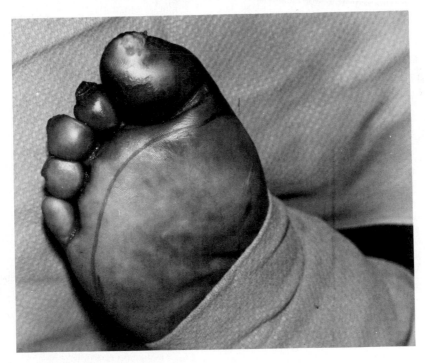

Fig. 11-34. Plantar skin incision for transmetatarsal amputation.

transverse (Fig. 11-35). The line should not be curved because a longer second or third metatarsal shaft may be left with a severe pressure point beneath its end. With distal traction on the toes and metatarsal heads, the plantar flap is separated from the metatarsals obliquely down to the skin edge (Figs. 11-36 and 11-37). All tendon slips are removed (Fig. 11-38). The inferior edges of the metatarsals are rounded. This effectively relieves most of the plantar pressure at the ends of the metatarsals (Fig. 11-39).

Pinpoint electrocoagulation and fine ligatures are used for hemostasis. The skin and subcutaneous tissue are closed in one layer. A wound irrigation system is used for 48 hours to remove debris and hematoma (Kritter, 1973) (Figs. 11-16, 11-17, and 11-40). A walking cast is applied at 10 to 12 days, and the patient is allowed to walk until maturation of the stump is complete. A rocker bottom shoe with a stiff sole has aided in removing much of the pressure from under the metatarsal necks.

Chopart, Lisfranc, Boyd, and Pirogoff amputations. These levels are mentioned mainly for historical interest. In a well-substantiated study by Harris and Silverstein (1964), the optimum site was distal to the tarsometatarsal joint.

Occasional superb results are seen at these levels, but our amputation clinic has had to revise many to the Syme level. Skin grafts over traumatic amputations at the Chopart and Lisfranc levels are especially prone to breakdown. Progressive equinus deformity is the usual end result, with ulceration at the lowest bone edge. Patients with skin grafts have had repeated ulceration over the grafted areas. Jacobs (1977), at Albany Medical College, has reported success at these levels in diabetic patients with tenotomy of the tendo Achillis and postoperative use of a polypropylene ankle orthosis. Our trials, however, have not stood up; the patients have eventually required a Syme level reconstruction. In noninfected cases in children, late equinus

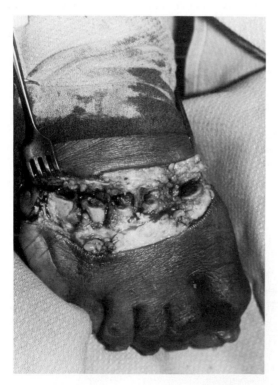

Fig. 11-35. Metatarsals divided about 15° from the transverse axis.

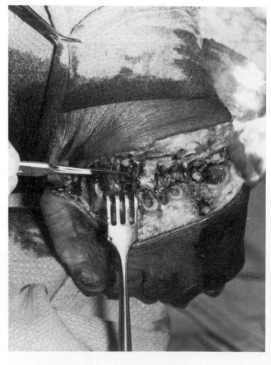

Fig. 11-36. Soft tissue divided from the metatarsal necks and heads.

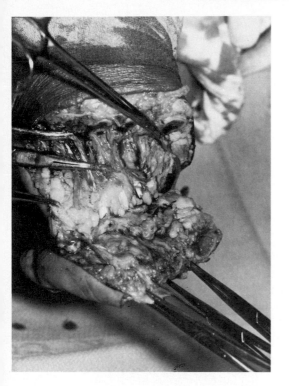

Fig. 11-37. Toes divided from the plantar flap.

can be avoided if the anterior tibial and extensor tendons are sutured into dorsal bony and fascial structures to provide dorsiflexion power.

An alleged advantage of Lisfranc and Chopart amputations is that ordinary shoes can be used. In general, we have found most patients require some sort of stiffening in the sole and/or a special toe block arrangement to wear ordinary shoes. A polypropylene ankle-foot orthosis has been of great help.

Syme's amputation. Since the heel pad is part of the foot and the function of a Syme amputee approximates more closely that of a partial-foot amputee (Syme, 1843; Waters et al., 1976), the Syme amputation is considered a partial foot in our clinic.

Indications. Any patient with a deformed, traumatized, dysvascular, or infected foot is a possible candidate for a Syme amputation. Congenital defects that produce shortened limbs and equinus deformity of the foot frequently do better with an amputation than with multiple attempts at reconstruction. A Syme prosthesis is far more functional and cosmetic than a shoe with a 5- or 6-inch plat-

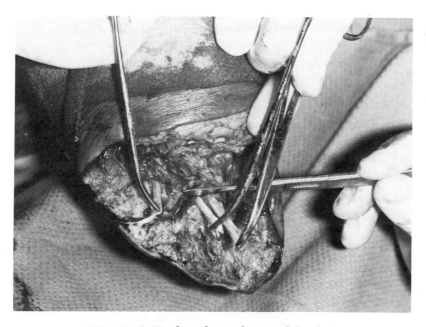

Fig. 11-38. Tendons drawn down and divided.

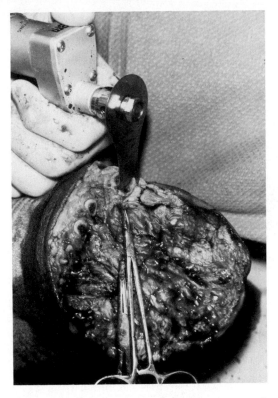

Fig. 11-39. Inferior edges of the metatarsals rounded to relieve pressure.

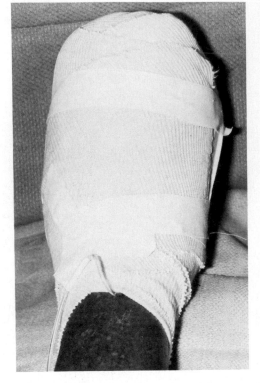

Fig. 11-40. A soft dressing is used until the wound has healed.

form and a severe equinus built in to gain length. Patients with fibular hemimelia, proximal focal femoral deficiencies, and congenital pseudarthrosis of the tibia frequently benefit from a Syme amputation.

Surgical technique. In noninfected cases the surgical technique should be that described by Harris (1956, 1961). In children the malleoli are not removed unless pressure problems occur (Wood et al., 1965). Then they are removed below the epiphyseal lines so as not to cause growth disturbances.

Spittler et al. (1954) described a two-stage method for infected forefeet following war wounds. This method has been modified with a simpler second stage for diabetic and dysvascular gangrene and infection (Wagner, 1977). Doppler transcutaneous ultrasound is used to obtain an ischemic index. If the index is above 0.45 in diabetics and 0.35 in arteriosclerotics, over 93% of the amputations have healed.

With one exception, the Syme amputation

technique is the same for a single-stage procedure as for the first stage of a two-stage method. In the two-stage method the incisions are 1 to 1.5 cm more anterior and distal than described by Syme to allow for the extra volume of the malleoli, which are not removed in the first stage. The incision starts medially 1 to 1.5 cm below and anterior to the midpoint of the medial malleolus (Fig. 11-41).

The incision then swings dorsally directly over the ankle joint to a point about 1.5 cm below and anterior to the lateral malleolus. The two malleolar points are connected by an incision directly across the sole. This incision goes down to bone usually across the os calcis or near the calcaneocuboid joint. On the dorsum the incision is carried down to the dome of the talus (Fig. 11-42).

Tendons are pulled down, severed, and allowed to retract. Vascular structures are identified and ligated or electrocoagulated.

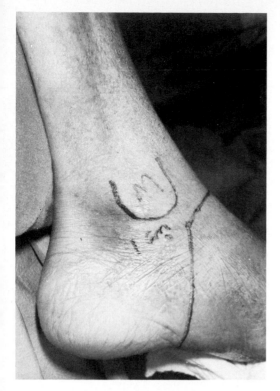

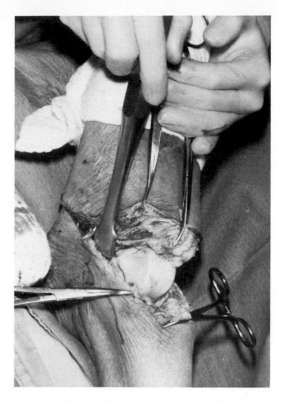

Fig. 11-41. Syme's two-stage amputation; skin incision 1 cm anterior and 1 cm distal to the midpoint of the malleoli.

Fig. 11-42. Incision carried directly to bone; subperiosteal dissection of the os calcis begun.

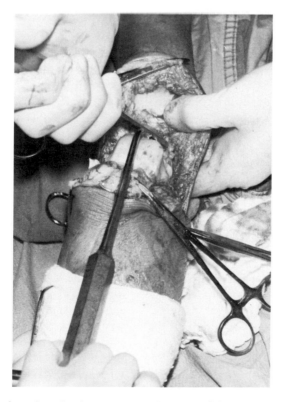

Fig. 11-43. Bone hook in the talus for traction. Subperiosteal dissection to the os calcis continues.

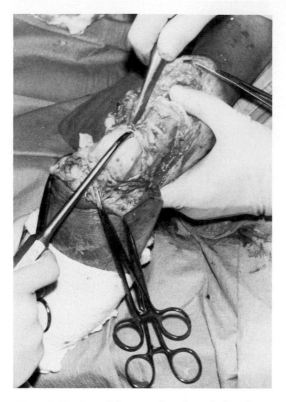

Fig. 11-44. Top of the os calcis denuded. A bone hook in the talus aids in control of the foot.

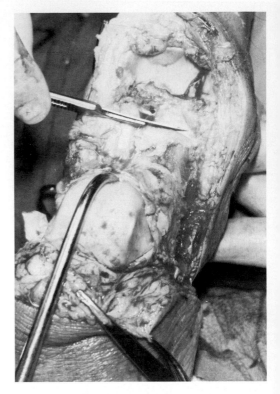

Fig. 11-45. Attachment of the Achilles tendon sectioned with a scalpel; dome of the ankle joint just above the scalpel.

The medial and lateral ligaments are severed from the body of the talus, allowing the talus to be dislocated anteriorly and downward. There is no preferred sequence of cutting; the exact method differs in each patient depending on which structures are tightest. Division of the collateral ligaments is alternated from side to side. Dissection of the body of the calcaneus is started subperiosteally on the lateral side (Figs. 11-42 to 11-44).

The superior surface of the os calcis is denuded subperiosteally. Traction through a bone hook in the talus aids as the dissection is continued around the os calcis (Fig. 11-45).

The two major danger points were well described by Syme. (1) The *neurovascular bundle* courses between the flexor hallucis longus and the flexor digitorum longus (Fig. 11-46). It is at danger when the knife is pushed in medially to sever the medial collateral ligaments. The flexor hallucis longus is first iden-

tified and used to protect the nerve and artery until the medial surface of the os calcis is dissected free. (2) The second danger point is at the immediate *subcutaneous attachment of the tendo Achillis*. Piercing of the posterior skin at this thin point jeopardizes healing. The operation failed in most of the few cases in which skin was inadvertently cut. Careful sharp dissection of the tendon and further subperiosteal dissection allow complete removal of the os calcis and talus. Minor bits of debris are removed, and hemostasis secured.

A Shirley drain is drawn into the cavity through a separate stab wound made over the tip of a hemostat pushed out posterolaterally (Fig. 11-15). The air filter is removed to allow antibiotic solution to be irrigated through the wound by gravity drainage (Wagner, 1977). This is done for 48 hours unless there is further sign of infection in the wound. Late removal is based on clinical appearance of the

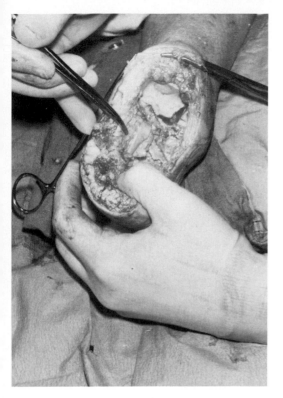

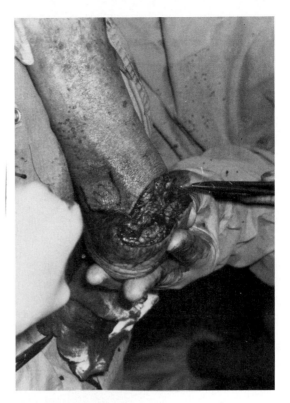

Fig. 11-46. Neurovascular bundle at the tip of the clamp; dome of the ankle just above the clamp.

Fig. 11-47. Closure of the deep fascia to the plantar aponeurosis.

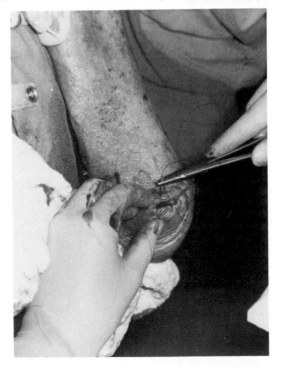

Fig. 11-48. Skin closure with nylon or other nonabsorbable suture.

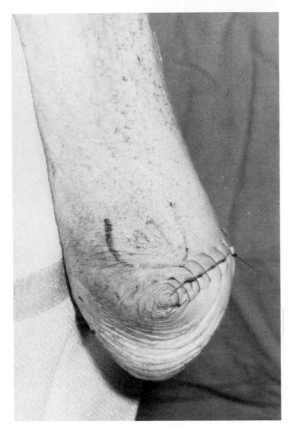

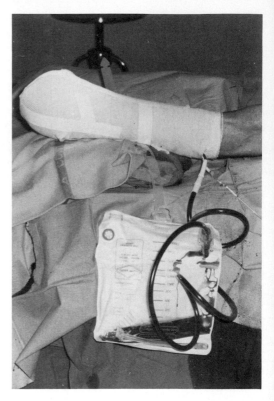

Fig. 11-50. Soft dressing applied in surgery. Wound irrigation is to gravity drainage.

Fig. 11-49. Closed incision with dog ears; good base of posterior skin. This would be sacrificed if dog ears were removed.

wound. At removal the tip of the tube is cut off aseptically and sent for culture. Closure of the wound is begun by suturing the plantar aponeurosis to the deep fascia over the front of the tibia (Fig. 11-47).

If either malleolus produces skin pressure, a stab incision into the fat pad produces a cavity that allows nesting of the malleolus into the fat and relief of the pressure. The skin is closed with nylon or similar suture (Figs. 11-48 and 11-49).

A soft dressing is used for 7 to 10 days (Fig. 11-50). A plaster cast is then applied, and the patient discharged if general health permits. If the heel pad is especially tough, a walking heel is added and the patient allowed to walk (Fig. 11-51).

Felt pads are cut out in the center and placed over the dog ears to protect them from pressure in the cast.

In noninfected and traumatic cases the procedure is performed in one stage. The incisions start at the midpoint of each malleolus and go directly to and through the sole. They then course obliquely across the ankle joint anteriorly. After disarticulation is complete, the malleoli and 1.5 cm of the distal tibia are exposed. The tibia must not be cut too short. Transection is done so a circle of about 3 cm of cartilage is left in the center of the plafond. Several drill holes are made around the periphery and the pad sutured in place. If the medial and lateral flares are too prominent or sharp, they are rounded. Closed irrigation and drainage are carried out for 48 hours. A cast is applied after the drain is removed. Walking is started at 10 to 12 days.

In two-stage procedures the second stage is performed at 6 weeks if healing is secure (Fig. 11-52). The dog ears are removed through medial and lateral elliptical incisions (Fig. 11-53). The malleoli are eliminate flush with the

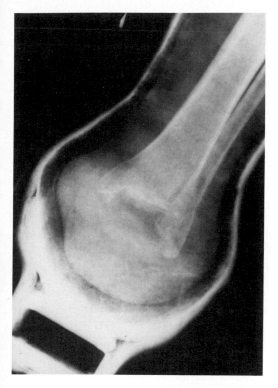

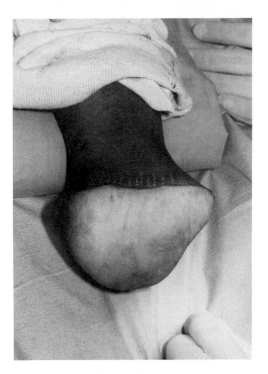

Fig. 11-51. First-stage Syme's amputation in a weight-bearing cast. Felt pads with the center cut out are used over the malleoli and dog ears to relieve pressure.

Fig. 11-52. Second-stage Syme's; healed first stage ready to have the dog ears and malleoli removed.

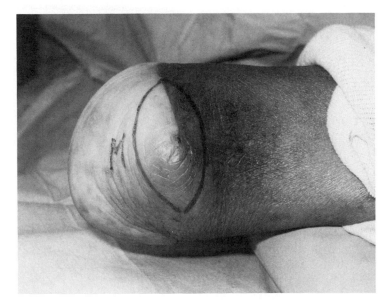

Fig. 11-53. Second-stage Syme's; elliptical incision over the medial malleolus. The volume of this wedge should equal the volume of the malleolus.

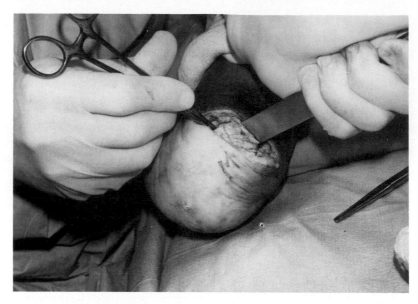

Fig. 11-54. Second-stage Syme's; removal of the medial malleolus flush with the dome of the ankle joint. Articular cartilage is not removed.

ankle joint (Fig. 11-54). A small portion of the flare is removed from the tibia and fibula to narrow the stump and eliminate pressure points (Fig. 11-55). If the pad is loose at this stage, more soft tissue is removed from the elliptical incision. We have not found it necessary to remove the articular cartilage because the pad has already begun to fibrose in place. For further fixation the fascia of the pad is sutured to the bone through drill holes (Fig. 11-56). Skin closure is with nylon or similar suture (Fig. 11-57). At 7 to 10 days the patient is placed in a walking cast (Fig. 11-58). The patient is usually ready for prosthetic fitting in about 6 weeks.

Syme's stumps have been long lasting and relatively free of trouble. Very few have become loose as atrophy progressed. These were returned to surgery and tightened up by removal of appropriate tissue wedges and suturing of the pad to the bone through drill holes. Late complications have been mainly related to progression of arteriosclerotic vascular lesions and have resulted in whole leg gangrene unrelated to any local problem in the Syme stump.

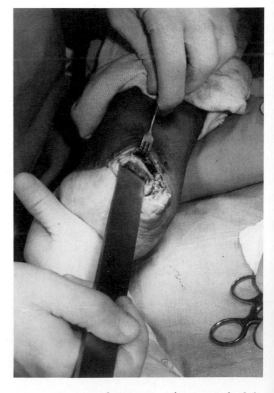

Fig. 11-55. Second-stage Syme's; removal of the flare of the tibia to relieve the bony prominence.

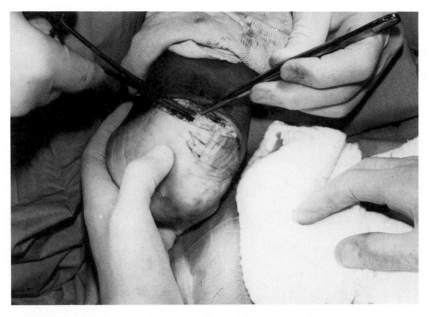

Fig. 11-56. Deep fascia drawn together to test the stability of the pad. More soft tissue is excised if the pad is too loose.

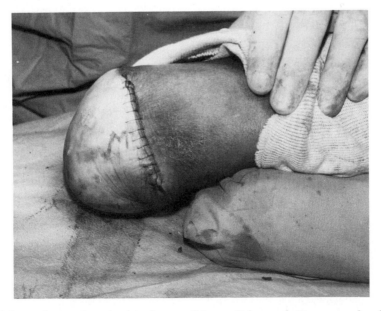

Fig. 11-57. Second-stage Syme's; skin closure of the medial wound. Dog ears and malleoli have been removed.

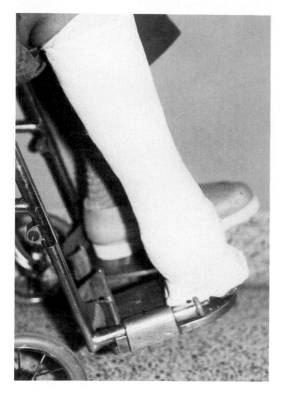

Fig. 11-58. Second-stage Syme's in a walking cast. This cast is used until the stump has matured enough for a definitive prosthesis.

In patients amputated at the Syme level for breakdown of Charcot joints in the foot, hypertrophic jointlike tissues have formed resulting in hypermobile pads. Removal of the excess tissue through wedge incisions has resulted in firm pads.

Syme's amputation in two stages for diabetic and dysvascular gangrene and infection. There has been some criticism of the two-stage technique, which requires a second hospitalization and a second anesthetic and surgical procedure. Other centers have not performed many Syme amputations in this type of patient due to the relatively high failure rate when performed in a single stage (Sarmiento and Warren, 1969). We believe that the articular cartilage left by disarticulation acts as a barrier to the spread of infection from the forefoot through cancellous bone channels. The irrigation drainage system also appears to aid in removal of potentially infected hematoma from the cavity left by disarticulation.

Studies show the Syme amputation to be superior in function to below-knee and above-knee levels in velocity, stride length, cadence, and oxygen-per-meter consumption (Waters et al., 1976). This is of importance because the diabetic patient is especially prone to amputation of the opposite limb within 18 to 36 months (Goldner, 1960). Approximately 50% of our amputees are bilateral. Most with a Syme amputation on one side and a higher level on the opposite state their wish to have had both at the Syme level.

Syme's amputation for crushing injuries. Heel pain has been a late disabling factor in a large group of nondiabetic patients with industrial crushing injuries of the foot. They have been unable to wear standard prostheses, and a substantial number have required further amputation to a below knee level. Review of these cases has disclosed the presence of preamputation heel pain in all. The postamputation pain was not that of the usual amputation neuroma or phantom pain but appeared more like that of a tarsal tunnel or a sympathetic dystrophy.

The amputation surgeon is urged to watch preoperatively for this type of heel pain in crushing foot injuries which may otherwise be suitable for a Syme amputation. If there is such pain, a low calf level should be chosen.

PROSTHETIC CARE

Toe and partial foot amputations rarely require prosthetic replacement. Shoe correction in the form of sole stiffeners and rocker bottoms appear to be of more value. Room temperature–vulcanizing foam is an excellent material for filling a shoe. It is especially valuable when all of the lateral toes and rays have been removed and the first metatarsal and great toe remain. Plastizote and similar foams can be shaped easily for shoe fillers.

Syme's prosthesis

Prostheses with windows, straps, buckles, and other loose pieces tend to break down faster and require more maintenance than do those with no loose structures. The double-wall prosthesis, with an elastic inner wall to provide suspension, appears to be most satisfactory. The SACH foot (single-action cushion heel) allows near normal gait. In bilateral amputees in whom length is not a problem, five-way ankles and similar mechanisms can be installed to aid in torque and other pressure relief.

Physical therapy

The Syme amputee appears to walk as a partial-foot amputee in his prosthesis. Most require no training except in the procedures for donning and doffing. Most have used a walking cast between stages, and all have done so following the second stage. The transition to a prosthesis is smooth. Most require no instruction and their daily use rapidly habituates them to their new relatively "stiff foot."

REFERENCES

Barnes, R. W., Shanik, G. D., and Slaymaker, E. E.: An index of healing in below-knee amputation: leg blood pressure by Doppler ultrasound, Surgery **79:**13, 1976.

Bessman, A. N., and Wagner, F. W.: Nonclostridial gas gangrene: report of 48 cases and review of the literature, J.A.M.A. **233:**958, 1975.

Burgess, E. M., and Marsden, F. W.: Major lower extremity amputation following arterial reconstruction, Arch. Surg. **108:**655, 1974.

Carter, S. A.: The relationship of distal systolic pressures to healing of skin lesions with arterial occlusive disease with special reference to diabetes mellitus, Scand. J. Clin. Lab. Invest. (supp. 128) **31:**239, 1973.

Chopra, J. A., Hurwitz, L. J., and Montgomery, D. A. D.: The pathogenesis of sural nerve changes in diabetes mellitus, Brain **92:**391, 1969.

Collens, W. S., Vlahos, E., Dobkin, G. B., Neuman, E., Rakow, R. K., Altman, M., and Siegman, F.: Conservative management of gangrene in the diabetic patient, J.A.M.A. **181:**692, 1962.

Di Gioia, R. A., Kane, J. G., and Parker, R. H.: Crepitant cellulitis and myonecrosis caused by Klebsiella, J.A.M.A. **237:**2097, 1977.

Ecker, M. D., and Jacobs, B. S.: Lower extremity amputations in diabetic patients, Diabetes **19:**189, 1970.

Goldner, M.: The fate of the second leg in diabetic amputees, Diabetes **9:**100, 1960.

Glattly, H.: A statistical study of 12,000 new amputees, South. Med. J. **57:**1373, 1964.

Greenbaum, D., Richardson, P. C., Salmon, M. V., and Urich, H.: Pathological observations on six cases of diabetic neuropathy, Brain **87:**201, 1964.

Gundersen, J.: Diagnosis of arterial insufficiency with measurement of blood pressure in fingers and toes, Angiology **22:**191, 1971.

Harris, R. I.: Syme's amputation; the technical details essential for success, J. Bone Joint Surg. **38B:**614, 1956.

Harris, R. I.: The history and development of Syme's amputation, Artif. Limbs **6:**4, 1961.

Harris, W. R., and Silverstein, E. A.: Partial amputations of the foot: a follow-up study, Can. J. Surg. **7:**6, 1964.

Holstein, P.: Distal blood pressure. A guidance in choice of amputation level, Scand. J. Clin. Lab. Invest. (supp. 123) **31:**245, 1973.

Jacobs, R.: Personal communication, 1977.

Kahn, O., Wagner, F. W., and Bessman, A. N.: Mortality of diabetic patients treated surgically for lower limb infection and/or gangrene, Diabetes **23:**287, 1974.

Kirkendall, W. M., Burton, A. C., Epstein P. H., and Freis, E. D.: Recommendations for human blood pressure determination by sphygmomanometers, Circulation **36:**980, 1967.

Kramer, D. W., and Perilstein, P. K.: Peripheral vascular complications in diabetes mellitus. A survey of 3,600 cases, Diabetes **7:**384, 1958.

Kritter, A. E.: A technique for salvage of the infected diabetic gangrenous foot, Orthop. Clin. North Am. **4:**21, 1973.

Kunin, C. M.: Urinary tract infections flow charts (algorithms) for detection and treatment, J.A.M.A. **233:**458, 1975.

Lamontagne, A., and Buchtal, F.: Electrophysiological studies in diabetic neuropathy, J. Neurol. Neurosurg. Psychiatry **33:**442, 1970.

Louie, T. J., Bartlett, J. G., Tally, F. P., and Gorbach, S. L.: Anaerobic bacteria in diabetic foot ulcers, Ann. Intern. Med. **85:**461, 1975.

Mackereth, M., and Lennihan, R.: Ultrasound as an aid in the diagnosis and management of intermittent claudication, Angiology **21:**704, 1970.

McKittrick, L. S., McKittrick, J. B., and Risley, T. S.: Transmetatarsal amputation for infection of gangrene in patients with diabetes mellitus, Ann. Surg. **130:**826, 1949.

Medical Staff Conference, University of California, San Francisco: Diabetic micro-angiopathy, West. J. Med. **121:**404, 1974.

Mooney, V., Wagner, F. W., Jr.: Neurocirculatory disorders of the foot, Clin. Orthop. **122:**53, 1977.

Moore, W. S.: Determination of amputation level measurement of skin blood flow with xenon (Xe133), Arch. Surg. **107:**798, 1973.

Pratt, T. C.: Gangrene and infection in the diabetic, Med. Clin. North Am. **49:**987, 1975.

Romano, R. L., and Burgess, E. M.: Level selection in lower extremity amputations, Clin. Orthop. **74:**177, 1971.

Rossini, A. A., and Hare, J. W.: How to control the blood glucose level in the surgical diabetic patient, Arch. Surg. **111:**945, 1976.

Sarmiento, A., and Warren, W. D.: A re-evaluation of lower extremity amputations, Surg. Gynecol. Obstet. **129:**799, 1969.

Senn, N.: Principles of surgery, Philadelphia, 1890, F. A. Davis & Co.

Spittler, A. W., Brenner, J. J., and Payne, J. W.: Syme amputation performed in two stages, J. Bone Joint Surg. 36A:37, 1954.

Stabile, B. E., and Wilson, S. E.: The profunda femoris-popliteal artery bypass, Arch. Surg. 112:913, 1977.

Syme, J.: Amputation at the ankle joint, Mon. J. Med. Sci. 2:93, 1843.

Wagner, F. W., Jr.· Amputation of the foot and ankle— current status, Clin. Orthop. 122:62, 1977.

Waters, R. L., Perry, J., Antonelli, D., and Hislop, H.: Energy costs of walking of amputees: the influence of level of amputation, J. Bone Joint Surg. 58A:42, 1976.

Williams, H. T. G., Hutchinson, K. J., and Brown, G. D.: Gangrene of the feet in diabetics, Arch. Surg. 108:609, 1974.

Wood, W. L., Zlotsky, N., and Westin, G. W.: Congenital absence of the fibula. Treatment by Syme amputation—indication and techniques, J. Bone Joint Surg. 47A:1159, 1965.

Yao, S. T.: Haemodynamic studies in peripheral arterial disease, Br. J. Surg. 57:761, 1970.

12

INFECTIOUS DISORDERS OF THE FOOT

Stanford F. Pollock

An understanding of infectious disorders of the foot is important for two reasons:

1. Foot infections are among the most common conditions seen in the practice of medicine and podiatry.
2. A patient with generalized systemic illness, which makes him more susceptible to any infection, may first seek medical attention because of the symptoms of that infection.

Thus the patient with unrecognized diabetes mellitus, arterial insufficiency, venous insufficiency, or systemic mycobacterial or fungal infection may have presenting complaints referable only to an infection of the foot.

The following outline offers a convenient guide for considering infections of the foot.

1. Bacterial infections
   a. Infections of soft tissues
      (1) Cellulitis
      (2) Lymphangitis
      (3) Felon
      (4) Tenosynovitis
      (5) Bursitis
   b. Infections involving bone
      (1) Pyogenic osteomyelitis
         (a) Acute
         (b) Chronic
         (c) Special types
            (i) Brodie's abcess
            (ii) Garré's osteomyelitis

      (2) Mycobacterial infection
         (a) Tuberculosis
         (b) Leprosy
      (3) Clostridial infection
      (4) Syphilis
2. Fungal infections
   a. Infections of skin and nails
      (1) Tinea pedis
      (2) Onychomycosis
   b. Infections involving deep structures including bone
      (1) Coccidioidomycosis
      (2) Mycetoma (madura foot)
         (a) Actinomycotic mycetoma
         (b) Maduromycosis

BACTERIAL INFECTIONS
Infections of soft tissues

Superficial pyogenic infections are often induced or aggravated by footwear. The distal portion or segment of the toe is susceptible to a felon similar to that which occurs in the finger. The troublesome, ubiquitous, tinea pedis organisms may combine with other bacterial organisms to infect the foot by means of neglected minor scratches, irritations caused by friction, or injury from such instruments as scissors. In the presence of such infection, continued wearing of shoes and weight bearing may lead to extension of the infection into the fascial planes, tendon sheaths, or lymphatic channels. Pyogenic organisms may invade any part of the foot through an abrasion in the skin surface. The abrasion may be microscopic and the patient may be completely unaware of its presence.

Cellulitis. Cellulitis can result from the entrance of pyogenic bacteria to the tissues underlying the epidermis. The most commonly encountered organism is *Staphylococcus* and the most common sites of entry of the organism are the numerous hair follicles. Continued irritation such as that caused by the eyelets of the shoe over the dorsum of the first metatarsocuneiform joint, generally the highest point on the dorsum of the midfoot, may aggravate the condition.

Cellulitis is best treated by complete bed rest, elevation of the foot, continual hot compresses, and appropriate systemic antibiotics. If pus is allowed to accumulate in a localized area, adequate drainage is mandatory.

Lymphangitis. Lymphangitis is generally caused by staphylococcal or streptococcal organisms that penetrate small wounds or abrasions.

The onset of symptoms of lymphangitis is sudden; a history of injury or abrasion may or may not be present. Pain and tenderness are experienced over a local point; chills often occur, followed by a rapidly rising tempera-

ture. Within 12 to 24 hours, bright red streaks may appear along the course of the lymphatic channels; inflammation and edema surround the streaks. The lymph glands proximal to the focus of infection become swollen, painful, and inflamed. Symptoms of general toxicity may be severe, out of all proportion to the appearance of the local lesion. In a few cases, organization of pus takes place at the focus of infection. Occasionally the infection spreads rapidly despite treatment until general septicemia develops. Koch (1934) has contributed a long study of the disease as it applies to the hand.

Treatment. Patients with lymphangitis should be hospitalized and kept at complete bed rest. The leg should be elevated, and moist hot compresses should be applied to the entire foot and leg continuously. High blood levels of appropriate antibiotics should be maintained. Close attention should be paid to such complications of toxemia as dehydration and electrolyte imbalance. Incision and drainage are rarely indicated and may even be harmful (Koch, 1929; Kanavel, 1939). Even if there is evidence of partial organization, it is better to err on the conservative side by not incising. The only indication for incision and drainage is the presence of localized loculated

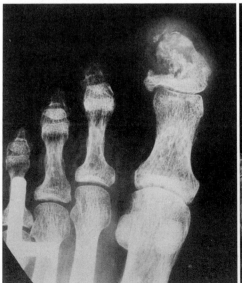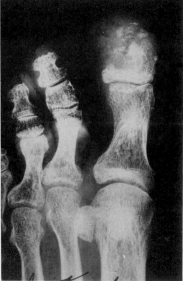

Fig. 12-1. Felon of the great toe with involvement of the distal phalanx.

areas of material. That condition is manifested by the presence of a blister or fluctuant mass directly under the skin, which ordinarily occurs at the focal point of infection but occasionally appears along the course of the lymphatic channels or in the area of the regional lymph nodes.

Felon. A felon, or whitlow, is a septic infection of the pulp space of the distal phalanx of the finger or toe (Fig. 12-1). Purulent material collects in the pulp space and may develop considerable pressure, causing accompanying severe throbbing pain. The pressure may cause decrease or obliteration of the blood supply to bone, which results in necrosis and sequestration. Osteomyelitis of the distal phalanx and the interphalangeal joint is a common complication of a felon (Fig. 12-2).

The distal segment of the toe becomes indurated, swollen, and throbbing 24 to 48 hours following the onset of infection. Pain may be severe, with sleep impossible. The discrepancy between objective observations and the severity of the pain is characteristic of

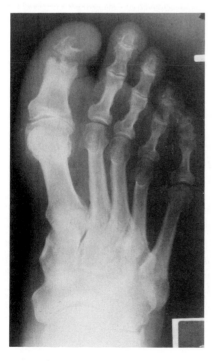

Fig. 12-2. Osteomyelitis of the first distal phalanx and heads of the proximal phalanges after injury.

a felon. After several days the pain diminishes as necrosis of bone progresses. Radiographic examination at the time may disclose early osteomyelitis of the distal phalanx.

Treatment. Local and systemic measures, which include bed rest, elevation of the foot, and warm compresses, should be instituted immediately. Appropriate systemic antibiotics tend to localize the infectious process and should also be started immediately.

Except during the early stages in the development of a felon, incision and drainage are mandatory under general anesthesia or adequate regional block. The pulp space should be opened widely by a semicircular (fishmouth) incision extending from one side of the toe to the other and encircling the distal half of the distal phalanx. Secondary vertical incisions may be made into the pulp space to facilitate drainage. If sequestrae are present, they may be removed. In most cases the process subsides in 2 to 3 weeks and the bone regenerates. If the bone of the distal phalanx has sequestered completely, the sequestrum is occasionally better left in position in the hope that it will serve as a scaffold for the new bone formation and thereby conserve the contour of the toe. In most cases, however, the entire sequestered bone should be removed.

On occasion, the infection will progress so rapidly and with such local destruction of bone and tissues that amputation of the distal phalanx or of the entire digit is necessary. This destructive process is generally seen in diabetes or peripheral small-vessel disease. When amputation is necessary, the skin flaps should be left open for free drainage and subsequent secondary closure.

Infectious tenosynovitis. Infectious tenosynovitis is a bacterial inflammation of tendon sheaths which may be acute or chronic. It is always caused by invasion of the bacteria into the involved tendon sheaths. The course of the disease depends largely on the virulence of the invading organism and the extent of invasion of the tendon sheaths.

Acute infectious tenosynovitis (Christie, 1956) is caused by a spread of infection from adjacent tissues by accidental laceration (direct inoculation) or by contamination from an incision made because of a subcutaneous infection. The laceration or puncture may be microscopic. Occasionally the infection spreads to other parts of the body.

The invader in most cases is one of the common pyogenic organisms, although infections from other more unusual organisms have been reported.

Diagnosis is based on the classic signs of inflammation along the course of the tendon. The inflammation produces extreme pain, especially severe at the insertion of the tendon (even though the active infection may be distant from it) because the infected tendon is immobilized. Any tendon or tendon sheath may be involved, but the extensor tendons of the foot are most commonly affected. Sliding of the tendon or tendons is a complication that may lead to extreme contracture.

Treatment consists of complete bed rest and prompt administration of appropriate antibiotics. Continuous, hot, moist compresses should be applied; and when fluctuation gives evidence of the organization or localization of purulent material, surgical drainage should be carried out promptly. The local injection of antibiotics into the tendon sheath will occasionally reduce the necessity for incision and drainage but should not be relied on to the exclusion of surgical drainage.

Chronic infectious tenosynovitis is caused by a specific disease such as syphilis or tuberculosis. It may be the only manifestation of active tuberculosis. Chronic infectious tenosynovitis is rare, but when it occurs it involves the sheaths of the extensors and peroneal tendons around the ankle joint.

Treatment consists of immobilization of the affected tendons and general treatment of the underlying systemic disease. Surgical repair of the gliding mechanism may be necessary when injury to the tendon and its sheath is severe.

Bursitis. Infectious bursitis includes two types: acute septic and retrocalcaneal.

Acute septic bursitis is inflammation of an adventitial bursa caused by the invasion of pyogenic organisms. It is often accompanied by pus formation. Usually a wound such as a small abrasion or laceration in the vicinity of the bursa causes acute septic bursitis. The condition may also follow a simple acute or traumatic bursitis due to the implantation of organisms from the circulatory system during a period of transient bacteremia.

Treatment consists of complete rest, hot compresses, appropriate antibiotics, and incision and drainage if localization or loculation has occurred. After the acute stage subsides, the patient may be ambulatory, provided pressure has been completely removed from the affected area.

Retrocalcaneal bursitis is an inflammation of the only consistent anatomic bursa of the foot. This bursa is situated between the posterosuperior surface of the calcaneus and the tendo Achillis. The condition is usually acute but may be chronic and may or may not suppurate.

Etiology. Tension from a tight heel, friction, and pressure from the shoe counter, with ensuing secondary infection, are ordinarily the causative factors. Infection may be metastatic. Because the bursa is enclosed in a limited area, the infected area is under pressure. The symptoms of swelling and inflammation above the posterosuperior portion of the calcaneus, pain, and tenderness to touch may be acute. Dorsiflexion of the foot increases the pain.

Treatment. In the acute stage of retrocalcaneal bursitis, treatment is the same as for acute cellulitis: complete rest, hot packs, and antibiotics. If the infection becomes organized, drainage should be instituted. In chronic or recurrent cases the heel cords must be stretched or lengthened and the bursa may need to be excised; however, such excision is at times followed by lengthy and painful convalescence because of the difficulty of occluding the dead space left by removal of the bursa.

For a more complete discussion of the surgical procedures done in cases of infectious bursitis, see Chapter 19.

Infections involving bone

Pyogenic osteomyelitis. The term "osteomyelitis" implies infection of bone. Particular subtypes, based on objectively determined variations, are placed within this broad definition and include acute, subacute, and chronic osteomyelitis, as well as special types of infectious diseases, such as mycotic infections of bone.

Acute osteomyelitis. This acute infection of bone may occur at any age by means of either local bacterial invasion or bacteremia with secondary seeding.

An intact bone in a healthy individual is resistant to infection, and although bacterial infection of soft tissues will often spare the skeleton, massive tissue injury may lower resistance to bacterial invasion. In some cases this lowered resistance is accompanied by a decreased blood supply to the bones as well. Many systemic illnesses lower intrinsic resistance; and subsequent infection of bone, which necessitates radical treatment, may occur.

Acute hematogenous osteomyelitis was encountered more frequently during the preantibiotic era than it is today. Antibiotics have significantly diminished the problems of osteomyelitis.

In 1936 Wilson and McKeever reported that they had found ten out of ninety foci of infection caused by hematogenous osteomyelitis in the bones of the foot. In the ten cases the infection was distributed among the following sites: calcaneus, five; metatarsals, three; phalanges, two.

The use of antibiotics may alter an acute osteomyelitis. For example, when antibiotics are administered in a random manner, a chronic smoldering infection may result and bypass the acute stage of the condition. The most common source of blood-borne bacterial seeding is *Staphylococcus aureus* (Clawson and Dunn, 1967).

The clinical picture of acute osteomyelitis varies according to the causative factors involved. Local bacterial invasion by hematogenous seeding produces a regional tissue response, with adjacent thrombosis, leukocytosis, and an attempted walling of the inoculum. The peculiarity of bone and its resistance to physical deformation render spontaneous drainage and tissue contractability impossible; consequently the infectious process will develop rapidly by means of intramedullary extension until the entire bone may become involved. Acute hematogenous spread is associated with localized pain, erythema, edema, fever, and systemic signs of toxicity. A positive blood culture will confirm the diagnosis.

Infection caused by local inoculation, or contamination caused by the loss of bony integrity due to a compound fracture, may not produce the extreme picture of acute hematogenous osteomyelitis because an immediate drainage pathway is available in these instances. However, the attendant tissue destruction and decreased vascularity do provide a medium that perpetuates the acute infection.

The radiographic picture of acute osteomyelitis can change. At the time of onset, no positive findings may appear; later, rarefaction caused by hyperemia and disuse, as well as soft-tissue swelling, periosteal thickening, medullary cloudiness, and loss of trabeculation may be evident. Radiographic findings are sometimes suggestive of greater bone destruction than actually exists (Fig. 12-3).

If left untreated, acute osteomyelitis will ultimately lead to chronic osteomyelitis or, in some instances, to one of the variant forms of osteomyelitis. The complementary relationship of the resistance of the host and the virulence of the invading agent bear a direct relationship to the ultimate resolution of the condition.

Treatment. The principles of treatment for acute bacterial osteomyelitis are basically the same as for pyogenic infection in other tissues of the body. Prompt identification of the infecting agent and antibiotic treatment, with correctly timed surgical drainage, are paramount. Needle aspiration through aseptically prepared skin into the suspected area, with immediate culture implantation, has proved to be the most successful technique for identifying the agent of infection. Selection of the antibiotic is best determined by the use of in vitro sensitivity studies and is confirmed by checking bactericidal serum levels with subcultures in the laboratory (Jawetz, 1962).

It should be mentioned that in many instances an effective concentration of the

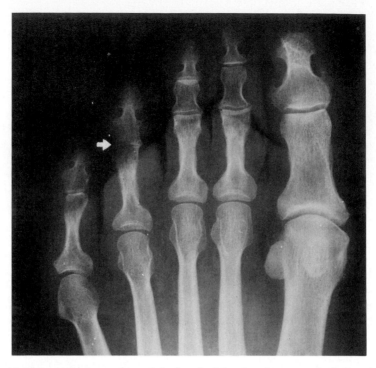

Fig. 12-3. Acute osteomyelitis of the head of the fourth proximal phalanx (arrow).

antibiotic of choice may be hazardous to other organ systems of the body. Care must be taken to anticipate this danger and detect such damage promptly (Benner, 1967). Studies of renal function, as well as electrolytic and audiometric studies, may be indicated for debilitated patients before antibiotic treatment is initiated.

Surgical drainage may be accomplished by direct incision of the abscess, with open packing and delayed closure, or by the insertion of a tube for aspiration. In most areas of infection, tubal aspiration may be performed alternately with topical instillation of the antibiotic (Jergesen and Jawetz, 1963). The primary goals of drainage are to relieve the pressure of the pus and to curtail the spread of the infectious process. Once adequate drainage is established the systemic findings will regress (Fig. 12-4).

Chronic osteomyelitis. An acute osteomyelitis that is inadequately treated or is untreated, in most cases, will develop into chronic osteomyelitis.

At this later stage of bacterial invasion, soft tissue change, bone destruction, vascular insufficiency, and new bone formation (with or without chronic drainage) characterize the clinical picture. Pain is present but is not as severe and incapacitating as in the acute form. In the blood smear, leukocytosis may be a finding, but the smear will show relative lymphocytosis or monocytosis, with a normal number of polymorphonuclear leukocytes. Clinically, sites of drainage will appear and a brawny edema will be present. A radiograph may show areas of dense sclerotic dead bone, as well as areas of reactive new bone at the periphery.

If chronic osteomyelitis is left untreated, drainage through one or more sinus tracts will eventually occur. Often small bits of dead bone (sequestra) can be seen in the drainage or may be picked out of the sinus tract. In response to the death of bone, the host creates peripheral new bone (involucrum) in order to maintain skeletal integrity. Rarely the epithelium of the chronic sinus tract undergoes malignant transformation.

Treatment. The treatment of chronic osteo-

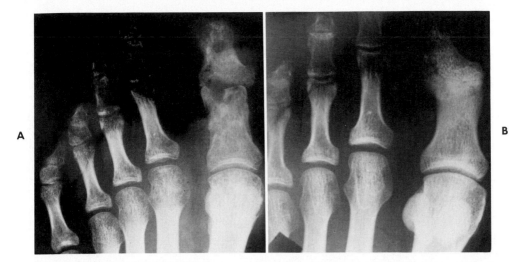

Fig. 12-4. A, Osteomyelitis of the entire hallux. B, After healing.

myelitis is inevitably surgical. Bacterial identification, repeated cultures, and prolonged antibiotic therapy, combined with various forms of surgical debridement, may provide arrest of the condition and expedite the return of normal function. Excision of the dead sequestrations as well as the local devitalized soft tissues should be carried out. Local irrigation and suction after debridement may provide good results; muscle pedicle grafts with saucerization may enhance healing (Rowling, 1959). Amputation remains the treatment of choice in some cases involving debility, continued progression of the disease, or both.

Before surgical procedures are performed, contrast studies of the sinus tract (sinograms) should be done to expose areas of necrotic tissue not evident on the radiograph. After surgical procedures have been carried out, the foot should be immobilized until the involucrum is able to withstand strain.

The regenerative power of bone in children is extraordinary; a bone that is nearly destroyed often will become completely regenerated and remodeled, but damage to the growth plate will result in shortening (Trueta, 1959).

Special types of osteomyelitis. Special types of osteomyelitis include Brodie's abscess and Garré's osteomyelitis.

Brodie's abscess. Under particular condi-

tions of host resistance and altered bacterial virulence, the patient with hematogenous osteomyelitis may develop a localized intramedullary abscess that is walled off by reactive bone. Pain is associated with this developing abscess, but little systemic involvement exists. The condition, named Brodie's abscess, is encountered five times as frequently in adolescent males as in the general population. In most of the reported cases the abscess shows a predilection for the distal tibia. Radiographs demonstrate a well-demarcated, punched-out lesion of the involved bone with increased cortical density and periosteal thickening (Greenfield, 1969). Radiographic findings may not differentiate Brodie's abscess from enchondroma, osteoid osteoma, and bone cyst (Fig. 12-5).

The patient may have acute symptoms, or may complain of having had mild discomfort for months. In long-standing cases a fusiform swelling sometimes develops adjacent to the bone; the abscess may be sterile at the time of culture. Symptoms can persist for years and then gradually subside with the death of the invading bacteria. No statistics are available on untreated cases inasmuch as the diagnosis is confirmed only by treatment.

Treatment of Brodie's abscess should include culture studies, excision of all necrotic material, and curettage of the bone. When no abscess is present, primary closure may be

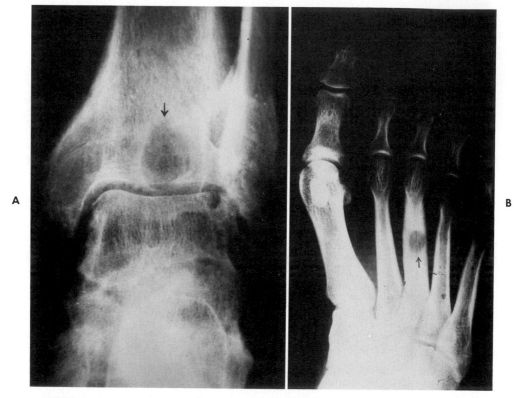

Fig. 12-5. Brodie's abscess. **A,** In the lower end of the tibia (arrow). **B,** In the third metatarsal. Note the increased density and periosteal thickening of the entire metatarsal shaft.

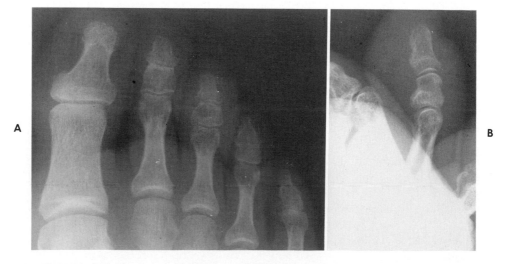

Fig. 12-6. Brodie's abscess involving the middle phalanx in the foot of a 17-year-old boy. **A,** Anteroposterior view; **B,** lateral view.

considered; but more often excision biopsy with delayed secondary closure is most effective. If only a minor phalanx is involved, total phalangectomy may be advisable (Fig. 12-6).

Garré's osteomyelitis. In this form of subliminal osteomyelitis, a dense bone reaction occurs without abscess formation or suppura-tion. The exact reason for this occurrence is unknown. Some authors deny its existence in the antibiotic era (Aegerter and Kirkpatrick, 1968). A low-grade embolic seeding transmitted by means of the blood or the lymphatic vessels is thought to be the cause. More often the tibia is involved, but the tubular bones of the foot may be affected (Fig. 12-7).

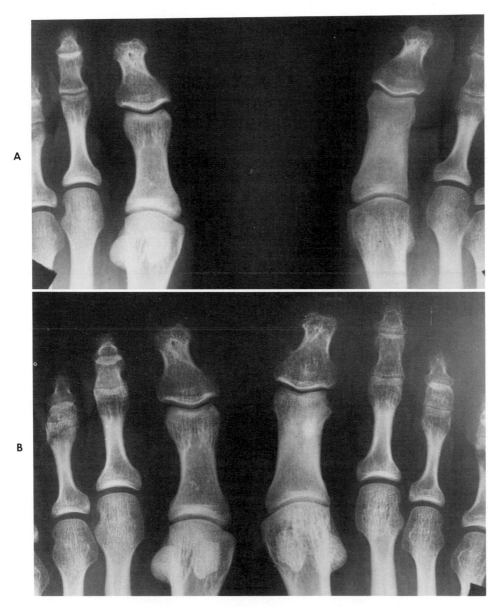

Fig. 12-7. Garré's osteomyelitis. **A,** Left, Normal foot for comparison. Right, Sclerosing and periosteal thickening of the first proximal phalanx. **B,** One year later. Note the decrease in bone density and the disappearance of periosteal thickening.

The onset of this form of osteomyelitis is either insidious, with pain and edema over the involved bone, or acute, with severe pain and systemic signs of toxicity. If only small bones are involved, the findings may be minimal.

Radiographic examination shows an increase in the density of bone trabeculation, as well as cortical thickening caused by periosteal new bone (Greenfield, 1969). A small tubular bone of the foot may become entirely involved in the process. This disease must be differentiated from osteoid osteoma and Paget's disease if the infectious process is localized to an area of a long tubular bone.

The treatment of Garré's osteomyelitis consists of surgical excision of the dense cortical bone (to allow for medullary exposure) with curettement of any devitalized areas. In order to avoid exacerbation or the spread of infection, cultures should be obtained and antibiotic therapy initiated at the time surgical procedures are performed. Initial closure of the wound has been advised by some surgeons who have reported success with this method.

Mycobacterial infection

Osseous tuberculosis of the foot. The bones of the foot are seldom sites of tuberculous lesions, but in establishing a diagnosis the surgeon must not overlook the possibility of tuberculous lesions (Fig. 12-8). Since the advent of antimicrobial agents, especially isonicotinic acid hydrazide, tuberculosis of the bone has decreased in severity. It may be difficult to diagnose because it often simulates other diseases of bone.

Tuberculosis of bone and joints is a slow, unrelenting, destructive manifestation of a systemic disease induced by the tubercle bacillus. Since the lesion is always secondary to a tuberculous focus elsewhere in the body, this focus should be located.

Tuberculosis of the bones of the foot may occur at any age. As a rule, the chronic infection is fairly widespread although isolated foci may be found, particularly in the calcaneus and talus.

According to Miltner and Fang (1936), the most important weight-bearing bones are affected in cases of multiple infection. The order of incidence, from highest to lowest, is

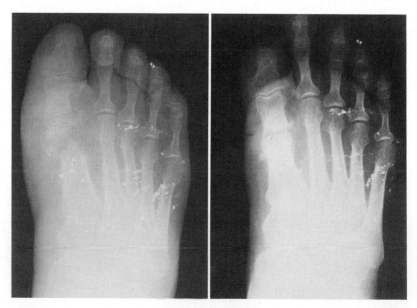

Fig. 12-8. Tuberculosis of the first metatarsal. Buckshot wounds antedated the onset of this involvement. Infection was proved by biopsy and guinea pig inoculation. (Courtesy Dr. D. D. Dickson.)

as follows: calcaneus, talus, first metatarsal, navicular, and first and second cuneiform bones.

Tuberculosis should generally be suspected in the presence of an unrelenting, prolonged chronic destructive process of bone with recurring acute exacerbations. Skin tests for tuberculosis should be performed, since this disease is apt to be present in such cases.

Reeves (1958) presented a thorough discussion of differential diagnosis of tuberculosis of the talus in a case in which the clinical diagnostic impressions included arthritis, degenerative disease, and granulomatous proliferation. Reeves emphasized a sign that is almost pathognomonic: radiographic evidence of partial sclerotic reaction, indicating unsuccessful healing, the fragmented talus being more severely diseased in one part than another. He also called attention to the need for follow-up radiographs, because the first ones might show no abnormality.

Whereas in the past surgery played a prominent role in the management of tuberculosis of bones and joints, the advent of triple therapy including para-aminosalicylic acid, isonicotinic acid hydrazide, and streptomycin has drastically reduced the need for surgical intervention.

Friedman and Kapur (1973) discussed the use of rifampin and ethambutol in combination with isoniazid, and it would appear that these three drugs administered in combination systemically constitute the current first line treatment of osseous tuberculosis. Such drugs as viomycin sulfate and cycloserine may be considered in particularly resistant infections.

Surgical intervention may now be limited to arthrodesis of severely deformed painful weight-bearing joints found to be destroyed by the disease before chemotherapy can be instituted, biopsies for diagnosis when material cannot be obtained by nonoperative means, occasional evacuation of a large collection of pus and debris if still evident clinically or radiographically after several months of chemotherapy, and, of course dural decompression for paralytic spine tuberculosis.

Leprosy (Hansen's disease). Leprosy is a specific chronic disease of man. It is thought to be caused by *Mycobacterium leprae*, because until recently cultivation of this organism and the production of subsequent disease in inoculated animals had not been accomplished. However, a relatively recent and successful effort to cultivate the organism and produce the disease in the armadillo has opened avenues for research in this area that were hitherto impossible.

The mode of transmission of leprosy is unknown, but direct and prolonged contact appears to be necessary. Once in the body, the bacilli are probably spread through the lymphatics and the bloodstream. Localization occurs in the skin, nerves, or both, but in advanced cases bacilli are found in all parts of the body with the exception of smooth muscle.

Feldman and Sturdivant (1976) have reported an epidemologic study of leprosy in the United States, pointing out that approximately 1,900 cases of leprosy existed between 1950 and 1969.

Clinical course and types of lesions. Jacobson and Trautman (1976) have outlined the classification of forms of leprosy as follows: An individual coming in contact with *M. leprae* may develop no disease or may develop an indeterminate form of leprosy. This form is characterized by a macular skin lesion with or without sensory nerve loss. From the indeterminate form the patient may, in the absence of treatment, go on to develop the tuberculoid form, the lepromatous form, or the borderline form existing in various mixtures of the tuberculoid and lepromatous forms.

TUBERCULOID. The lesions in tuberculoid leprosy consist of areas of asymmetric lesions from tubercles containing epithelial cells, giant cells, lymphocytes and plasma cells with few or no bacilli present. The lepromin skin test is positive in patients with this form of leprosy.

LEPROMATOUS. The lesions in lepromatous leprosy are characterized by the formation of lepromas, nodules that are made up of large macrophages which contain numerous bacilli and fat droplets. This is considered the most advanced stage of the disease, and the lepromin skin test is negative in individuals with this form of leprosy.

BORDERLINE. Borderline leprosy (known in the United States as intermediate or dimorphous) is characterized by the presence of lesions which demonstrate mixtures of both the tuberculoid and the lepromatous types, and an entire spectrum of pathology between the two types may be encountered. The skin test is variable, tending to be positive in patients exhibiting lesions of the tuberculoid type and negative in patients exhibiting lesions more consistent with the lepromatous type.

It would appear that the cellular immunity to *M. leprae* is highest in the tuberculoid form and lowest in the lepromatous form.

Effects of leprosy upon the feet. The foot may be affected in several ways: (1) leprous lesions may develop in the feet directly; (2) lepromatous involvement of the peripheral nerves may result in anesthetic feet; and (3) involvement of the peroneal nerve may result in foot drop.

Harris and Brand (1966) indicated two distinct methods of destruction of the foot once pain sensibility is lost. The first is slow erosion and shortening associated with perforating ulcers under the distal, weight-bearing, end of the foot. The second is a proximal disintegration of the tarsus in which mechanical forces often determine the onset and progress of the condition.

The treatment of such feet is as follows:

1. The patient must be educated to use the feet only for gentle walking.

2. Immobilization of the feet in plaster or complete bed rest is necessary for the treatment of ulcers.

3. One should be alert to signs of tarsal disintegration. The earliest signs may be local warmth, swelling, or both. When these signs occur, gait analysis should be carried out and suitable shoe adjustment should be made until the patient can walk a limited distance without developing abnormal tarsal heat at points of stress.

4. When definite bone damage is seen, full immobilization is imperative.

5. In cases in which joints are disintegrating, surgical fusion should be performed without delay.

Warren (1971), in a study of tarsal bone disintegration in over 1,500 leprosy patients treated at the Hong Kong Leprosarium during a twelve-year period, found that early detection and treatment by immobilization permitted healing with minimal deformity or disability and that feet with advanced lesions could be similarly treated without amputation.

Involvement of the common peroneal nerve frequently results in foot drop. Carayon et al. (1967) described promising results in the correction of this deformity with a dual transfer of the posterior tibial and flexor digitorum longus tendons.

Treatment. The current management of leprosy is primarily by chemotherapeutic means with dapsone (DDS, diaminodiphenylsulfone), clofazimine, and rifampin used in combination or alone as the drugs of choice.

Jacobson and Trautman (1976) have reviewed the use of these drugs and the reactions that may be seen to the treatment of leprosy. The reactions to treatment include the (1) reversal reaction, in which a more lepromatous form tends to revert to a more tuberculoid form accompanied by fever, edema, and ulceration, and (2) erythema nodosum leprosum. The reversal reaction is best treated by the administration of systemic corticosteroids and erythema nodosum leprosum by the administration of thalidomide.

Surgical procedures continued to play an important role in the treatment of neurologic manifestations of leprosy.

Clostridial infection (gas gangrene). Anaerobic bacteria of the genus *Clostridia* may be found in wounds in three situations: as saprophytic contaminants, in clostridial cellulitis, and in clostridial myonecrosis (true gas gangrene).

Sim (1975) has pointed out that examination of stained smears of nearly all fresh wounds caused by violent trauma reveals clostridial organisms. Despite the high incidents of contamination, clostridial infections do not occur often. When the anaerobic clostridial organism multiplies in tissues devitalized by wounding without significant production of toxin, saprophytic contamination is felt to be present and no specific treatment other than the general measures applicable to all contaminated wounds is necessary.

Clostridial cellulitis is a septic process usually caused by *Clostridium perfringens* and is often mistakenly diagnosed as gas gangrene (clostridial myonecrosis). It is an infection of the subcutaneous tissues and fascial planes rendered susceptible by ischemia or crush injury. In this case, muscle is generally not affected; the patient exhibits only mild toxemia and profuse crepitation in the subcutaneous tissues of the involved areas.

Gas gangrene or clostridial myonecrosis is characterized by clostridial invasion of normal uninjured muscle with necrosis of muscle cells rapidly extending in every direction from the site of injury. The patient is extremely toxic, due probably to the production by the clostridia of the alpha toxin or lecithinase. Gas production may be minimal in myonecrosis, and the course of the disease may be extremely rapid. In the foot clostridial cellulitis

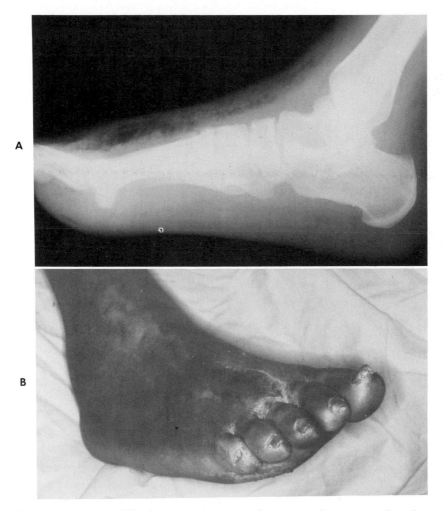

Fig. 12-9. Gas gangrene of the foot. **A,** Lateral view showing gas formation in the subcutaneous tissue on the dorsum as a result of clostridial cellulitis. **B,** Clostridial cellulitis of the dorsum of the foot. Note the fluctuant swelling of subcutaneous tissue.   *Continued.*

is more commonly encountered because, compared with the leg or thigh, the foot has relatively little muscle tissue (Fig. 12-9). The most common causative organisms are *Clostridium perfringens*, *C. novyi*, and *C. septicum*.

Diagnosis. The possibility of a clostridial infection should be considered whenever there is a crush injury with devitalized tissue of even a small amount. This is especially true if there has been the possibility of contamination by foreign body, soil, or feces.

The diagnosis is made essentially by physical examination. The characteristic picture of gas gangrene is tissue edema, necrosis, discoloration, characteristic autopsy room odor, brown exudate, and crepitation due to gas formation in the soft tissues. Care should be taken, however, not to assume that any infection associated with gas formation is clostridial; many other organisms can produce gas, or

air can be trapped in the soft tissues as a result of open injury. Diagnosis is confirmed by the findings of characteristic gram-positive bacilli on exudate or debrided soft tissue. Cultures are rarely of value in making the diagnosis because of the prolonged delay.

Treatment. Gas gangrene is almost always preventable. The most important single aspect in the prevention of gas gangrene is thorough, adequate debridement of all dead avascular tissue. The wound must be debrided back to bleeding tissue and, in the case of muscle, to the point at which the muscle contracts when gently pinched. Prophylactic use of antibiotics is of some value; generally penicillin in very high doses is the drug of choice. It must be pointed out, however, that no antibiotic can prevent gas gangrene in the absence of thorough surgical debridement.

The use of polyvalent gas gangrene antitoxin is controversial; probably it should not

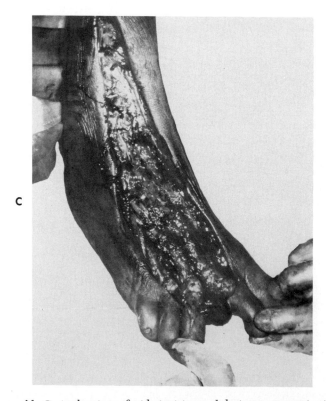

Fig. 12-9, cont'd. C, At the time of wide incision and drainage; necrotic tissue excised.

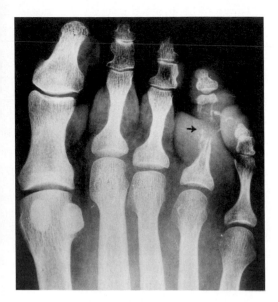

Fig. 12-10. Necrosis of the fourth digit in latent syphilis.

be used prophylactically. Its value in treatment remains questionable. Also used in treatment is hyperbaric oxygen (3 atmospheres), which is probably a helpful adjunct. However, hyperbaric oxygen should not be considered a substitute for adequate thorough surgical treatment. Despite adequate local debridement and the use of antibiotics and hyperbaric oxygen, occasionally the infection cannot be controlled without amputating the involved limb.

Syphilis

Syphilitic neuropathy. Until the advent of antibiotics, latent syphilis was the most common destroyer of the joints of the body (Figs. 12-10 and 12-11). Although the late manifestations of syphilis have now become rare, the venereal disease rate for both syphilis and gonorrhea has continually increased throughout the world. Charcot's joint was frequently encountered as a result of syphilis; but its predilection was for the knee rather than the foot, although the ankle was often affected and other joints were not unaffected. Antibiotics

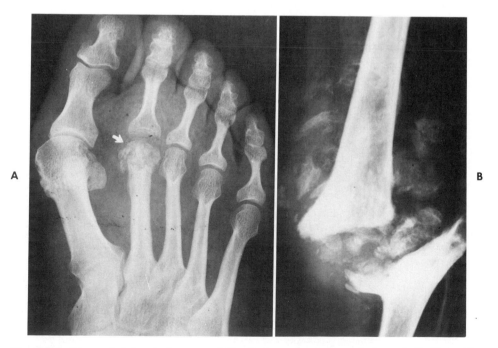

Fig. 12-11. Charcot's joints in latent syphilis. **A,** Second metatarsophalangeal. **B,** Knee. Note the bizarre destruction and new bone formation.

and antianemia therapy have greatly diminished the incidence of arthropathies caused by syphilis and anemia.

FUNGAL INFECTIONS
Infections of the skin and nails

Tinea pedis (athlete's foot, dermatophytosis, ringworm). Tinea pedis is perhaps the most common infection of the foot. Spores of one or more strains of trichophytes are commonly harbored between the toes and under the nails, but they may also invade any part of the foot. Chronicity and recurrence are common. The spores of the organism may lie dormant for months or years before they mature and multiply under favorable conditions such as excessive moisture, friction, pressure, or trauma either accidentally or iatrogenically.

When the disease is active, it assumes various forms and degrees from minute fissures between the toes to a vesicular scaly dermatitis over large areas on the entire foot (Fig. 12-12). It varies from a low-grade inflammatory process to a violent infection, although serious illness is rare. The most common causative organisms is *Trichophyton menta-grophytes* and *T. rubrum*. In severe cases secondary bacterial infection may be present.

Treatment is directed at relieving the severe itching and other signs of local irritation. Frequent changes of dry socks, use of foot powders, and drying thoroughly between toes after bathing are of importance. For severe cases an article in *Medical Letter* recommends the drugs clotrimazole and miconazole applied locally ("Drugs for Athlete's Foot," 1976). Griseofulvin taken systemically for many months has been useful in suppressing the infection but is probably *not* indicated since there is some question as to the carcinogenicity of griseofulvin.

The condition known as pustular acrodermatitis enters into the differential diagnosis, for it may have an identical appearance. Microscopic examination of potassium hydroxide–treated scrapings from suspected lesions, however, will show the typical mycelia of a true fungal infection.

Onychomycosis. Onychomycosis represents a condition in which there is fungal infection of the toenail and nail bed. This is most commonly due to *Trichophyton rubrum* and secondly to *T. mentagrophytes*. Other

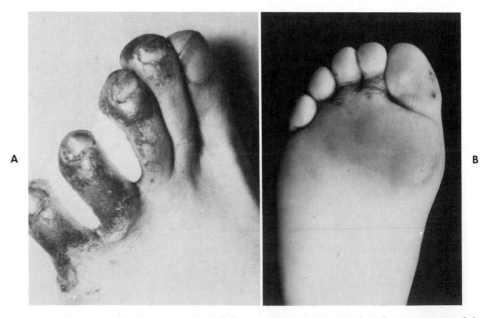

Fig. 12-12. Dermatophytosis. **A,** Acute, of the toes. **B,** Chronic, in the plantar creases of the toes.

cases have been due to *Candida albicans*. In this condition thick accumulations of keratinous material appear under the nail; the nail is often discolored to a yellowish tint and grows eradically.

Treatment is generally with keratolytic agents. Topical treatments such as Castellani's paint and gentian violet along with nail debridement appear to be the most useful in controlling but not eradicating the condition. In cases due to *Candida albicans*, underlying systemic illness may be suspected. In severe cases nail avulsion is indicated.

Infections involving the deep structures including bone

Coccidioidomycosis. *Coccidioides immitis*, a specific fungus, gains entrance through the respiratory tract or skin and is disseminated through the blood or lymph channels or is spread by direct extension. Spores settle in cancellous bone and bone lesions form. The resulting infection is usually chronic and shows clinical and radiographic changes similar to those in chronic osteomyelitis.

McMaster and Gilfillan (1939) reported twenty-four cases of coccidioidal osteomyelitis with multiple foci involving various parts of the body, including the foot. The average age of their patients, who were predominantly men, was 32 years. Thirteen of the patients died; all were proved to have had an associated active pulmonary involvement.

Grebe (1954) reported a case of monostotic coccidioidal infection in which the bone lesion occurred in the left calcaneus. Evidence of disease or injury had not been observed. There was no response to wide excision of the bone lesion, but rapid healing was accomplished by treatment with hydroxystilbamidine isethionate.

More recently, the use of amphotericin B as described by Winn (1955, 1963) has produced encouraging results in cases which might previously have been fatal. Amphotericin B has been particularly useful in preventing massive dissemination of the disease in patients who undergo surgical procedures for coccidioidal lesions. A fall in the coccidioidal complement fixation titer indicates successful treatment and may occur after surgical removal of the infected tissue. Although treatment with amphotericin B has effectively reduced the toxicity of the disease, it should also be noted that amphotericin B is an extremely toxic drug and that *Coccidioides immitis* is among the most resistant of fungal infections to the drug.

Mycetoma (madura foot)

Actinomycotic mycetoma and maduromycosis. Mycetoma is a chronic granulomatous disease (Fig. 12-13) found mainly in tropical

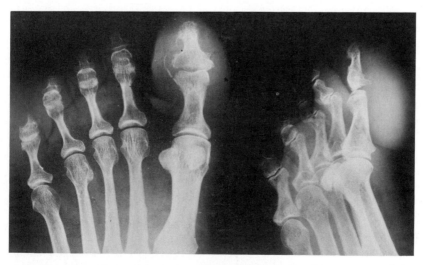

Fig. 12-13. Massive granuloma of the great toe; result of a mycotic infection acquired in a tropical country.

countries, especially in some districts of India. Etiologically mycetoma can be separated into actinomycotic mycetoma, caused by several species of *Streptomyces* and *Nocardia*, and maduromycosis, caused by large filament-producing species of higher fungi such as *Madurella*, *Leptosphaeria senegalensis*, *Allescheria boydii*, *Monosporium apiospermum*, and others.

The clinical picture is the same whether the condition is actinomycotic in origin or produced by the higher fungi. The disease begins as a granuloma, generally subcutaneous in location (Fig. 12-14). The deep structures are involved only late in the course of the disease (Oyston, 1961). New tumors form while old ones soften, and the foot increases enormously in size, becoming deformed.

Franz and Albertini (1954) found extensive osteoporosis of the tarsal bones in one of their patients. Primary mycetoma of bone is a more uncommon condition. According to Majid et al. (1964), all primary intraosseous infections that have been studied mycolog-

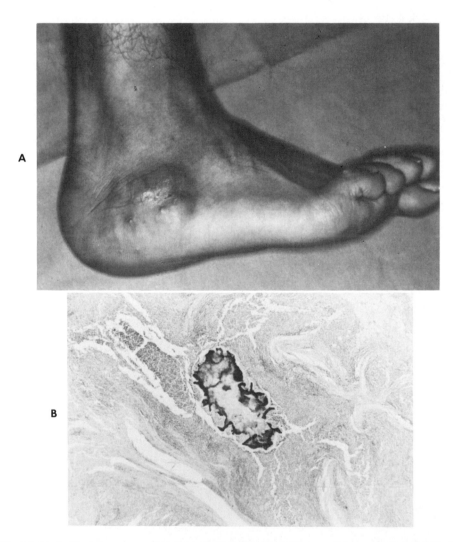

Fig. 12-14. **A,** Draining sinus of the lateral side of the heel. Biopsy of the extensive nodular lesion of the soft tissues revealed *Nocardia*. **B,** *Nocardia* colony with chronic inflammation; sulfur granule of the lesion in **A.**

ically are caused by *Madurella mycetomi*.

A similar condition indigenous to the United States is caused by *Actinomyces bovis*, a gram-positive, non–acid-fast, nonmotile filamentous organism related to true bacteria but resembling fungi.

The characteristic lesion in this condition is a firm, relatively nontender, abscess with central necrosis that may drain to the surface. Consequently, the sinus track produced has little tendency to heal spontaneously.

Identification of the organisms and appropriate antimicrobial sensitivity studies are important, since treatment may depend to some degree on the use of antimicrobial agents. Actinomycotic mycetoma may be sensitive to penicillin, tetracycline, erythromycin, and chloramphenicol and sulfones. Even restoration of diseased and partially destroyed bones has been reported with chemotherapy in the treatment of mycetoma caused by *Streptomyces madurae* by Kamalam et al. (1975).

Mycetomas caused by *Madurella* types of organisms are fairly resistant to antimicrobial therapy. Although Neuhauser (1955) reported promising therapeutic results with diaminodiphenylsulfone, Wilson (1975) has stated that he knows of no chemotherapeutic agent, including amphotericin B, effective against infections with such organisms as *Allescheria boydii*. In spite of the results of antimicrobial treatment, surgery often is necessary. In all these conditions early excision of superficial lesions leads fairly often to cure. In advanced cases amputation above the diseased area may be necessary.

REFERENCES

Aegerter, E., and Kirkpatrick, J. A., Jr.: Orthopedic diseases, ed. 3, Philadelphia, 1968, W. B. Saunders Co.

Benner, E. J.: Use and abuse of antibiotics J. Bone Joint Surg. **49A:**977, 1967.

Carayon, A., Bourrel, P., Bourges, M., and Touzé, M.: Dual transfer of the posterior tibial and flexor digitorum longus tendons for drop foot: report of thirty-one cases, J. Bone Joint Surg. **49A:**144, 1967.

Christie, B. G. B.: The diagnosis and treatment of tenosynovitis, Br. J. Clin. Pract. **10:**677, 1956.

Clawson, D. K., and Dunn, A. W.: Management of common bacterial infections of bones and joints, J. Bone Joint Surg. **49A:**164, 1967.

Drugs for athlete's foot and tinea cruris, Med. Lett. Drugs Ther. **18:**101, 1976.

Feldman, R. A., and Sturdivant, M.: Leprosy in the United States 1950-1969: an epidemiologic review, South. Med. J. **69:**970, 1976.

Franz, A., and Albertini, B.: Sul micetoma primitivo del piede: piede di Madura, Chir. Organi Mov. **40:**412-430, 1954.

Friedman, B., and Kapur, V. N.: Newer knowledge of chemotherapy in the treatment of tuberculosis of bones and joints, Clin. Orthop. **97:**5, 1973.

Grebe, A. A.: Monostotic coccidioidal infection: Report of a case successfully treated with 2-hydroxystilbamidine, J. Bone Joint Surg. **36A:**859, 1954.

Greenfield, G. B.: Radiology of bone diseases, Philadelphia, 1969, J. B. Lippincott Co.

Harris, J. R., and Brand, P. W.: Patterns of disintegration of the tarsus in the anaesthetic foot, J. Bone Joint Surg. **48B:**4, 1966.

Jacobson, R. R., and Trautman, J. R.: The diagnosis and treatment of leprosy, South. Med. J. **69:**979, 1976.

Jawetz, E.: Assay of antibacterial activity in serum, Am. J. Dis. Child. **103:**81, 1962.

Jergesen, F., and Jawetz, E.: Pyogenic infections in orthopedic surgery: combined antibiotic and closed wound treatment, Am. J. Surg. **106:**152, 1963.

Kamalam, A., Premalatha, S., Augustine, S. M., and Saravanamuthu, A.: Restoration of bones in mycetoma, Arch. Dematol. **111:**1178, 1975.

Kanavel, A. B.: Infections of the hand, ed. 7, Philadelphia, 1939, Lea & Febiger.

Koch, S. L.: Felons, acute lymphangitis and tendon sheath infections: differential diagnosis and treatment, J.A.M.A. **92:**1171, 1929.

Koch, S. L.: Acute rapidly spreading infections following trivial injuries of the hand, Surg. Gynecol. Obstet. **59:**277, 1934.

Majid, M. A., Mathias, P. F., Seth, H. N., and Thirumalachar, M. J.: Primary mycetoma of the patella, J. Bone Joint Surg. **46A:**1283, 1964.

McMaster, P. E., and Gilfillan, C.: Coccidioidal osteomyelitis, J.A.M.A. **112:**1233, 1939.

Miltner, L. J., and Fang, H. C.: Prognosis and treatment of tuberculosis of the bones of the foot, J. Bone Joint Surg. **18:**287, 1936.

Neuhauser, I.: Black grain maduromycosis caused by *Madurella grisea*, Arch. Dermatol. **72:**550, 1955.

Oyston, J. K.: Madura foot: a study of twenty cases, J. Bone Joint Surg. **43B:**259, 1961.

Reeves, J. D.: Differential diagnosis in case 44122: presentation of the case, N. Engl. J. Med. **258:**612, 1958.

Rowling, D. E.: The positive approach to chronic osteomyelitis, J. Bone Joint Surg. **41B:**681, 1959.

Sim, F. H.: Anaerobic infections, Orthop. Clin. North Am. **6:**1049, 1975.

Trueta, J.: The three types of acute haematogenous osteomyelitis: a clinical and vascular study, J. Bone Joint Surg. **41B:**671, 1959.

Warren, G.: Tarsal bone disintegration in leprosy, J. Bone Joint Surg. **53B:**688, 1971.

Wilson, J. C., and McKeever, F. M.: Bone growth disturbance following hematogenous osteomyelitis, J.A.M.A. **107:**1188, 1936.

Wilson, J. W.: Discussion of Transactions of the Los Angeles Dermatological Society. *Nocardia brasiliensis* mycetoma, Arch. Dermatol. **11:**1371, 1975.

Winn, W. A.: The use of amphotericin B in the treatment of coccidioidal disease, Am. J. Med. **27:**617, 1955.

Winn, W. A.: Coccidioidomycosis and amphotericin B, Med. Clin. North Am. **47:**1131, 1963.

13

KERATOTIC DISORDERS OF THE PLANTAR SKIN

Roger A. Mann and Henri L. DuVries

Disorders of the skin to which the foot is especially susceptible are either excrescences caused by friction and pressure over a bony prominence, which are by far the most common lesions of the foot, or diseases of the skin itself, which may be intrinsic or extrinsic and are covered in all texts on dermatology. Friction or pressure may result in hard or soft corns, calluses, keratoses, suppurating sinuses, ulcers, or fibromatoses. Keloids and hypertrophic scars are usually secondary to the healing of lacerations, burns, or surgical wounds. Some intrinsic diseases of the skin are verrucae, dermatoses (especially tinea infections), epidermal cysts, and the rare diastasis of the fifth toe known as ainhum.

The various types of solitary lesions appearing on the plantar surface of the foot are (1) common diffuse calluses, (2) small, deep-seated, circumscribed nucleated calluses, (3) solitary or multiple verrucae plantares, (4) circumscribed fungating areas, (5) epidermal cysts, and (6) intractable plantar keratoses. These conditions are frequently misdiagnosed and are often treated as though they were verrucae plantares.

EXCRESCENCES CAUSED PRIMARILY BY FRICTION, PRESSURE, OR FAULTY WEIGHT BEARING

Corns and calluses are common disorders of this type. They are essentially localized keratoses caused by intermittent pressure from without and solid resistance from within; the outside pressure is produced by the shoe, which is resisted from within by the bones. Therefore one rarely sees corns or calluses over the shafts of long bones. They occur either on the condyles of the epiphyses of long bones or on the prominent projections of short bones.

A hard corn (heloma durum) will form primarily on the exposed surfaces of the toes. The fibular side of the fifth toe is by far the most common site of the hard corn; occasionally it will develop on the fibular side of the fifth metatarsal head. A soft corn (heloma molle) forms over a condyle of a phalanx between the toes. A callus (tyloma) may form over or under any bony prominence of the foot but commonly does so on the plantar surface of the foot and heel.

The terms *heloma* and *tyloma* are considerably misleading because they imply that the lesion is neoplastic, whereas the lesion may actually be a reactive proliferation of dead epithelium secondary to pressure. The findings of an extensive study of corns by Bonavilla (1968) support this hypothesis.

Corn (heloma, clavus)

A corn is an accumulation of horny layers of skin over a bony prominence.

Etiology. The outline of the bones of the

foot is irregular; the bones have numerous projections, especially over the condyles of the heads and bases of the metatarsals and phalanges. The shoe presses on these prominent condylar processes, and the soft tissues over the prominences bear the brunt of pressure and friction exerted on the foot by the shoe. Nature attempts to protect the irritated part by accumulating horny epithelium, but the accumulation so elevates the prominence that the shoe increases the pressure on the underlying live tissues. Excrescences and numerous other morbid changes are inevitable over such pressured areas.

That the prominences under excrescences represent proliferative changes in bone is an erroneous concept. Galland (1933) and McElvenny (1940) spoke of exostosis under corns. A study of 5,000 radiographs of such cases disclosed that only in rare instances are there cortical changes of bone in the condyle.

General treatment. Palliative measures such as reduction of the horny accumulation, changing the patient into a broad-toed soft-soled shoe, and padding the area to distribute the pressure give relief in most cases, especially if the site of the corn is a non—weight-bearing area. In many cases the patient can be taught to care for the callus himself by using a pumice stone after bathing. Excrescences on a weight-bearing surface call for orthopaedic appliances. (See Chapter 17.)

Intractable conditions over a non—weight-bearing area respond to excision of the condylar prominence immediately under the excrescence (Billing, 1956; Rutledge and Green, 1957). Excrescences on the weight-bearing areas usually occur under a metatarsal head and are caused by the deforming restriction of the shoe on the forepart of the foot, or they are associated with some degree of deformity or anomaly of the anatomic structures or alignment of the bones of the foot. They will be discussed later in this chapter.

Corn on lateral side of fifth toe. These are common, because the fifth toe receives the maximal pressure of the curve of the outer border of the forepart of standard shoes. Ordinarily the head of the proximal phalanx of the fifth toe is the most prominent surface at that point, which is why the corn is nearly always over the fibular condyle of the head of the proximal phalanx.

Operative treatment. The following procedure for condylectomy of the phalanges under a corn on the fibular side of the fifth toe usually involves the head of the proximal phalanx but may also involve condyles of the middle phalanx:

1. After a digital block with 1% procaine hydrochloride, make an incision over the dorsolateral aspect of the toe, medial to the corn, extending it from proximal to the nail to about the base of the proximal phalanx (Fig. 13-1, *A*). The corn itself should not be incised because the scar would be exposed to further friction; moreover, callus tissues are devitalized and therefore healing is poor.

2. Retract the lateral margin of the skin and subcutaneous tissue to expose the condylar projection covered by capsule and fascia.

3. Carry the line of the skin incision into the capsule; denude the bone over the lateral margin of the capsule and retract with the skin (Fig. 13-1, *B*).

4. Excise the condyle which has been exposed (Fig. 13-1, *C*).

5. Smooth the surface with a small rongeur.

6. Close the skin and capsule in one layer with mattress sutures (Fig. 13-1, *D*).

Postoperative pain is usually slight. Ordinarily healing is rapid, and walking can begin immediately with a shoe whose lateral aspect has been cut out. The toe need never be deformed by this operation.

In cases comprising the 2% incidence of recurrence, the head of the proximal phalanx may be amputated or the middle phalanx may be excised as an alternative procedure, depending on which structure lies under the corn. If the patient also has a soft corn in the forth web (usually caused by pressure of the head of the proximal phalanx), amputation of the head should be done initially. However, a flail toe deformity does occasionally result (Fig. 13-2), sometimes making syndactylization of the fourth and fifth toes necessary.

Excision of head of fifth proximal phalanx. The technique for excising the head of the fifth proximal phalanx is as follows:

1. Make an incision over the dorsum of the

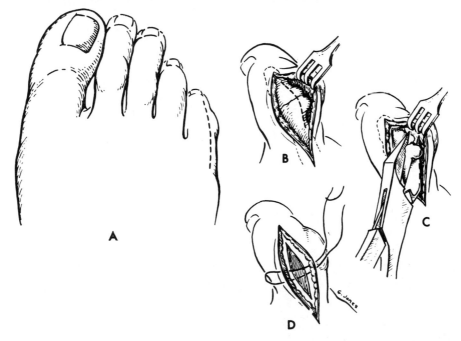

Fig. 13-1. DuVries' technique for condylectomy of a corn on the fifth toe. **A,** Longitudinal incision over the dorsolateral aspect of the fifth toe. **B,** Skin and capsule retracted. **C,** Fibular condyles of the phalanges amputated. **D,** Skin and capsule closed by mattress sutures.

fifth toe, extending from the distal interphalangeal joint to about the middle of the shaft of the proximal phalanx.

2. Retract the skin, continue the original incision through the capsule, and retract its margins together with the skin and the extensor tendon.

3. Cut the medial and lateral collateral ligaments of the proximal interphalangeal joint.

4. Flex the distal end of the toe to expose the head of the proximal phalanx. Excise it at its neck.

5. Close the skin and capsule with a single layer of sutures. Apply a compression dressing to occlude the dead space.

6. Remove the sutures on about the tenth day. The corn will usually lift off in about a month.

7. Keep the fifth toe taped to the fourth toe for 6 weeks to help minimize any floppiness of the toe.

Corn on dorsum of middle three toes and great toe. These corns are, for the most part, secondary to hammertoe (Chapter 20).

Soft corn in web between fourth and fifth toes. These are caused by long-continued compression of the skin between the head of the fifth proximal phalanx and the base of the fourth proximal phalanx (Fig. 13-3). Corns in this area are a common disability. A sinus leading into the metatarsal interspace may produce recurrent episodes of acute infection, which often complicate this lesion.

Treatment by condylectomy. Condylectomy of the tibial side of the head of the fifth proximal phalanx gives relief. The procedure is similar to that described for hard corn of the fifth toe, except the incision is made on the dorsomedial aspect of this toe. When a corn on the fibular side of the fifth toe is also present, excision of the head of the fifth proximal phalanx is the treatment of choice. Amputation of the condyle on the fibular side of the base of the fourth proximal phalanx also gives relief (Fig. 13-4). This more traumatic procedure is outlined here; it is only occasionally indicated.

1. Make an incision over the dorsolateral

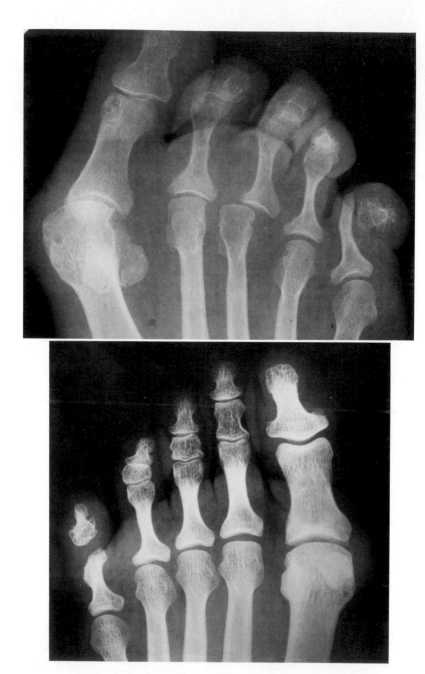

Fig. 13-2. Flail toes produced by phalangectomy.

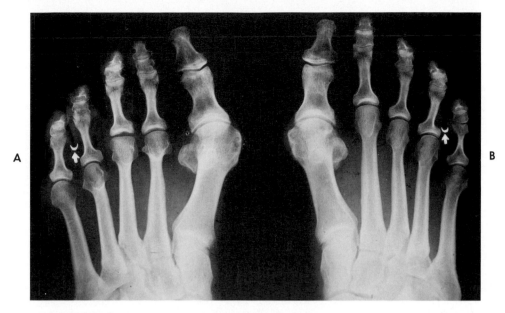

Fig. 13-3. A, No impingement. **B,** Head of the fifth proximal phalanx adjacent to the base of the fourth proximal phalanx impinging on the soft tissue in the fourth web and causing a soft corn.

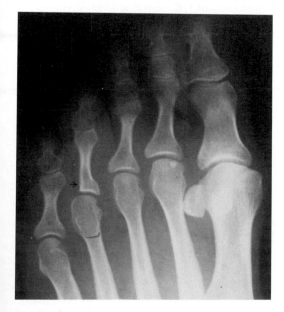

Fig. 13-4. Postoperative appearance of excision of the condyle at the base of the fourth proximal phalanx.

aspect of the fourth proximal phalanx, extending from the middle of the shaft of this phalanx to a point just proximal to the head of the fourth metatarsal (Fig. 13-5, *A*).

2. Open and retract the capsule of the metatarsophalangeal joint to expose the offending condyle for removal by a nasal saw (Fig. 13-5, *B*).

3. Close the skin and capsule by a single layer of sutures (Fig. 13-5, *C*).

Soft corn on lesser toes. A soft corn on the lesser toes may form over any condylar process of the phalanges. Condylectomy immediately under the excrescence by a procedure similar to that described for a corn of the fifth toe is effective.

Corn over tibial side of great toe. A large corn may develop over the tibial side of the interphalangeal joint of the great toe. It is often associated with a hallux valgus deformity and rotation of the great toe; the condyle is so rotated as to cause pressure against the skin in this area. It can, however, occur in people with normal feet, particularly those who participate in sports like tennis and squash.

In most cases self-care of the callus can be taught to the patient, and no other treatment

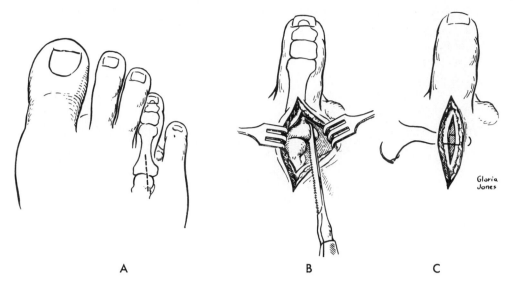

A   B   C

Fig. 13-5. Technique for excision of the base of the fourth proximal phalanx for a soft corn in the fourth web. **A,** Incision over the dorsolateral aspect of the fourth metatarsophalangeal joint. **B,** Skin and capsule retracted; fibular condyle of base of fourth proximal phalanx excised with a nasal saw. **C,** Skin and capsule closed with single layer of sutures.

is indicated. Occasionally the medial and plantar condyles of the base of the distal phalanx and head of the proximal phalanx must be excised in order to relieve the pressure by these bones against the skin. If there is a concomitant hallux valgus deformity with rotation of the great toe, unless the great toe deformity is corrected the callus will continue to recur.

Corn over base of fifth metatarsal. This corn is caused by an unusual prominence of the bone and is often associated with pes cavus, metatarsus adductus, or a residual of an old clubfoot deformity. In most cases correction is possible by the use of padding to shield the area and by wearing shoes that do not exert pressure over the area. When this corn occurs because of a major deformity of the foot, the deformity must be corrected to relieve the condition. Occasionally, when the condition is the result of an abnormally prominent bone as an entity by itself, reduction of this bony prominence is indicated.

Technique for reduction. The following steps accomplish reduction:

1. Make a linear incision over the dorsolateral aspect of the base of the fifth metatarsal, extending from the proximal third of the fifth metatarsal to the lateral aspect of the calcaneocuboid articulation.

2. Retract skin and incise down into the fascia.

3. Detach the fascia from the base of the fifth metatarsal, which includes a portion of the insertion of the peroneus brevis tendon.

4. With an osteotome, excise the lateral and occasionally the plantar prominence of the base of the fifth metatarsal.

5. Repair the tendon and fascia with fine chromic catgut, and close the skin in the usual manner.

6. Apply a compression bandage that may be released in 24 hours. The patient may bear weight in 48 hours, in a shoe that has been cut out over the area of operation.

Neurovascular corn. These are extremely painful lesions encountered most often on the ball of the foot. They may occur on the fifth toe but rarely on other parts of the foot. Often they are mistaken for a wart.

The neurovascular corn may be secondary to an old, deeply nucleated, corn under a metatarsal head or on the fifth toe. After paring and/or enucleating the corn (a considerably more painful procedure), one uncovers a glossy surface which contains fibers and small vessels. Occasionally a minute area appears at the periphery that under magnification seems to be loosened. When this area is even lightly touched with a sharp instrument, the patient experiences violent and excruciating pain. The condition is caused by an invagination of live epithelium with nerves and blood vessels along the border of the hard dead epithelium of a callus.

Treatment. Because a neurovascular corn is usually caused by prolonged trauma from shoe pressure, the live epithelium underneath it is relatively devitalized and as a result does not respond readily to therapy.

If a localized painful area at the periphery of the corn is found, stab it and permit it to bleed (which it will do profusely). The small vessels will then collapse. To destroy the neurovascular bundle of the peripheral portion, apply 95% phenol. Destruction of the major portion of the lesion may be accomplished by repeated applications of the escharotics commonly used for the eradication of small skin growths.

First and foremost, take care to avoid any additional friction and pressure over the area.

Callus (tyloma)

Calluses are large keratotic masses that form on the plantar surface of the foot and are histologically similar to corns. A certain amount of callus formation on the plantar aspect of the foot is normal, particularly in individuals who are active in various forms of athletics. In these people the callus formation is generalized, particularly in the forefoot area. When the callus formation is localized underneath a metatarsal head, the condition will often become symptomatic and require treatment.

The symptomatic usually well-localized callosity is referred to as an intractable plantar keratosis.

Etiology. The etiology of intractable plantar keratoses generally can be divided into three groups:

1. If the *overall structure* of the forefoot produces a *varus* or *valgus tilt*, excessive weight will be borne on one area of the forefoot and not another resulting in a keratotic lesion under the area bearing the maximum weight. The varus or valgus may also be produced by a residual paralysis of the foot secondary to old trauma or a neuromuscular imbalance.

2. *Osseous abnormalities* can lead to localized pressure and hence to plantar keratoses (Fig. 13-6). These include plantar flexion abnormalities such as plantar flexion of the first ray so the excessive pressure is carried on the first metatarsal head, a long metatarsal, or a plantar-flexed metatarsal (either due to an old fracture or on a congenital basis); or the abnormalities may be secondary to enlargement of a sesamoid bone.

3. *Faulty footwear* can also produce sufficient pressure on the toes to cause an intractable plantar keratotic lesion. The narrow pointed shoe with a high heel is usually incriminated in the etiology of a plantar keratosis (Fig. 13-7).

General treatment. The general treatment of intractable plantar keratoses consists of local treatment of the keratotic lesion by trimming and obtaining an adequate shoe, preferably one with a soft sole and adequate padding, to relieve the area of pressure. If after conservative treatment the keratotic lesion continues to be symptomatic, consideration should be given to surgical correction.

Intractable plantar keratosis under first metatarsal head. The most common type of keratotic lesion under the first metatarsal head is secondary to a lesion under the tibial sesamoid. In rare cases the fibular sesamoid is the offender, and this is usually secondary to abnormality of the fibular sesamoid (Fig. 13-8).

The tibial sesamoid normally assumes most of the weight-bearing function transmitted to the head of the first metatarsal. At times due to enlargement of the tibial sesamoid and at times due to a mild forefoot varus deformity or plantar flexion of the first ray, a localized keratotic lesion will occur underneath the tibial sesamoid. Occasionally, as a hallux valgus

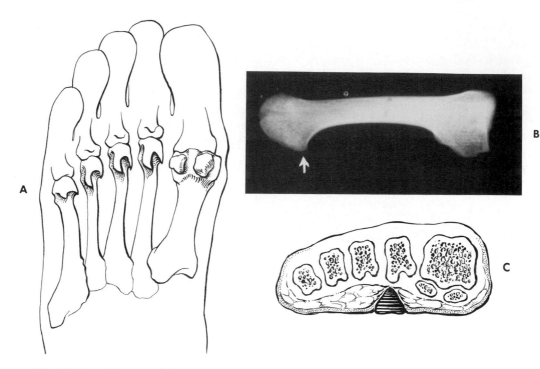

Fig. 13-6. **A,** Sharp condylar process of the three middle metatarsals (plantar aspect). **B,** One metatarsal. Note the sharp condylar process. **C,** Cross section of metatarsal heads; hyperkeratosis under the sharp condylar process of the second metatarsal head.

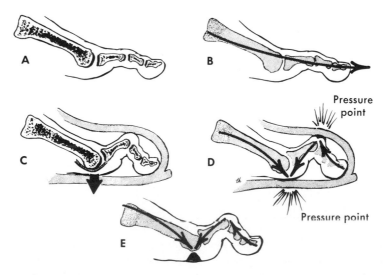

Fig. 13-7. **A** and **B,** Normal escape of force from body weight. **C,** Contraction of the intrinsic muscles as toes strike against the end of the shoe. (These muscles are inserted into the bases of the proximal and middle phalanges.) **D** and **E,** Counterforce on the plantar surface of the metatarsal heads with each step.

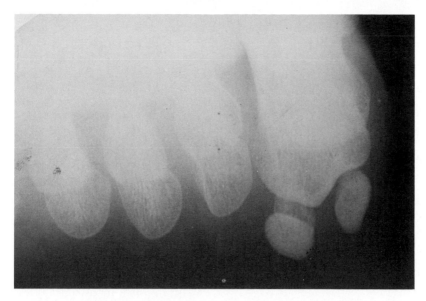

Fig. 13-8. Hyperkeratosis under the fibular sesamoid.

deformity develops and the first metatarsal head slips off the sesamoids, the tibial sesamoid becomes a weight-bearing focus and causes a keratotic lesion.

The keratotic lesion caused by the tibial sesamoid is a discrete localized keratotic lesion with a dense keratotic center. When this type of lesion is trimmed down with a scalpel, a punctate keratotic focus is identified. In the diagnosis, weight-bearing projections are most helpful as well as axial views of the sesamoids. If one measures the center of the keratotic lesion on the patient's foot, it should be centered underneath the involved sesamoid on the weight-bearing AP projection of the foot. If the lesion is not well localized under the tibial sesamoid, another diagnosis should be strongly considered.

Treatment. The treatment of an intractable plantar keratosis underneath the tibial sesamoid should be conservative. The proper regimen has just been outlined and is discussed again in Chapter 17. If, however, conservative treatment does not produce adequate symptomatic relief, surgical excision of the sesamoid must be considered. Only one sesamoid should ever be excised at a time or a cock-up deformity of the metatarsophalangeal joint will result.

Excision of tibial sesamoid. The technique for excising the tibial sesamoid is as follows:

1. Under hemostatis make a semielliptical incision along the contour of the medioplantar border of the metatarsophalangeal joint of the great toe. Extend the incision from the middle third of the metatarsal to the middle of the proximal phalanx (Fig. 13-9, *A*).

2. Carry the incision directly down to the capsule of the metatarsophalangeal joint and retract the plantar skin along with the medial plantar nerve plantarward.

3. Place the index finger against the plantar surface of the sesamoid while the great toe is dorsiflexed. This will outline the tibial sesamoid (Fig. 13-9, *B*).

4. Make a 1 cm incision just plantar to the abductor hallucis along the medial aspect of the sesamoid (Fig. 13-9, *C*).

5. Remove the sesamoid by sharp dissection, using its own outline as a guide (Fig. 13-9, *D*).

6. Close the capsule and fascia with interrupted chromic sutures and close the skin in the usual manner (Fig. 13-9, *E*).

7. Apply a compression bandage for 24 hours. The patient may begin walking in a wooden shoe the day after surgery.

Occasionally a large diffuse intractable

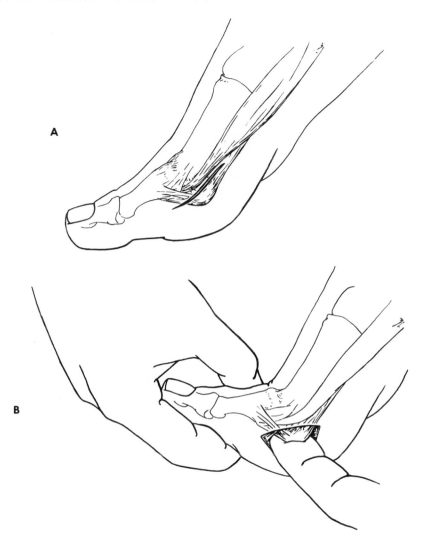

Fig. 13-9. Technique for excision of the tibial sesamoid. **A,** Semielliptical incision following the medioplantar border of the first metatarsophalangeal joint. **B,** Retraction of the skin margin and insertion of the surgeon's right index finger into the wound. When the great toe is dorsiflexed, the sesamoid glides over the index finger, pinpointing the sesamoid. **C,** Incision into the capsule along the mediosuperior surface of the sesamoid. **D,** Grasping the periosteum of the sesamoid with Allis forceps. The sesamoid is excised by sharp dissection. **E,** Closing the capsule and fascia with interrupted catgut sutures. Skin is closed in layers as usual.

plantar keratosis is seen under the first metatarsal head. In this condition the etiology is plantar flexion of the first metatarsal, as can be determined by observing the forefoot with the hindfoot in a neutral position and noting that the first metatarsal head is significantly depressed. Gentle pressure against the bottom of the foot will reveal increased resistance of the first metatarsal head. The conservative

treatment of adequate padding often is not successful in this problem.

The surgical treatment of choice is an osteotomy of the first metatarsal carried out at the metatarsal base to allow the first metatarsal to rise. The surgeon must be extremely cautious during this procedure so as not to overcorrect the first metatarsal and thus transfer pressure to the lesser metatarsals. I believe it better to

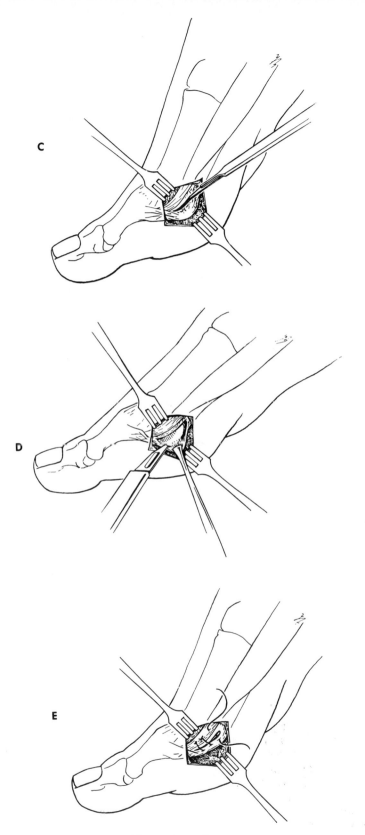

Fig. 13-9, cont'd. For legend see opposite page.

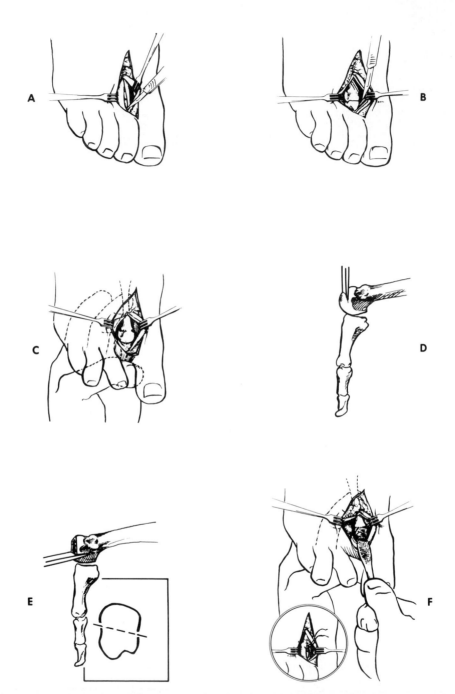

Fig. 13-10. Procedure for arthroplasty and plantar condylectomy for intractable keratosis under the lesser metatarsal heads. **A,** Hockey stick–shaped incision from the middle of the metatarsal shaft to the web; skin and extensor tendon retracted and capsule incised longitudinally. **B,** Capsule sectioned on both sides of the metatarsal head vertically. **C,** Involved toe plantar flexed with the thumb of the left hand while pressure is applied against the metatarsal shaft with the index finger. **D,** About 2 mm of articular surface removed. **E,** Plantar condyle removed with an osteotome. Note the angulation to facilitate removal of more of the fibular aspect. **F,** Surface smoothed with a nasal rasp; capsule and skin closed.

undercorrect slightly in this condition rather than take a chance at overcorrecting.

Intractable plantar keratoses under middle three metatarsal heads. Intractable plantar keratoses under the middle three metatarsal heads generally should be divided into two basic groups: those with a small discrete plantar keratosis and those with a large diffuse keratosis. This division is extremely important since the etiology is different and the correct diagnosis is imperative for proper treatment of the lesion.

The *small discrete* plantar keratotic lesion is caused by the sharp condylar process present under the metatarsal head. The condylar projection on the fibular side is always the larger of the two (Fig. 13-6). The condition becomes symptomatic for various reasons. The metatarsal may be slightly plantar flexed, which will cause the condyle to be pushed into the plantar skin and thereby produce a keratotic lesion; the condition may follow a metatarsal that has healed in a slightly plantar-flexed position; or the condition may be caused by a tight shoe. In the last condition the buckling of the toes would force the metatarsal heads into the plantar aspect of the foot, causing the keratotic lesion (Fig. 13-7).

Regardless of the etiology of the small punctate lesion, conservative treatment should be initially undertaken. The conservative treatment consists of trimming of the keratotic lesion and placing the patient in a proper soft-soled shoe with adequate padding to relieve the pressure on the keratotic area. The treatment of choice for this localized keratotic lesion is an arthroplasty as described by Du Vries (1953) and modified (1965) to include an arthroplasty. A long-term follow-up of the procedure has been reported by Mann and Du Vries (1973).

The technique for the arthroplasty is as follows:

1. Make a hockey stick–shaped incision, starting in the web space, and carry it down over the metatarsal head and distal third of the metatarsal shaft (Fig. 13-10, *A*).

2. Identify the transverse metatarsal ligament on the medial and lateral sides of the involved metatarsal head and cut the transverse metatarsal ligament.

3. Make an incision next to the extensor tendon through the dorsal capsule to expose the metatarsophalangeal joint.

4. Cut the collateral ligament and plantar flex the involved toe with the thumb of the left hand while applying pressure against the metatarsal shaft with the index finger of the same hand (Fig. 13-10, *B* and *C*).

5. Remove about 2 mm of the distal portion of the metatarsal head (Fig. 13-10, *D*).

6. Remove at least half the plantar condyle with an osteotome, angulating the osteotome slightly toward the fibular side (Fig. 13-10, *E*).

7. Round off the metatarsal head with a rasp, irrigate, and reduce the metatarsophalangeal joint. Close the skin in a routine manner (Fig. 13-10, *F*).

8. Apply a compression dressing for 24 hours postoperatively, following which the patient can walk in a supportive dressing and wooden shoe for a period of 3 weeks.

This type of arthroplasty will produce a satisfactory result 85% of the time. In approximately 5% of cases, the lesion will not be helped by the surgical procedure; and in about 10% a transfer lesion will result. Following an arthroplasty of the metatarsophalangeal joint of a lesser toe, roughly 25% of the motion of the metatarsophalangeal joint is lost; but I do not believe the loss is of any real clinical significance.

The *large diffuse* plantar keratosis, which is an intractable lesion, is caused by an elongated or plantar flexed metatarsal. It usually occurs under the second metatarsal but occasionally develops under the third and rarely under the fourth or fifth metatarsal. The plantar lesion is diffuse, generally measuring 1 to 1.5 cm across, and does not have a small keratotic core as is found in the lesion caused by prominence of the plantar metatarsal condyle.

If after adequate conservative treatment the lesion persists, surgical intervention is indicated. The procedure of choice is a metatarsal osteotomy as described by Giannestras (1954) (Figs. 13-11 and 13-12). I personally (R.A.M.) do not do the metatarsal osteotomy as described by Giannestras in his article but prefer to make a long oblique cut of the meta-

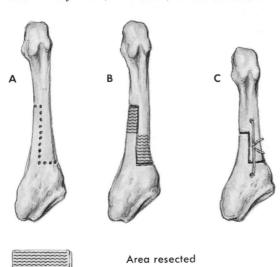

Fig. 13-11. Giannestras' step-down osteostomy. The metatarsal is shortened to alleviate plantar keratosis.

Area resected

Fig. 13-12. Foot of a 24-year-old woman. Severe hyperkeratosis had occurred under the second metatarsal head after the first metatarsal had been shortened by osteotomy for hallux valgus. The second metatarsal was forced to carry an abnormal part of the body weight. Giannestras' operation relieved the problem.

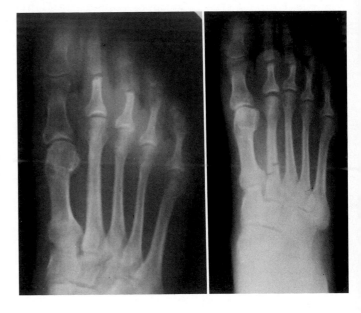

tarsal shaft. I then shorten the metatarsal enough to produce a smooth metatarsal arch. If the metatarsal is overshortened, a transfer lesion will result; it is therefore important to individualize the treatment and be able to shorten the metatarsal as close to the precise amount as technically possible. Postoperatively the patient is treated in a wooden shoe with the foot supported in a dressing for a period of 6 weeks.

In my experience the success rate for the Giannestras-type procedure in eliminating the callus under the involved metatarsal head is essentially 100%; but 5% to 10% of patients will develop a transfer lesion under an adjacent metatarsal head. This is probably due in part to the fact that it is unusual to have only one metatarsal which is too long; rather, not infrequently the second and third metatarsals are longer than the first, fourth, and fifth.

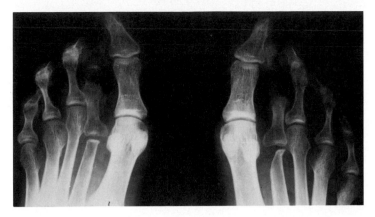

Fig. 13-13. Feet of a 42-year-old man who complained of disability from previous surgical procedures.

Thus, even though the second metatarsal may be shortened back to the level of the first metatarsal, the third metatarsal head can then become symptomatic.

There are other procedures described for treatment of intractable plantar keratoses which involve a proximal or distal osteotomy of the metatarsal shaft. Most of these are dorsal wedge osteotomies that allow the metatarsal to rise. The osteotomy at the base of the metatarsal, I believe, has a place in the treatment of intractable plantar keratoses although I personally do not use the procedure frequently. The osteotomy at the neck of the metatarsal to allow the metatarsal head to angulate dorsally causes, in my opinion, too much scarring and loss of motion about the metatarsophalangeal joint to be used in lieu of the previously mentioned more successful procedures.

I believe that in most cases only one metatarsal should be shortened at a single procedure although occasionally I have shortened two metatarsals on the same foot simultaneously. More than two metatarsals should never be shortened at a single procedure on the same foot.

There are other procedures reported in the literature for treatment of intractable plantar keratoses. I previously have mentioned the procedures I believe to be most successful. Excision of a metatarsal head for the treatment of an intractable plantar keratosis is mentioned just to condemn it. This procedure will only lead to more difficulty, secondary transfer lesions, and shortening of the involved toe (Figs. 13-13 to 13-16).

At times the intractable keratosis has been misdiagnosed as a verruca plantaris and the keratotic lesion has been treated by various modalities which produce severe dense scarring on the plantar aspect of the foot. When there is a severe dense scar on the plantar aspect of the foot under a metatarsal head, none of the aforementioned procedures is successful in relieving the keratotic lesion. In such cases consideration should be given to excising the lesion at the same time the metatarsal procedure is done. The skin margins are then sutured so they are not under any tension (Fig. 13-17). These patients treated with excision of the plantar skin should be kept non–weight bearing for a total of 6 weeks to allow the plantar skin to heal with minimal scar formation.

Suppurating sinuses of the foot

Suppurating sinuses of the foot are newly formed channels lined with granulation tissue. They discharge a serosanguineous material which may become purulent from secondary infection. The sinus may form in a corn or callus over a bony prominence. Such suppurating sinuses ordinarily are chronic, but acute exacerbations are typical.

Etiology. A suppurating sinus of the foot is

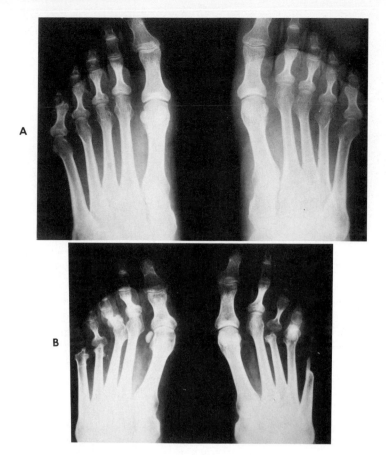

Fig. 13-14. Feet of a 28-year-old woman who had sought help for keratosis under the metatarsal heads. **A,** Preoperative; **B,** postoperative.

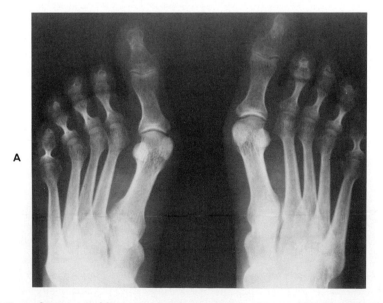

Fig. 13-15. Feet of a 51-year-old woman who had sought my advice in 1961 for calluses under the metatarsal heads caused by moderate clawtoes. She then sought help for severe disability after surgical procedures performed elsewhere in 1963. **A,** Preoperative, 1961; **B,** postoperative, 1964.

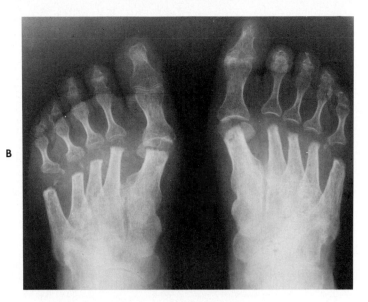

B

Fig. 13-15. cont'd. For legend see opposite page.

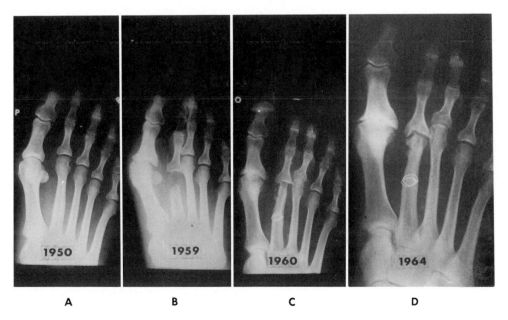

A   B   C   D

Fig. 13-16. Intractable keratosis under the right second metatarsal head in a 30-year-old woman. A, Preoperative, 1950. B, Postoperative, 1959. A surgical procedure had been performed elsewhere eight years previously. She now sought help because of disability, especially because the second toe was lying on the dorsum of the foot. Note that the first metatarsophalangeal joint had also been surgically treated. A fibular graft on the second metatarsal remnant was implanted, and the first metatarsophalangeal joint was repaired. C, One year postoperative. D, Four years postoperative.

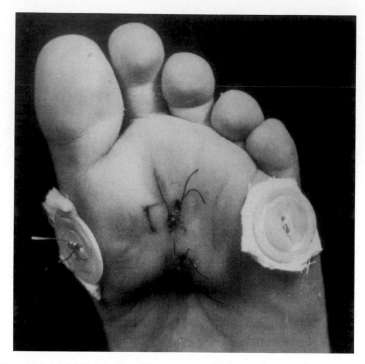

Fig. 13-17. Coaptation of skin margins after excision of a plantar lesion. The margins are held by a retention wire suture deep below the incision.

produced in the same way as are corns and calluses—by persistent sharp pressure over a bony prominence that devitalizes the tissue under the excrescence and, in some cases, causes necrosis of the central portion. The presence of a debilitating disease worsens the degenerative process.

Lusskin (1961) reported a case of serpentine sinus of the foot which led to a dead end; the disorder proved to be a congenital dermal defect.

Site. Suppurating sinuses of the foot occur in the following areas: under a hard corn on the lesser toes; in the center of a soft corn, generally in the web between the fourth and fifth toes; and on the tibial side of the great toe joint, usually over the tibial condyle of the first metatarsal head and occasionally associated with a hallux valgus deformity, especially if there is a sharp projection on the tibial side of the head. On the fibular side of the fifth metatarsal head, it is often associated with a tailor's bunion.

A degenerative sinus may occur under any of the metatarsal heads, especially the middle three. In the young and middle-aged they are often secondary to unusually large condylar processes on the plantar surface of the head of the metatarsals. When they are situated under the first metatarsal, they are usually caused by an uncommonly large or malshaped sesamoid. Clawtoe or clawfoot may produce such a sinus under a metatarsal head. In older persons, this type of sinus is often associated with a degenerative disease, such as diabetes. Trophic changes as a result of peripheral nerve disease also produce this kind of sinus, typically under the head of the first metatarsal, and usually retrogress to produce extensive ulceration. Under the head of the second metatarsal a degenerative sinus often results from the static dislocation of the second metatarsophalangeal joint.

Treatment. When the sinus is present over a non–weight-bearing area and is not complicated by a debilitating disease, excision of the

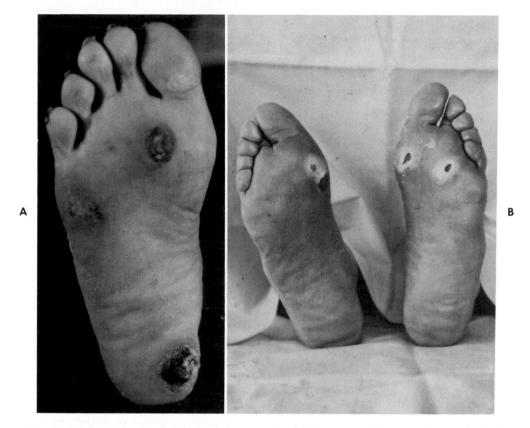

Fig. 13-18. A, Traumatic ulcers under the second and fifth metatarsal heads and under the heel. **B,** Traumatic (pressure) ulcers. Right foot, First metatarsal head. Left foot, First and third metatarsal heads.

condyle or bony prominence beneath the sinus, without excision of the necrotic tissue, disposes of the problem in most cases. Excision to eliminate the sinus itself may or may not be required.

On the plantar surface, in cases such as hammertoe or metatarsophalangeal dislocation in which debilitating disease is not a complication, healing usually takes place after open reduction of the deformity underlying the sinus or excision of the offending plantar condyle or sesamoid is performed.

Patients in whom there is an underlying debilitating disease should be treated conservatively to achieve balanced weight distribution through such mechanical measures as shoe inlays, metatarsal bars, shoe wedging, and padding. Total weight bearing should be reduced as much as possible. Close coopera-

tion with the internist to improve the general medical status is important. The sinus itself must be kept clean. Rough handling or the application of chemical irritants is likely to worsen the degenerative process. Only the most conservative surgical procedure is ever indicated, and then only in extreme cases.

Traumatic ulcer

Traumatic ulcers are usually caused by excessive pressure on a weight-bearing area over a long period of time. Degeneration of the skin surface and the underlying soft structures leads to ulceration. Traumatic ulcers most commonly occur under the metatarsal heads, but they may appear over any bony prominence (Figs. 13-18 and 13-19). They are often seen in older persons, because in these people the general tissue vitality is reduced

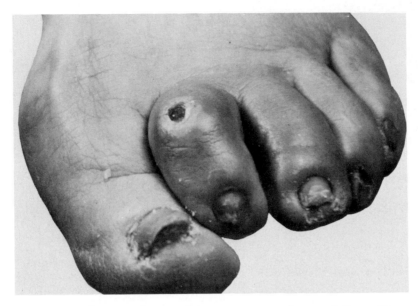

Fig. 13-19. Traumatic ulcer over the second toe. Acute tinea infection of all toes. (Courtesy Dr. Ned Pickett.)

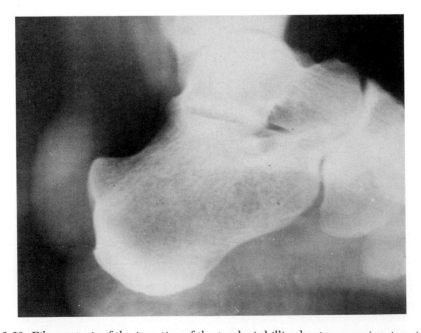

Fig. 13-20. Fibromatosis of the insertion of the tendo Achillis; due to a prominent posterosuperior tuberosity of the calcaneus.

and the irritation has been long standing. General disease, such as diabetes and peripheral neuritis, can accelerate the process.

Such ulcers are characterized by large amounts of granulation tissue surrounding a small orifice that exudes a nonpurulent discharge; they are subject to recurrent secondary infection that may become intractable.

To treat these ulcers:

1. Excise all the surrounding overlying callus.

2. Cauterize the granulation tissue with 90% phenol or 10% silver nitrate.

3. Paint the ulcer with a dye such as carbolfuchsin or gentian violet.

4. Protect the area from further pressure by the use of padding or a foot appliance.

Hypertrophy of the skin and soft tissues over the tendo Achillis

Hypertrophy of the skin and soft tissues over the tendo Achillis is an accumulation of connective tissue immediately above the tendon's insertion. The condition, often referred to as tendo Achillis bursitis, develops in persons in whom the upper posterior border of the calcaneus juts out acutely posteriorly. This enlargement is sometimes referred to as Haglund's disease (p. 285). A calcaneus thus shaped makes the contour of the back of the heel a straight line (Fig. 13-20). The shoe counter is always convex; therefore, its upper margin exerts an abnormal amount of friction and pressure on the prominence. The condition is more common in women as a result of wearing pumps and high heels. The growth is solid connective tissue in which a cavity appears only if the tissue breaks down, producing a draining sinus. Occasionally an adventitious bursa forms.

The growth may be excised through an incision on either side of the tendon. Great care must be taken in dissection since the mass is not encapsulated and the skin may be irreparably injured. The skin should be sutured subdermally to prevent dead space and consequent hematoma formation. A walking plaster cast should be applied with the foot in mild plantar flexion to avoid movement of the wounded area, which might interfere with healing. It should be borne in mind that this area is notoriously poor in healing. A window in the cast over the field of operation permits redressing. The cast is removed in about 3 weeks. Dorsiflexion is begun gradually.

REFERENCES

Billig, H. E., Jr.: Condylectomy for metatarsalgia: indications and results, J. Int. Coll. Surgeons 25:220, 1956.

Bonavilla, E. J.: Histopathology of the heloma durum: some significant features and their implications, J. Am. Podiatry Assoc. 58:423, 1968.

DuVries, H. L.: New approach to the treatment of intractable verruca plantaris (plantar wart), J.A.M.A. 152:1202, 1953.

DuVries, H. L.: Surgery of the foot, ed. 2, St. Louis, 1965, The C. V. Mosby Co.

Galland, W. I.: An operative treatment for corns, J.A.M.A. 100:880, 1933.

Giannestras, N. J.: Shortening of the metatarsal shaft for the correction of plantar keratosis, Clin. Orthop. 4:225, 1954.

Lusskin, R.: Serpentine sinus— a tract leading nowhere, J. Bone Joint Surg. 43A:118, 1961.

McElvenny, R. T.: Corns: their etiology and treatment, Am. J. Surg. 50:761, 1940.

Mann, R. A., and DuVries, H. L.: Intractable plantar keratosis, Orthop. Clin. North Am. 41:67, 1973.

Rutledge, B. A., and Green, A. L.: Surgical treatment of plantar corns, U. S. Armed Services Med. J. 8:219, 1957.

14

AFFECTIONS OF THE FOOT

James O. Johnston

TUMOROUS CONDITIONS OF THE SOFT TISSUES AND BONES OF THE FOOT

In this discussion of tumor and tumorlike conditions occurring in the foot and ankle area, it should first be stated that malignant tumors of the foot (and incidentally of the hand) are rare conditions and that soft tissue tumors are more common. Therefore, when one is uncertain whether a lesion is benign or malignant, it is better to assume the benign condition and treat accordingly rather than perform an unnecessary amputation for a pseudomalignant condition.

Generally most of the neoplastic conditions occurring in the foot are seen more typically in other parts of the body and are not specific problems of the foot. There is, however, an important difference in clinical prognostication of like tumors located in different parts of the body. For example, when one considers cartilaginous tumors in the pelvis or proximal large bones of the extremity, one must be extremely cautious because of the known potential of these tumors for malignancy and tendency to metastasize. By contrast, the same type of cartilaginous tumor located in the foot is almost always benign. This has a direct bearing on treatment: cartilaginous tumors in the proximal part of the body should be aggressively resected whereas smaller lesions in the hand or foot can usually be handled by conservative resection. The giant cell tumor is another good example of a tumor with variable prognosis depending on its location. Surgical treatment for the giant cell tumor can therefore also vary.

Benign tumors of the soft tissues

Fibroma. Fibromas are benign soft tissue lesions seen in all parts of the body, in soft tissue as well as in bone. They are well-localized lesions in most cases with well-defined borders. Fibromas are frequently subcutaneous in location and firm to palpation. They grow very slowly and are usually asymptomatic and nontender to palpation.

Fig. 14-1 shows a typical, firm, and well-circumscribed subcutaneous fibroma resected from the tarsal sinus area of the foot. The lesion can be cut like a piece of hard rubber, and the exposed surfaces are white with the gross appearance of a cut Achilles tendon.

Microscopically this tumor is composed of well-differentiated fibroblasts producing large amounts of dense collagen fiber that contributes to its physical characteristics.

A fibroma can be easily resected, and there is very little chance of local recurrence.

Fig. 14-2 shows a patient with surfer's knobs. These fibromatous lesions are found on the dorsum of the foot as the result of repeated physical trauma to this area (e.g., many hours spent on a surfboard).

Keloid. Keloid is the clinical name given to

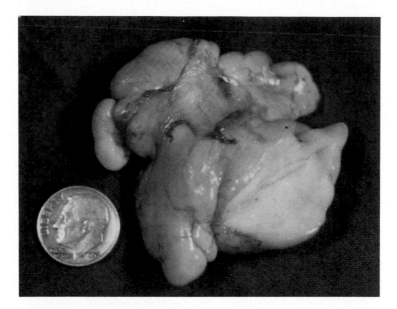

Fig. 14-1. Well-circumscribed firm subcutaneous fibroma removed from the foot.

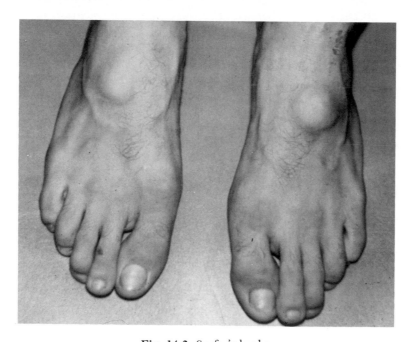

Fig. 14-2. Surfer's knobs.

dense hypertrophic dermal fibrous tissue that forms in excess as a response to skin lacerations or surgical incisions. Keloids are familial and are firmly fixed in the genetic makeup of fibroblasts all through the body. It is difficult therefore to avoid keloid formation in certain patients when making surgical wounds for reconstructive purposes.

To reduce the chance of a disfiguring or disabling scar, one should at least be aware of this potential before performing surgery. It is well known that dark-skinned people are generally more prone to keloid formation whereas light-skinned races or individuals with hyperelastic skin rarely form keloids but instead tend to form flat scars which spread.

The best treatment for keloid formation is prevention if possible. For this reason it is best to make surgical incisions parallel with skin creases or skin lines (in the extremities, a transverse incision). It is also wise to use good subcutaneous closures and avoid surface stitches completely. Skin tapes left in place for several weeks and splinting of wounds near joints are helpful. The use of gamma irradiation or steroids to inhibit fibrosis is considered controversial and is probably best left in the hands of a plastic surgeon who has experience with these modalities.

Fig. 14-69 is a classic picture of a keloid scar formed as the result of a longitudinal incision made along the heel cord and across the ankle joint (p. 461).

Plantar fibromatosis (Keller and Baez-Giangreco, 1975). Plantar fibromatosis is a locally aggressive idiopathic proliferative fasciitis of the plantar aponeurosis that is usually bilateral and frequently seen in children and young adults. In older people it is often associated with Dupuytren's contracture of the palmar fascia of the hand. The basic microscopic pathology of Dupuytren's and plantar fibromas is about the same. However, in children the microscopic picture is much more worrisome and can be misdiagnosed as a malignant fibrosarcoma. Fig. 14-3 shows the typical nodularity of this fibroma in the long plantar ligament.

If the nodules are small and cause little trouble, they can be left alone. If they grow large and cause pain or pressure on an adjacent nerve, however, it is best to perform aggressive resection. Pedersen and Day (1954) advised a longitudinal incision along the medial plantar aspect of the first metatarsal proximally to the tarsal navicular. Skin flaps are developed to expose the fibroma and plantar fascia. The fibrotic lesion is aggressively excised, with removal of much of the normal-appearing adjacent plantar fascia. It is important to perform aggressive resection

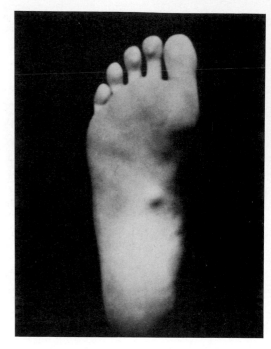

Fig. 14-3. Fibromatosis of plantar fascia in an adolescent.

because of the high incidence of local recurrence when only the fibroma is removed. The skin flaps are then tacked down to prevent hematoma, and Hemovac brand suction tubes are placed beneath the skin as well. A firm compression dressing is also helpful in preventing hematoma formation.

Neurilemoma. The neurilemoma is a benign neurogenic tumor of nerve sheath origin that is well encapsulated, usually solitary, and found on the surface of a peripheral nerve. Fig. 14-4 shows a typical lesion resected from the surface of the medial plantar nerve. This tumor is easy to resect and rarely causes damage to its nerve of origin because of its eccentric location. It rarely recurs or becomes malignant.

Neurofibroma. The most common neurogenic tumor is the neurofibroma. This tumor can be solitary (Fig. 14-5) or multicentric and quite diffusely invasive, as in the plexiform type seen in the dysplastic condition known as von Recklinghausen's disease (neurofibromatosis) with associated tan-pigmented café-au-

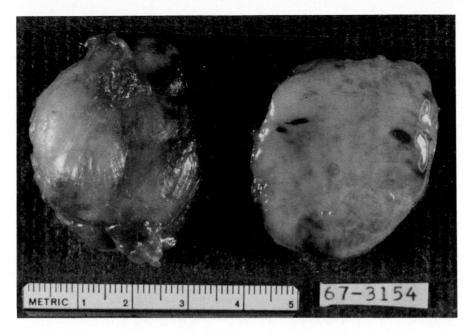

Fig. 14-4. Neurilemoma shelled off the surface of the medial plantar nerve.

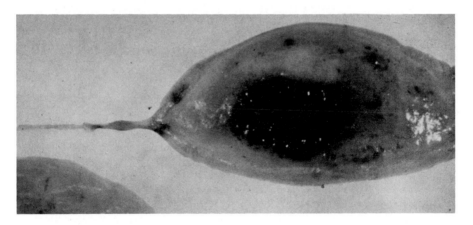

Fig. 14-5. Localized neurofibroma of a small peripheral nerve.

lait spots on the skin. The neurofibroma is more disabling because of its central location in a peripheral nerve. As a result it interferes with nerve function and, if resected, the entire nerve is frequently removed with the tumor. The neurofibroma, by contrast with the neurilemoma, is more prone to become malignant. This usually occurs in larger more proximal nerves, however, and not in the hand or foot.

In *neurofibromatosis* many peripheral nerves are involved. Associated with the dyplastic condition, severe deformity of the subadjacent bones of the feet is not unusual (Fig. 14-6). One may also find extensive soft tissue hypertrophy and localized gigantism in neurofibromatosis.

Lipoma. In the extremities the subcutaneous lipoma is a common tumor. It can also be found in muscle bellies and, on rare occa-

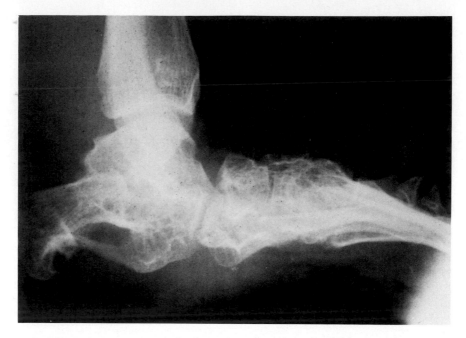

Fig. 14-6. Associated bone defect seen in a foot affected with neurofibromatosis.

sion, in medullary bone. In the foot, however, lipomas usually are located just beneath the skin. These are soft nontender lesions that are asymptomatic. They are usually well encapsulated and easy to excise surgically, with very little chance for local recurrence or malignant transformation.

Ganglion (Soren, 1966). Another common tumorous condition of the extremities is the ganglion cyst. This lesion should not really be considered a tumor, mainly because it is not the product of proliferating cells. In fact, the ganglion is the product of mucoid cystic degeneration in the area of a dense collagen structure such as a joint capsule or thick collagenous tendon sheath. Ganglions are usually located in an area where such structures are under continuous physical stress, for example, around the wrist and ankle joints. With repeated activity across these areas, the collagen tissue undergoes mucoid degeneration with the formation of amorphous gelatinous material. If its point of origin is near the skin surface, as is usual around the ankle and dorsal aspect of the foot, the gelatinous material may form a firm subcutaneous nodule. In the case of a ganglion arising from a joint

capsule, the cyst can rupture into the joint space and thus be converted to a synovial cyst filled with synovial fluid instead of gelatinous material.

Many small ganglions may appear spontaneously and grow gradually for a time and then rupture internally into subcutaneous tissues and be absorbed, without many symptoms or disability to the patient. If the cyst becomes unsightly or causes pains because of pressure against a shoe, the treating physician may elect to aspirate it and thus solve the immediate problem. However, there is a 70% chance of local recurrence with this conservative approach. If one wishes a more definitive cure, a surgical excision is required. Then the surgeon must remove the entire cyst wall. Perhaps even more important, to prevent local recurrence, the surgeon must excise most of the surrounding degenerative capsular or tendon sheath collagen tissue which frequently contains small microscopic foci for potential additional lesions.

At times one will see a patient with multiple ganglion-like lesions involving multiple tendon sheaths across the dorsum of the ankle. In this case the diagnosis of a rheumatoid process

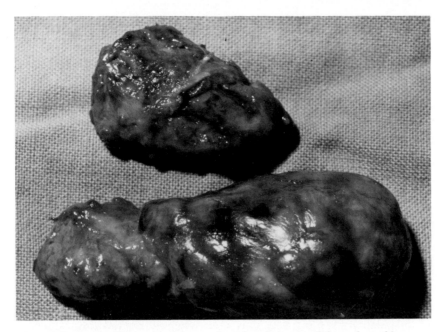

Fig. 14-7. Giant cell tumor of the tendon sheath removed from the ankle area.

should be strongly suspected and the appropriate studies begun to confirm the impression.

Giant cell tumor of tendon sheath (Eisenstein, 1968). Along with the ganglion cyst and lipoma, the so-called giant cell tumor of tendon sheath is a common tumor found subcutaneously in the hand and foot. It has been named because of its common relations to tendon sheaths and tenosynovial tissues but can also be located in subcutaneous areas far removed from a synovial membrane. In this case it should probably be assigned a different name such as "benign fibrous histiocytoma."

These lesions are well circumscribed and relatively easy to resect (Jones et al., 1969). They are considered by most surgeons to be a benign neoplastic process composed histologically of giant cells, reticulum cells, and cholesterol-laden histiocytes (foam cells) dispersed throughout a fairly dense fibrotic stroma. In the early stages these lesions take on a reddish brown coloration because of the large amount of hemosiderin found in the tissue. At this time they are usually growing in size and may be painful. As time passes, they

tend to involute spontaneously and become more xanthomatous and fibrotic which accounts for another pathologic name frequently assigned these lesions (xanthofibroma).

The giant cell tumor of tendon sheath can assume a considerable size around the ankle area and usually originates from a major tendon sheath, such as the one seen in Fig. 14-7 which measured 3 inches in length. This ankle lesion demonstrates the well-circumscribed and nodular appearance of the tumors, which may recur locally after resection but rarely if ever become malignant.

Pigmented villonodular synovitis. The same basic pathologic condition just described can also occur in subsynovial tissues of joints and then the histology is identical to that of the giant cell tumor of tendon sheath. This condition usually occurs in the knee joint or the major joint of the lower extremity in young men as a monoarticular form of hemorrhagic synovitis. The joint synovium has a characteristic brown discoloration and is thickened with a coarse villonodular pattern. The treatment for the benign process is to perform as complete a synovectomy as possible. Recurrences are not unusual, and occasionally low-dosage radiotherapy will be called for to combat multiple recurrences.

Sometimes these synovial lesions, and tenosynovial lesions as well, will invade adjacent bony structures (Fig. 14-8)

Vascular tumor (McNeill and Ray, 1974). The most common vascular tumor seen in the extremity is the port-wine capillary type of hemangioma. These are hamartomatous dysplastic lesions of a benign nature and rarely have serious clinical consequences. They can result in localized erosive ulcerations that occasionally require surgical excision.

More extensive lesions located subcutaneously or in muscle tissue may infiltrate diffusely over large areas. The characteristic radiographic appearance of these larger cavernous lesions is visible evidence of many small spherical calcific phleboliths (Fig. 14-9). This is a diffuse dysplastic condition similar to neurofibromatosis insofar as it can cause subadjacent bony deformity and even disappearance of the bone (disappearing bone disease). Also, as seen in neurofibromatosis, there may be associated localized gigantism of adjacent bone and soft tissue (Fig. 14-10),

e.g., enlargement and deformity of the second and third toes. Treatment for these larger lesions is surgical, and whether one resects locally or amputates for severe local mechanical disability will depend on the extensiveness of the tumor. These lesions never become malignant.

Glomus tumor (Smyth, 1971). Another benign vascular tumor found in the hand or foot is a very small but frequently very painful one, the glomus tumor. The glomus tumor is usually located in a subungual location in the hand or foot but may also arise in subcutaneous locations, such as the one seen in Fig. 14-11 in the web space between the toes. These tumors are usually bright red and assume the size of a small pea. Simple surgical excision brings on a dramatic relief of symptoms.

Ectopic ossification. Areas of soft tissue calcification or ossification in the hand or foot are usually the result of ischemia of tissues, secondary to either an old injury with scar formation or a generalized disease process associated with vasculitis such as scleroderma or Raynaud's disease.

Fig. 14-12 shows an example of heterotopic

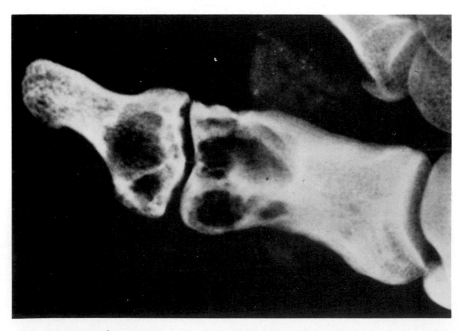

Fig. 14-8. Juxta-articular erosion in the interphalangeal joint of the great toe secondary to pigmented villonodular synovitis.

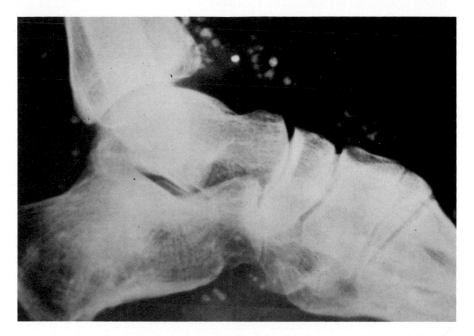

Fig. 14-9. Extensive hemangiomatosis of the foot with diagnostic calcific phleboliths.

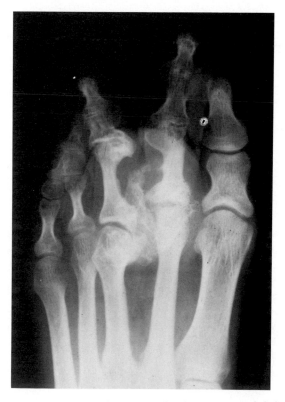

Fig. 14-10. Hemangioma of the foot with associated enlargement and deformity of the second and third toes.

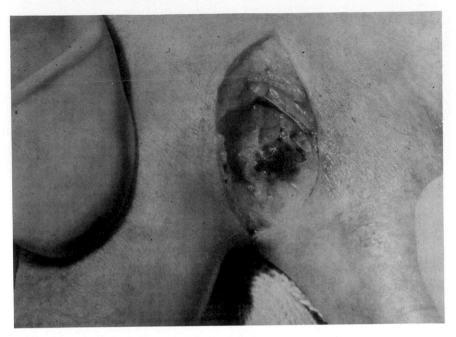

Fig. 14-11. Glomus tumor in a subcutaneous location in the dorsal web space between the toes.

bone formation in the heel cord as the very late sequelae of an old heel cord rupture. This resulted in fibrosis and ischemia which progressed to calcification. Then with gradual vascular ingrowth, bone was formed in the dense traumatized scar tissue.

Malignant tumors of the soft tissues

Fibrosarcoma (Simon and Enneking, 1976). The soft tissue fibrosarcoma is an extremely rare tumor of the hand or foot. One should always consider a benign diagnosis for this tumor. If it does occur, it will do so in older individuals. The lesion may be slow growing with a fairly well-differentiated fibroblast as the tumor cell that forms a fair amount of collagen fiber. In this case the tumor might be resected by a radical *en-bloc* resection without amputation. However, if the tumor is quite anaplastic, with poorly differentiated fibroblasts and minimal collagen formation, amputation is usually best.

Synovial cell sarcoma. The synovial cell sarcoma is also a rare tumor of the foot. It is most commonly seen about the knee area in young adults. Stening (1968) pointed out the

frequency of its occurrence about the ankle and tarsal area. Fig. 14-13 is a radiograph of the ankle area of a 10-year-old girl with a synovial cell sarcoma. These tumors grow slowly at first and may initially be confused with a benign process such as the ganglion cyst or lipoma. They are firm on palpation and may present with mild symptoms of pain. The cell of origin is the synovioblast, which produces proteoglycan (hyaluronic acid).

The synovial cell sarcoma rarely occurs inside a joint cavity. It may calcify as do fibrosarcomas. The most characteristic feature of the lesion, which is almost necessary to make the microscopic diagnosis, is the presence of a pseudoglandular epithelium that gives the tumor the appearance of an adenocarcinoma. However, there is no basement membrane beneath this pseudoepithelium as there would be in the true adenocarcinoma. The tumor is bimorphic (i.e., composed of fibroblastic cells as well). Both cell populations are felt to be of synovioblastic origin.

This tumor carries about the same prognosis as a malignant fibrosarcoma, with a 25% chance of five-year survival (Cameron and

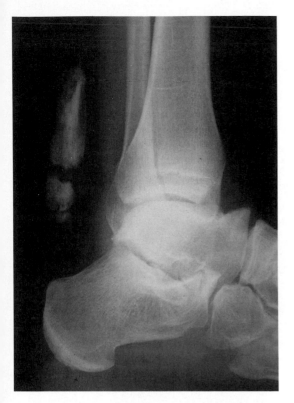

Fig. 14-12. Heterotopic bone formation of the heel cord as a late result of trauma.

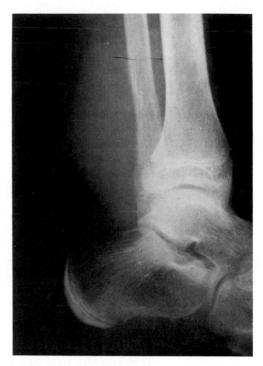

Fig. 14-13. Synovial cell sarcoma in the heel cord area of a 10-year-old girl.

Kostuik, 1974). The treatment of choice is amputation. Lymph-node metastasis often occurs, which demands careful examination of the inguinal area prior to surgery.

Kaposi's sarcoma (angiosarcoma). The angiosarcoma of Kaposi deserves attention because of its predilection for the skin of the hands and feet, particularly of the great toe (Lewis, 1967). This tumor initially appears as multiple painful red or purple subcutaneous nodules that measure up to 1 cm in diameter (Fig. 14-14). The lesions may be telangiectatic or verrucous. The tumor enlarges slowly and may cause lymphatic obstruction and edema. Because of the slow growth of this tumor, wide resection with grafting and radiotherapy successfully arrests it.

Malignant melanoma. The malignant melanoma is an adult skin tumor that frequently occurs in the lower extremity, especially on the plantar surface of the foot. Nearly 50% of

these lesions arise out of benign junctional nevi (Ackerman, 1968). The junctional nevus is usually flat, tan, and nonhairy. Signs to alert the surgeon to a malignant transformation from junctional nevus to malignant melanoma include enlargement, deepening pigmentation, ulceration, and halo pigmentation in the skin around the nevus. Less than 1% of junctional nevi on the sole of the foot become malignant, which does not justify routine prophylactic removal of all junctional nevi in this location. An ulcerating neoplasm on the plantar surface of the foot, however, is almost certain to be a truly malignant melanoma, even if not pigmented.

The *subungual melanoma* (seen in Fig. 14-15) is another localized clinical entity that usually requires early amputation of the toe. A blue nevus, which is very dark and flat and can easily be confused with the melanoma, is, in fact, usually benign and rarely metastasizes.

Treatment of malignant melanomas of the foot other than the toe just mentioned usually

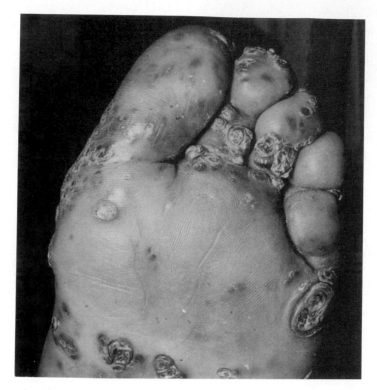

Fig. 14-14. Kaposi's sarcoma of the foot. (Courtesy Dr. Marcus Caro.)

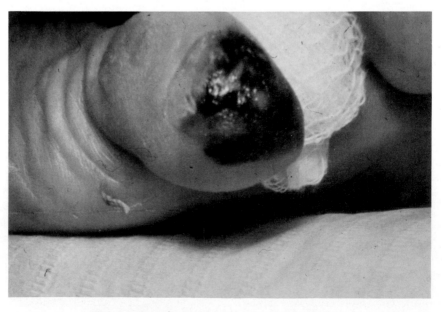

Fig. 14-15. Subungual melanoma of the fifth toe.

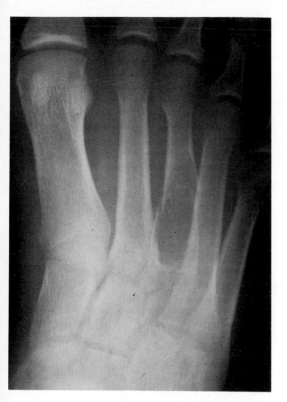

Fig. 14-16. Pathologic fracture through a solitary bone cyst at the base of the third metatarsal.

consists of widely excising the entire lesion and surrounding skin with a cold knife (noncautery). In some cases removal of the inguinal lymph nodes and even the deeper iliac nodes is advised. With this proper therapy the five-year survival rate is 30%. Radiation treatment is of no value, however.

Benign tumors and cysts of bone

Solitary bone cyst (Smith and Smith, 1974). This simple or unicameral bone cyst is a common defect found typically in growing bone on the diaphyseal side of the growth plate. It is a cystic lesion, usually filled with serous liquid and lined by a thin membrane containing fibrous tissue and giant cells. It may be asymptomatic until the acute episode of a painful pathologic fracture such as seen in the third metatarsal in Fig. 14-16.

A common location for the simple cyst is the larger tarsal bones such as the os calcis or talus. An example of a talar lesion in a 10-year-old child is seen in Fig. 14-17, *A*; appropriate curettage was performed, with bone grafting. The postoperative radiographic appearance is seen in Fig. 14-17, *B*. The younger the patient

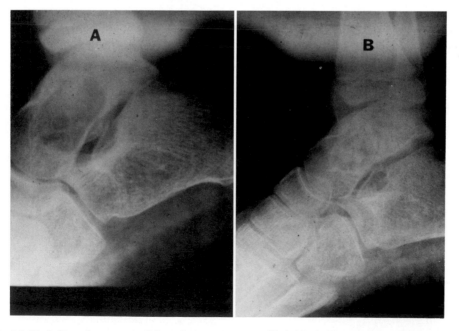

Fig. 14-17. Solitary bone cyst of the talus in a 10-year-old child. **A,** Preoperative. **B,** Postoperative, following a successful bone grafting procedure.

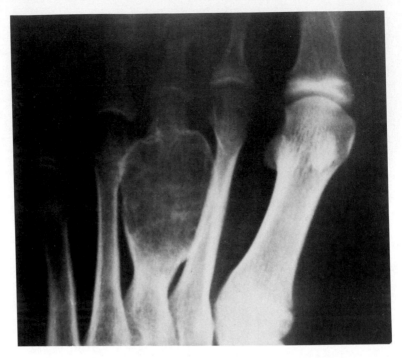

Fig. 14-18. Aneurysmal bone cyst of the third metatarsal.

at the time of grafting, the more likelihood there is that the cyst will recur. For this reason, if possible, it is best to wait till the age of 13 or 14 years before performing a definitive graft.

Epidermoid cyst. The epidermoid cyst is seen typically in the distal phalanx of the finger or toe, beneath the nail bed. It presents as a bulbous enlargement of the tip of the digit; on radiographs a geographic cystic lesion in the subungual area of the terminal phalanx is seen. The cyst will transilluminate and is filled with serous fluid, like the solitary cyst, but its lining is made up of nail-bed matrix and contains keratin. The cyst is usually the product of an old crushing injury to the tip of the toe which drives nail matrix down into the phalanx, where it continues to grow in an ectopic location to form a keratin-lined cyst. The treatment is simple curettement and grafting.

Aneurysmal bone cyst. A benign cystic lesion of bone which may occur in the foot is the hemorrhagic or aneurysmal bone cyst. It is a lesion seen in growing metaphyseal bone of children and is characterized by its dilated

and thin-shelled appearance on radiographs (as viewed in the third metatarsal, Fig. 14-18). This lesion is in a quiescent stage compared with the cyst seen in Fig. 14-19, in which there are very advanced hyperemic destructive changes in the talonavicular area that might suggest a malignant process or infectious disease.

At time of biopsy, the cyst was filled mainly by unclotted blood and lined by a mossy friable layer of reddish brown material. Microscopically the cyst was loaded with large giant cells that might suggest the diagnosis of a giant cell tumor. The giant cell tumor can also be aneurysmal in nature and fairly hemorrhagic. However, it is a more solid, fleshy tumor of bone, with more malignant potential. In the case of a foot lesion, the prognosis is very good following a simple curettement and bone grafting, the same treatment used for a simple bone cyst.

Osteochondroma. The osteochondroma is a common benign tumor located in the metaphyseal area of long bones in children. It may be solitary or multiple and probably results when small peripheral portions of the growth plate

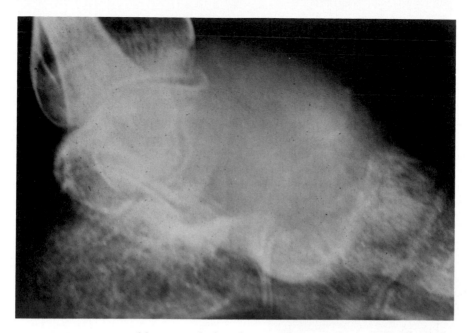

Fig. 14-19. Aneurysmal bone cyst before the typical reactive bony shell is formed.

separate from the main plate and continue as separate localized growth centers on the surface of the metaphyseal cortex. Osteochondromas do not usually occur in the hand or foot. Fig. 14-20 shows a typical sessile osteochondroma in the distal tibia, where it has interfered with the normal development of the adjacent fibula. Treatment consists of simple resection at the base of the bony stock, making sure to remove the entire cartilaginous cap, which on rare occasion can slowly develop into a secondary chondrosarcoma.

Bone spur. The bone spur is a reactive lesion that commonly occurs in the foot. It is usually secondary to repeated irritation of the foot bone at the point of attachment of a ligament or joint capsule. The spurs forming from the tuberosity of the os calcis are typical examples of reactive bone spurs and should not be confused with the osteochondroma, which has a cartilaginous cap and is never present at the tip of a spur.

Subungual exostosis. A special type of reactive bone spur is the type found beneath the

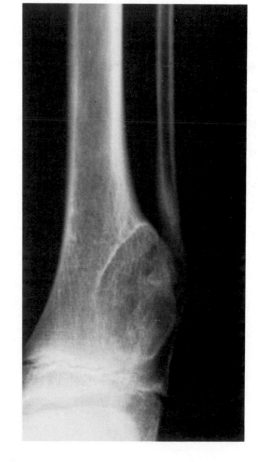

Fig. 14-20. Sessile osteochondroma of the distal tibia.

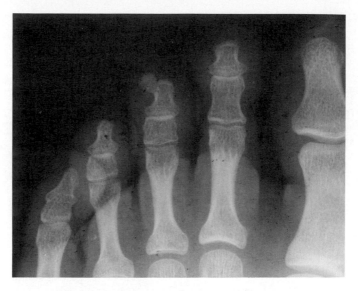

Fig. 14-21. Exostosis of the third distal phalanx.

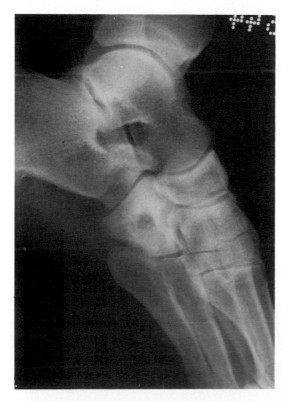

Fig. 14-22. Typical appearance of an osteoid osteoma of the cuboid.

nail of a toe such as the one seen in Fig. 14-21 on the tip of the third toe. The great toe is the most common site for this lesion, which on rare occasion will present with a cartilaginous cap and, in fact, represents a very small osteochondroma. The pearly mass growing through the nail may be misdiagnosed as a malignant tumor. All these benign lesions can be easily resected. However, in the case of a reactive spur, one might anticipate a recurrence unless the source of irritation were removed.

Osteoid osteoma. The osteoid osteoma is a small but painful neoplasm of the bone that occurs in children and is frequently observed in the lower extremities. The metaphyses of the long bones are the most frequent location; however, the tarsal bones of the foot are not unusual locations for this benign osteoid-forming lesion. The radiograph (Fig. 14-22) of a typical lesion in the cuboid area shows dense osteoblastic reaction surrounding the small osteolytic nidus that takes on the appearance of an inflammatory granuloma such as a Brodie abscess.

Osteoid osteomas will spontaneously resolve over a period of several years as the nidus is gradually replaced by dense reactive

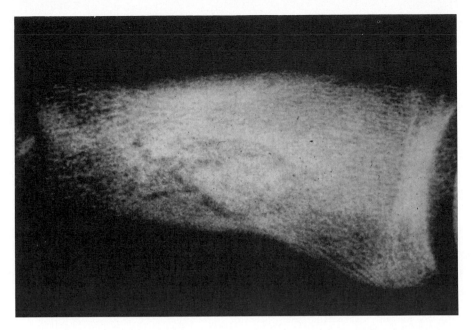

Fig. 14-23. Dense osteoid osteoma in the proximal phalanx of the great toe.

bone similar to that seen in Fig. 14-23, where there remains only a thin shell of inflammatory tissue around a centrally dense osteoma. When the lytic portion is completely filled in, the pain will stop. If pain necessitates an early operation, the critical portion of the lesion to remove is the hyperemic and painful nidus. The surrounding dense bone may be left intact. Local recurrence is almost nonexistent.

Osteoblastoma (Giannestras and Diamond, 1958; Cowie, 1966). The large form of the osteoid osteoma is the osteoblastoma, also called the "giant osteoid osteoma." It is found in the same locations as the osteoid osteoma, including the tarsal bones. Its central nidus must be larger than 1 cm, and it is a great deal more hemorrhagic in nature. The radiograph (Fig. 14-24) is of a typical lesion of the talar neck which required a second curettement after a recurrence from previous surgery.

Enchondroma. A common benign tumor of bone in the hand or foot is the well-known enchondroma. This dysplastic, hamartomatous, cartilaginous lesion—like the simple bone cyst—is asymptomatic unless a pathologic fracture occurs through it. Fig. 14-25

shows the typical radiograph appearance of an enchondroma with geographic punched-out appearance, a sharp reactive edge, and characteristic flocculated calcification in its central area. These lesions may be treated by simple curettement and bone grafting. Only on rare occasion do they turn malignant.

Dysplastic cartilaginous lesions can also occur on the surface of a bone, in which case it is referred to as a juxtacortical chondroma; this lesion gives the radiograph appearance of a blister on the surface of the cortex.

Even more unusual is the occurrence of a dysplastic cartilaginous lesion in the lining of a joint or tendon sheath. Fig. 14-26 presents an example of a benign tumor of cartilage arising from the anterior capsule of the ankle joint. In this case the lesion is referred to as a juxtaarticular chondroma and treatment is by simple surgical excision.

Chondroblastoma. The chondroblastoma is a benign giant cell lesion found typically in the epiphyseal areas of long bones in children. Fig. 14-27 shows the radiographic appearance of a lesion located in the distal fibular epiphysis of a 12-year-old boy. Notice the characteristic flocculated calcification in the lytic le-

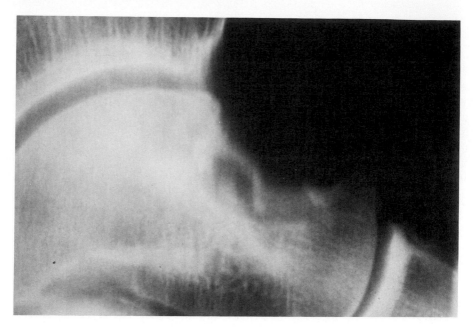

Fig. 14-24. Osteoblastoma in the neck of the talus of a 30-year-old woman.

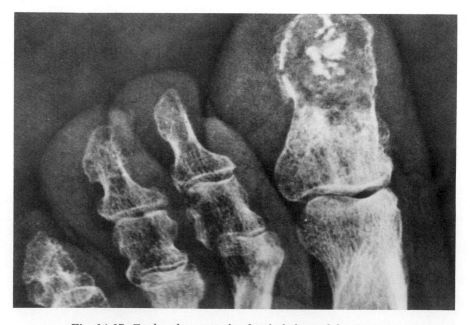

Fig. 14-25. Enchondroma in the distal phalanx of the great toe.

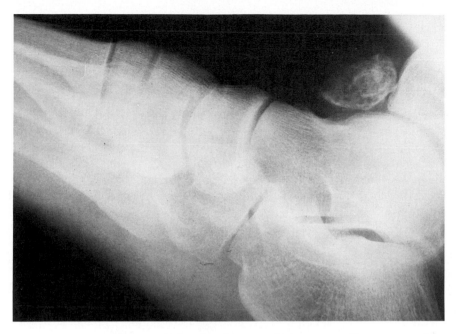

Fig. 14-26. Typical juxta-articular chondroma in the anterior ankle joint capsule.

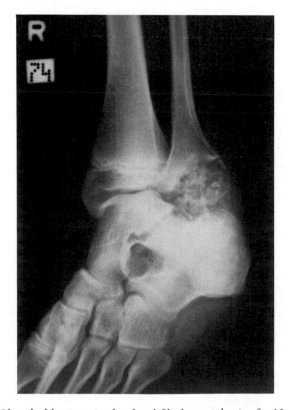

Fig. 14-27. Chondroblastoma in the distal fibular epiphysis of a 12-year-old boy.

sion, which suggests chondroid elements. This tumor is sometimes referred to as an epiphyseal giant cell tumor of adolescence. However, its prognosis is much better than for the adult giant cell tumor. Treatment consists of simple curettement and possible grafting. The os calcis and talus are targets for this tumor in the foot.

Fibroma of bone. Dysplastic fibroma of bone is a common condition of the skeletal system and can be found in all parts of the body, including the foot. These fibromas have a similar radiographic appearance to the solitary cyst and may in fact have a similar pathologic origin. Fig. 14-28 is a radiograph of a typical fibroma of bone seen in the os calcis. Notice the sharp geographic appearance, which suggests a benign condition. These lesions are usually asymptomatic until the time of a possible pathologic fracture. They are frequently seen in children and young adults in metaphyseal bone. If treatment is necessary because of recurrent fracture or threat of fracture, it consists of simple curettement and grafting.

At times a patient is found to have multiple bony involvement with fibromas of bone in the feet; this condition is referred to as *polyostotic fibrous dysplasia* (Fig. 14-29). There is chronic dilatation of the first and fourth metatarsal shafts. The condition tends to amplify on one side of the body more than on the other, with a resultant leg length discrepancy due to bowing of the femur.

Another benign variation of fibrous defects in bone is the so-called *chondromyxoid fibroma* (Fig. 14-30). This tumor has about the same radiographic appearance as the nonossifying fibroma and can be treated the same way, i.e., with simple curettement and possible grafting. The distinguishing histologic characteristic of this rare lesion is the presence of myxoid and chondroid tissue.

Sarcoidosis. Sarcoidosis is a generalized systemic granulomatous disease of unknown etiology that acts in many ways like a low-grade lymphoma. It involves structures of the lymphoid system (including bone marrow), especially in blacks. Bones most typically involved are located in the hands and feet. Fig. 14-31 is a typical radiograph of a sarcoid foot with granulomatous changes in the distal first metatarsal that might suggest gout. However, the smaller more centrally located

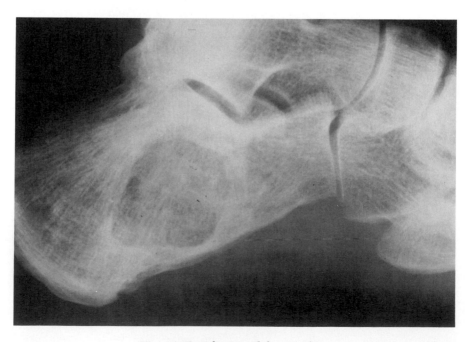

Fig. 14-28. Fibroma of the os calcis.

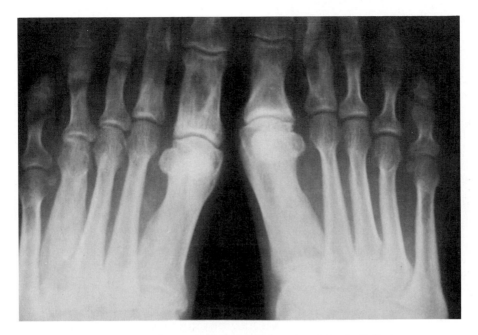

Fig. 14-29. Polyostotic fibrous dysplasia involving both feet.

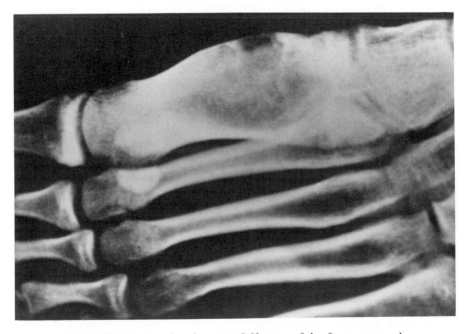

Fig. 14-30. Benign chondromyxoid fibroma of the first metatarsal.

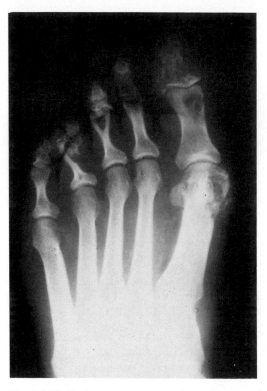

Fig. 14-31. Lytic-appearing granulomas in sarcoidosis of the foot.

lesions in the phalanges suggest sarcoidosis. These patients present with subcutaneous nodularities overlying the bony changes that could suggest a rheumatoid process.

Melorheostosis. Melorheostosis is an idiopathic condition seen typically in the bones of the lower extremities. It is usually picked up as an incidental finding from a radiograph obtained for some other reason. Fig. 14-32 provides an example of this abnormality of enchondral ossification involving the tibia, talus, and first ray to the tip of the great toe. The flowing appearance on the radiograph accounts for the name given this condition, which can sometimes occur across joints and result in stiffening.

Tarsoepiphyseal aclasis. This condition is a rare and localized epiphyseal dysplasia of a hypertrophic nature seen usually in bones about the ankle of one leg only. Its characteristic deformed enlargement of the talus is well demonstrated in Fig. 14-33, where it might suggest other conditions such as fibrous dysplasia or neurofibromatosis. The talus is the most common place to find this defect; but it can occur in a growing child on the medial side of the knee, with enlargement of the medial

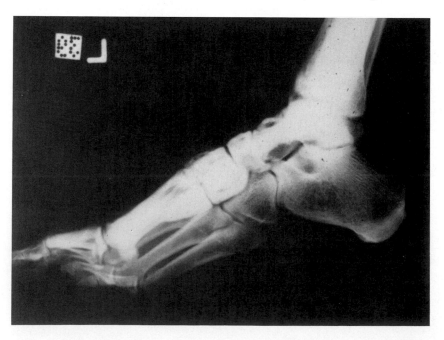

Fig. 14-32. Melorheostosis; flowing hyperostosis down the inner aspect of the foot and ankle.

femoral condyle. Early recognition should lead to early surgical treatment.

Stippled epiphyses. Conradi's disease (chondrodysplasia punctata) is a rare form of congenital dwarfism presenting at birth with the clinical manifestations of achondroplastic dwarfism. However, on radiographic examination, the diagnostic features of stippled epiphyses appear (Fig. 14-34). There is extensive calcific stippling around the major epiphyseal ossification centers of the tarsal areas of the foot. This is a dystrophic form of calcifica-

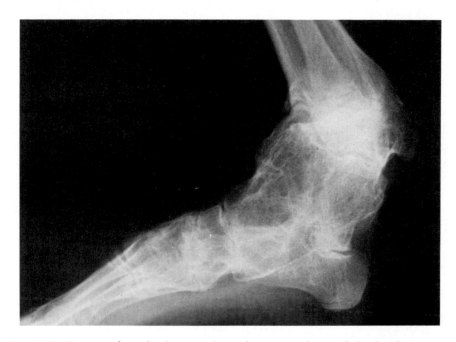

Fig. 14-33. Tarsoepiphyseal aclasis involving the entire talus, with localized gigantism.

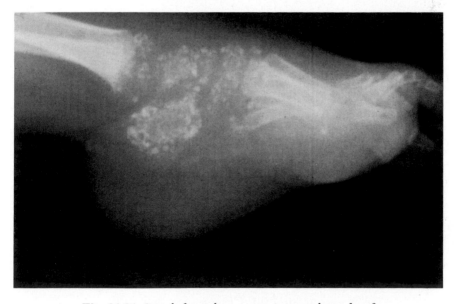

Fig. 14-34. Stippled epiphyses seen in a newborn dwarf.

tion in the germinal cartilage which gradually disappears with time and growth. In many cases the dwarfism clears up, and the older child may enjoy a fairly normal physical appearance.

Bone islands. Bone islands are common findings on bone radiographs. These represent small well-circumscribed areas of increased bone density secondary to a failure of proper remodeling of bone in the metaphyseal areas of the growing skeleton. If multiple lesions are seen (Fig. 14-35), the condition is referred to as osteopoikilosis; it is usually observed in radiographs of the asymptomatic hands and feet. Lesions located more proximally may suggest the possibility of osteoblastic metastatic disease. An isotopic bone scan can help clear this differential diagnostic point in most cases.

Malignant tumors of bone

Malignant tumors of the hand or foot are unusual; and when they do occur, they tend to behave less aggressively than the same tumor in a more proximal portion of the extremity in larger bones. For this reason, when the pathologist is uncertain as to the exact nature of a lesion of the hand or foot at biopsy, it is frequently good judgment on the part of the clinician to assume a benign diagnosis and elect conservative local resection. The general statement can also be made that malignant tumors of the hand and foot will tend to metastasize rather late in the course of the disease.

Osteosarcoma. The osteogenic sarcoma is a highly malignant tumor, usually seen in the metaphyseal areas of fast-growing bones in children such as the tibia or femur. Most of these are seen in boys and are common about the knee joint. Bones of the feet are involved in less than 1% of all cases, which makes this diagnosis rare. Fig. 14-36 shows one of these rare cases of an osteosarcoma in the first metatarsal of a young man. The combination of lytic destruction of the subadjacent cortex and exuberant and chaotic production of neoplastic osteoid around the entire shaft of the metatarsal points strongly toward a malignant diagnosis of a bone-forming sarcoma.

At the present time the best method of treatment is amputation. Since about 1972, however, adjunctive chemotherapy has greatly improved the prognosis. The drugs

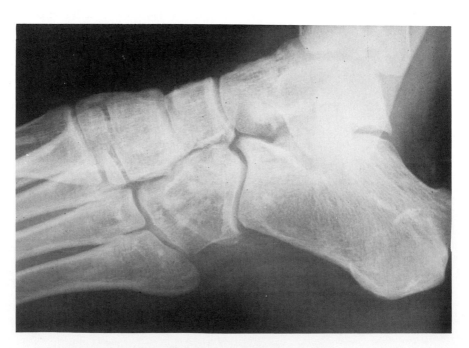

Fig. 14-35. Osteopoikilosis or multiple bone islands in the foot.

used most commonly include high-dosage methotrexate with citrovorum factor rescue and adriamycin in combination with other chemotherapeutics such as vincristine. Jaffe and Watts (1976) have been able to report a 60% cure rate for this tumor through the use of chemotherapy after amputation.

Pulmonary metastasis from this tumor was at one time considered a fatal condition, and nothing further was done for the patient. However, Spanos et al. (1976) have presented encouraging results with resection of metastatic lesions. They report a 28% five-year survival without recurrence. The new chemotherapy programs may well improve this figure.

It should be mentioned that radiotherapy has been dropped as a therapeutic modality for this tumor. Immunotherapy may hold some promise for the future.

Because the osteosarcoma is such a rare lesion in the foot, it might be wise to include a few pseudotumors that masquerade as malignant lesions. Fig. 14-37 is a radiograph of such a pseudotumor in the third metatarsal of a 19-year-old track runner which demonstrates the typical callus formation seen in a stress fracture. These lesions frequently show no fracture line across the involved bone, and the patient may give no definite history of any single injury to the foot. Biopsy generally shows aggressive osteoid production that might suggest to the pathologist a malignant diagnosis. Such a mistaken diagnosis could then tragically lead to treatment by amputation for a benign process.

Another example of a pseudotumor is seen in Fig. 14-38 in a young patient with factor VIII–type hemophilia. This occurs in the form of a highly lytic and aneurysmal lesion of the os calcis which could easily pass for an aggressive sarcoma of some type.

Ewing's sarcoma. Ewing's sarcoma is also a childhood tumor seen more typically in long

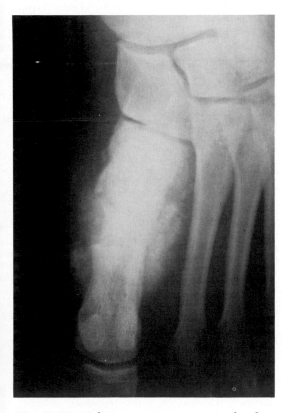

Fig. 14-36. Malignant osteosarcoma in the first metatarsal of a young man.

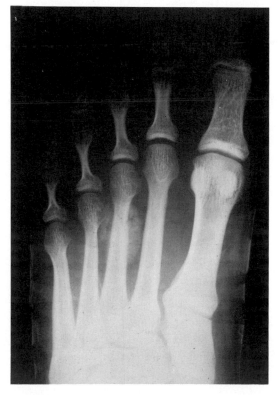

Fig. 14-37. Stress fracture in the third metatarsal, presenting as a pseudotumor.

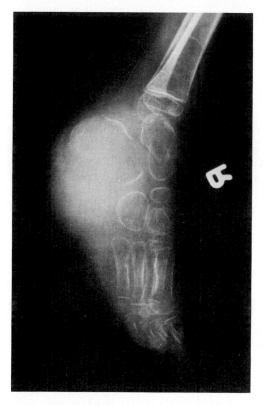

Fig. 14-38. Pseudotumor of hemophilia in the os calcis of a young boy.

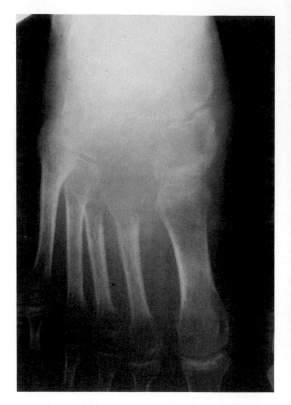

Fig. 14-39. Ewing's sarcoma in the midtarsal area of a young man.

bones of the lower extremities or in the pelvis. However, according to Pritchard et al. (1975) at the Mayo Clinic, about 5% are located in the foot area. It carries the worst prognosis for survival of any of the primary sarcomas of bone. It probably is a very primitive mesenchymal tumor of the round cell variety, similar to the reticulum cell tumor seen in adults.

Fig. 14-39 shows the typical radiographic appearance of Ewing's sarcoma seen in the midtarsal area of a young man. This lesion is purely lytic in nature, and its high degree of bony permeation suggests an infectious process such as tuberculosis. It is also quite necrotic and, when cut into, may drain a liquid necrotic material that suggests purulence to the operating surgeon.

Fig. 14-40 illustrates another Ewing sarcoma in the area of the first cuneiform bone of a 35-year-old man that displays extensive lytic

destructive changes which might also suggest an infectious process. This patient was treated by amputation.

In the past, the traditional therapy for Ewing's sarcoma has been irradiation therapy with 5,000 to 6,500 rads to the entire bone. There is a current trend away from this, however, because of the advent of the newer chemotherapeutic programs which have increased the short-term prognosis for survival up to 60% (Lewis et al., 1977).

At the Mayo Clinic, Pritchard et al. (1975) have reported a 45% five-year survival following amputation, compared with a 13% survival after irradiation therapy alone. They therefore are suggesting amputation with adjunctive chemotherapy for extremity lesions. Lewis et al. (1977) also advise amputation for extremity lesions, especially those of the foot and ankle.

Chondrosarcoma. Like the osteosarcoma,

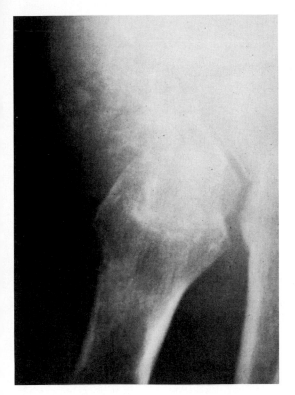

Fig. 14-40. Ewing's sarcoma of the first cuneiform.

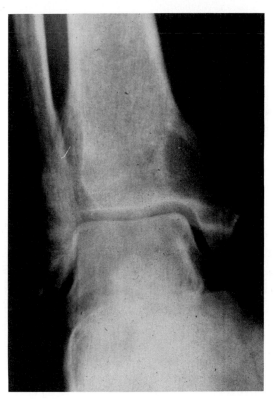

Fig. 14-41. Chondrosarcoma in the medial malleolus of a middle-aged man.

chondrosarcoma is rare in the foot. About 1% of all cases are seen in the foot or tarsal area and usually occur as primary lesions in middle-aged adults. The usual site for this tumor is the pelvis. The tumor is slow growing and late to metastasize to the lung. Fig. 14-41 is a radiographic film of a chondrosarcoma seen in the medial malleolus of a 50-year-old man. Unlike the benign cartilage tumors, the malignant chondrosarcoma usually presents with symptoms of pain. In the large study of these tumors of the foot by Dahlin and Salvador (1974), it was shown that local curettement is not beneficial. Treatment is by excision of the entire bone involved with the tumor. This gives very little chance of recurrence or metastasis.

Giant cell tumors (Goldenberg et al., 1970). Giant cell tumors are low-grade malignant lesions that are rarely seen in the hand or foot. If discovered in the foot, this tumor may,

in fact, be an aneurysmal bone cyst (which has a similar clinical appearance). Fig. 14-42 shows a giant cell tumor in the os calcis with typical lytic appearance and fairly aggressive permeative edge suggesting malignancy. Fig. 14-43 presents a more benign-appearing giant cell tumor of the fifth metatarsal in a 16-year-old boy; this tumor has the slightly aneurysmal appearance typical of giant cell tumors. Most experts agree that giant cell lesions in the hand or foot carry a much better prognosis than do giant cell tumors of long bones. For this reason the accepted treatment for the first occurrence is usually local curettement and bone grafting, if needed. Radiotherapy is contraindicated due to possible transformation into an irradiation sarcoma.

Fibrosarcoma (Larsson et al., 1976). The fibrosarcoma as a primary bone tumor of the foot is extremely rare. Fig. 14-44 is an example of the fibrosarcoma seen in the fifth meta-

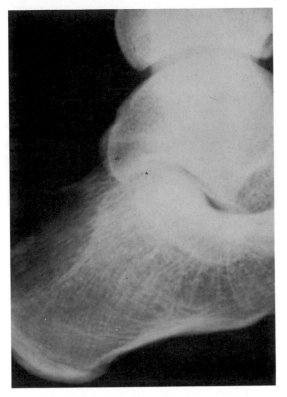

Fig. 14-42. Giant cell tumor of the os calcis.

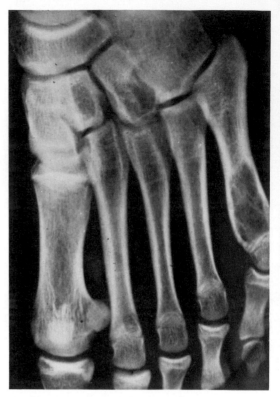

Fig. 14-43. Giant cell tumor of the fifth metatarsal.

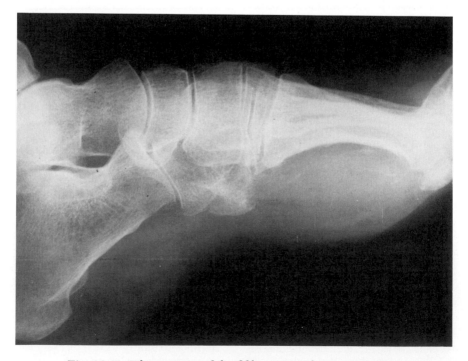

Fig. 14-44. Fibrosarcoma of the fifth metatarsal in a young man.

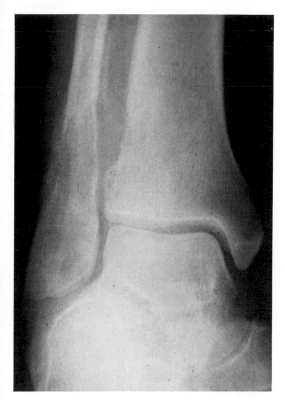

Fig. 14-45. Metastatic lung carcinoma to the lateral malleolus.

tarsal of a young adult male. This tumor occurs in about the same locations as the osteosarcoma, and the recommended treatment is amputation of the entire foot. Adjunctive chemotherapy could be considered for grade 3 to 4 lesions.

Metastatic tumors to foot. It is generally unusual to find a metastatic carcinoma in the bones of the hand or foot, or even distal to the elbow or knee. Of the metastatic group in this rare location, the bronchogenic carcinoma of the lung is perhaps the most common. Fig. 14-45 is a radiograph of a metastatic carcinoma of the lung to the lateral malleolus with lytic destructive changes as well as periosteal lifting that might well suggest a primary sarcoma such as the Ewing tumor seen more typically in this location. Another example of a metastatic lesion in the foot is seen in Fig. 14-46, where a carcinoma of the colon has metastasized to the second toe, with a pathologic fracture through the proximal phalanx. Conservative treatment for these lesions must be considered, with local resection followed by irradiation of the part to prevent local recurrence.

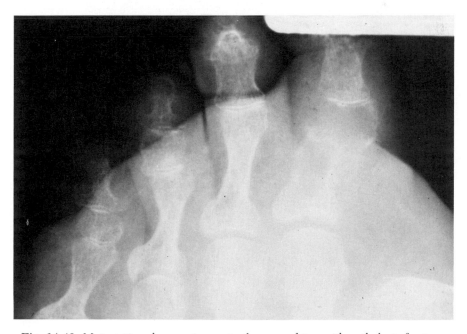

Fig. 14-46. Metastatic colon carcinoma to the second toe with pathologic fracture.

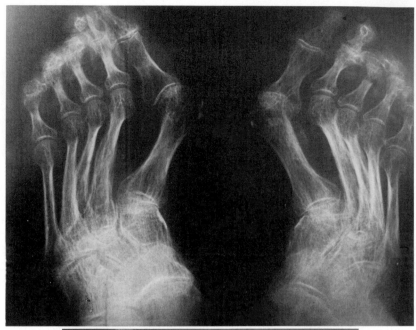

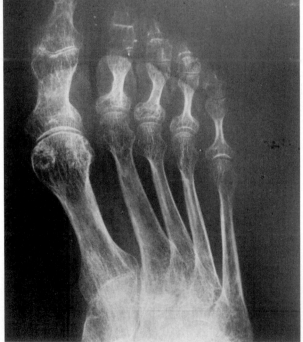

Fig. 14-47. Extensive osteoporosis; generalized decalcification.

METABOLIC BONE DISEASE

Just as an internist looks at the chest radiograph for evidence of generalized disease process, a physician who deals with hand or foot problems should become familiar with generalized radiographic changes in the structure of bone. Much can be learned about the general metabolic state of the entire patient based on the various changes that take place in bone for one reason or another. In this section I will introduce some of the major categories of metabolic bone disease and present examples of these disease states as we recognize them on routine radiographs of the foot.

Osteoporosis. Osteoporosis is not a disease state but, in fact, is a condition of bone seen in many diseases in which there occurs a total decrease in bone volume that results in a decreased bone density and an increased bone porosity associated with decreased physical strength.

The most common cause for an osteoporotic change in normal bone is through the simple process of disuse. Just as muscle loses its volume with lack of exercise, so bone decreases in volume by weight if not physically stressed with activity. A good example of disuse osteoporosis is seen in Fig. 14-47, a radiograph of a foot that has been in a non–weight-bearing cast for 6 weeks. The greatest degree of bone loss occurs in the metaphyseal-epiphyseal areas, where metabolic changes are seen early, as opposed to cortical bone, in which more time is needed to show thinning or increased porosity. The simple solution to this form of osteoporosis is removal of the cast as soon as possible to begin stressing the bone once again. Even weight bearing in a cast will help avoid unnecessary osteoporosis from inactivity.

Another example of osteoporosis related to the disuse type is *Sudeck's atrophy* (reflex sympathetic dystrophy) (Arieff et al., 1963), sometimes referred to as sympathetic dystrophy of bone. This is a painful type of osteoporosis frequently seen in (often neurotic) women who sustain a minor injury to their foot which causes them to overreact to their injury by not using the foot for a prolonged period of time. The result is a radiographic

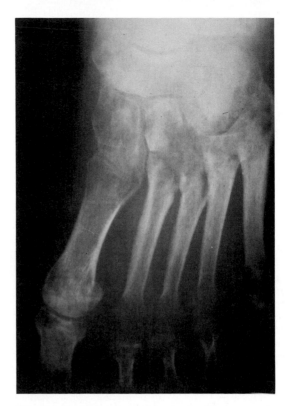

Fig. 14-48. Sudeck's atrophy in the foot as manifested by spotty osteoporosis

picture like that seen in Fig. 14-48, with characteristic spotty porosis throughout the midtarsal area. At first, the radiograph might suggest the infiltrative process of an inflammatory disease such as osteomyelitis. The foot may look cold and sweaty or at other times hot and swollen. These appearances have been attributed to some reflex instability of the autonomic system controlling the capillary flow of blood through the tissues of the foot. The best treatment for this chronic painful condition is to motivate the patient to exercise the foot and begin weight bearing as soon as possible. Sometimes lumbar sympathetic blocks are useful to decrease the pain so weight bearing can begin.

There are several hormonal abnormalities associated with osteoporosis. In *hypothyroidism* the general body metabolism slows down and, as a result, bone volume decreases. Fig. 14-49 is a radiograph of the foot of a hypothyroid patient. Note the relative accentuation of the major stress trabeculae due to excessive loss of the finer transverse trabeculae. The bone takes on a coarsened vertical trabecular pattern, and there is thinning of the cortical anatomy of the tibia. The enlarged calcaneal spur is the by-product of any long-standing osteoporotic or osteomalacic process of bone. Other well-known hormonal causes of osteoporosis include *hyperthyroid osteoporosis* (high-turnover disease) and *steroid osteoporosis* (low-turnover disease); both diseases have a similar radiographic appearance (Fig. 14-49). The most common of all porotic states in the hormone class is *postmenopausal osteoporosis*, which results from decreased blood estrogens at menopause and is seen mainly in Caucasian women. The treatment is aimed primarily at correction of the underlying hormone defect, if possible, and an attempt to stress the bone through exercise as much as possible.

It is well known that at least 30% of bone volume must be lost before osteoporotic changes can be detected on a simple clinical x-ray examination of the foot. Presently there are several commercial gamma-emitting bone scanners with the technical capacity to detect a 3% or 4% loss in bone density. This can be helpful in early detection of osteoporosis or for following a given patient under treatment. Fig. 14-50 is a photograph of the ^{125}I bone scanner used in our laboratory to determine bone density at the wrist. Similar units are designed to scan the os calcis in the foot.

A well-known cause of osteoporosis in children is scurvy. Vitamin C is required by the body to produce collagen fiber needed to form osteoid by osteoblasts on the surface of bony trabeculae. When this vitamin is deficient, the radiograph is like Fig. 14-51, of a child with scurvy. The thinned femoral cortex and the radiolucent scorbutic band running across the distal femoral metaphysis just above the increased radiodense markings of the zone of

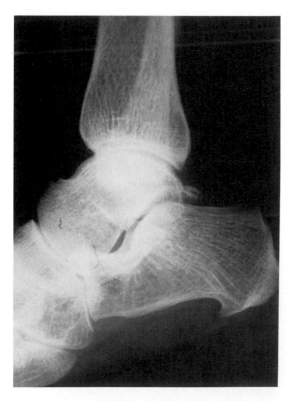

Fig. 14-49. Hypothyroid osteoporosis.

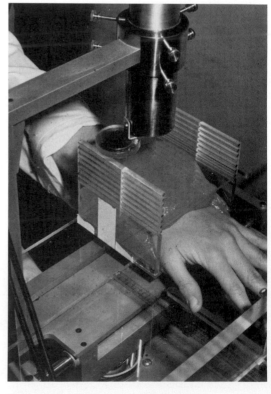

Fig. 14-50. ^{125}I gamma-emitting bone scanner to detect minute changes in bone density.

provisional calcification are characteristic.

Osteomalacia. Osteomalacic bone differs from osteoporotic bone insofar as there is a disproportionate loss of bone mineral compared with bone osteoid. The result is a decrease in bone rigidity: the bone becomes more like hard rubber. In the early stages, the bone volume is affected only slightly; but if the condition persists, bone volume also decreases and osteoporosis results as a terminal state. Numerous disease states exist which produce osteomalacia. The major ones include any intestinal disease in which there is a failure to transport calcium, phosphorus, or vitamin D across the gut wall into the bloodstream or renal disease in which there is a failure to activate vitamin D or there is a loss of too much calcium or phosphorus in the urine. Fig. 14-52 is the radiograph of a typical osteomalacic ankle in an adult patient with a chronic malabsorptive syndrome of the intestinal tract. The coarsened trabecular pattern is similar to that seen in osteoporosis. Fig. 14-53 is another example of the radiographic appearance of osteomalacia, in an adult with chronic pancreatic insufficiency. Characteris-

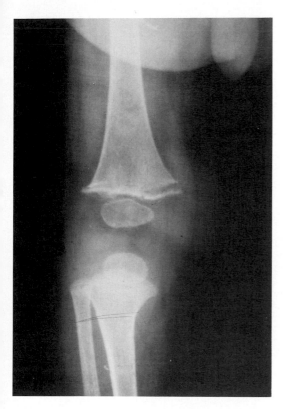

Fig. 14-51. Osteoporosis in a child with scurvy.

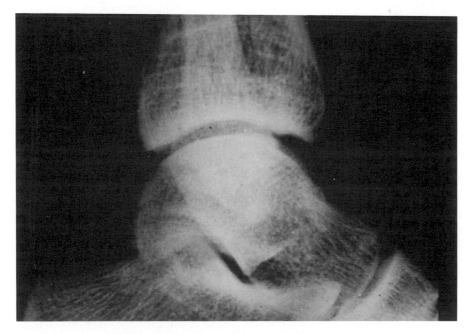

Fig. 14-52. Osteomalacia in an adult ankle.

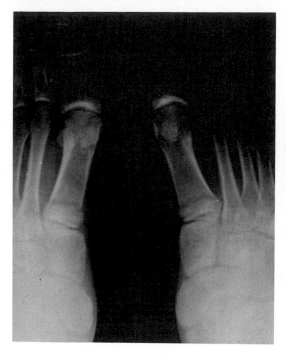

Fig. 14-53. Looser's zones in the first metatarsals of an osteomalacic bone.

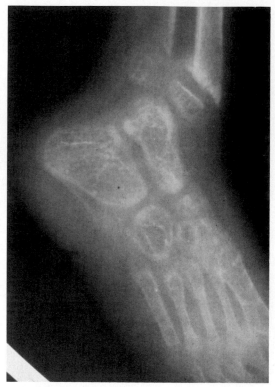

Fig. 14-54. Severe rachitic state in a child with renal osteodystrophy.

tic Looser's zones in the proximal areas of both first metatarsals are apparent. These transverse radiolucent bands have been attributed to vessels circumventing the malacic bone. Other physicians, including me, believe the bands represent stress fractures or fatigued areas from ordinary activity on weakened bone.

The osteomalacic state in children is referred to as *rickets*, which also is a mineral-deficient state of bone created by many diseases affecting the intestinal tract or kidneys. Fig. 14-54 is a radiograph of a child's foot that demonstrates severe rachitic changes secondary to a disease state known as *renal osteodystrophy*. In osteodystrophy, there are severe osteomalacic changes in bone as well as slipping of the epiphyses and calcification of the plantar ligaments not usually seen in ordinary vitamin-D–deficient rickets; in ordinary rickets there is merely a widening of the growth plate. Renal osteodystrophy is another name for rickets secondary to renal failure and is usually the end result of severe tubular glomerulonephritis in children. The ultimate

cure for this condition is to have a renal transplant performed.

A familial condition with the physical and radiographic appearance of rickets in children is the *Schmid form* of metaphyseal chondrodysplasia (previously called metaphyseal dysostosis). Fig. 14-55 is the radiograph of a child with the Schmid form of this heritable growth dysplasia, which has a widened and cupped growth plate but no evidence of the decreased bone density seen in rickets. The serum phosphorus level is normal in the Schmid syndrome and depressed in most rachitic states.

Because of a chronically suppressed serum calcium level, many forms of rickets demonstrate secondary states of hyperparathyroidism. However, there is a primary form of *hyperparathyroidism* seem secondary to an adenoma of the parathyroid gland causing it to put out excessive amounts of parathormone. The parathormone stimulates bone cells to destroy bony structure so as to mobilize large

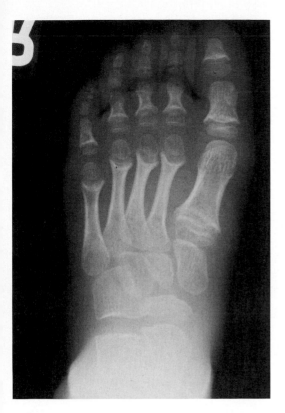

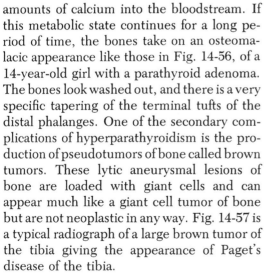

Fig. 14-55. Schmid form of metaphyseal chondrodysplasia that mimics rickets.

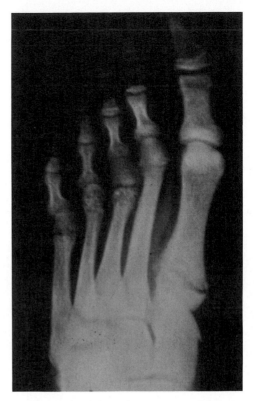

Fig. 14-56. Osteomalacic bone in an adolescent with primary hyperparathyroidism.

amounts of calcium into the bloodstream. If this metabolic state continues for a long period of time, the bones take on an osteomalacic appearance like those in Fig. 14-56, of a 14-year-old girl with a parathyroid adenoma. The bones look washed out, and there is a very specific tapering of the terminal tufts of the distal phalanges. One of the secondary complications of hyperparathyroidism is the production of pseudotumors of bone called brown tumors. These lytic aneurysmal lesions of bone are loaded with giant cells and can appear much like a giant cell tumor of bone but are not neoplastic in any way. Fig. 14-57 is a typical radiograph of a large brown tumor of the tibia giving the appearance of Paget's disease of the tibia.

Another interesting parathyroid disease of bone that frequently presents the radiographic appearance of hyperparathyroidism but exhibits low serum calcium levels is a

disease known as *pseudohypoparathyroidism*. Fig. 14-58 is the radiograph of a patient with this disease. Metatarsals two through five are short, with hypoplastic distal phalanges. Subcutaneous ectopic bone also is seen. This disease results because of a heritable defect in the renal tubule which is resistant to the normal or elevated levels of parathormone in these patients.

Paget's disease. Most people still consider Paget's disease of bone to be an idiopathic inflammatory disease state which initially produces a spotty hyperemic osteolysis associated with pain and an elevated alkaline phosphatase level in the blood. The bone becomes weakened because of the lytic process, and deformity results (e.g., bowing of the legs and widening of the skull). Then as a healing response by the patient, osteoblastic activity occurs and the involved bones become very dense-appearing on x-ray examina-

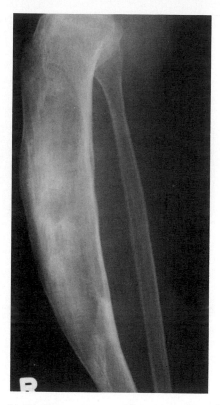

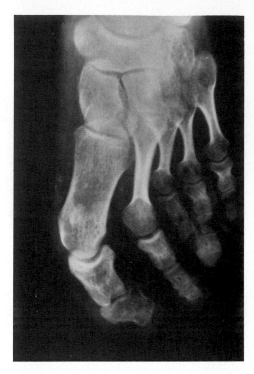

Fig. 14-58. Pseudohypoparathyroidism.

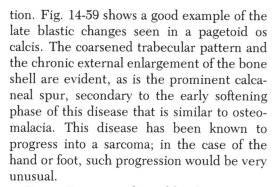

Fig. 14-57. Brown tumor of hyperparathyroidism giving the appearance of Paget's disease.

tion. Fig. 14-59 shows a good example of the late blastic changes seen in a pagetoid os calcis. The coarsened trabecular pattern and the chronic external enlargement of the bone shell are evident, as is the prominent calcaneal spur, secondary to the early softening phase of this disease that is similar to osteomalacia. This disease has been known to progress into a sarcoma; in the case of the hand or foot, such progression would be very unusual.

Gout. Gout is a heritable disease seen mostly in older men with a clinical picture of hyperuricemia associated with synovitis and the presence of urate deposits in soft tissue. The exact cause for the peripheral tissue production of excessive uric acid is still unknown. The condition frequently appears for the first time in the area of the first metatarsal heads with an acute intermittent cellulitis that eventually turns into a granulomatous process involving the juxta-articular structures about

the first metatarsophalangeal joint (Fig. 14-60). There is geographic erosion on the medial aspect of the first metatarsal head and on the base of the proximal phalanx. As time progresses, the arthritic process develops into a tophaceous condition with accumulation of urate deposits around the joint like those seen in the macroscopic section (Fig. 14-61). Extensive destructive changes can be seen in the first metatarsophalangeal joint. Sometimes the presence of small cutaneous ulcerations with uric acid crystals at the center that can be scraped with a knife and viewed under the microscope confirm the clinical diagnosis of gout. Fig. 14-62 shows a gouty foot with two diagnostic ulcers on the dorsum of the third toe. Fig. 14-63 shows more extensive gouty arthritic changes throughout the entire midtarsal area and first ray. Tophaceous gout can produce extensive soft tissue tumor masses beneath the skin which might suggest neurofibromatosis (as seen in Fig. 14-64 in a 45-

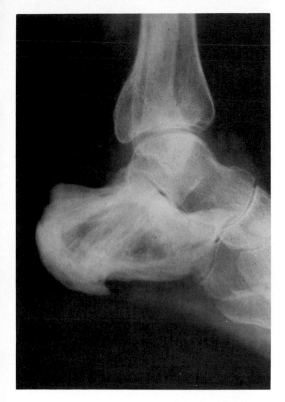

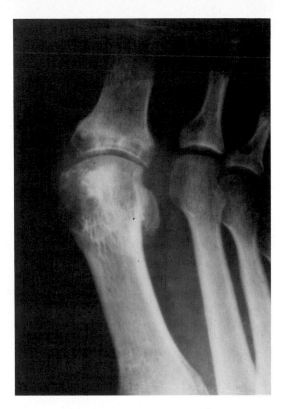

Fig. 14-59. Paget's disease of the os calcis.

Fig. 14-60. Gouty arthropathy of the first metatarsophalangeal joint.

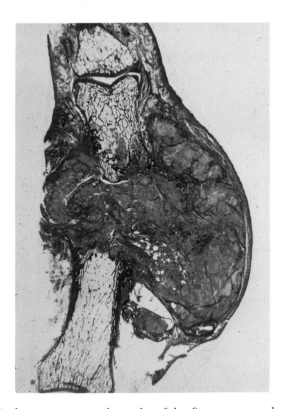

Fig. 14-61. Tophaceous gouty arthropathy of the first metatarsophalangeal joint.

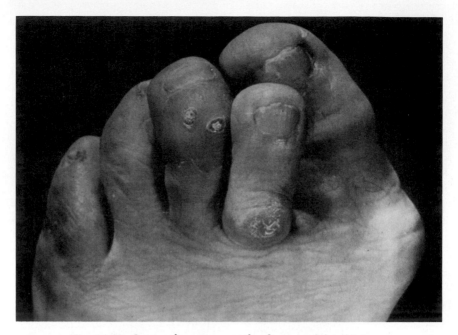

Fig. 14-62. Gouty ulcerations on the dorsum of the third toe.

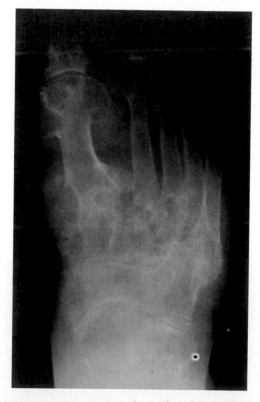

Fig. 14-63. Extensive gouty arthropathy of the midtarsal area.

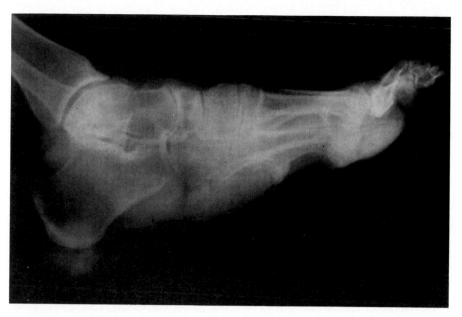

Fig. 14-64. Early tophaceous gout involving mainly subcutaneous tissues.

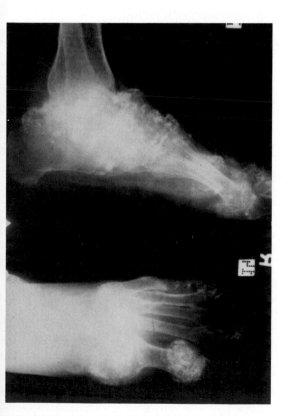

Fig. 14-65. Advanced calcific tophaceous gout in an older patient.

year-old with minimal arthritic changes). However, as time passes, the joints also become involved and the tophaceous material calcifies as seen in Fig. 14-65 in a much older patient. This radiograph takes on the appearance of the radiograph of a neuropathic foot. Balasubramanian and Silva (1971) suggest debridement of the tophi and bone grafting, if necessary.

Acromegaly. In acromegaly there is an overproduction of pituitary hormone after adult life is reached. This produces generalized hypertrophy of all somatic tissues, including bone as well as soft tissues overlying the bones. Fig. 14-66 shows an example of the thickening seen in the heel pad of such a patient. More characteristic of this disease state is the generalized hypertrophy of bone about the face and jaw (Fig. 14-67). Large air sinuses and a "Dick Tracy" mandible are evident, and the sella turcica is enlarged as a result of the pituitary adenoma.

Hypercholesterolemia. Another metabolic disease state relating to the foot and ankle area is hypercholesterolemia, which can lead to the life-threatening problems of coronary artery disease and myocardial infarction. In the ankle area, however, one commonly sees

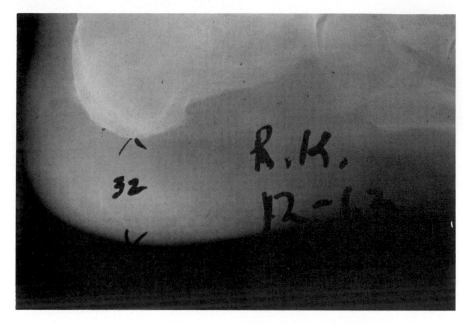

Fig. 14-66. Thickened heel pad in an acromegalic patient.

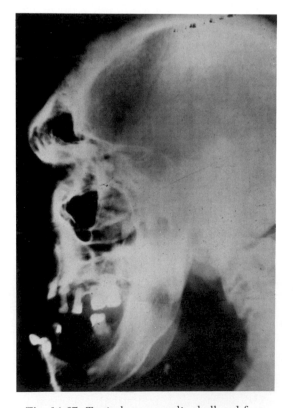

Fig. 14-67. Typical acromegalic skull and face.

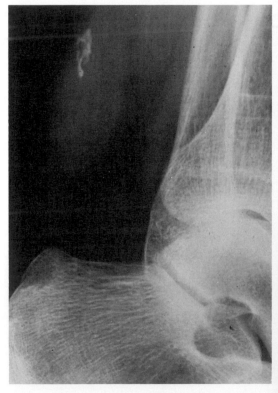

Fig. 14-68. Dystrophic calcification in the heel cord of a patient with hypercholesterolemia.

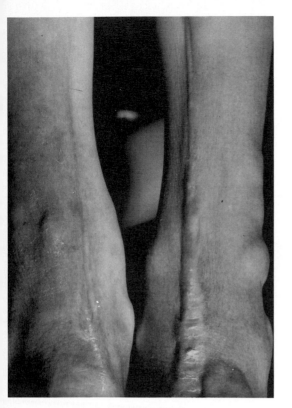

Fig. 14-69. Heel area in a hypercholesterolemic patient after complete debridement of both heel cords.

evidence of dystrophic calcification in the heel cord associated with weakening of the cord, pain, and microscopic tearing in the weakened structure. Fig. 14-68 shows the typical radiographic appearance of the calcification seen in a patient's heel cord associated with a fusiform enlargement of the cord that could even suggest a tumor mass.

These tendons should never be injected with cortisone, for this could increase the possibility of the pathologic rupture which occurs in a fair number of such patients. In one of my own patients both heel cords ruptured; and large deposits of cholesterol were found in and around the area, requiring multiple debridements. It was eventually necessary to completely remove both heel cords because of advanced degenerative changes that frustrated any attempt at a reconstructive approach to her mechanical problem. Fig. 14-69 is a photograph of this patient's heels after multiple surgical procedures.

REFERENCES
General

Ackerman, L. V., and Spjut, H. J.: Tumors of bone and cartilage, Washington D.C., 1962, Armed Forces Institute of Pathology.

Aegerter, E., and Kirkpatrick, J. A., Jr.: Orthopedic diseases, ed. 4, Philadelphia, 1975, W. B. Saunders Co.

Dahlin, D. C.: Bone tumors, ed. 2, Springfield, Ill., 1967, Charles C Thomas, Publisher.

Geiser, M., and Trueta, J.: Muscle action, bone rarefaction and bone formation, J. Bone Joint Surg. **40B:**282, 1958.

Greenfield, G. B.: Radiology of bone diseases, Philadelphia, 1969, J.B. Lippincott Co.

Jaffe, H. L.: Tumors and tumorous conditions of the bones and joints, Phildelphia, 1958, Lea & Febiger.

Spjut, H. J., Dorfman, H. D., Fechner, R. E., and Ackerman, L. V.: Tumors of bone and cartilage. Atlas of tumor pathology, Ser. 2, Fasc. 5, Washington, D.C., 1971, Armed Forces Institute of Pathology.

Stout, A. P., and Lattes, R.: Tumors of the soft tissues. Atlas of tumor pathology, Ser. 2, Fasc. 1, Washington, D.C., 1967, Armed Forces Institute of Pathology.

Specific

Ackerman, L. V.: Surgical pathology, ed. 4, St. Louis, 1968, The C. V. Mosby Co.

Arieff, A. J., Bell, J. L., Tigay, E. L., and Kurtz, J. F.: Reflex physiopathic disturbances, J. Bone Joint Surg. **45A:**1329, 1963.

Balasubramanian, P., and Silva, J. F.: Tophectomy and bone-grafting for extensive tophi of the feet, J. Bone Joint Surg. **53A:**133, 1971.

Cameron, H. U., and Kostuik, J. P.: A long-term follow-up of synovial sarcoma, J. Bone Joint Surg. **56B:**613, 1974.

Cowie, R. S.: Benign osteoblastoma of the talus, J. Bone Joint Surg. **48B:**582, 1966.

Dahlin, D. C., and Salvador, A. H.: Chondrosarcoma of bones of the hands and feet: a study of 30 cases, Cancer **34:**755, 1974.

Eisenstein, R.: Giant-cell tumor of tendon sheath, J. Bone Joint Surg. **50A:**476, 1968.

Giannestras, N. J., and Diamond, J. R.: Benign osteoblastoma of the talus: a review of the literature and report of a case, J. Bone Joint Surg. **40A:**469, 1958.

Goldenberg, R. R., Campbell, C. J., and Bonfiglio, M.: Giant cell tumor of bone, J. Bone Joint Surg. **52A:**619, 1970.

Jaffe, N., and Watts, H. G.: Multidrug chemotherapy in primary treatment of osteosarcoma: an editorial commentary, J. Bone Joint Surg. **58A:**634, 1976.

Jones, F. E., Soule, E. H., and Coventry, M. D.: Fibrous xanthoma of synovium (giant-cell tumor of tendon sheath, pigmented nodular synovitis), J. Bone Joint Surg. **51A:**76, 1969.

Keller, R. B., and Baez-Giangreco, A.: Juvenile aponeu-rotic fibroma: Report of three cases and a review of the literature, Clin. Orthop. **106**:198, 1975.

Larsson, S. E., Lorentzon, R., and Boquist, L.: Fibro-sarcoma of bone: a demographic, clinical and histopath-ological study of all cases recorded in the Swedish Cancer Registry from 1958 to 1968, J. Bone Joint Surg. **58B**:412, 1976.

Lewis, G. M.: Practical dermatology, ed. 3, Philadelphia, 1967, W. B. Saunders Co.

Lewis, R. J., Marcove, R. C., and Rosen, G.: Ewing's sarcoma-functional effects of radiation therapy, J. Bone Joint Surg. **59A**:325, 1977.

McNeill, T. W., and Ray, R. D.: Hemangioma of the extremities: a review of 35 cases, Clin. Orthop. **101**:154, 1974.

Pedersen, H. E., and Day, A. J., Dupuytren's disease of the foot, J.A.M.A. **154**:33, 1954.

Pritchard, D. J., Dahlin, D. C., Dauphine, R. T., Taylor, W. F., and Beabout, J. W.: Ewing's sarcoma: a clini-copathological and statistical analysis of patients surviv-ing five years or longer, J. Bone Joint Surg. **57A**:10, 1975.

Simon, M. A., and Enneking, W. F: The management of soft tissue sarcomas of the extremities, J. Bone Joint Surg. **58A**:317, 1976.

Smith, R. W., and Smith, C. F: Solitary unicameral bone cyst of the calcaneus: a review of twenty cases, J. Bone Joint Surg. **56A**:49, 1974.

Smyth, M: Glomus-cell tumors in the lower extremity: report of two cases, J. Bone Joint Surg. **53A**:157, 1971.

Soren, A: Pathogenesis and treatment of ganglion, Clin. Orthop. **48**:17, 1966.

Spanos, P. K., Payne, W. S., Ivins, J. C., and Pritchard, D. J.: Pulmonary resection for metastatic osteogenic sarcoma, J. Bone Joint Surg. **58A**:624, 1976.

Stening, W. S.: Primary malignant tumours of calcaneal tendon, J. Bone Joint Surg. **50B**:676, 1968.

15

DISEASES OF THE NERVES OF THE FOOT

Roger A. Mann

Most neurologic disorders of the foot stem from changes in the cerebrospinal system, with secondary changes in the lower extremity. Except for connective-tissue changes in the digital branches of the plantar nerve, intrinsic diseases of the nerves of the foot are rare. Some discussion of them, however, is pertinent here.

INTERDIGITAL PLANTAR NEUROMA

Histologically a plantar neuroma is a neurofibroma, which is an accumulation of collagenous material in the neurilemma (sheath of Schwann). Neurilemma is present only in peripheral nerves; therefore, such changes occur only in peripheral nerves, as pointed out by both Ewing (1942) and Boyd (1943).

Winkler et al. (1948) reviewed microscopic sections of twenty specimens of presumed neurofibroma of the foot but did not find evidence of active proliferation of either nerve or neurilemma. They found instead that the enlargement was caused by a deposition of hyaline and collagenous material.

In 1876 Thomas George Morton described the entity known as Morton's neuralgia or Morton's metatarsalgia. He suggested that the condition was probably caused by neuritis of the third branch of the medial plantar nerve. Textbooks on anatomy describe the medial plantar nerve as having four digital branches. The most medial branch is the proper digital nerve to the medial aspect of the great toe. The next three branches are named the first, second, and third common digital nerves and are distributed to both the medial and lateral aspects of the first, second, and third interspaces respectively. The lateral plantar nerve gives off a superficial branch, which splits into a proper digital nerve to the lateral side of the small toe, and it also gives off a common digital nerve to the fourth interspace. The common digital nerve frequently gives rise to a communicating branch, which passes to the third digital branch of the medial plantar nerve in the third interspace (Fig. 15-1).

Tubby (1912) treated a series of patients who had so-called Morton's neuralgia by excising the head of the fourth metatarsal. He stated: "On occasion when the nerve was seen, it was resected and it often showed small nodular masses." Betts (1940) was the first to demonstrate histologically the extensive connective tissue enlargement of the third digital branch of the medial plantar nerve. He observed this enlargement in nineteen cases in which he and his colleagues performed resections of the nerve because of so-called Morton's neuralgia. Nissen (1948) remarked that before 1940 several English surgeons who had noticed nodular masses on the plan-

463

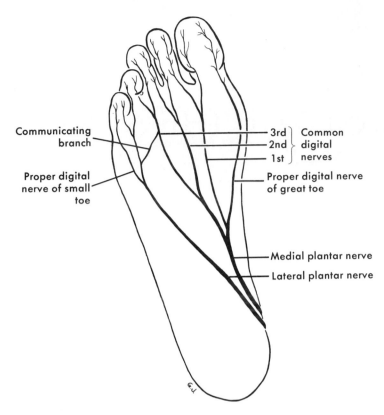

Fig. 15-1. Plantar nerves of the right foot.

tar digital nerve in the course of surgical procedures involving the plantar surface thought that fibrous changes were taking place.

McElvenny (1943) and McKeever (1952) reported independently that they had found a thickened digital nerve in the third metatarsal interspace about the same time as Betts (1940). Then Baker and Kuhn (1944), Bickel and Dockerty (1947), Watson-Jones (1949), and others all substantiated Betts' observations.

An interdigitial neuroma is more prevalent in women by a ratio of approximately 4 to 1 (Bovill, 1965; Bradley et al., 1976). The condition can occur at any age but most commonly between 40 and 60 years. Generally it is unilateral, but bilateral neuromas are seen 10% to 15% of the time. Two neuromas in the same foot rarely occur simultaneously. The third digital nerve is by far the most frequently affected. The second is next most commonly, and the first and fourth are rarely, affected.

Etiology. The cause of neuroma as related to the foot is not entirely clear. Nissen (1948) believed it to be a result of degeneration of the digital vessels in the cleft between the third and fourth toes. Winkler et al. (1948) postulated that the predisposition of the third digital nerve to the disease was related to its receiving a filament from the lateral plantar nerve (Fig. 15-1), although the third digital nerve is essentially a branch of the medial plantar nerve. Possibly neuromas of the digital plantar nerve branches result from chronic irritation. Irritating factors include the wearing of faulty footwear, walking on hard floors, standing for long periods, the proximity or touching of metatarsal heads due to metatarsal fractures, and anatomic variations of bones and nerves on the plantar surface.

From the standpoint of the biomechanics of

the foot, more motion appears to occur in the third interspace than in the other interspaces—probably because of the joining of the medial and longitudinal arch systems at the third interspace. DuVries believes that of the five metatarsals, the fourth is the least securely anchored at its base. This weak attachment permits a floating action of the distal end of the fourth metatarsal when the foot is in motion. The anatomic instability of the fourth metatarsal head may well be a source of irritation and trauma to the terminal portion of the third digital nerve. Prolonged irritation of living tissue by mechanical friction can induce proliferation of connective tissue or collagenous material in the involved area.

Furthermore, the three digital branches of the medial plantar nerve lie between the heads and shafts of the metatarsals and are subject to constant friction. In response to this friction, collagenous connective tissue accumulates in the neurilemma. Increased thickness subjects the nerve to greater friction. The overwhelming predilection to thickening of the third digital branch seems to give credence to the fact that the contributing causes of neuroma are increased motion and friction in the area of the third interspace.

An extensive review of Morton's neuroma by Reed and Bliss (1973) has concluded that the changes in Morton's neuroma are related to trauma secondary to impingement of the intermetatarsal bursa and neurovascular bundle between the heads of the metatarsal bones. The authors divide the histopathologic findings into five categories: (1) The intermetatarsal nerve demonstrates atrophy with demyelinization and endoneurial fibrosis. (2) The intermetatarsal artery demonstrates intimal thickening. The fibrous matrix of the thickened intima is hyalinized and poorly cellular. This produces a fibrous endarteritis which can partially or completely occlude the lumen of the artery. (3) The intermetatarsal bursa (not present in all specimens) demonstrates hyalinized fronds covered with fibrinoid. (4) The fibrous matrix surrounding the nerve and forming the clinical neuroma varies from dense hyaline fibrous tissue to edematous fibrous tissue. (5) The surrounding fi-

broadipose tissue demonstrates elastic fibers that are both increased in number and abnormally arranged.

Dissection and sectioning of digital plantar nerves taken at random from cadavers and from freshly amputated feet show microscopically that asymptomatic nerves and neuromas may have a similar appearance.

Symptoms. The most common symptom of an interdigital neuroma is pain localized to the plantar aspect of the foot between the metatarsal heads. The pain is aggravated by activities and relieved by resting the foot, particularly rubbing it with the shoe off. At times a person will note that he feels no symptoms when walking barefooted on a soft surface but develops pain promptly when putting on a tight-fitting shoe. The pain is usually fairly well localized to the plantar aspect of the foot but occasionally radiates toward the tip of the toes of the involved interspace. On rare occasion the pain radiates toward the dorsum of the foot or more proximally into the plantar aspect of the foot.

The pain itself is usually described as burning in nature but without a sharp component to it. Occasionally the patient will have the feeling that there is something moving around in the bottom of the foot which when caught in the right position causes an acute sharp pain. I believe these symptoms are probably caused by the patient's actually stepping on the enlarged tissue about the nerve.

Diagnosis. Palpation of the plantar aspect of the involved interspace often causes a sharp stabbing pain similar to that occurring when the patient bears weight on the foot. The involved nerve can be palpated in about one third of the patients. When palpated, a mass can be felt beneath the examiner's finger and can actually be rolled back and forth. If the examiner then squeezes the mass against the metatarsal head, the patient experiences a moderate amount of discomfort and will usually note the pain beneath the examining finger as well as radiating out toward the toes of the involved interspace (Fig. 15-2). The diagnosis must be made on the basis of the history and physical examination since neither radiographs nor laboratory tests offer

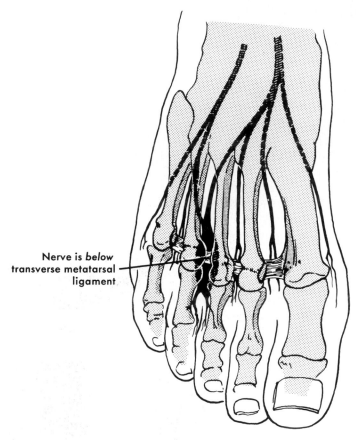

Nerve is *below* transverse metatarsal ligament

Fig. 15-2. Schematic view of the third branch of the medial plantar nerve. Note that it courses plantarward, under the transverse metatarsal ligament.

clues. Occasionally the toes associated with the involved interspace demonstrate hyperesthesia to pinprick.

In the differential diagnosis of plantar neuroma, the possibility of tarsal tunnel syndrome should always be kept in mind. Sometimes bony abnormalities involving the lesser metatarsophalangeal joints produce similar symptoms (Fig. 15-3).

Treatment. Conservative treatment includes such palliative measures as metatarsal bars and pads, but these appliances usually afford only temporary relief. Injection of the involved interspace with a local anesthetic and steroid preparation is occasionally useful as a diagnostic tool, particularly if there is tenderness in two interspaces in the same foot when the examiner attempts to determine which interspace is involved. Intractable pain in the interspace between the second and third and the third and fourth metatarsal heads that cannot be relieved by mechanical measures justifies a diagnosis of operable neuroma.

Excision of the entire nerve gives complete relief. European surgeons excise the nerve of the second or third digital branch through a plantar approach, as described by Betts (1940) and Nissen (1948). In the United States the approach generally is through the dorsum, as described by McElvenny (1943) and by McKeever (1952). The American approach has advantages, the most important being prevention of scar formation on the plantar surface. Furthermore, this approach does not pass through important fascial planes as does the plantar incision. The nerve is easily identified in the metatarsal interspace, and the dorsal approach does not present any obstacle to observing or excising the nerve.

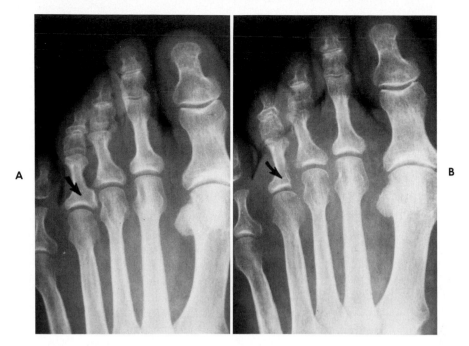

Fig. 15-3. A, Anomalous relation of the base of the fourth proximal phalanx to the third metatarsal head in the foot of a 54-year-old woman. Twice she had undergone surgical procedures for neuroma, without relief. **B,** Correction of the anomaly. Symptoms were alleviated.

Technique for excising an interdigital neuroma

1. Under tourniquet control, make an incision on the dorsal aspect of the foot starting in the web space between the involved toes. Carry the incision proximally about 1 inch to the level of the metatarsal head. It is important to keep the incision directly in the web space because deviation to either side may result in cutting one of the fine dorsal digital nerves, which would cause a painful neuroma within the scar.

2. Carry the incision down directly between the metatarsal heads. Place a Weitlander between the metatarsal heads to spread them apart. This will put the transverse metatarsal ligament under tension.

3. Using a neurologic freer, dissect out the common digital nerve and identify the transverse metatarsal ligament. Carefully transect the transverse metatarsal ligament, being careful not to cut the underlying structures. Once this has been accomplished, the nerve can be readily freed from the surrounding vessels and fat.

4. The common digital nerve is now lying free in the base of the wound. Grasp it with the forceps, pull distally, and cut it as proximal as possible. It should be cut just proximal to the level of the metatarsal head. This having been accomplished, the nerve is then easily dissected distally and cut just past the bifurcation into its terminal branches. Dorsiflex the ankle to pull the stump more proximally into the foot.

5. Suture only the skin and apply a compression bandage for 18 to 24 hours. After this time the compression bandage is released and another firm dressing is applied. Ambulation is then begun in a wooden shoe.

6. The foot is kept wrapped with a firm dressing for 3 weeks following the procedure.

After excision of an interdigital neuroma, approximately 95% of our patients are clinically asymptomatic. Recurrence of the neuroma following proper resection is less than 1%. It is interesting to note that although the nerve is completely excised the majority of patients retain nearly normal sensation in the involved web space. An occasional patient, however, will note numbness in the web space.

Recurrent neuroma

Some patients will have a recurrence of symptoms in the foot after resection of the interdigital neuroma, occurring usually two to three years after the initial operative procedure. These people should be treated conservatively at first.

If conservative measures fail and the symptoms persist, reexploration of the interspace is necessary. Prior to exploring the interspace, the surgeon should carefully examine the plantar aspect of the foot in order to accurately localize the neuroma, which is usually adjacent to the metatarsal head. Careful localization preoperatively makes finding the neuroma much simpler at the time of surgical exploration. Reexploration of the interspace is done as described earlier for the original neuroma, but a great deal of care and patience must be exercised to identify the tumor. Once identified, the neuroma is freed from its adhesions and transected as proximal to the metatarsal head as possible; this is rarely more than 1 cm proximal to the metatarsal head. Reexploration of the foot for a recurrent neuroma gives a satisfactory result in about 75% of cases.

Occasionally the pain cannot be relieved, even by excision of the recurrent neuroma. These patients present a most difficult management problem.

REFLEX SYMPATHETIC DYSTROPHY (CAUSALGIA)

Reflex sympathetic dystrophy is a clinical entity in which the patient after major or minor trauma or surgery develops a symptom complex and burning pain, swelling, and motor dysfunction which can be extremely disabling. The condition has been called Sudek's atrophy and causalgia, but reflex sympathetic dystrophy is the preferred term.

Reflex sympathetic dystrophy has been divided into several categories by Lankford and Thompson (1977). In their clinical classi-fication, trauma to a purely sensory nerve is "minor causalgia"; when caused by a non-nerve injury, "minor traumatic dystrophy"; when caused by more severe trauma, "major traumatic dystrophy"; and when caused by trauma to a major mixed nerve, "major causalgia."

Insofar as the foot is concerned, a minor causalgia or minor traumatic dystrophy is usually seen after foot surgery, lacerations of the foot, minor trauma such as a twisting injury to the foot and ankle, or fracture of a metatarsal bone. Major traumatic dystrophy is seen after a severe crash injury to the lower extremity; major causalgia can be seen after trauma to the sciatic nerve or its terminal trunks—common peroneal and posterior tibial nerves.

Etiology. The etiology of reflex sympathetic dystrophy is poorly understood, although the condition is generally thought to be secondary to an abnormal autonomic response to trauma.

In their review Lankford and Thompson (1977) pointed out that three factors must be present at the same time for reflex sympathetic dystrophy to occur: a painful lesion secondary to trauma (either major or minor), a diathesis or susceptibility of the patient, and an abnormal autonomic reflex.

Symptoms. Symptoms vary somewhat depending on the type of reflex sympathetic dystrophy the patient may manifest.

Minor causalgia, affecting a purely sensory nerve, will involve only the foot. The patient describes the pain as burning in nature and experiences marked dysesthesias. The pain usually follows the course of a sensory nerve.

Minor traumatic dystrophy is the most common type seen and usually involves the toes, often following a crush injury to the toes. The patient manifests fairly well localized pain, mild to moderate generalized edema of the affected foot and ankle, some motor dysfunction, and vasomotor changes indicated by cool moist skin.

Major traumatic dystrophy follows a more extensive injury to the foot and ankle. The symptoms are similar to those seen in minor traumatic dystrophy although the changes may be more extensive and marked demineralization of the bone is noted radiographically.

Major causalgia, which follows an injury to a major mixed nerve—namely the sciatic, posterior tibial, or common peroneal—is not common; but the symptoms may be extremely severe and disabling. The patient manifests an intense burning pain generally following the sensory distribution of the nerve but which cannot be well localized. The clinical findings are again the marked sensitivity of the extremity to any type of touch, increased vasomotor response in the form of cool moist skin, and marked motor dysfunction.

Treatment. The most critical factor in the treatment of reflex sympathetic dystrophy is early recognition of the problem. This is particularly important in the minor causalgic and minor traumatic forms of the condition. In these two entities the problem can be thwarted early in its clinical course before more severe changes occur.

Initial treatment should be directed toward vigorous physical therapy in the form of range-of-motion exercises and using the ex-

tremity, whirlpool exercises, and control of the edema by an elastic stocking. Approximately 90% of these patients respond favorably when such treatment is started early.

Once the condition has become more severe, it is much more difficult to treat. In the more chronic cases there may be permanent changes in the soft tissues and joints. In the later stages treatment consists of lumbar sympathetic blocks (preferrably by an anesthesiologist), which will interrupt the abnormal sympathetic reflex. These can be repeated on three or four occasions to provide complete relief. If after successful sympathetic block the symptoms continue to recur, a sympathectomy should be considered.

In the treatment of major traumatic dystrophy or major causalgia, it may be necessary to do a neurolysis of the involved nerve as well as the other treatment modalities mentioned.

TARSAL TUNNEL SYNDROME

The tarsal tunnel syndrome is caused by pressure exerted on the posterior tibial nerve or one of its terminal branches as it passes beneath the flexor retinaculum at the level of the ankle or more distally as it divides into its terminal branches—medial plantar nerve,

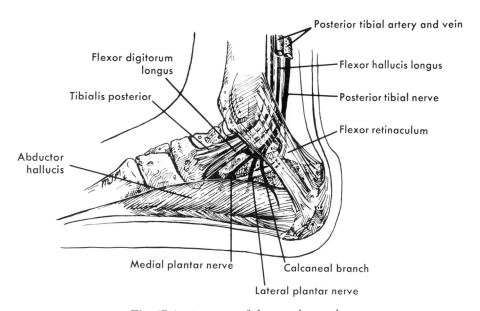

Fig. 15-4. Anatomy of the tarsal tunnel.

lateral plantar nerve, and medial calcaneal branch (Fig. 15-4). The condition is analogous to the carpal tunnel syndrome in the wrist and was first described by Keck (1962) and later in the same year by Lam.

Etiology. The tarsal tunnel syndrome may follow a twisting injury to the ankle, fracture of the calcaneus, fracture of the distal tibia, or crush injury to the ankle region; at times no etiology is identified.

Symptoms. The patient usually complains of a burning pain in the plantar aspect of the foot often aggravated by activities but also present at rest. Some patients note a burning pain while in bed at night. Others complain of a tingling feeling in the plantar aspect of the foot. Occasionally the pain will radiate up the medial aspect of the calf toward the knee.

Physical findings. The examination of the patient will demonstrate a positive Tinel sign over the tarsal tunnel area, located behind the medial malleolus. It is important to percuss the entire course of the posterior tibial nerve and terminal branches, looking for a positive Tinel sign which may indicate the area of pathology. Percussion of the nerve will cause localized discomfort as well as pain radiating out toward the distribution of the medial or lateral plantar nerve. Motor dysfunction and a sensory deficit are rarely associated with the tarsal tunnel syndrome, but occasionally a slight decrease in sensation can be found.

The diagnosis is confirmed by electrodiagnostic studies of the posterior tibial nerve and branches. The terminal latency to the abductor hallucis should be less than 6.2 msec, and that to the abductor digiti minimi less than 7.0 msec. Attempts should be made to identify fibrillation potentials within the abductor hallucis and abductor digiti minimi.

Treatment. Conservative management of the true tarsal tunnel syndrome rarely results in any clinical relief. An attempt can be made to infiltrate the area with local anesthetics and steroids, but this has rarely been helpful in my hands. If the clinical symptoms are present and are confirmed by electrodiagnostic studies, release of the posterior tibial nerve and its three terminal branches is indicated. I have found that approximately 75% of patients are relieved by the surgery and 25% obtain little or no relief (Mann, 1974). A symptomatic patient is rarely made worse by having a tarsal tunnel release performed.

As mentioned previously, it is important to carefully percuss preoperatively the course of the posterior tibial nerve and medial and lateral plantar branches to note where the most sensitive area of the nerve is located. This will enable the surgeon to explore the particular area for any type of unexpected pathology such as a ganglion of the tendon sheath compressing the nerve or possibly localized scar tissue.

Surgical technique

1. The tarsal tunnel is approached through a curved incision. Begin about 1 cm posterior to the medial margin of the tibial shaft and carry it downward parallel with the tibia and behind the medial malleolus.

2. Once the incision passes the plane of the tip of the medial malleolus, curve it gradually plantarward.

3. Identify the retinaculum and carefully release it in its entirety. The posterior tibial nerve can be identified in the proximal portion of the dissection and traced distally. Care must be taken to avoid cutting the small (and sometimes multiple) medial calcaneal branch which arises from the lateral plantar nerve and is surrounded by fatty tissue.

4. Identify and trace the medial and lateral plantar nerves distally. The medial plantar branch should be followed along the superior margin of the abductor hallucis and flexor sheath of the flexor hallucis longus. The lateral plantar nerve is followed into the substance of the abductor hallucis. Any fibrous bands within this muscle that seem to be constricting the nerve should be released. At the conclusion of the dissection, the three terminal branches of the posterior tibial nerve should be lying free.

5. Instill 1 ml of hydrocortisone into the wound around the nerve and close the wound in layers (not the retinaculum). Apply a sterile compression dressing.

6. The patient is then kept non–weight bearing on crutches for a period of 3 weeks, after which weight bearing is permitted.

PERIPHERAL NERVE ENTRAPMENTS ABOUT THE FOOT

The major cutaneous nerve trunks about the dorsal aspect of the foot are close to the surface; therefore any superficial trauma can cause entrapment of a cutaneous nerve and produce a rather painful localized condition or at times be the precipitating cause of a reflex sympathetic dystrophy. The etiology of the injury may be secondary to blunt trauma, lacerations, and/or deep abrasions, or may be iatrogenic.

Symptoms. The patient usually complains of a localized pain over the area of the peripheral nerve entrapment. Any type of pressure against the area will often cause an increase in the symptoms which at times make wearing a shoe most difficult.

Diagnosis. The diagnosis is made by palpation of the involved area and by eliciting a positive Tinel sign over the involved nerve.

Treatment. The treatment is usually directed toward relieving the local symptoms. Injection of the area with local anesthetic and steroids may afford the patient some relief and occasionally will bring complete relief. If this fails, surgical exploration of the area should be carried out; the nerve must be resected sufficiently proximally that the cut end and the eventual traumatic neuroma will be located in an area of soft fatty tissue and localized pressure will not be exerted upon it. At times treatment of this condition is most difficult and the results less than optimal.

REFERENCES
Interdigital plantar neuroma

Baker, L. D., and Kuhn, H. H.: Morton's metatarsalgia: localized degenerative fibrosis with neuromatous proliferation of the fourth plantar nerve, South. Med. J. 37:123, 1944.

Betts, L. O.: Morton's metatarsalgia: Neuritis of the fourth digital nerve, Med. J. Aust. 1:514, 1940.

Bickel, W. H., and Dockerty, M. B.: Plantar neuromas, Morton's toe, Surg. Gynecol. Obstet. 84:111, 1947.

Bovill, E. G., Jr.: Diseases of nerves. In DuVries, H. L.: Surgery of the foot, ed. 2, St. Louis, 1965, The C. V. Mosby Co.

Boyd, W.: A textbook of pathology, ed. 4, Philadelphia, 1943, Lea & Febiger.

Bradley, N., Miller, W. A., and Evans, J. P.: Plantar neuroma: analysis of results following surgical excision in 145 patients, South. Med. J. 69:853, 1976.

Ewing, J.: Neoplastic diseases, Philadelphia, 1942, W. B. Saunders Co.

McElvenny, R. T.: The etiology and surgical treatment of intractable pain about the fourth metatarsophalangeal joint (Morton's toe), J. Bone Joint Surg. 25:675, 1943.

McKeever, D. C.: Surgical approach for neuroma of plantar digital nerve (Morton's metatarsalgia), J. Bone Joint Surg. 34A:490, 1952.

Morton, T. G.: A peculiar and painful affection of fourth metatarsophalangeal articulation, Am. J. Med. Sci. 71:37, 1876.

Nissen, K. I.: Plantar digital neuritis: Morton's metatarsalgia, J. Bone Joint Surg. 30B:84, 1948.

Reed, R. J., and Bliss, B. O.: Morton's neuroma, Arch. Pathol. 95:123, 1973.

Tubby, A. H.: Deformities, including diseases of the bones and joints, ed. 2, vol. 1, London, 1912, Macmillan & Co., Ltd.

Watson-Jones, R.: Leri's pleonosteosis, carpal tunnel compression of the median nerves and Morton's metatarsalgia, J. Bone Joint Surg. 31B:560, 1949.

Winkler, H., Feltner, J. B., and Kimmelstiel, P.: Morton's metatarsalgia, J. Bone Joint Surg. 30A:496, 1948.

Reflex sympathetic dystrophy (causalgia)

Lankford, L. L., and Thompson, J. E.: Reflex sympathetic dystrophy, upper and lower extremity: diagnosis and management, In Instructional Course Lectures, American Academy of Orthopaedic Surgeons, vol. 26, St. Louis, 1977, The C. V. Mosby Co.

Tarsal tunnel syndrome

Keck, C.: The tarsal-tunnel syndrome, J. Bone Joint Surg. 44A:180, 1962.

Lam, S. J. S.: A tarsal-tunnel syndrome, Lancet 2:1354, 1962.

Mann, R. A.: The tarsal tunnel syndrome, Orthop. Clin. North Am. 5:109, 1974.

16

DERMATOLOGY AND DISORDERS OF THE TOENAILS

Jerral S. Seibert and Roger A. Mann

In many specialties of medicine, there is overlapping of subject matter; such is the case concerning orthopaedic and skin foot problems. It behooves the practitioner to have some knowledge of the allied fields because frequently patients unknowingly will seek advice concerning symptoms and conditions of the other specialty. The following cutaneous entities commonly found on the feet are discussed. By no means is this listing complete for all the dermatologic conditions affecting the feet. That is beyond the scope of the present chapter; the reader is referred to further complete treatises such as those of Costello and Gibbs (1967) and Gibbs (1974).

An important corollary should be reemphasized for examining skin lesions of the feet: the clinician should always check the hands and occasionally other parts of the integument because many afflictions involving the feet will also be present on the palms or other areas of the skin.

CORNS, CALLUSES, AND WARTS

Discrete hyperkeratotic skin lesions on the feet are perhaps the most common complaint and it is important to distinguish the exact identity of the lesion for successful therapy.

Calluses develop at sites of pressure usually under the bony prominences of the feet. They tend to be the largest, and corns the smallest, of the hyperkeratotic lesions. To differentiate these plantar lesions, one must pare away the hyperkeratotic covering so the distinguishing clinical characteristics are evident. Calluses have wide papillary lines that do not diverge from their normal direction. The margins of calluses are rather diffuse whereas those of corns and warts are sharply demarcated. Corns and warts have deviating papillary lines or lines that are interrupted by a sharply marginated lesion. Calluses have no cores and no visible blood vessels. Corns have papillary lines diverging around a sharply marginated translucent core devoid of blood vessels. Warts have the fine capillaries which diagnostically rise perpendicularly to the surface. Pain may be a distinguishing feature with the various lesions. Calluses are usually not painful until they become large and extensive. Corns, particularly the neurovascular and soft types, are quite painful. Warts may be painful, depending on the type and location (Fig. 16-1). Lateral pressure elicits pain in the wart; direct pressure causes pain in the corn.

Treatment of a callus usually requires that the pressure causing it be removed. This requires the patient to wear correctly fitted shoes or use corrective protective pads to distribute the body weight evenly over the

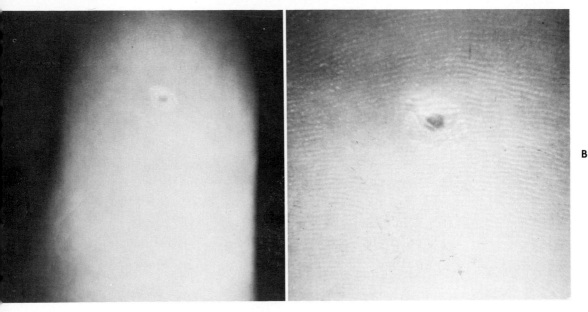

B

Fig. 16-1. Plantar clavus (corn). This painful lesion developed on the heel of an adolescent girl who suspected a wart. Inspection of her "everyday shoes" revealed a protruding nail at the site of the hyperkeratosis.

weight-bearing portions of the foot. To reduce the callus formation, periodic paring plus use of 40% salicylic acid plasters is effective.

Corns also result from friction and pressure localizing especially on the bulb of the great toe or on the sides, tips, and tops of other toes; under bony prominences; and in the metatarsal area. Treatment consists of paring periodically plus application of a 40% salicylic acid plaster with a felt pad fashioned to fit around the corn to relieve the pressure. Protective padding is required to keep the corn from recurring; the padding or cushion can be incorporated into a supportive insole in the shoe. Again, it is important to emphasize that properly fitted shoes should be worn to prevent recurrences. In this regard, as Montgomery points out, properly fitted shoes are an important part in the treatment of any plantar keratotic lesions. Too narrow a shoe squeezes the toes together and may cause soft corns; too short a shoe may cause corns to form on the tips and tops of the toes; too high a heel interferes with the proper distribution of the body weight across the foot and may cause painful calluses, corns, or warts.

The second type of corn, neurovascular corn, is notable for it is usually painful and frequently mistaken as a verruca. It is usually situated on the plantar surface under the first or fifth metatarsal head and appears as a small (1 to 3 mm) lesion with a diffuse translucent core which fades into the surrounding tissues. At the periphery of the corn, small dried up capillaries appear, some of which lie parallel with the skin rather than perpendicular as do the vessels in warts. Treatment of the neurovascular corn consists of weekly paring and application of a caustic such as 50% silver nitrate. Further thinning by application of keratolytic such as 40% salicylic acid plaster can further thin down this tissue. Adequate padding, again, is essential. Excising these painful lesions is inadvisable, for a resolving scar may occur that is more painful than the original corn. Orthopaedic surgery is sometimes required for removal of the plantar condyle of the metatarsal head for resistant cases.

A third type of corn affects the intertriginous aspects of the toes and is sometimes misdiagnosed as tinea pedis. The soft corn is painful and appears as a flat white soggy area on the opposing surfaces of adjacent toes usually in the fourth interdigital web. Other interdigital spaces may be involved, for the condition occurs whenever the condyle of a phalanx of one toe presses against the condyle of the head of the adjacent metatarsal. Paring away the superficial material reveals two small cores opposing each other. Sometimes for chronic cases a sinus track with purulent exudate will be present. Treatment of the soft corn may be simply separating the toes with a cushion such as lambs wool or a thin piece of foam rubber, or other measures may be tried such as keeping the corn thin by paring and by application of a keratolytic such as salicylic acid plaster. Again, proper fitting shoes that give the toes room to spread apart should be

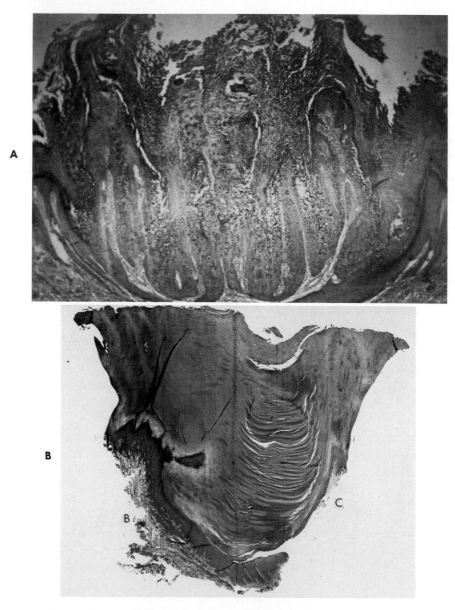

Fig. 16-2. Microscopic sections of a verruca. **A,** Typical mushrooming of the entire epidermis. Note the thickening of the rete pegs with some fusion at the base and degeneration at the top. **B,** Compression of subdermal living epithelium. Hyperkeratinization of the uppermost layers of epidermis, with flushing of the rete Malpighi (*B* and *C*), is shown.

worn. If these conservative measures fail, excision of the prominent condyle will effect a cure.

Plantar warts or "papillomas of the sole" are frequent lesions seen in a dermatology office. They can occur on any part of the foot; and when they occur under pressure points, they give rise to tenderness and localized pain. Fig. 16-2 presents the histologic difference between a wart and a keratotic lesion (e.g., a callus). Warts are caused by a DNA virus belonging to the papovavirus group. The first step in treatment is to pare away the superficial keratin surface. A sharply marginated lesion appears with many capillary dots which rise perpendicular to the surface of the skin.

Plantar warts are usually grouped into one of three types:

1. A single or solitary wart surrounded by callus tissue with the papillary lines diverging around it. Depending on its location, if it is located under a bony prominence, it may be painful (Fig. 16-3).

2. Multiple warts, a second type, characterized by a large "mother" wart surrounded by tiny "daughter" warts which appear as blister satellites nearby (Fig. -16-4). When these tiny lesions are pared, a minute capillary usually is found.

3. The mosaic wart, which is usually painless and is commonly mistaken for a callus. These warts may be quite large (several centimeters in diameter) and may be present for years appearing as patches of individually coalescent cores resembling a mosaic (Fig. 16-5).

Treatment of plantar warts vexes most dermatologists since these viral lesions show a strong tendency to recur. Nonscarring measures are preferable because of the tendency

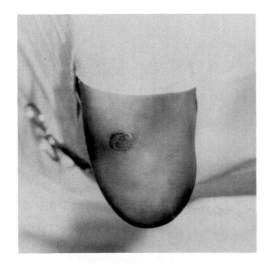

Fig. 16-3. Typical verruca plantaris on the heel.

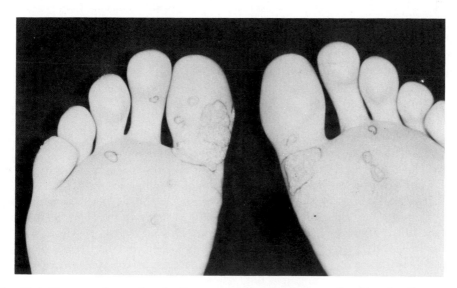

Fig. 16-4. Verrucae; larger "mother" warts and their satellite smaller "daughter" warts.

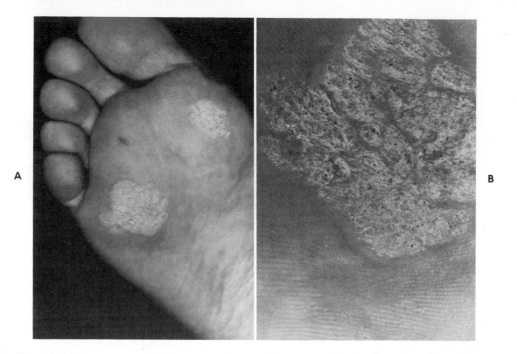

Fig. 16-5. Mosaic verrucae. **A,** Large colonies of wart tissue localized on the sole. **B,** Mosaic pattern of this viral lesion.

of the scars to be painful. Use of 40% salicylic acid plaster when applicable sometimes reduces the warts and occasionally cures them. Other measures, like the application of 10% formalin and then covering with 40% acid plaster and tape nightly, a measure devised by Tromovitch and Kay (1973), will cure many plantar warts. Cryosurgery with liquid nitrogen is frequently effective for small plantar warts. Blunt dissection of the plantar warts (Pringle and Helms, 1973) is another popular method for treating multiple and single warts. In this method, the tissue about the wart is anesthetized and the wart is dissected out with a blunt dissector and scissors, care being exercised not to go too deeply in the dermis. A pressure dressing or mild caustic such as trichloroacetic acid or silver nitrate is applied to the base. Deep electrosurgery and surgical excision should be avoided on all plantar warts because of the resultant scar. Acid therapy with use of the 40% salicylic acid plaster is one of the best overall forms of treatment for most plantar warts. It is conservative, usually non-painful, and does not cause scarring; and the plaster cut to the size and shape of the wart is held in close apposition by plastic nonporous tape changed daily or at longer intervals depending on the case. Sometimes a combination of other acids such as trichloroacetic acid or even the stronger bichloracetic acid is swabbed on the warts. These other acids are quite painful, but together with paring and repeated 40% sal acid plasters application the acid methods produce good results. Weeks or even months may be required for eradication, however.

Friction blisters. Everyone at some time in his life has had a blister develop on the feet from wearing a new pair of shoes or exercising strenuously when the feet have not been accustomed to such activity. A typical clear fluid blister develops that, with proper rest, goes on toward complete healing. If a patient develops recurrent blisters on the feet, consideration should be given to an entity called Weber-Cockayne type of epidermolysis bullosa. This acquired form was first described in soldiers who developed blisters after taking long marches. The vesicles or bullae appeared on the soles although the weight-bearing areas were predominantly affected.

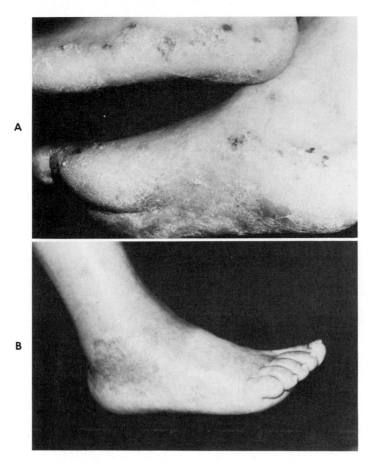

Fig. 16-6. Tinea pedis. Two patterns of chronic *Trichophyton rubrum* infection of the feet. **A,** Diffuse red scaly pattern of a moccasin which had been present for two decades. **B,** Note the annular serpiginous character of the fungus on the lateral side of the foot.

COMMON INFECTIONS OF THE FEET
Tinea (superficial fungal infections, tinea pedis)

"Athlete's foot," the term used often to designate a superficial fungal infection of the feet, is frequently misdiagnosed and mistreated. Fungal infections of the feet are chronic in a high proportion of American men. Women show a lower frequency of infection because generally their feet are cooler, drier, and cleaner. Warmth and moisture are the factors that lead to increased maceration and penetration of the causative fungal organisms. The two most common organisms causing tinea pedis are *Tricophyton rubrum* and *Tricophyton mentagrophytes*.

The characteristic scaling and maceration between the toes, a sign of tinea infection of the feet, usually involves the fourth and fifth interdigital webs. The *T. rubrum* infections tend to be chronic and often show a low-grade dry salmon-colored scaly inflammation on the sole of the foot, such as the instep and the sides, sometimes enveloping the foot like a moccasin (Fig. 16-6). The *T. mentagrophytes* fungal infection frequently shows clusters of blisters about the toes or in the area of the transverse arch (Fig. 16-7). Diagnosis of this type of infection can be made by performing a 10% potassium hydroxide examination of skin scrapings and discovering the mycelial elements as long branch forms. Fungus culture can pinpoint the pathogen but requires 2 to 4 weeks for final diagnosis. Besides involving

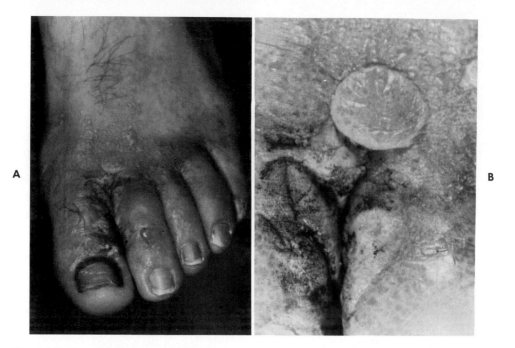

Fig. 16-7. Tinea pedis. **A,** Vesicular form, most often caused by the organism *Trichophyton mentagrophytes*. **B,** Close-up of vesicle.

the toes and soles, tinea may affect the dorsum of the foot; the most common site is the base of the fourth and fifth toes. On the dorsum of the foot, the fungal infection assumes the more typical "ringworm" pattern—central clearing and extension of the lesions with an annular configuration. Fungal infections of the feet are rare in children before puberty although they do occur.

In the differential diagnosis of tinea of the feet, one must consider various forms of eczema (e.g., atopic, contact, dyshidrosis) and other entities like psoriasis and soft corns. In high school boys a not rare complication involves the progression of a tinea infection. Impetiginization and cellulitis occur and occasionally ascending lymphangitis. Use of proprietary irritant medication often causes a severe contact dermatitis.

Treatment of the fungal infection depends on the type of infection. For the acute blistering tinea pedis caused by *T. mentagrophytes*, one should not overtreat with antifungal agents but should first treat the raw oozing surface of the skin as an acute dermatitis with antiseptic soaks like Burow's solution and

soothing ointments like vioform-HC cream. There are a number of excellent local fungistatic agents that are beneficial—miconazole nitrate cream and clotrimazole cream. Advice should be given to the patient to keep the skin of the feet exposed to the air to dry out. Griseofulvin should not be used as a routine measure in the therapy of most tinea pedis infections.

Mycotic infection of the toenails frequently accompanies tinea pedis or on occasion involves one or more of the toenails. Zaias (1972) has grouped four types of onychomycosis:

1. Distal subungual onychomycosis, primarily involving the distal nail bed and hyponychium with secondary involvement of the underside of the nail plate.

2. White superficial onychomycosis. This is invasion of the toenail plate on the surface of the nail by such organisms as *T. mentagrophytes*, *Cephalosporium*, and *Aspergillus*.

3. Proximal subungual onychomycosis, very rare.

4. *Candida* onychomycosis involving the entire nail plate.

The distal subungual onychomycosis is

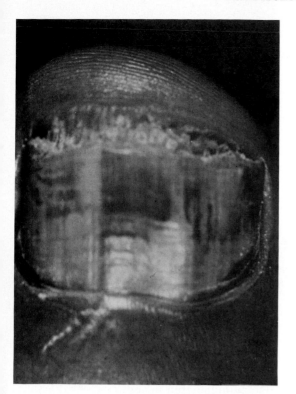

Fig. 16-8. Onychomycosis toenail. An advanced example of distal subungual onychomycosis. Involved nails are thickened and opaque with distal crumbly material. In the toe web spaces, the interdigital psoriasis appears white and is frequently mistaken for fungal infection.

most common. This deeply seated form of onychomycosis is seen as yellowish longitudinal streaks within the nail, the parasite invading progressively from the free edge toward the root, thickening the nail bed and deforming the plate.

The second type, white superficial onychomycosis, appears as opaque white well-demarcated islands on the surface of toenail plates. Of this type there are various etiologic agents, but the commonest is *T. mentagrophytes*. The abnormal whitish crumbly material can be easily scraped off with a glass slide.

The third type, proximal subungual onychomycosis, is uncommon and consists of white areas extending distally from underneath the proximal nail fold. *T. rubrum* and others have been found to produce this type of onychomycosis.

The fourth type of nail onychomycosis, *Candida*, appears as opaque noncrumbly nails which have longitudinal white strands within the nail plate (Fig. 16-8). The nail bed thickens and the distal digit appears bulbous and pseudoclubbed. Diagnosis of toenail mycosis is either by potassium hydroxide examination of nail scrapings with identification of the fungal elements or by fungus culture. Treatment of the dermatophytic onychomycosis resides unquestionably with oral griseofulvin in adequate dosage, usually 1 gm of microcrystalline griseofulvin daily for toenail infection. This therapy may need to be continued for 8 to 12 months. There is a high rate of failure, however, usually evident in a few months after the patient has been on the drug. Recently glutaraldehyde solution 10% buffered to a final pH of 7.8 has been used as an ancillary form of toenail mycotic therapy. For nondermatophytic onychomycosis such as *Scopulariopsis brevicaulis*, avulsion of the involved nails is perhaps the best treatment and is curative in the majority of cases. There is no effective drug for this organism.

Bacterial infections occur frequently on the feet and are conveniently divided into primary and secondary pyodermas. Impetigo is a superficial skin infection that may be caused by *Staphylococcus* or *Streptococcus* or both and usually affects grade school children. Lesions consist of thin-walled vesicles on an erythematous base. The vesicles form yellow crusts, and peripheral extension results in irregular serpiginous lesions. The lesions are common on the face but can occur everywhere on the body except the palms and the soles. Ecthyma is a form of pyoderma which begins as small vesicles or pustules on an erythematous base and quickly develops a purulent, irregular ulcer. These lesions are common on the lower extremities and like impetigo readily respond to systemic antibiotics. Burow's compresses are helpful in removing the crusts, and topical antibiotic ointment should be applied several times daily.

Paronychia is a cellulitis of the nail folds characterized by swelling, erythema, pain, tenderness, and often a purulent discharge from beneath the nail fold. Secondary dystrophic changes of the nail are frequently seen, and chronic paronychia involvement with *Candida* may occur. Therapy consists of treating any underlying predisposing systemic disease such as diabetes and systemic antibiotics as indicated by culture and sensitivities. If *Candida* infection is present, specific antiyeast therapy with nystatin or amphotericin B topically may be instituted. Secondary pyodermas which may affect the feet can be grouped into the following categories:

1. Infectious eczematoid dermatitis, resulting from a discharge of wet drainage seeping over the skin from an underlying cellulitis or pyogenic infection. Autoinoculation often occurs, and the infection spreads by contiguous drainage.

2. Infected intertrigo, resulting from the effects of friction, moisture, and sweat retention, and common between the toes, where it has often been diagnosed as tinea infection. Treatment consists of promoting dryness by cool drying compresses and a bland absorbent powder. Secondary infection is treated by the appropriate topical antibiotic.

3. Miscellaneous pyogenic infections of the toe webs by gram-negative bacteria, such as *Pseudomonas* and *Proteus*, producing clinical pyodermic infections which are resistant to the usual forms of antibacterial therapy. The organisms and therapy should be determined by culture and sensitivities. Careful investigation to determine the presence of any underlying systemic disorders such as diabetes, lymphoma, or immunoglobulin defect that could predispose to the establishment of such cutaneous infections should be made. Amonette and Rosenberg (1973) found topical management with a combination of bed rest, exposure to air, and application of silver nitrate solution, Castellani's paint, and gentamicin sulfate cream to be the best solution to therapy.

4. Erythrasma, frequently seen in the intertriginous areas such as the toe webs. The causative organism is a tiny bacterium called *Corynebacterium minutissimum* producing a well-demarcated reddish brown fine desquamation that fluoresces orange-red or coral pink under the Woods lamp. Wearing loose clothing and using antibacterial soaps will usually prevent this infection or eliminate it once established, but some cases require oral erythromycin.

Not every form of intertrigo of the toe webs is linked to an infection as by a fungus or a bacterium (e.g., psoriasis) that when it has extensive involvement of the skin, involving the feet, usually also infects the web areas, where the eruption appears white and soggy. Confirmation of the entity is by therapeutic trial of a topical steroid cream which is effective in eliminating this form of intertrigo.

SPECIFIC DISCRETE SKIN LESIONS OF THE FEET
Benign pigmented nevus

Melanocytic nevi are the most common "skin tumor" in human beings, an estimated average of twenty or more nevi occurring per adult (Lerner, 1972), although for various reasons this count may be inaccurate. Suffice it that everyone has several nevi. More nevi occur on the upper part of the body than on the lower; but some appear on the foot, and hence the physician may be asked concerning opinions for management of a particular lesion. Most people have no pigmented lesions at birth; fewer than 3% of infants are born with pigmented nevi, the nevi appearing a few years after birth like small dark dots which gradually enlarge as the person grows.

The varieties of nevi, named as to the histologic appearance of their "nevus cells," fall into three general types—junctional, intradermal, and compound. Since 50% of melanomas arise from preexisting nevi, it is important to know which nevi should be excised. Junctional and compound nevi are subjected to constant rubbing or trauma and should be excised. Small, flat, light brown lesions on the palms and soles should be left alone. Approximately 12% of people have pigmented lesions on their palms and soles, and it is not practical to excise all these lesions. The infrequently encountered large, elevated, dark nevus of the palm or sole, however, should be removed. Increase in size, darkening of color, itching, inflammation, and trauma are events which arouse concern in the patient regarding previously ignored nevi. In children and young adults nevi enlarge as the person grows. Bleeding into a nevus results in a blue to black discoloration. Changes vary according to the depth and extent of the bleeding. Most bleeding occurs following trauma. The injury may have been mild and is often forgotten by the patient. At times the examiner cannot tell whether the darkening is due to melanin or to blood; hence the lesion must be excised.

The blue nevus is another variety of melanocytic nevus that is so called because of the dark blue-black color of the lesion which results from the melanin pigment deep in the dermis. These nevi may be distributed anywhere on the body and not infrequently appear on the feet. Although generally benign, blue nevi can show malignant transformation so they will have to be evaluated with regard to change in size, irritation, etc. as discussed earlier (Fig. 16-9).

Glomus tumor. The glomus tumor is most frequently encountered on the acral portions of the extremities. The lesion is often subungual and consists of a purplish nodule measuring only a few millimeters in diameter. It is tender and gives rise to severe paroxysmal pains. Glomus tumors rarely ulcerate or bleed, and excision usually results in a cure although subungual lesions are more difficult to eradicate. Differential diagnoses include ordinary hemangiomas as well as neuroma, Kaposi's sarcoma, hemangiopericytoma and granuloma telangiectaticum. There is another type of glomus tumor characterized by multiple painless hemangiomas and frequently a familial pattern (Conant and Wisenfeld, 1971). The multiple lesions are usually asymptomatic.

Eccrine poroma. Eccrine poroma was first described by Pinkus et al. in 1956 as a fairly common solitary tumor two thirds of which occur on the soles or sides of the feet. This benign tumor derived from the eccrine sweat ducts usually arises in the young or in middle-aged adults. It has a rather firm

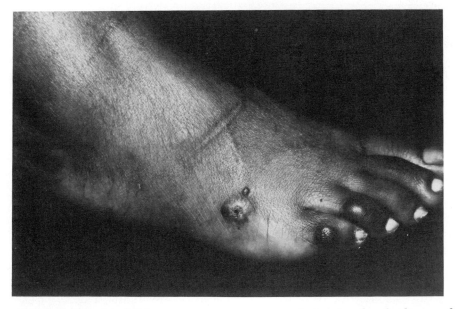

Fig. 16-9. Nevi of the feet. A blue nevus is not an uncommon lesion, found on the dorsum of the foot. It is characterized by a dark blue-black color and often simulates a melanoma.

consistency, is often raised and slightly pedunculated, is usually asymptomatic, and measures less than 2 cm in diameter (Fig. 16-10). Treatment by excision is curative in any location.

Epidermal inclusion cyst. Epidermal cysts are common skin lesions on the scalp, face, trunk, and extremities; infrequently they occur on the palms and rarely on the soles. When an epidermal cyst arises on the sole, it is probably a result of traumatic implantation of the epidermis. The lesions are often misdiagnosed as callus or verruca and appear as an elevated nodule of up to 2 cm diameter that is movable and tender. The differential diagnoses include synovial lesion, fibroma, xanthoma, and tumors of the appendages. Surgical removal usually is curative (Greer, 1974).

Pyogenic granuloma. The pyogenic granuloma, sometimes called granuloma telangiectaticum, resembles proud flesh and occurs as a single lesion of dull red color that is soft to moderately firm, raised, and slightly pedunculated. It usually grows rapidly to 0.5 cm; occasionally, however, it reaches a size of 2 cm and remains unchanged. The surface of the lesion shows ulceration and crusting, and the patient relates that the lesion bleeds easily when only slightly touched. It may appear on the foot but most commonly is located on the fingers and face. Staphylococcal infection appears to have a role in the development of pyogenic granulomas, and they not uncommonly are seen on the lateral nail folds of the toes in conjunction with ingrown toenails. Differential diagnosis includes hemangioma, epithelioma, eccrine poroma, malignant melanoma, or foreign body granuloma. The treatment is surgical by excision, although on the soles simple electrodesiccation and curettage can be relied on to effect a consistent cure.

Dermatofibroma. Dermatofibromas occur in the skin as firm, indolent, single or multiple nodules usually situated on the extremities, but they may occur anywhere. There are several synonyms for this lesion: nodular subepidermal fibrosis, sclerosing hemangioma, histiocytoma; basically the lesion represents a reactive fibrosis consequent to some idiopathic inflammatory process.

The firm papules measure a few millimeters in size but may get as large as 2 to 3 cm. Most have a reddish brown color but occasionally become bluish black, even suggesting a malignant melanoma. In the histiocytomas, because of the cellular composition of the tumor, frequently the color is yellow due to lipid composition. Treatment is by surgical excision, although, if the lesions are asymptomatic and not enlarging, they may be observed.

Foreign body of the sole. Frequently foreign bodies of the sole are mistaken for warts or corns because of the protective callus which has formed. When this covering is pared away, some pus may exude and further shaving will reveal a foreign body such as a stiff hair, a rose thorn, a piece of glass, a shell particle, or anything that may have invaded the skin. Once it has been extracted, a cure

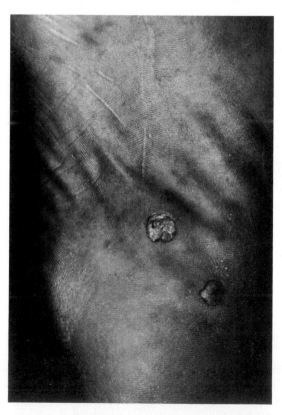

Fig. 16-10. Eccrine poroma; an adnexal papillomatous tumor frequently arising on the feet. Here, two poromas near the heel appear almost like verrucae. They are pedunculated friable lesions which bleed easily.

quickly results. When confronted with small calluses of the feet not overlying bony prominences, the physician should always consider the possibility of the presence of an imbedded hair (Morrell, 1957).

Keloids. Of the three types of scar—the ordinary flat scar, elevated hypertrophic scar, and keloid—only the keloid shows extension of the scarring process beyond the borders of the initial injury; the hypertrophic and ordinary scars conform almost exactly to the area of injury. There is probably a predisposing genetic factor in the production of keloids, and certainly a racial factor, since blacks are more susceptible. Moreover, certain areas such as the V area of the chest and the ear lobes, especially in women, are prone to develop keloids.

The keloid presents as a brawny elevated lesion that is usually hyperemic or hyperpigmented in the early stages and later becomes hard and stony white. Hypertrophic scars and keloids are frequently pruritic and sensitive to pressure. Because they may regress spontaneously, hypertrophic scars have a better prognosis than do keloids. Treatment of keloids involves intralesional injection with corticosteroids or radiotherapy; plastic surgery may be necessary with concomitant medical therapy including administration of systemic corticosteroids.

Black heel. Black heel is a curious entity, usually affecting the sole, first described by Crissey and Peachey in 1961 under the title of "Calcaneal Petechiae." The lesion presents as an irregular black or bluish black plaque, oval or circular in shape, on the posterior or posterolateral aspect of one or both heels (Fig. 16-11).

Usually only a single lesion is present that at first glance may represent a melanoma or a large verruca with capillary tufts. However, paring the lesion with a scalpel reveals the true nature in successive layers of reddish brown punctate specks of dry blood which arise because of a sudden shearing force such as encountered in active sports (e.g., weight lifting, basketball, jogging, tennis). This condition, which is completely asymptomatic, almost invariably affects adolescents and

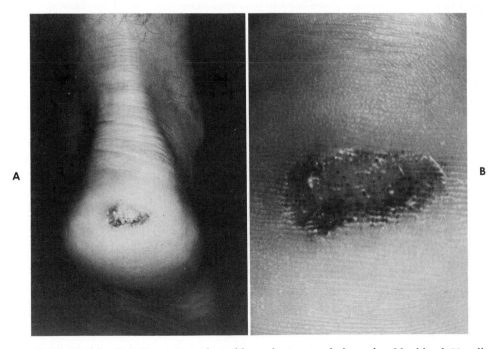

A

B

Fig. 16-11. Black heel. **A,** Keratotic and wartlike with pinpoint dark specks of dry blood. Usually situated on the posterior heel, it characterizes the black heel (seen in athletes). **B,** Close-up of the lesion.

young adults; after a diagnosis has been made, no treatment is required although paring can remove the entire lesion.

Arteriovenous fistula. An uncommon skin lesion, usually on the foot or ankle, that simulates Kaposi's sarcoma, the arteriovenous fistula is seen in patients who are young (under 30) as opposed to the older age of patients affected by Kaposi's sarcoma.

The skin lesions are soft reddish purple nodules and plaques which frequently ulcerate. Other characteristics include hyperpigmentation and a fibrous verrucoid eruption. The lesion results because of an arteriovenous communication without an intervening capillary bed. Such fistulas are either traumatically acquired or congenital in origin. Other manifestations include enlargement of the limb, pain, bruit, increased warmth, stasis changes, edema, paresthesias, and increased sweating. Diagnosis is made by appreciation of the clinical signs and symptoms along with skin biopsy. Therapy, of course, is surgical.

Chromoblastomycosis and mycetoma. These deep fungal infections are included in the present discussion because, although uncommon clinically, they characteristically and typically affect the foot. The chromoblastomycosis is caused by several morphologically similar fungi, of which the chief offenders are *Fonsecaea pedrosi, F. compactum,* and *Phialophora verrucosa.*

The lesion is slow growing and wartlike, occasionally developing an ulcerative papilloma with a tendency to spread along the lymphatic channels. Lymphedema and secondary infection may occur later. There is a high incidence of this infection among workers who are exposed to injury with wood. Usually the infection remains localized without dissemination. To be considered in the differential diagnosis are other verrucoid ulcerative diseases such as blastomycosis, madura foot, and bromoderma. Treatment depends on the organism; amphotericin B has been recommended for some cases.

Mycetoma (also called maduromycosis or madura foot). This deforming deep fungal infection usually affects the foot but may involve the hand and invade the skin, subcutaneous tissue, and bone. Again, several organisms are involved and the type of infection depends on the geographic area.

The infection starts as a small indurated subcutaneous papular nodule presumably from the site of trauma on the foot. The overlying skin breaks down, forming a sinus track; then exudates appear containing the characteristic white, yellow, red, pink, or black granules according to the particular fungus involved. The "granules" are actually small hyphae produced by species of *Nocardia* or *Streptomyces;* granules with larger hyphae are produced by *Allescheria boydii* or other fungi. The infection continues for months or years penetrating into the deep fascia, muscle, or bone with abscess and sinus formation and overgrowth of granulation tissue. The result is grotesque enlargement of the foot and deformity which is usually relatively painless (Fig. 16-12). Therapy depends on the organism. Some of the mycetomas caused by the actinomycetes respond to large doses of penicillin. Other drugs are being used, including the sulfas, but sometimes mycetomas are unresponsive and amputation of the foot becomes necessary.

Malignant discrete skin lesions of the feet

Malignant melanoma. Often referred to as melanocarcinoma or the black cancer, this lesion can occur anywhere on the cutaneous surface or mucous membranes yet is frequently encountered on the soles. In the majority of instances melanomas probably originate from preexisting nevi or pigmented lesions. This highly malignant disease is rarely seen in blacks; but when it occurs in blacks, the lesions are usually on the soles of the feet (Fig. 16-13). Clinically the lesion presents as a jet black mottled junctional nevus with the following history:

1. Increase in size
2. Increase in pigmentation
3. Formation of crusts
4. Formation of nodules within the lesion
5. Bleeding and ulceration

There is a wide range of clinical appearances of melanomas since almost any color

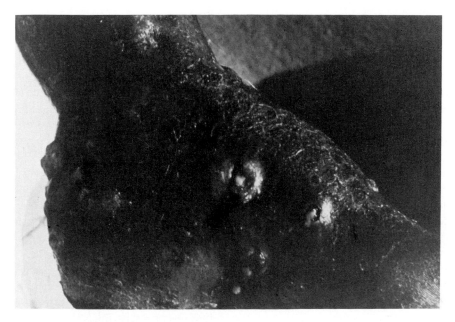

Fig. 16-12. Maduromycosis. This long-standing deep fungal infection of the subcutaneous tissues results in marked deformity of the foot with sinus tracks, fibrosis, and papulonodules. Exudates containing the characteristic "granules" drain from the multiple sinuses and abscesses.

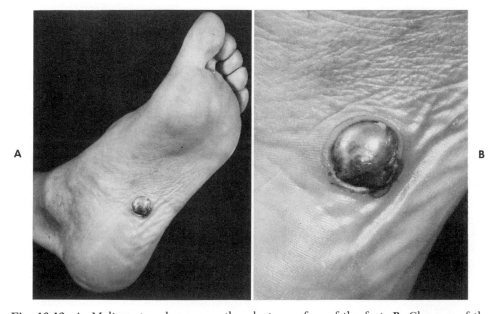

Fig. 16-13. A, Malignant melanoma on the plantar surface of the foot. **B,** Close-up of the lesion.

change can be seen. Even the amelanotic melanomas, those lacking any melanin pigment, are deadly. Differential diagnosis of melanoma includes very active junctional nevus, prickle cell epithelioma, pyogenic granuloma, Kaposi's sarcoma, seborrheic keratosis, and angiokeratoma. Treatment includes wide surgical excision and, depending on the type of melanoma (superficial spreading or nodular) and its depth of penetration, possible lymph node surgery.

Kaposi's sarcoma. Multiple idiopathic hemorrhagic sarcoma or Kaposi's sarcoma has a predilection for the feet and affects predominantly men, especially those in the fifth to seventh decades (Fig. 16-14). There are some interesting racial incidences: in the United States the majority of cases occur in people who have immigrated from eastern Europe or who are of Jewish origin; in certain areas of Africa, the condition is endemic.

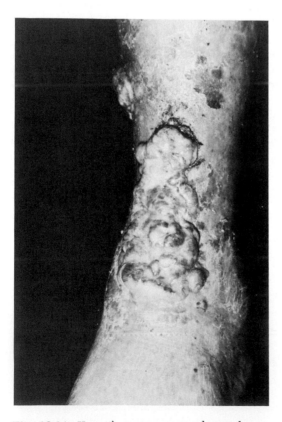

Fig. 16-14. Kaposi's sarcoma; an advanced case with ulceration and beginning fungating tumors.

The earliest clinical lesion appears as a pyogenic granuloma–like papule usually on the soles, less commonly on the palms. Sometimes the bluish, violaceous, semihard millet seed tumor gradually occurs with a tendency to coalesce; other times it seems to form verrucoid plaques resembling those of lichen planus. Lymphostasis is a common occurrence in advanced Kaposi's sarcoma and may result in considerable brawny edema of the leg. Untreated, the verrucoid papules grow to huge fungating tumors with ulceration. The disease is systemic in many cases with involvement of the gastrointestinal tract and other internal organs. Differential diagnosis includes stasis dermatitis, hypertrophic lichen planus, malignant melanoma, arteriovenous fistula, and deep mycoses. Treatment includes several modalities such as chemotherapy, radiotherapy, electrocautery, excision, and cryosurgery. Profusion with radioactive elements has also been employed.

Squamous cell carcinoma. This malignant tumor of the skin uncommonly affects the feet but is important because of its tendency to metastasize. The squamous cell carcinoma, sometimes called "prickle cell epithelioma," develops on the feet in association with previously damaged or diseased skin (Fig. 16-15). It may arise on the sites of burned out lupus vulgaris or discoid lupus erythematosus after a long period of time; it is also seen on skin that is chronically scarred or ulcerated by a previous injury such as a severe burn, the malignant ulceration being called a "Marjolin ulcer."

The squamous cell carcinoma itself is not distinctive and presents as a friable ulcerated tumor with a granular surface. It may be mistaken for a pyogenic granuloma, basal cell carcinoma, eccrine poroma, verruca, foreign body granuloma, or deep fungal infection such as chromoblastomycosis. Keratoacanthomas are another lesion which mimic the squamous cell carcinoma; but they develop quickly, in a matter of weeks or months, whereas a squamous carcinoma usually develops slowly. Differentiation between these two lesions histologically is often difficult. Early treatment by surgical excision or, if small, by electrodesiccation and curettage prevents further complications.

Bowen's disease is a form of squamous cell carcinoma that because of its histology is often referred to as intraepithelial epithelioma or squamous cell carcinoma in situ (Fig. 16-16). The tumor usually does not present as a growth but more often resembles a plaque of psoriasis, eczema, or even tinea. It is usually erythematous and scaly, and the patient will remark that this "sore does not heal" but persists and enlarges. There is an association of Bowen's disease with internal malignancies, especially carcinoma of the respiratory and gastrointestinal tract (Graham and Helwig). Management of Bowen's disease consists of diagnosis and biopsy followed by local excision. An alternate surgical technique, if the lesion is very small, is destruction of the superficial tumor by electodesiccation and curettage.

Epithelioma cuniculatum is another variant of the squamous cell carcinoma; it occurs on the sole and is very rare. This malignant lesion consists of a bulbous mass that is deeply involuted and perforated by numerous sinus tracks. Undoubtedly its appearance is influenced by the pressure effects of weight bearing. Metastases are not seen, for the tumor is only locally malignant. Treatment consists of surgical excision. In some cases, because of the extent of the lesion, amputation of the foot has been required.

Arsenic introduced into the body through industrial chemicals, medicinals, or hidden sources may be the cause of squamous cell carcinoma on the skin of the feet and on other portions of the integument. Inorganic arsenic

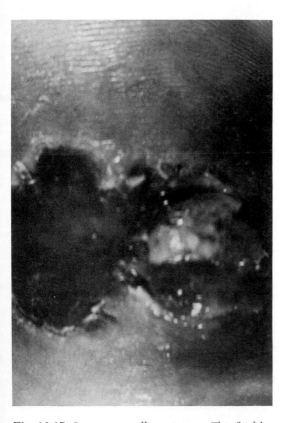

Fig. 16-15. Squamous cell carcinoma. This friable persistent ulceration developed on the foot of a 65-year-old man who also had multiple arsenical keratoses on the palms and soles.

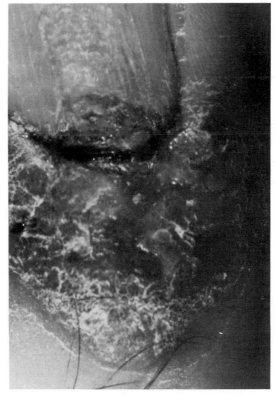

Fig. 16-16. Bowen's disease. This carcinoma-in-situ is frequently mistaken for tinea infection or eczema and presents as a red, scaly, oozing, persistent patch of abnormal skin on the digits.

in such medications as Fowler's solution, from sources like insecticides, and through industrial exposure as in mining and paints constitutes another form of this poisoning. There is a long latent period after introduction of the heavy metal into the system. Decades later discrete keratoses develop on the palms and soles along with epitheliomas on the torso and extremities. A peculiar diagnostic hyperpigmentation may occur in chronic arsenic poisoning and is seen as a "raindrop" form on the back or chest. Bowen's disease develops in cases of arsenic intoxication on the palms and soles as well as the extremities and torso. If the earlier squamous cell lesions are ignored, frank invasive squamous cell carcinomas may be seen on the acral areas of the extremities. Treatment consists of surgical excision of the carcinoma.

Basal cell carcinoma also goes by the term basal cell epithelioma or "rodent ulcer." This tumor, which is the most common malignant tumor usually affecting the exposed areas of the body where sunlight hits, is extremely rare on the sole of the foot. Basal cell carcinoma is locally malignant and as a rule does not metastasize. The lesion may show a pearly border, although on the foot it appears more like a pyogenic granuloma. Treatment is by surgical excision.

INFLAMMATORY SKIN PROBLEMS OF THE FEET

Eczema is a common inflammatory condition of the skin in which the rash shows vesicles, erythema and subsequent fissuring, crusting, and marked itching. Dermatitis is used as a synonym for the older *eczema* term. There are other manifestations of eczema in the more chronic form—like hyperpigmentation and thickening of the skin with hyperkeratinization, sometimes called lichenification. Various forms of eczema are localized to the feet.

Atopic dermatitis may involve the palms and soles and in some cases other characteristic body areas (Fig. 16-17). It often has the familial background of the so-called atopic diseases—allergic rhinitis, asthma, urticaria, or migraine headache. Frequently this intrin-

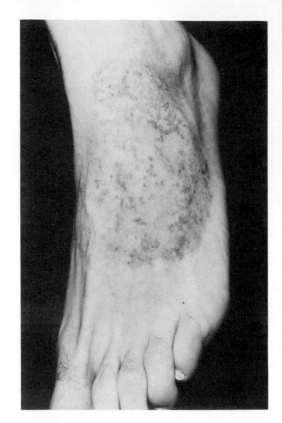

Fig. 16-17. Atopic dermatitis. This patch of eczematoid rash could be confused with tinea or contact dermatitis from shoes. Involvement of the flexural folds plus the chronic history supports the diagnosis of atopic dermatitis.

sic form of eczema begins in infancy or childhood, and the patients may be misdiagnosed as having fungal infection of the skin of the hands and feet and treated with antifungal medications without response. The diagnosis of atopic dermatitis involving the feet is difficult at times because of (1) the impression derived from a background of atopic diseases in the patient's history or family history and (2) the chronicity of the process without other factors such as contact being present.

Dyshidrotic eczema, also sometimes called pompholyx, is an eczematoid reaction affecting the soles and the palms. Usually only these areas of the skin are affected; clinically there are deep-seated noninflammatory vesicles or even large bullae which develop singly or in groups. The blisters are clear at first and then become cloudy or even pustular. Although the palms and soles are the usual sites of involvement, other areas such as the sides of the fingers and the backs of the hands may be affected. Since hyperhidrosis sometimes is an accompanying symptom, these vesicles were formerly thought to be evidence of sweat retention. This thought is no longer held, however, and current research indicates that dyshidrosis is simply an eczematoid reaction pattern of the skin. The dyshidrotic pattern is unique only by virtue of the anatomy of the hands and feet. Current thought as to etiology includes atopic dermatitis, a form of neuro-dermatitis, and an allergic reaction akin to dermatophytids.

Contact dermatitis or eczema may be of two basic types: a primary irritant and an allergic variety. Examples of substances used on the feet that can cause primary irritant reaction are soaps, detergents, and acids such as salicylic, benzoic, and trichloroacetic. By contrast, there is a whole range of potential allergenic substances included in dermatologic medications employed in everyday practice. Such proprietary medications as benzocaine along with topical antibiotics and topical antihistamines are examples of these cutaneous sensitizers. The picture of a contact dermatitis secondary to topical medications shows the agent localized to a certain part of the skin of the foot. Here there may be erythema, edema, vesiculation, or even frank bullae. Patch testing may be helpful in cases of allergic contact dermatitis after the initial acute episode has subsided.

Shoe dermatitis is another, not uncommon, form of allergic contact dermatitis (Fig. 16-18). Many ingredients are responsible for this type of allergy, the most common being the rubber as well as the various glues that are used in cementing the outer leather to the usual inner cloth lining of shoes. The picture of shoe dermatitis shows a dermatitis involving the dorsal aspects of the feet and toes and as a rule bilateral. The patient may have recently purchased a new pair of shoes, which further incriminates his footwear as the cause of the skin problem. Patch testing to the several ingredients used in the manufacture of

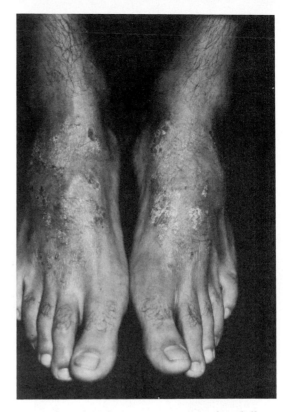

Fig. 16-18. Shoe dermatitis; two examples of allergic contact dermatitis, a reaction to one of the ingredients of new shoes. The clinical picture is of bilateral rashes involving the dorsa of the feet.

shoes may reveal the culprit to be mercapto-benzothiazol, one of the thiurams or mono-benzyl ether of hydroquinone, or rarely a chromate. Differential diagnosis of a shoe contact dermatitis involves atopic dermatitis and tinea pedis

Treatment of all forms of eczema of the feet usually involves application of corticosteroid creams and lotions as well as cool astringent compresses or foot soaks when the process is in the acute vesicular stage. Vioform sometimes combined with steroid cream and tar preparations also is helpful in treating the more chronic cases. Oral medications such as systemic corticosteroids are sometimes required if the process is severe; and likewise if secondary infection or cellulitis is present, antibiotics should be given orally.

Psoriasis. Psoriasis is a skin disease affecting an estimated 1% to 2% of the population. There are many varieties of this dermatosis; but suffice it that the usual varieties involve the sites of predilection, such as the elbows, knees, scalp, and the more severe cases show lesions on the extremities and torso. In all forms, no matter how severe, there may be psoriatic lesions on the feet and palms (Fig. 16-19). Sometimes a form of the disease called "inverse psoriasis" appears in which the psoriatic lesions are on the opposite skin areas such as the flexor regions rather than the extensor. Another form of psoriasis, so-called pustular psoriasis, involves the palms and soles. On the feet the lesions of pustular psoriasis are characterized by patches of erythematous skin studded with small discrete pustules. On culture of these pustular lesions, the report comes back sterile.

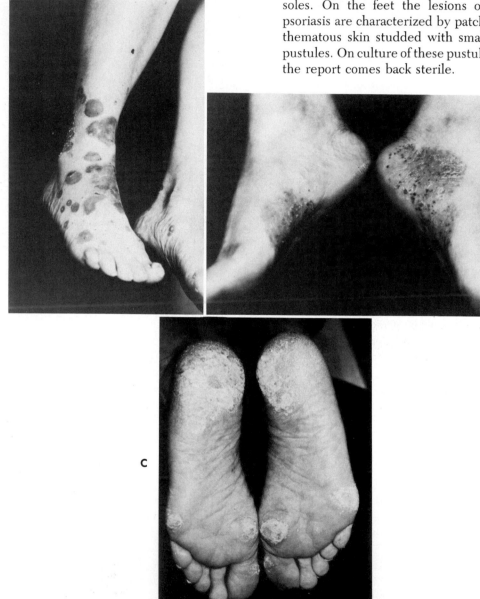

Fig. 16-19. Psoriasis. Three variations on the theme of psoriasis. **A,** Discrete red plaques on the right foot. There were also similar typical psoriatic lesions on the elbow and knees. **B,** Pustules involving characteristically the soles. The rash consists of confluent erythematous patches with scaling and pustules. **C,** Marked discrete keratoderma on the weight-bearing surfaces of the feet.

Psoriasis usually is manifested by an erythematous plaque covered by a white silvery scale that is adherent and when removed leaves a tiny bleeding site. The lesions are discrete and sharply demarcated from the normal skin. When the soles are involved, there is a marked tendency for the psoriatic lesions to be more hyperkeratotic and fissured. Frequently the lesions of psoriasis involving the palms and soles are mistaken for "eczema." Another variant in the clinical picture of psoriasis involving the feet is so-called "white psoriasis" seen in the toe webs. This abnormality, manifested by macerated white skin, may be misdiagnosed as tinea infection because of negative microscopic scrapings, negative fungus cultures, and the presence of psoriasis elsewhere on the body. Treatment of psoriasis on the feet is similar to treatment of the condition elsewhere on the body: reliance on topical potent steroid creams usually with occlusive technique at night to promote greater absorption. Occasionally, topical tar preparations and soaking the feet in bath oils and the use of keratolytic agents are helpful.

Lichen planus. This is another papulosquamous disease of the skin characterized by flat-topped shiny violaceous papules which are usually distinctive in their location (Fig. 16-20). The volar aspects of the wrists, sacral area of the back, and mucous membranes such as the buccal areas in the mouth and the vulva or penis are involved. This dermatosis is usually pruritic, yet one does not see many excoriations from scratching. The cause is unknown although flareups occur with nervous tension.

There are various forms of this disease, such as the hypertrophic form (which may be seen as thicker infiltrated plaques on the shins of the legs) and the erosive lichen planus form (which can affect the feet with extensive ulceration and may involve the mucous membranes). Diagnosis of lichen planus is usually subjective* by the typical polygonal viola-

ceous skin lesions with a slight scale called Wickham's striae; but, on occasion, skin biopsy can be performed to substantiate the diagnosis. In the differential diagnosis of lichen planus, one must consider lichen simplex chronicus, also called localized neurodermatitis and also showing a marked hyperkeratotic element, Kaposi's sarcoma, drug eruption, and even secondary lues. Treatment consists of topical steroids, usually the fluorinated or potent ones, with occlusion technique. Sometimes, intralesional or even short low-dosage courses of systemic steroids are necessary.

Granuloma annulare. This is a papular skin eruption with annular configurations of lesions, especially on the annular aspects of the extremities such as the elbows, knees, feet, and hands (Fig. 16-21). The disease is of unknown etiology and has no serious systemic

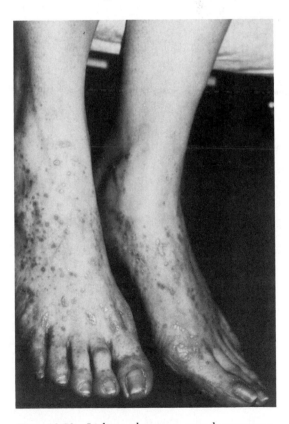

Fig. 16-20. Lichen planus; a papulosquamous eruption showing flat polygonal shiny violaceous papules. Linear lesions resulting from scratch marks, the so-called Koebner phenomenon, are frequently seen.

---

*The spectrum of lichen planus is great. Rarely does a classic case appear. Usually the case involved is not a textbook example, so considerable leeway in the diagnosis is called for.

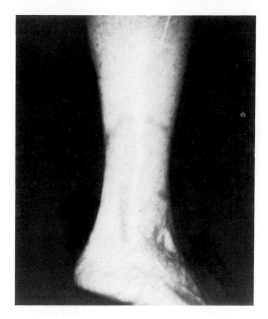

Fig. 16-21. Granuloma annulare; an unusually large plaque on the right foot extending up the lower leg. The lesion had been present for years. Its raised nonscaly annular border is fairly typical. A more typical case is represented by the faint round barely perceptible patch on the posterior aspect of the foot. The border of this lesion is raised, but there was no scaling.

complications; it frequently occurs in children and in adults. Often there are typical lesions on the dorsal areas of the feet consisting of red to flesh-colored papules without surface change. The papules are not prone to ulceration. Inflammation and the lack of scaling distinguish granuloma annulare from tinea; the two are often confused. There are other forms: a so-called disseminated papular form which is more widespread and involves the torso and a deep subcutaneous variety which is seen on the shin, particularly in children. Differential diagnosis ranges from larva migrans to sarcoidosis and rheumatoid arthritis. Biopsy of the skin lesion reveals a noncaseating granuloma; interestingly, the procedure of biopsy sometimes seems to speed the resolution of the process. Other therapy consists of topical steroid cream with occlusion and intralesional injection of steroid. Since the disease is frequently asymptomatic and not progressive, often no therapy is necessary.

TOENAIL PROBLEMS

Diseases and deformities of the great toenail are among the most common and disabling of foot problems; about 5% result from general diseases such as psoriases, endocrine disorders, or trophic changes. Intrinsic factors account for 95%; and of these, 15% are directly or indirectly related to tinea infection. The rest stem from mechanical causes and constitute the most trying groups of foot problems.

Psoriasis. Psoriasis of the toenails is a frequent accompaniment of the cutaneous disease and is often mistaken for fungal involvement of the nail by the lay population (Fig. 16-22). The most severe form of nail involvement with psoriasis, which sometimes goes to the point of shedding the nails, is associated with so-called psoriatic arthritis; however, many patients without arthritic changes, having psoriasis show the following abnormal findings:

1. Stippling or geographic pitting (tiny often grouped depressions in the surface of the nail plate). This change is not unique for psoriasis but can also be seen in alopecia areata.
2. Onycholysis, especially lateral and distal (sometimes with yellowing and opacity of the nail plate, which becomes separated from the nail bed). This change is frequently confused with onychomycosis. Scrapings of the nails for microscopic examination and fungus cultures should be made before therapy is instituted.

Treatment of psoriatic nail changes of the feet are generally unsatisfactory. Intralesional injection of corticosteroid may be effective for treating fingernails afflicted with psoriasis, but similar therapy on involved toenails is less often performed.

Onychogryposis. Onychogryposis refers to hypertrophy of the nail plate, especially the great toe, so the nail appears much like a claw or horn. This is seen primarily in elderly patients. Frequently there is doubt whether any nail care, e.g., proper trimming, has ever

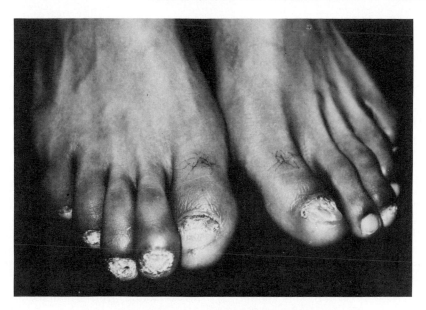

Fig. 16-22. Psoriatic toenail dystrophy. Severe destruction of the nail plates is occasionally seen in psoriasis associated with arthritis. The crumbly appearance of the nails may be identical with that of onychomycosis, which should be ruled out by appropriate tests.

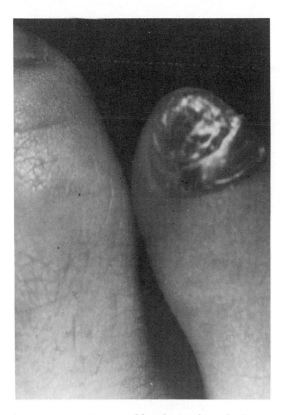

Fig. 16-23. Subungual exostosis. A 16-year-old girl complained of a painful enlarging "wart" under the fifth toenail. However, clinical examination failed to reveal any wart tissue; radiographic examination confirmed the diagnosis.

been performed. Sometimes in extreme cases the nail measures as much as 8 to 10 cm and curves upon itself, resembling a ram's horn. Treatment of onychogryposis consists of trimming the dystrophic nail and periodic clipping.

Subungual exostosis. Subungual exostosis is a bony growth that pushes up the nail plate, thereby causing pain. The lesion usually affects girls in adolescence, and the great toe is most commonly involved (Fig. 16-23). A frequent finding is the predilection of the exostosis for the inner border of the terminal phalanx of the great toe. The patient reports pain aggravated by walking due to encroachment of the expanding exostosis against the nail plate. Differential diagnosis includes subungual verruca, pyogenic granuloma, glomus tumor, carcinoma of the nail bed, melanotic whitlow, keratoacanthoma, and enchondroma. Diagnosis is easily made by radiographic examination of the involved digit. Treatment is excision or curettage.

Tennis toe. This term refers to the hemorrhagic discoloration that occurs under the

toenail of the great toe due to trauma, usually while playing tennis. Stopping quickly, with resultant bending of the toe, causes hemorrhage underneath the nail. Treatment consists of hot soaks and rest from activity.

Subungual hemorrhage. Crushing or shearing trauma to the nails produces a painful subungual hemorrhage manifested by a dusky swelling of the nail plate. Within hours pressure builds up because of bleeding underneath the nail and a throbbing pain brings the patient to the physician for relief. Use of a nail drill or burning through the nail plate with a red hot paper clip is effective in releasing the increased pressure. Radiographs may be necessary to rule out fracture; further therapy may include oral antibiotics.

Melanotic whitlow. Melanomas which involve the nails are termed melanotic whitlows. Blackish discoloration develops, especially in the nail bed. These malignant tumors are more common on the fingers than on the toes (Fig. 16-24). Besides the most frequent cause of darkening of the nails, trauma—other causes are Addison's disease and Peutz-Jeghers syndrome. Once the diagnosis of melanotic whitlow has been made by biopsy, amputation of the digit is the usual therapy.

MISCELLANEOUS SKIN PROBLEMS OF THE FEET

A marked and thickened hyperkeratosis involving the soles and palms may be encountered and frequently is of hereditary origin (Fig. 16-25). The prototype for any diffuse keratoderma is keratosis palmaris et plantaris or Unna-Thost. This thickening of the palmar-plantar skin begins early in life and is sharply demarcated from the normal skin on the sides of the feet. Painful fissuring may develop and also discrete keratoses on the dorsal surface of the digit as well as on the knees and elbows. Differential diagnosis is not usually a problem insomuch as the hyperkeratotic picture of psoriasis or tinea infection involving the soles is usually quite different. Treatment of the hereditary hyperkeratosis is, at best, unsatisfactory with the use of keratolytics such as salicylic acid or propylene glycol under occlusion (e.g., Saran wrap).

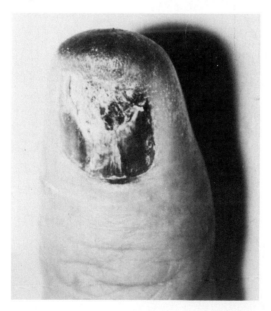

Fig. 16-24. Melanotic whitlow. A black discoloration of the nail of long duration which cannot be explained by trauma (hemorrhage), fungal involvement, or systemic disease (Addison's disease) should point to a malignant melanoma of the nail.

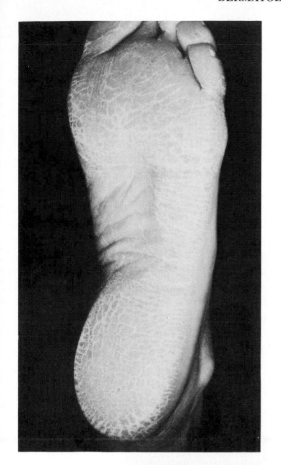

Ainhum. Ainhum refers to the constriction of the fifth toes of blacks who have walked barefoot for years (Fig. 16-26). The trauma related to walking barefoot causes the resultant fibrosis on the fifth toe with constriction and may eventually end with spontaneous painless amputation. The condition is sometimes seen in patients who have had the fifth toe severely traumatized and the resultant scar tissue distorts the toe sufficiently to produce constriction. Ainhum must be differentiated from the so-called pseudoainhum, which consists of annular constrictions or amniotic bands that may affect the great toe and lower portions of both legs. The constrictive bands, when excised, have broad fingerlike projections of collagenous and coarse elastic bundles penetrating deeply into the subcutaneous fat. Othe diseases to consider in the differential diagnosis of ainhum are leprosy and syringomyelia. Treatment of ainhum and pseudoainhum is surgical.

Fig. 16-25. Keratosis plantaris; a marked keratoderma of hereditary origin with sharp margination of the process at the periphery of the acral areas. The thick keratin masses on the feet may be prone to painful fissures.

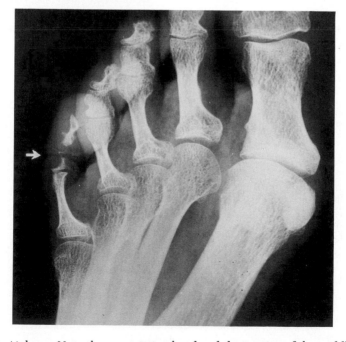

Fig. 16-26. Ainhum. Note the constricting band and destruction of the middle phalanx.

DISEASES AND DEFORMITIES OF THE TOENAILS

Diseases of the nail may be local or constitutional affections or may be the result of congenital malformations. The nails are cutaneous appendages; therefore diseases of the skin and constitutional diseases affecting the skin often involve the nails.

White and Laipply (1958) classified diseases of the nail as caused by (1) infection, (2) psoriasis, (3) contact, (4) eczema (atopic dermatitis), (5) hypovitaminosis, (6) tumor, (7) trauma, or (8) general disease.

Pardo-Castello (1960) published what is probably the most exhaustive review of diseases of the nails. His classification covers divisions according to (1) affections peculiar to the nails, (2) onychodystrophies, (3) ungual manifestations of dermatosis and of systemic disease, and (4) congenital affections of the nails.

Congenital nail deviations are errors of development that produce such anomalies of the nail as pachyonychia (hypertrophy of the nail and nail bed), polyonychia (Fig. 16-27), and anonychia. Tauber and associates (1936) reported a case of pachyonychia congenita and reviewed the published reports of the disease. It is a rare disease involving the nails and is accompanied by palmar and plantar keratoses, among other symptoms. Krausz (1970), in a review of 6,754 cases of disorders of the nail, reported 81% to be caused by local factors, such as trauma or *Candida albicans* infection.

Constitutional diseases involving the nails are in the province of the internist; skin diseases involving the nails are in the domain of the dermatologist. Only local and surgical nail problems are considered in this discussion.

Onychia. Onychia is an inflammation of the matrix. It usually extends into the nail grooves (paronychia). If the disturbance involves multiple digits, it is often caused by systemic disease. In some instances local tinea infection leads to onychia in multiple nails. Onychia affects the great toe most frequently, where trauma from pressure of the shoe and from superimposed secondary infection is the cause.

Treatment consists of relief of all pressure and daily application of a germicide and a fungicide dressing. In rare instances the condition may become acute, requiring antibiotic therapy, chemotherapy, or both.

Paronychia. Paronychia is an inflammation of the nail groove that commonly affects the great toe but may affect the lesser toes; at times it extends to the matrix (in which case it is called onychia). Unlike onychia, however, paronychia is by itself rarely due to constitutional or skin diseases.

Paronychia varies in its severity. It may

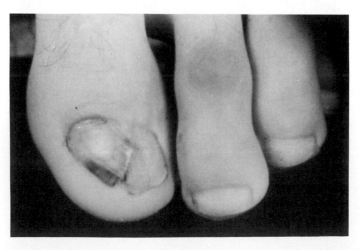

Fig. 16-27. Congenital double nail of the great toe. (Courtesy Dr. C. E. Krausz.)

occur as a mild cellulitis; but mechanical pressure (e.g., from the boxing of the shoe) has crowded the tissue on the side of the nail, a severe state of suppuration may be present. Granulation tissue and extensive ulceration in the groove are characteristic. Paronychia is either accompanied by or the forerunner of unguis incarnatus.

Treatment consists of the following steps:

1. Relieve all pressure from the shoes.

2. Excise a linear portion, about 2 mm of the nail margin, to relieve the cutting effect on the edematous nail groove.

3. Paint the granulation tissue with 10% silver nitrate or 90% phenol.

4. Apply a fungicide dye and cover with a sterile dressing.

Onychauxis (clubnail). The hypertrophied nail, termed onychauxis, or, popularly, clubnail, for the most part involves the great toenails; but the nails of the lesser toes may be affected (Fig. 16-28). The deformity may be caused by constitutional conditions such as nutritional deficiencies or psoriasis. Most cases, however, are the result of local conditions: trauma to the matrix and nail bed, tinea infection; indeed, tinea infection is the most frequent cause. In most "ringworm fungi" infections of the nail, the undersurface of the nail can become tremendously thickened from the accumulation of debris from the infection (Zaias, 1972).

The affected nail and its bed are thickened and deformed. When the disorder is caused by tinea gypsum, the surface of the nail may have white dead streaks or patches which can be readily excised. When the undersurface of the nail contains a yellowish or brown powdery substance, destruction of the nail bed has been by tinea purpureum.

In about 10% of cases of clubnail the nail bed and the dorsal distal surface of the distal phalanx undergo hypertrophic bone changes.

Three methods of treatment are available. In the first, the hypertrophied nail and bed are gradually reduced by grinding and then applying antifungal dressings. In the second, which is reserved for severely deformed clubnails, avulsion of the nail is advised. The third method is ablation of the nail matrix and allowing the nail bed to epithelialize over or carrying out a terminal Syme (p. 365).

Onychogryposis (ram's horn nail, hostler's toe). Onychogryposis is uncommon. It was known also as ram's horn nail and hostler's toe because of its occurrence in men who tended horses. The great toe alone or several toes may be affected (Fig. 16-29). The massive

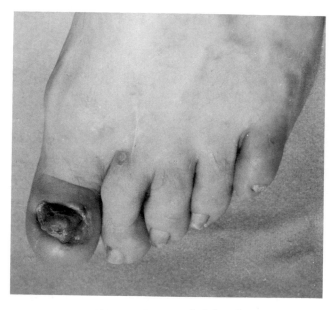

Fig. 16-28. Typical clubnail.

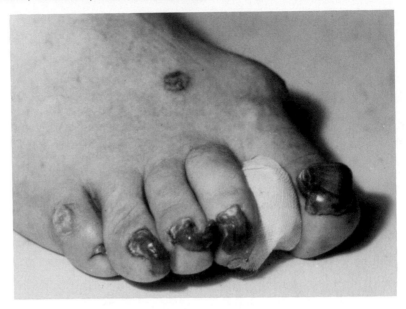

Fig. 16-29. Ram's horn nails of the first four toes.

growth folds over the anterior surface of the toe, often terminating on the plantar surface. The condition does not appear to have any relation to tinea infection. In most cases it is the result of a congenital tendency and repeated trauma to the matrix associated with poor hygiene. For this last reason it is more likely to be seen in derelicts than in people who are careful of cleanliness.

The entire horn up to the nail bed and to the matrix is readily removable with a pair of strong nail nippers. By frequent subsequent trimming the condition becomes asymptomatic. Treatment as outlined for onychauxis is indicated when there is pain with recurrent infection.

Onychoma: neoplasms of and around nail. Verrucae, periungual fibromas, and subungual exostoses are common tumors about the nail. Verrucae and periungual fibromas usually appear in the nail groove but may occur in the nail bed under the nail. They respond readily to fulguration or excision. Subungual exostosis is discussed on p. 494.

Malignancy of the nail bed has been encountered, and its possibility should not be overlooked. Ashby (1956) found reports of twenty-five cases of primary carcinoma of the nail bed and added two proved cases of his

own. Subungual melanoma, or melanotic whitlow, is a malignancy in aged people that is often unrecognized (Gibson et al., 1957). Nevertheless, certain signs should arouse diagnostic interest: increasing pigmentation, chronic painless granular excrescences, and persistent splitting of the nail. Differential diagnosis is essential. Treatment should be studied in each case with the advice of a competent consultants.

Unguis incarnatus. Diseases and deformities of the great toenail are generally grouped under the lowly term "ingrown nail" and are treated empirically. Because of the lack of differential diagnosis and understanding of the diagnosis, in numerous instances these patients are subjected to a series of unsuccessful operative procedures which often produce more complicated problems than the original disease, including recurrence and consequent iatrogenic deformity. I have seen patients who were subjected to ten operative procedures for "ingrown nail," often with a result worse than the original complaint.

The terms "ingrown nail" and "onychocryptosis" are misleading because they imply that the side of the nail grows down into the nail groove. The unfortunate terminology has given rise to misinformation regarding this

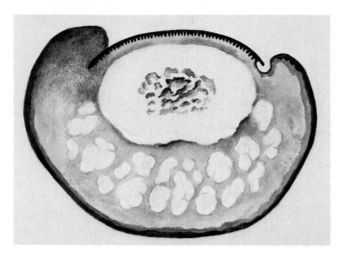

Fig. 16-30. Left, Hypertrophy of the nail lip and occlusion of the nail groove. Right, Normal relation of the nail margin to the nail groove.

common disability; but because of its common usage, the term will be used in the following discussion.

All evidence points to the fact that the growth of nails in vertebrates depends on the matrix and that the width of the nail is in direct relation to the width of the matrix (Pardo-Castello, 1960; Bean, 1963; Bloom and Fawcett, 1968). There is no evidence that the matrix becomes wider in persons suffering from ingrown nail. The old term "ingrown nail" was chosen on the assumption that ingrowth of the nail, or growing down of the nail into the nail groove, was caused by increasing width of the convexity of the nail. Therefore, at first surgeons aimed at destroying the growth of the nail margin; but their attempts at correction failed (DuVries, 1933, 1944). Bartlett (1937) also concluded that the terms "ingrown nail" and "ingrowing nails" are misnomers. The coined term "hypertrophy of the ungualabia" (DuVries, 1933, 1944) is more descriptive of the true pathologic condition in most of these cases.

Frost (1950) recognized three types of ingrown nails: (1) a normal nail plate, but as a result of improper nail trimming, a fish hook or spur remains in the nail groove; (2) an inward distortion of one or both lateral margins of the nail plate (incurvated nail); (3) a normal nail plate, but the lip is hypertrophied (Fig. 16-30).

Lloyd-Davies and Brill (1963) suggest that avulsion of the nail, which is commonly practiced as a treatment for ingrown nail, is probably the cause of hypertrophy of the lip distal to the nail and causes the entire nail to become embedded and clubbed (Fig. 16-31). Unlike the fingernails, if the nail of the great toe has been taken off, the new nail frequently becomes deformed as it grows out because of the upward pressure placed on it during weight bearing.

There are two distinct conditions that produce the symptoms. The first, which accounts for about 75% of cases, is primarily hyperplasia of the nail groove and nail lip (hypertrophy of the ungualabia). The second, which accounts for 25% is essentially a deformity of the nail plate. It is caused by a malformation of the dorsum of the distal phalanx or by hypertrophy and irregular thickening of the nail bed, often the result of tinea unguium. The normal nail plate and its bed are 2 or 3 mm thick; the contour is determined largely by the shape of the dorsum of the distal phalanx. The shape and contour of the dorsum of this bone may vary widely because of secondary changes in the bone from irritation and pressure. Such variations often produce nail deformities, whose symptoms are grouped and diagnosed as ingrown nail. The most common type is an incurvation of the nail margins.

Etiology. Normally the space between the

Normal toe

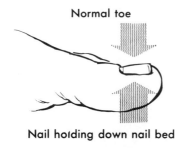

Nail holding down nail bed

After nail avulsion

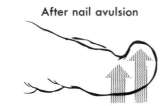

Upward pressure forces causing upward
deformation of distal nail bed

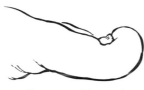

Regrowing nail approaching soft tissue wall

Fig. 16-31. Avulsion of the nail as treatment for "ingrown toenail" causing hypertrophy of the nail lip and resulting in an embedded and clubbed nail. (Modified from Lloyd-Davies, R. W., and Brill, G. C.: Br. J. Surg. **50:**592, 1963.)

nail margin and the nail groove is about 1 mm. The groove is lined with a thin layer of epithelium and lies immediately under and on the sides of the nail margin (Fig. 16-30). Under normal conditions this space is sufficient to protect the groove from irritation. The boxing of shoes, however, often exerts a downward pressure on the nail plate or on the nail lip on the side of the toe; that pressure obliterates the space between the nail margin and nail groove, producing constant irritation to the groove. The reactive swelling in the groove

creates a cycle which leads to gradual hyperplasia of the groove and nail lip and ultimately to permanent hypertrophy (Fig. 16-32).

As the process continues, the nail groove is finally incised by the nail margin, often with ensuing suppuration and secondary infection. To relieve the acute symptoms, the surgeon excises a triangular section of the nail margin; however, the area left by excision is the forerunner of the fishhook formation (Fig. 16-33), about which Frost (1950) speaks. Hypertrophy of the groove fills the space of the excised nail margin. As the nail continues its growth distally, it impinges on the elevated nail groove and gives rise to recurrent episodes of infection and massive formation of granulation tissue.

Congenitally thick nail lips predispose to ingrown nail. This congenital factor explains why ingrown nails are sometimes seen in infants or even in neonates who have thick nail lips and/or an absence of freedom between the nail groove and nail margin. In adults the condition is acquired.

The size, shape, and contour of the nail plate and bed are usually normal. Hyperplastic changes of the nail groove and lip are accompanied by formation of granulation tissue on the lip and groove. The granulation tissue bleeds freely on slight provocation. Hypertrophy may mask a large part or even most of the nail.

Treatment. The variety of procedures reported for the cure of the so-called ingrown nail indicates that none is completely satisfactory; indeed, postoperative recurrence is frequent. Keyes (1934) reviewed 110 cases in which five different procedures resulted in fifteen recurrences.

The procedures generally practiced fall into two distinct groups: (1) excision of the nail margin, matrix, and nail groove as illustrated by Graham (1929), Winograd (1929), and Jansey (1955), among others (Fig. 16-34), and (2) reduction of the hypertrophied lip as recommended by Ney (1923), Bartlett (1937), and DuVries (1944).

Recommended procedure. The treatment for the different stages of hypertrophied ungualabia is as follows.

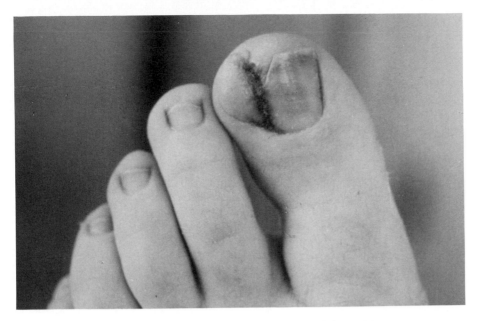

Fig. 16-32. Hypertrophy and overlapping of the nail lip.

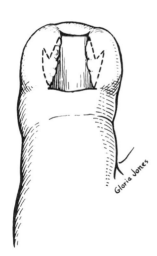

Fig. 16-33. Consequence of repeated cutting of the distal end of the nail margin; "fishhook."

Fig. 16-34. A, Nail margin, groove, and part of the nail lip excised. B, Eponychium sutured over the matrix.

A

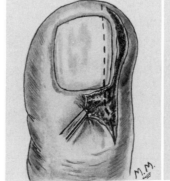

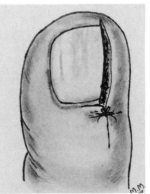

B

MILD CASES

1. Relief may be obtained by inserting a few loose strands of cotton in the nail groove and applying an astringent such as 10% silver nitrate.

2. Permit the nail to grow out freely over the distal end of the nail groove. The wearing of footwear that does not exert constant pressure against the great toe is required.

3. In the presence of acute cellulitis (with or without infection) the offending nail margin must be excised, the granulation tissue cauterized with silver nitrate, the patient started on oral antibiotics, and the foot soaked 20 minutes three times a day until the acute process has subsided.

4. After the acute process has subsided, an attempt should be made to permit the nail to grow over and depress the ungualabia. If it is not successful, a Winograd procedure should be performed.

MODERATELY SEVERE CASES. Plastic reduction of the nail lip usually corrects moderately severe cases of hypertrophied nail lip.

1. Remove a spindle-shaped section, about 3 × 1 cm from the side of the nail lip, which is triangular on cross section (Fig. 16-35, A and B). The incisions extend from the most distal portion of the toe to about 0.5 cm proximal to the nail fold, meeting about 2 mm under the nail groove.

2. Excise the excess subdermal fat.

3. Coapt and suture the skin margins, drawing the nail groove downward (Fig. 16-35, C and D).

The wound heals by first intention, and the procedure results in a free space between the nail groove and margin.

ADVANCED HYPERTROPHY OF THE NAIL LIP. The technique of a Winograd (1929) procedure is as follows:

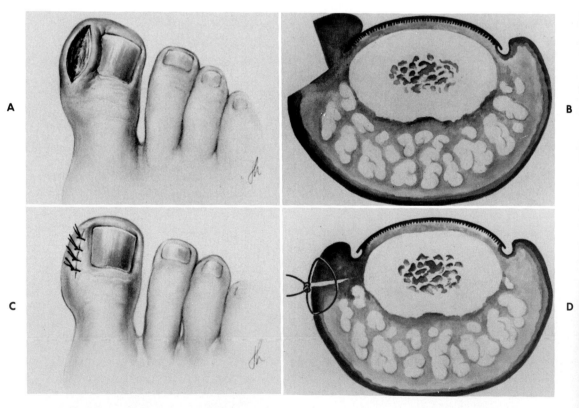

Fig. 16-35. A, Triangular section removed from the side of the toe. **B,** Cross section after excision. **C,** Nail lip and nail groove pulled down after suturing of the nail margins. **D,** Cross section after suturing.

1. Obtain an adequate digital block with 1% procaine hydrochloride; then use a ¼-inch Penrose drain as a tourniquet about the base of the great toe.

2. Make a 4 mm oblique incision in the corner of the nail bed, carrying it down to the nail.

3. Resect the appropriate width of nail margin (anywhere from 2 to 3 mm), starting distally and moving proximally to include the entire nail matrix. Once this incision has been made, the entire block of tissue with nail bed and matrix down to bone can be excised.

4. Carefully inspect the matrix area to be sure the entire matrix has been removed. If there is any doubt, the area may be curetted with a small curette.

5. Place a single suture in the skin incision and apply a compression dressing.

6. The compression dressing is left in place for 72 hours, following which a Band-Aid is applied. If the inflammation ensues after the procedure, the toe may be soaked in warm water 20 minutes, three times a day.

The Winograd procedure is about 95% successful in solving unguis incarnatus. Approximately 5% of the time, a nail horn will regrow, which if symptomatic can be re-excised.

Incurvated nail (inverted nail; involuted nail). Incurved nail is included ordinarily in the term "ingrown nail" and constitutes about 25% of such cases. The disorders are essentially deformities of the nail plate and nail bed; and they may vary widely—from deformity of the nail margins, which curve into the side of the distal phalanx, to deformity of the entire nail plate, which, on cross section, appears horseshoe shaped (Fig. 16-36). Generally the nail margins invert toward the sides of the distal phalanx. Because the contour of the nail depends largely on the contour of the dorsal surface of the distal phalanx, deformity of the nail often occurs secondary to an anomalous dorsal surface of that bone. It may also be caused by hypertrophy of the nail bed.

Treatment. No single surgical procedure can be recommended as being applicable to all the variations of the deformity.

When only the margin of the nail is

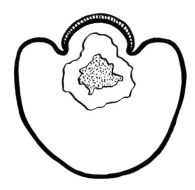

Fig. 16-36. Incurvation of nail margins.

deformed, excision of the nail margin and nail groove, including the matrix of the nail, gives relief. This can be performed by the procedures described by Winograd (1929) (Fig. 16-34).

When incurvation of the nail is too severe, ablation of the nail and matrix is the treatment of choice. The following is the technique for nail ablation:

1. Obtain a digital block using 1% procaine hydrochloride; then use a ¼-inch Penrose drain as a tourniquet around the base of the great toe.

2. Make an oblique incision in each corner of the nail and carry it proximally 4 mm down to the nail.

3. Avulse the nail.

4. Remove the matrix *en bloc* to ensure that none will be left. The matrix bed must be carefully inspected and curetted is necessary.

5. Place a suture in each corner of the skin incision and apply a petrolatum gauze dressing over the nail.

6. The compression dressing is left 72 hours, following which it can be removed and a Band-Aid applied. If inflammation follows the toe may be soaked for 20 minutes three times a day in warm water.

"Ingrown" nail of lesser toes. The lesser toes are subject to disease and deformity similar to those that affect the great toe but such disorders occur less frequently and rarely in severe form. Occasionally a Winograd procedure can be done on a lesser toe for an ingrown nail margin. In the majority of cases, however, I believe a nail ablation–type procedure leads to a better overall result.

REFERENCES

Amonette, R. A., and Rosenberg, E. W.: Infection of toe webs by gram-negative bacteria, Arch. Dermatol. **107**:71, 1973.

Ashby, B. S.: Primary carcinoma of the nail-bed, Br. J. Surg. **44**:216, 1956.

Bartlett, R. W.: A conservative operation for cure of so-called ingrown toenail, J.A.M.A. **108**:1257, 1937.

Bean, W. B.: Nail growth: A twenty-year study, Arch. Intern. Med. **111**:476, 1963.

Beneke, E. S.: Scope monograph on human mycoses, ed. 6, Kalamazoo, Mich., 1976, The Upjohn Co.

Bloom, W., and Fawcett, D. W.: A textbook of histology, Philadelphia, 1968, W. B. Saunders Co.

Bluefarb, S.: Kaposi's sarcoma, Springfield, Ill., 1964, Charles C Thomas, Publisher.

Brown, S. M., and Freeman, R. G.: Epithelioma cuniculatum, Arch. Dermatol. **112**:1295, 1976.

Caravati, C. M., Hudgins, E. M., and Kelly, L. W.: Tinea pedis in children, Cutis **17**:313, 1976.

Cohen, H. J., Frank, S. B., Minkin, W., and Gibbs, R. C.: Subungual exostoses, Arch. Dermatol. **107**:431, 1973.

Conant, M. A., and Wisenfeld, S. L.: Multiple glomus tumors of the skin, Arch. Dermatol. **103**:481, 1971.

Costello, M., and Gibbs, R.: The palms and soles in medicine, Springfield, Ill., 1967, Charles C Thomas, Publisher.

Crissey, J. T., and Peachey, J. C.: Calcaneal petechiae, Arch. Dermatol. **83**:501, 1961.

Dabrowa, N., Landau, J. W., and Newcomer, V. D.: Antifungal activity of glutaraldehyde in vitro, Arch. Dermatol. **105**:555, 1972.

DuVries, H. L.: Hypertrophy of ungual labia, Chiropody Rec. **16**:11, 1933.

DuVries, H. L.: Ingrown nail, Chiropody Rec. **27**:155, 164. 1944.

Fisher, A.: Contact dermatitis, Philadelphia, 1966, Lea & Febiger.

Frost, L.: Root resection for incurvated nail, J. Natl. Assoc. Chiropody **40**:19, 1950.

Gibbs, R.: Skin diseases of the feet, St. Louis, 1974, Warren H. Green, Inc.

Gibson, H. G., Montgomery, H., Woolner, L. B., and Brunsting, L. A.: Melanotic whitlow (subungual melanoma), J. Invest. Dermatol. **29**:119, 1957.

Graham, H. F.: Ingrown toe nail, Am. J. Surg. **6**:411, 1929.

Graham, J., and Helwig, E.: Bowen's disease and its relationship to systemic cancer, Arch. Dermatol. **80**:133, 1959.

Greer, K. E.: Epidermal inclusion cyst of the sole, Arch. Dermatol. **109**:251, 1974.

Jansey, F.: Etiologic therapy of ingrowing toe nail, Q. Bull. Northwestern Univ. Med. School **29**:358, 1955.

Keyes, E. L.: The surgical treatment of ingrown toenails, J.A.M.A. **102**:1458, 1934.

Krausz, C. E.: Nail survey: 28th October 1942, to 3rd April 1970, Br. J. Chiropody **35**:117, 1970.

Lathrop, R. G.: Ingrowing toenails: causes and treatment, Cutis **20**:119, 1977.

Lerner, A. B.: Pigmented nevi, Mod. Med. p. 131, 1972.

Lloyd-Davies, R. W., and Brill, G. C.: The aetiology and outpatient management of ingrowing toe-nails, Br. J. Surg. **50**:592, 1963.

Mann, R. A., and DuVries, H. L. Intractable plantar keratosis, Orthop. Clin. North Am. **41**:67, 1973.

Montgomery, R. M.: Painful plantar problems, Consultant, p. 45, October, 1977.

Morrell, J. F.: "Pilonidal" sinus of the sole, Arch. Dermatol. **75**:269, 1957.

Ney, G. C.: An operation for ingrowing toe nails, J.A.M.A. **80**:374, 1923.

Pardo-Castello, V.: Diseases of the nails, ed. 3, Springfield, Ill., 1960, Charles C Thomas, Publisher.

Pinkus, H., Rogin, J. R., and Goldman, P.: Eccrine poroma, Arch. Dermatol. **74**:511, 1956.

Pringle, W. M., and Helms, D. C.: Treatment of plantar warts by blunt dissection, Arch. Dermatol. **108**:79, 1973.

Raque, C. J., Stein, K. M., Lane, J. M., and Reese, E. C.: Pseudoainhum constricting bands of the extremities, Arch. Dermatol. **105**:434, 1972.

Resnik, S. S., Lewis, L. A., and Cohen, B. H.: The athlete's foot, Cutis **20**:353, 1977.

Rosin, L. J., and Harrell, E. R.: Arteriovenous fistula, Arch. Dermatol. **112**:1135, 1976.

Tauber, E. B., Goldman, L., and Claassen, H.: Pachyonychia congenita, J.A.M.A. **107**:29, 1936.

Tromovitch, T. A., and Kay, D. M.: Plantar warts, Cutis **12**:87, 1973.

White, C. J., and Laipply, T. C.: Diseases of the nails: 792 cases, Ind. Med. Surg. **27**:325, 1958.

Winograd, A. M.: A modification in the technic of operation for ingrown toe-nail, J.A.M.A. **92**:229, 1929.

Zaias, N.: Onychomycosis, Arch. Dermatol. **105**:263, 1972.

PART THREE

Treatment

17

CONSERVATIVE TREATMENT AND OFFICE PROCEDURES

Roger A. Mann

Prior to discussing conservative means of treating some disorders of the feet, I should like to say a word about footwear and its influence on the functioning of the feet. As emphasized in Chapter 8, shoes, especially women's shoes, have been responsible for a majority of the toe deformities physicians commonly encounter. Although men and women have worn and suffered the consequences of improper footwear since antiquity, contemporary society continues to perpetuate the use of ill-fitting shoes.

The deforming effects of improper shoes on a normal foot can cause hallux valgus, hammertoes, hard corns, and plantar keratoses. Properly fitted footwear should not crowd the forefoot but should allow the toes to extend fully as the person walks (Fig. 8-2, *C*). To ensure adequate length and width, shoes should always be fitted to the weight-bearing foot.

MODIFICATIONS OF THE SHOE

Numerous modifications can be made in the heel, shank, or sole areas of the basic shoe (separately or in combination) to correct specific disorders of the foot. Rather than recommend an "orthopaedic shoe" for all symptomatic feet, the clinician should prescribe shoe modifications that suit the individual needs of the patient.

Wedges and pads are used to accomplish shoe modifications. A wedge is usually made of leather and is placed on the exterior walking surface of the shoe or within the construction of the shoe. It is intended to alter the weight-bearing pattern of the foot. Unlike the wedge, the pad acts on a specific site. It is used for therapeutic purposes and is in direct contact with the foot. It is usually made of felt, leather, or plastic.

The heel

Thomas heel. The most common heel modification is the Thomas heel (Fig. 17-1). This heel was originally designed to bring the calcaneus from a valgus position to a more neutral one and to support the medial aspect of the foot. Its use is indicated in cases of symptomatic flatfoot. It produces a varus tilt of the calcaneus and gives mechanical support to the collapsing talonavicular joint as well. In cases of hindfoot valgus it can be used to keep the calcaneus in a less valgoid position. A Thomas heel should not be used if the calcaneus is in a varus position.

Unfortunately, today most Thomas heels are not properly fitted. To be effective, a Thomas heel should extend from the midportion of the navicular on the medial side to a line that intersects the longitudinal axis of the fibula on the lateral side. The Thomas heel

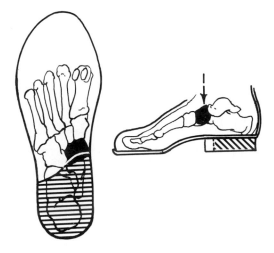

Fig. 17-1. Thomas heel; extends to the midportion of the navicular to provide support.

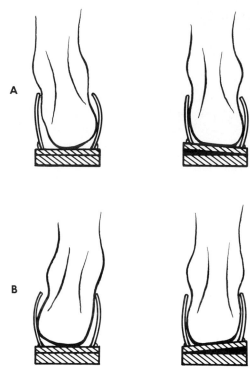

Fig. 17-2. Heel lifts. **A,** Medial heel wedge for correction of valgus heel deformity. **B,** Lateral heel wedge for correction of varus heel deformity.

may be combined with an inner heel lift to help accomplish inversion of the calcaneus.

Heel lifts. A medial or lateral lift of 0.3 to 0.6 cm may be used to bring the heel out of a varus or valgus position (Fig. 17-2). Such a lift will transfer weight to the medial or lateral aspect of the foot.

Widened heels. Heels that have been widened are used to stabilize and thereby diminish painful subtalar motion. They are beneficial in the treatment of degenerative changes in the subtalar joint.

The shank

The shank of the shoe can be either flexible or rigid. In attempting to correct a postural abnormality of the foot by means of an external modification of the heel or sole, one usually recommends that the shank be flexible so the foot can respond to the areas being corrected. Conversely, if an appliance is to be placed within the shoe, the shank should be more rigid.

The sole

The sole of the shoe can be modified through the use of lifts to affect the regions of the great toe, the metatarsals, and the medial and lateral aspects of the foot.

Lifts in region of great toe. Lifts in the region of the great toe make that toe less flex-

ible and restrict the motion of the joint. This modification is useful in the treatment of hallux rigidus (Fig. 17-3). A rocker bottom shoe will also diminish the motion in the metatarsophalangeal joint of the great toe as well as diminish pressure underneath the metatarsal heads.

Lifts in region of metatarsals. There are two devices for modifying shoes in the metatarsal area: a bar and an anterior heel.

The sole is often modified by a *metatarsal bar*, which transfers the weight usually borne by the metatarsal heads to a more proximal plantar area. The bar should be placed proximal to the metatarsal heads and may be either straight or curved (Fig. 17-4). Improper placement of the bar in relation to the metatarsal heads is the most common error made in using this type of appliance. If the bar is placed too far forward, the painful metatarsal condition will be aggravated. The insole of the

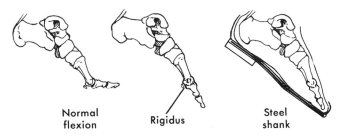

Fig. 17-3. Sole modification for treatment of hallux rigidus. A steel shank is incorporated to diminish motion at the metatarsophalangeal joint.

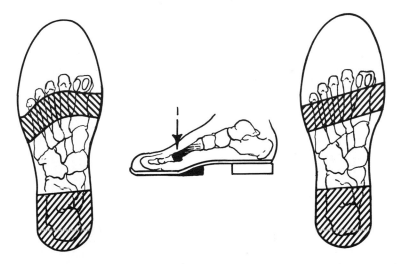

Fig. 17-4. Metatarsal bars. These appliances may be either straight or curved but must be placed proximal to the metatarsal heads.

patient's shoe should be examined to determine the weight-bearing area; marks should then be made on the sides of the sole just proximal to the metatarsal heads. In this way proper placement of the bar by the shoemaker is assured. The bar can be from 0.3 to 1 cm thick, depending on the clinical picture.

The anterior *heel* is also effective in relieving pressure on the metatarsal region and is preferred by some clinicians to the metatarsal bar.

Both these appliances are used to relieve metatarsalgia caused by atrophy of the plantar fat pad, intractable plantar keratosis, Morton's neuroma, trauma to the metatarsal heads, and other conditions that affect the metatarsal heads.

A great deal of progress has been made recently in the production of insole materials. There are now materials that will permit the clinician in his office to produce an insole which specifically relieves areas of pressure on the plantar aspect of the foot. Other materials, such as Plastizote, when placed in a shoe will mold to the pressure points exerted by the patient against the material and thus produce a total contact type of insole. When a total contact interface is established between the plantar skin and the insole, pressure is distributed over a broad area. A shoe known as the extra-depth shoe has an enlarged toe box area and should be used with the Plastizote insole to prevent the toes from being pushed against the top of the shoe.

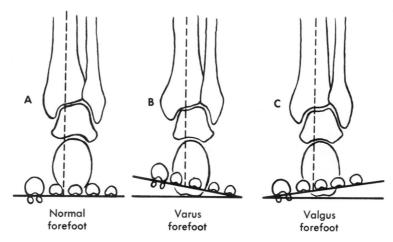

Fig. 17-5. Forefoot alignment. **A,** Normal forefoot. **B,** Fixed varus forefoot. The condition may be treated with a medial sole lift. **C,** Fixed valgus forefoot. The condition may be treated with a lateral sole lift. (From Sgarlato, T. E.: A compendium of podiatric biomechanics, San Francisco, 1971, California College of Podiatric Medicine.)

Lifts in medial and lateral regions of foot. Medial and lateral sole lifts (0.3 to 0.6 cm thick) may be used either alone or combined with a heel modification to help correct imbalances of the foot. A medial lift will transfer the weight to the outer border and can be used to accommodate forefoot varus or to help realign the foot after trauma. A lateral lift will transfer weight to the inner border of the foot, may be used to treat forefoot valgus, and will also help to realign the foot after trauma (Fig. 17-5). In the treatment of flatfoot, the lateral lift is used to help correct the forefoot varus that often accompanies hindfoot valgus. A lateral lift is also frequently combined with a Thomas heel to help support a flatfoot deformity (Fig. 17-6).

Appliances

Felt pads. Felt pads are used primarily to relieve areas of abnormal pressure, usually on the plantar aspect of the foot. They may also be used to support the longitudinal arch during the period when the clinician is attempting to determine which combination of supports is best suited to his patient. The pads may be cut by the physician (Fig. 17-7) or ready-made adhesive backed pads may be purchased in various sizes. In treating an area

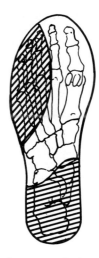

Fig. 17-6. Combination of Thomas heel, which corrects heel valgus and supports the navicular, and lateral sole lift, which corrects forefoot varus. This combination is used in the treatment of flatfoot deformity.

of abnormal wear or in attempting to ascertain exactly where to place permanent pads, we have found placing pads in the shoe or taping them to the patient's foot useful.

The main disadvantage of felt pads for permanent use is their tendency to pack down; to be most effective, they should be

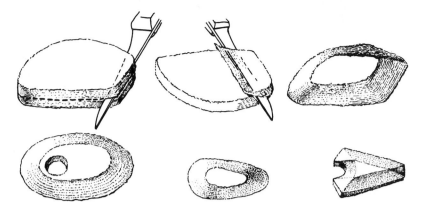

Fig. 17-7. Felt pads; may be shaped by the physician to relieve abnormal pressure on the plantar aspect of the foot.

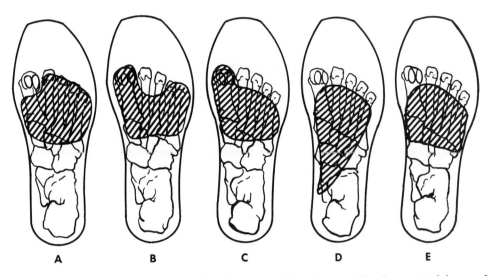

Fig. 17-8. Commonly used shoe pads for relief of painful conditions of the foot. **A,** Pad designed to relieve pressure on the sesamoids. **B,** Pad to support various metatarsal heads (in this case, for treatment of Morton's neuroma). **C,** Pad to support a short first metatarsal and relieve pressure on the lesser metatarsal heads. **D,** Pad to support the longitudinal arch and relieve pressure on the metatarsal heads. **E,** Pad to relieve pressure on the metatarsal heads.

used in a shoe that has a fairly rigid sole. Correct placement and the indications for the most commonly used shoe pads are illustrated in Fig. 17-8.

Once felt pads have provided relief to the patient, a more permanent type of insert can be substituted. Leather appliances, metal arch supports (e.g., the Whitman support), a UCBL type of insert, or a functional orthotic

appliance to correct imbalance of the foot may be prescribed.

Leather appliances. The leather appliance is well adapted simply to elevate a metatarsal in order to redistribute the weight on the plantar aspect of the foot. This type of modification will allow the affected area to carry less weight and will thus relieve the symptoms. Examples of commonly used leather ap-

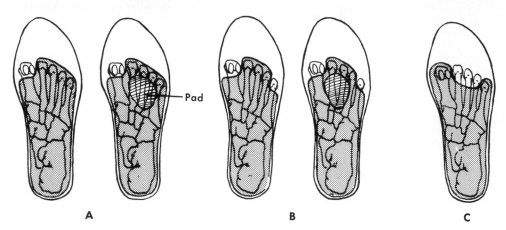

Fig. 17-9. Commonly used leather appliances for relief of painful conditions of the foot. A pad (striped area) may be incorporated into the appliance for greater support. **A,** For relief of painful sesamoids. **B,** For relief of painful callosities under the first and fifth metatarsal heads. **C,** For relief of metatarsalgia in the second, third, and fourth metatarsals.

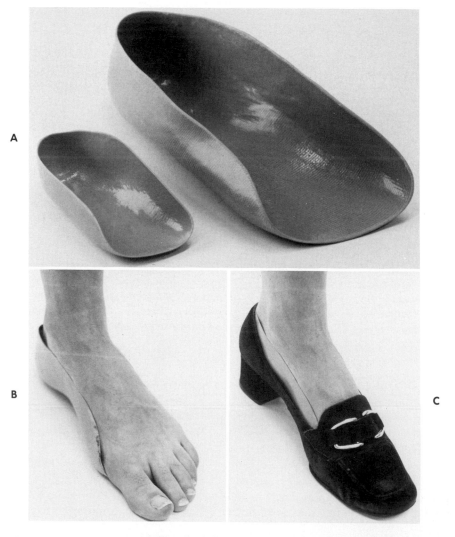

Fig. 17-10. UCBL inserts. **A,** Child and adult sizes. **B** and **C,** Insert on the foot and in the shoe.

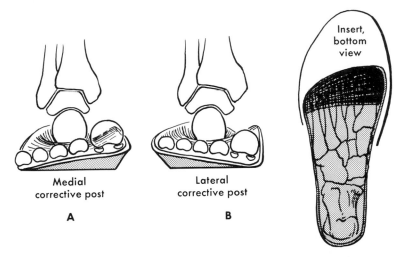

Fig. 17-11. Orthotic appliances. **A,** Fixed varus forefoot treated by supporting the medial side of the foot. **B,** Fixed valgus forefoot treated by supporting the lateral side of the foot.

pliances are shown in Fig. 17-9. These appliances are indicated in the treatment of plantar callosities, metatarsalgia, Morton's neuroma, and various afflictions of the metatarsal heads.

Metal appliances. Appliances made of metal are useful to support a symptomatic foot in which there is a structural weakness (e.g., flatfoot), distortion as by a fracture-dislocation, or an adult foot with a residual structural abnormality like a partially corrected clubfoot or with advanced arthritis. Such feet often require well-molded metal supports to achieve the mechanical stability that the ligamentous and bony structures cannot provide. This type of appliance must be fabricated over an accurate mold of the foot. Generally, however, metal appliances are being phased out as plastic material has become more reliable and simpler to handle.

UCBL insert. The UCBL insert helps to correct structural abnormalities of the foot through control of the hindfoot and is based on the premise that the hindfoot controls the forefoot. The heel is placed in a corrected position; the correction is maintained by a laminated fiberglass heel cup (Fig. 17-10). Although the applications of the UCBL insert are still being explored, it has proved to be useful in the treatment of symptomatic flatfoot, hallux valgus aggravated by an associated

flatfoot deformity, calcaneal spurs with associated fasciitis of the plantar aponeurosis, and various other postural problems of the foot concomitant with growing (Henderson and Campbell, 1967).

Orthotic appliances. Functional orthotic appliances are used in an attempt to balance a foot in which an anatomic disorder is present (e.g., forefoot varus or valgus as illustrated in Fig. 17-5, hindfoot varus or valgus, or a combination of these disorders). The appliances are fitted to a plaster mold of the foot held in a corrected position and are generally fabricated from a rigid plastic material (Fig. 17-11). Heel and forefoot posts are added to the appliance to give the needed correction.

FOOT STRAPPING

Foot strapping is advantageous for the treatment of specific disorders. Only those strappings used most commonly are discussed.

Acute injuries. Acute injuries which result in foot strain, sprain, or undisplaced fracture may be treated by foot strapping and a wooden shoe. The strapping consists of circular rings of tape that are wrapped around the forefoot and basically support it. When a fresh injury is being treated, care must be taken to allow for edema.

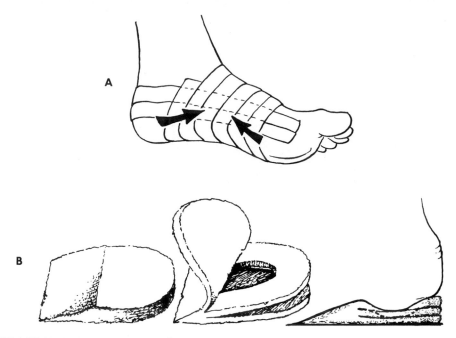

Fig. 17-12. **A,** Bow strapping; relieves pressure on the plantar fascia by shortening the medial side of the foot. **B,** Cut-out felt pad; relieves pressure on the plantar tubercle of the calcaneus.

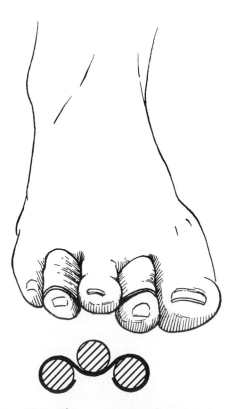

Fig. 17-13. Sling to support a hammered toe.

Symptomatic calcaneal spurs and plantar fasciitis. In these disorders, bow strapping (Fig. 17-12, *A*) relieves pressure, thereby reducing discomfort. A felt pad relieves pressure on the plantar tubercle of the calcaneus (Fig. 17-12, *B*).

Acute sesamoiditis. In the treatment of this disorder, the hallux should be taped in a plantar-flexed position to relax the tendons containing the sesamoids.

Symptomatic hammertoe. A hammered toe can often be treated by passing tape around the normal toe on each side of the hammered toe, thus making a sling of the tape (Fig. 17-13). In addition, pads placed underneath the toe are helpful (Fig. 17-14).

PHYSICAL THERAPY

Physical therapy of the foot and ankle is directed toward reestablishing full range of motion in the foot and strengthening its muscles. Physical therapy is indicated after the foot has been injured or after a surgical procedure has been performed on the foot.

Sprains and fractures of ankle. Extension and flexion exercises for the ankle and inver-

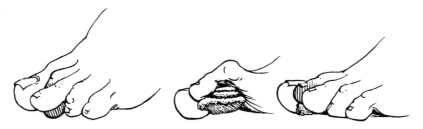

Fig. 17-14. Felt pad built up under a hammertoe; provides relief of pressure on the tip of the toe.

sion and eversion exercises for the subtalar joint may be prescribed for the treatment of healed ankle sprains or fractures. The patient should begin these exercises without bearing weight and then progress to bearing weight when functional motion has been reestablished.

Toes. Toe-gripping exercises using marbles and jacks help increase the range of motion of the toes.

Tendo Achillis. Stretching exercises for the tendo Achillis are best performed as follows: The patient stands erect, 60 to 90 cm away from the wall. He extends his arms to the wall and gently leans forward until his hands touch it, keeping his body erect and his heels firmly on the floor. When the patient first begins this exercise, his feet should be parallel; as progress is made, he should internally rotate his foot 15° to 30° in order to produce increased stretching of the tendon.

REFERENCES

Brachman, P. R.: Mechanical foot therapy, Danville, Ill., 1966, Interstate Printers & Publishers.

Cailliet, R.: Foot and ankle pain, Philadelphia, 1968, F. A. Davis Co.

Henderson, W. H., and Campbell, J. W.: UCBL shoe insert: casting and fabrication, Univ. Calif. Biomech. Lab. Tech. Rep. Ser. 53, August, 1967.

Lewin, P.: The foot and ankle: their injuries, diseases, deformities, and disabilities, ed. 4, Philadelphia, 1959, Lea & Febiger.

Swanson, M. J. M.: Textbook of chiropody, ed. 2, Baltimore, 1954, The Williams & Wilkins Co.

18

SURGICAL APPROACHES TO THE DEEP STRUCTURES OF THE FOOT AND ANKLE

Verne T. Inman and Roger A. Mann

Identical skin incisions may be employed for a variety of surgical procedures on the deep structures of the foot and ankle. The selection of a particular incision should have two objectives. The first and most important is to provide an adequate exposure of the anatomic parts so the surgeon can accomplish his task with dispatch and facility. The second objective is to select an incision that will minimize functional losses.

To achieve his objective, the surgeon should keep in mind the following principles:

1. Deprivation of the blood supply may cause a delay in healing and increase the probability of infection.

2 Contractures of surgical scars may limit motion if the scars are present across normal skin creases.

3. The presence of scars over bony prominences or weight-bearing surfaces where they are subjected to pressures may prove distressing to the patient.

4. The sectioning of small cutaneous nerves often produces areas of anesthesia. These may themselves be of little significance; but when a painful neuroma develops in the proximal end of the nerve, annoying and often incapacitating symptoms result. This is partic-

ularly true when the nerve is caught within the incision and the scar is subjected to the external pressure of a shoe or to distortion during the normal movements of walking.

5. Incisions on the weight-bearing surfaces of the foot should be avoided.

Principles. It appears proper at this time to enunciate several anatomic and physiologic principles:

1. Peripheral nerves and blood vessels generally are found to be contiguous. The larger nerves accompany arteries and their venae comitantes; the smaller nerves accompany veins. When clamping these vessels, the surgeon should be aware that there may be small nerves adjacent to them. If a nerve is included in the tie, the patient later may have complaints which will prove annoying to him and embarrassing to the surgeon.

2. Undermining the skin must be avoided. If flaps are to be extended, the superficial and, if possible, the deep fasciae should be included to preserve the blood supply.

3. It is preferable to make a longer incision than to employ forceful retraction on the skin. Remember that incisions heal from side to side and not from end to end.

4. Within a physiologic range, the metabolism of cells changes with temperature.

When operating without a tourniquet, the surgeon may employ warm wet sponges; but he should not use hot sponges, for the latter, with temperatures above 60° C (140° F), will kill cells. When operating under a tourniquet, the surgeon should use cold sponges exclusively. It is harmful to warm the tissues; to do so increases their metabolic requirements and simultaneously deprives them of circulation.

5. It may be redundant to emphasize that tissues should be handled atraumatically. However, it does no harm to emphasize that tissues should not be crushed, stretched, or permitted to dry or be burned with hot sponges.

6. Removal of the tourniquet and control of bleeding are advisable before closure. A "dry" operative wound will heal better than a "soupy" one.

In the following pages, various surgical approaches to the structures of the foot and ankle are briefly described. Some are classic approaches that have been employed routinely over many years; others are special incisions described by individual surgeons for specific purposes. An attempt will be made in the descriptions to present the advantages and disadvantages of each approach. In addition, the various reconstructive or surgical procedures that may be performed through a particular incision will be enumerated. For a more detailed description of each approach, the reader will find at the end of the chapter a list of references which includes material of the originating surgeons.

EXPOSURE OF THE ANKLE JOINT
Medial approaches

Simple medial approach. This approach may be employed for reduction and internal fixation of fractures of the medial malleolus. It provides only an exposure of the fracture. It is inadequate to permit exploration of the ankle joint or repair of the deltoid ligament, and it places the scar over a bony prominence. The tendon of the tibialis posterior grooves the malleolus; if the incision is made carelessly, the sheath of the tendon may be opened or the tendon may be cut. When care is not exer-

cised, the incision may divide the saphenous vein and nerve, which cross superficial to the malleolus. The saphenous nerve should be preserved.

A straight longitudinal incision is made that extends from a point 5 cm above the tip of the malleolus and is carried distally to the tip of the malleolus. The skin is retracted slightly to expose the malleolus extraperiosteally (Fig. 18-1, *A*).

Medial anterior approach (Jergesen, 1959). This incision not only permits exposure of the medial malleolus but also has the added advantage of permitting inspection of the medial side of the ankle joint. Such exposure is important in internal fixation of fractures of the medial malleolus. Using this approach, the surgeon can determine the adequacy of the reconstitution of the articular surfaces as well as detect the presence of small bone fragments or the interposition of soft tissue. Furthermore, one can check whether the fixation devices (screws or pins) have traversed the joint cavity. The deltoid ligament can be readily exposed for inspection or repair through this incision.

The incision begins anterior to the medial malleolus (5 to 6 cm above its tip), proceeds distally to the joint level, and then curves backward, passing 1 to 2 cm below the tip of the malleolus and stopping directly below the posterior margin of the malleolus. The saphenous vein and saphenous nerve are exposed and retracted posteriorly. The superficial fascia is divided in the direction of the skin incision. The fascia is undermined to expose the malleolus and the superficial fibers of the deltoid ligament. The sheath of the posterior tibial tendon, covered by the flexor retinaculum, is found deep in the distal extremity of the incision. A longitudinal incision of the anterior joint capsule along the anterior margin of the deltoid ligament generally permits adequate exposure of the anteromedial compartment of the ankle joint (Fig. 18-1, *B*).

Posteromedial approach (Jergesen, 1959). This is an excellent approach for the open reduction and internal fixation of fractures that involve both the medial malleolus and the posterior lip of the tibia, with or without

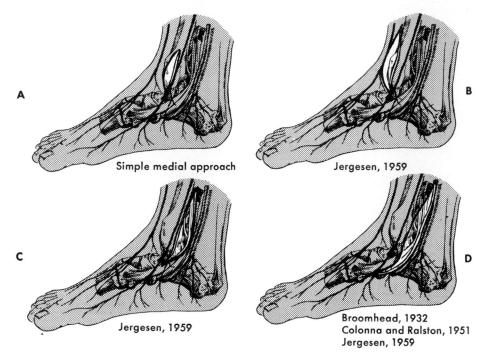

A   Simple medial approach

B   Jergesen, 1959

C   Jergesen, 1959

D   Broomhead, 1932
Colonna and Ralston, 1951
Jergesen, 1959

Fig. 18-1. Medial approaches to the ankle.

posterior displacement of the talus in the mortise.

The patient is placed in prone lateral decubitus. The longitudinal extent of the incision is determined by the location of the fracture. The incision parallels the posterior aspect of the tibia, curves forward gently to pass 2 cm below the tip of the malleolus, and ends at the level of the anterior margin of the malleolus. The tibial periosteum may be incised directly beneath the longitudinal component of the skin incision. In this way the posteromedial aspect of the distal extremity of the tibia is exposed subperiosteally without entering the deep portion of the muscle compartment. To preserve the periosteal attachment of the fracture fragments, one may accomplish extraperiosteal exposure by entering the deep posterior muscle compartment. Proximally the intermuscular septum is divided close to its attachment to the tibia. Distally the flexor retinaculum ligament and the sheath of the posterior tibial tendon are incised. The dissection should be developed close to the periosteum. The foot is plantar flexed to facilitate retraction of the posterior tibial tendon and to

expose the posterior talotibial ligament as well as the adjacent joint capsule (Fig. 18-1, *C*).

Posteromedial approach (Colonna and Ralston, 1951). The incision begins 6 cm proximal and 2 cm posterior to the medial malleolus. It curves anteriorly and inferiorly across the center of the medial malleolus. The medial malleolus is then exposed by reflecting the periosteum, care being taken to preserve the deltoid ligament. The flexor retinaculum is then divided, and the flexor hallucis longus tendon and the neurovascular bundle are retracted laterally. The tibialis posterior and flexor digitorum longus tendons are retracted medially and anteriorly to expose the posterior tibial fracture (Fig. 18-1, *D*).

Medial approach to posterior malleolus (Broomhead, 1932). This approach is of particular value in fractures of the medial tip of the posterior tibia. The incision begins midway between the posterior border of the tibia and the medial border of the tendo Achillis. It then curves inferior to the medial malleolus, continuing to the medial margin of the foot; thus, exposure of both the medial lip and the posterior lip of the tibia is accomplished. The

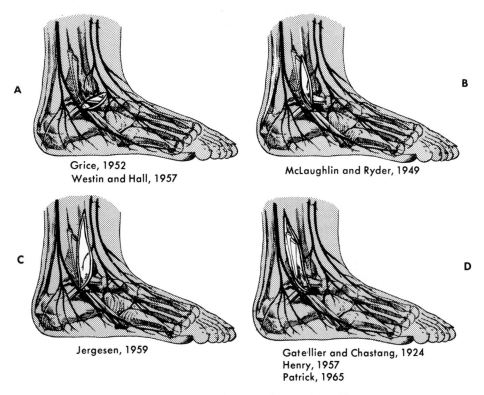

A

Grice, 1952
Westin and Hall, 1957

B

McLaughlin and Ryder, 1949

C

Jergesen, 1959

D

Gatellier and Chastang, 1924
Henry, 1957
Patrick, 1965

Fig. 18-2. Lateral approaches to the ankle.

distal tibia is exposed by reflecting the capsule and periosteum and then retracting posteriorly the tendons of the tibialis posterior, flexor digitorum longus, and flexor hallucis longus along with the neurovascular bundle (Fig. 18-1, *D*).

Exposure of medial aspect of ankle by osteotomy of medial malleolus (Banks and Laufman, 1953). Once the medial malleolus has been exposed through either an anterior or a posterior medial approach, it may be osteotomized at the level of its junction with the shaft of the tibia. By abducting the foot, one can expose the entire superior surface of the talus and the articular surface of the tibia.

In closure, the medial malleolus is accurately replaced and maintained by a screw or pin.

This addition to the medial or posteromedial approaches permits treatment of osteochondritis dissecans or other benign lesions within the ankle joint.

Lateral approaches

Simple lateral approach (McLaughlin and Ryder, 1949). The incision begins over the distal third of the fibula and curves gently forward to run just in front of the anterior end of the bone and to end just below the tip of the malleolus. The peroneal tendons are retracted posteriorly and the extensor digitorum longus tendon is retracted anteriorly to expose the tibiofibular syndesmosis and the lateral fibular lip. The distal end of the malleolus is exposed by longitudinally splitting the fibers of the fibular collateral ligament. The lateral malleolar fracture can be readily visualized and reduced with this approach; however, access to the joint itself is limited (Fig. 18-2, *B*).

Anterolateral approach (Jergesen, 1959). This approach gains access to the tibiofibular joint and the anterolateral aspect of the ankle joint. The proximal origin of the incision depends on the site and extent of the fracture.

The incision begins along the anterolateral margin of the distal fibular shaft, proceeds distally to the level of the ankle joint, curves back to pass a scant fingerbreadth below the malleolar tip, and ends at a point directly below the posterior margin of the malleolus. The lateral branch of the superficial peroneal nerve lies in the subcutaneous fat in the anterior portion of the incision. A smaller, inconstant, branch separates from the main trunk distal to the point at which it perforates the fascia in the middle third of the ligament. This small branch lies in fat and courses distally, parallel with the lower shaft of the fibula, to ramify in the area of the malleolus. Injury to this branch, after a longitudinal incision over the center of the lower fibula has been made, may lead to a sensitive scar.

Dissection of the skin posteriorly exposes the lateral malleolus. The fibular attachment of the transverse crural ligament and the crural fascia are divided to free the tendons of the peroneus tertius and the extensor digitorum longus. The sural nerve and the lesser saphenous vein are located in the lower part of the incision. To gain access to the calcaneal attachment of the calcaneofibular ligament, the inferior retinaculum is incised and the peroneal tendons are retracted (Fig. 18-2, *C*).

Posterolateral approach (Gatellier and Chastang, 1924). This approach makes use of the fact that the fibula in many cases is fractured. The incision begins at a point 10 to 12 cm proximal to the tip of the lateral malleolus and proceeds distally along the posterior margin of the fibula to the malleolar tip. Then it curves anteriorly for 2 to 5 cm, in line with the peroneal tendons. The fibula and the lateral malleolus are exposed subperiosteally; the sheaths of the peroneal retinacula and tendons are incised, and the tendons are displaced anteriorly. If no fibular fracture is present, the malleolus is osteotomized from 8 to 10 cm proximal to the malleolar tip. The interosseous membrane as well as the anterior and posterior malleolar ligaments is divided; the calcaneofibular and talofibular ligaments are preserved as a hinge. The distal fibula is

turned laterally on the hinge to expose the lateral and posterior distal tibia and the lateral ankle joint. Unsuspected fragments can be removed from the joint and anatomic reduction of the posterior fragment can be accomplished. This approach also permits access to the entire lateral surface of the talus.

To close, the fibula is replaced and fixed with a long screw into the tibia. The tendons are replaced and the tendon sheaths and retinacula are repaired. The cross screw is removed when the patient is ambulatory (Fig. 18-2, *D*). This approach has been reemphasized by Patrick (1965).

Posterolateral approach (Henry, 1957). Similar to the posterolateral approach described by Gatellier and Chastang (1924)—this approach has the patient prone with a sandbag beneath the instep, the knee bent, and the foot plantar flexed.

The incision begins about 2 cm below the lateral malleolus and extends 10 to 12 cm proximally and 1 cm anterior to the lateral border of the tendo Achillis. The fascia is incised in line with the incision. Approximately 3 cm above the calcaneus, a branch of the peroneal artery is encountered and the underlying fat is opened. The interval is then sought between the flexor hallucis longus and the peroneus brevis. By blunt dissection the interval is enlarged as far proximally as possible. The flexor hallucis longus is retracted medially to expose the posterolateral aspect of the tibia (Fig. 18-2, *D*).

Posterior approach

The posterior approach, originally described by Picot (1923), has now become a standard approach. A 12 cm incision begins along the posterolateral border of the tendo Achillis to the level of its insertion. The superficial and deep fasciae are divided. A Z-plasty division and reflection of the tendo Achillis is done. The fat and areolar tissue in the space between the flexor hallucis longus and the peroneus brevis tendon are retracted medially to expose the distal tibia, the posterior ankle joint, and the posterior surface of the talus (Fig. 18-3, *D*).

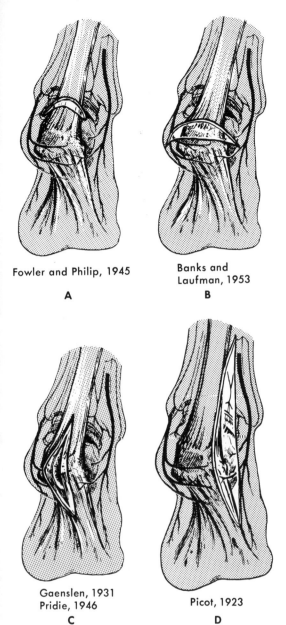

Fowler and Philip, 1945

A

Banks and
Laufman, 1953

B

Gaenslen, 1931
Pridie, 1946

C

Picot, 1923

D

Fig. 18-3. Posterior approaches to the calcaneus and its adjacent structures.

Anterior approach

In the approach described by Colonna and Ralston (1951), the incision begins along the anterior aspect of the ankle 8 to 10 cm proximal to the joint line; it continues distally to a point approximately 5 cm below the joint. The deep fascia is divided in line with the skin

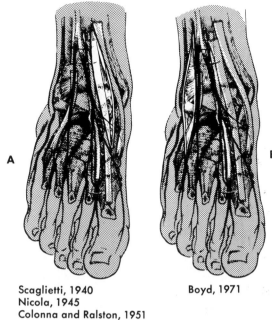

A

B

Scaglietti, 1940
Nicola, 1945
Colonna and Ralston, 1951

Boyd, 1971

Fig. 18-4. Anterior approaches to the ankle and its adjacent structures.

incision. The approach is usually developed in the interval between the extensor hallucis longus and extensor digitorum longus tendons; however, Scaglietti (1940) and Nicola (1945) advised using the interval between the tendons of the tibialis anterior and the extensor hallucis longus. The anterolateral, malleolar, and lateral tarsal arteries must be identified, isolated, and ligated. The dorsal artery of the foot and the deep peroneal nerve are carefully exposed and retracted. The periosteum, capsule, and synovium are incised in line with the skin incision, and the full anterior width of the ankle joint is exposed by subcapsular and subperiosteal dissection (Fig. 18-4, *A*).

EXPOSURE OF THE ANKLE JOINT INCLUDING THE SUBTALAR AND TRANSVERSE TARSAL ARTICULATIONS
Anterolateral approach

Exposure of the ankle, talocalcaneal, talonavicular, and calcaneocuboid articulations is best accomplished through an anterolateral approach. Boyd (1971), who has described this approach, has suggested that it may well be called a "universal incision" for many surgical procedures on the foot and ankle. It avoids major vessels and nerves, and it can be extended proximally to reveal the distal tibia or distally to expose the articulations between the cuboid and the fourth and fifth metatarsals. Through such an incision arthrodesis of the tarsal joints may be done and excision of the talus as well as various talar coalitions can be performed.

The skin incision extends distally from a point 5 cm above the ankle joint and 1 cm in front of the anterior edge of the fibula toward the base of the fourth metatarsal. Here there is an overlap area supplied by twigs from the intermediate dorsal cutaneous peroneal branch and the superficial branches of the sural nerve.

If the intermediate dorsal cutaneous branch is exposed, it should be carefully preserved and retracted medially. The anterolateral malleolar artery will be encountered proximally and the lateral tarsal artery distally in the incision. Both may be sacrificed. The fascia and crural ligaments are incised, exposing the capsule of the ankle. The extensor digitorum brevis may be detached from its origin and reflected to uncover the talonavicular and calcaneocuboid regions and the region of the sinus tarsi (Fig. 18-4, *B*).

Lateral approaches to the subtalar joint and adjacent structures

Approach to subtalar and talonavicular joints (Kocher, 1911). This is a classic approach to the subtalar and talonavicular joints for subtalar or triple arthrodesis.

The incision begins about 2 cm proximal to the tip of the lateral malleolus, proceeds in a gentle curve around and below the malleolus, and terminates at the level of the talonavicular joint. The small saphenous vein and nerve should lie posteriorly. The anterior portion of the incision crosses the intermediate dorsal cutaneous nerve. Both nerves should be protected. The deep fascia is incised to expose the peroneal tendons. They may be retracted posteriorly if necessary to gain a wider field, or they may be divided by a Z-plasty and later

resutured. To gain access to the posterior facet of the subtalar articulation, the calcaneofibular ligament must be cut. If the lateral side of the ankle is to be explored, the anterior talofibular ligament must also be cut to permit dislocation of the talus medially (Fig. 18-5, *C*).

The disadvantage of this incision is that it necessitates the cutting of tendons and ligaments. Also, it is notorious for its poor healing. An anterolateral incision is preferable.

Lateral approach to sinus tarsi (Grice, 1952; Westin and Hall, 1957). Exposure of the sinus tarsi is readily performed through a short lateral curvilinear incision. This is the approach typically used in extra-articular arthrodesis of the subtalar joint in children.

The incision is 3 to 4 cm in length. It follows the skin creases from the tip of the lateral malleolus upward and forward and lies directly over the sinus tarsi. The peroneal tendons are located in the posterior extremity of the incision. Care should be taken to avoid cutting the intermediate dorsal cutaneous branch of the superficial peroneal nerve, which lies just at the anterior end of the incision. The cruciate ligament is incised and preserved to facilitate closure. The fat and the loose connective tissue are removed to expose the upper bony borders of the sinus tarsi. The origin of the extensor digitorum brevis and the attachments of the interosseous talocalcaneal ligament appear at the floor of the sinus (Fig. 18-2, *A*).

Approach to subtalar joint (Ollier, 1891). This is an approach that essentially uses only the anterior portion of the Kocher incision. It is slightly longer than the limited approach employed by Grice (1952) and Westin and Hall (1957) for extra-articular arthrodesis (Fig. 18-2, *A*). The approach is adequate for a subtalar or triple arthrodesis.

The incision commences 1 cm below the tip of the lateral malleolus and curves gently upward to terminate over the talonavicular joint. The intermediate dorsal cutaneous nerve crosses the anterior extremity of the incision and should be preserved. The peroneus tertius and long extensor tendons are exposed and must be retracted medially. The

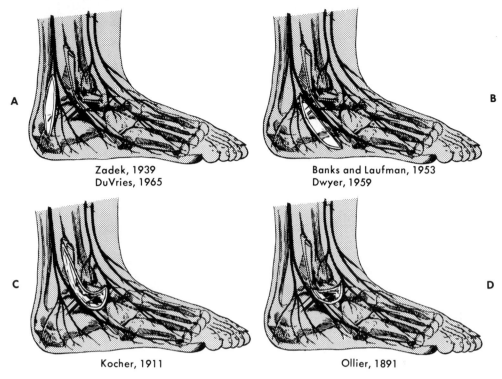

Zadek, 1939
DuVries, 1965

Banks and Laufman, 1953
Dwyer, 1959

Kocher, 1911

Ollier, 1891

Fig. 18-5. Lateral approaches to the calcaneus and subtalar joint.

peroneal tendons lie distal and posterior to the the lateral malleolus. They may be retracted inferiorly. The origin of the extensor digitorum brevis must be detached from its calcaneal attachment and is reflected distally (Fig. 18-5, *D*).

EXPOSURE OF THE CALCANEUS AND ADJACENT STRUCTURES
Medial approach to the calcaneus (Dwyer, 1959)

This approach can be used to expose the medial side of the calcaneus for osteotomy. It is also well suited for exposure of the soft tissue structures posterior to the medial malleolus and for decompression of the posterior tibial nerve in patients with tarsal tunnel syndrome or rupture of the posterior tibial tendon.

The incison begins at the superior aspect of the calcaneus and 1 cm posterior to the medial malleolus. It curves around and slightly distal to the malleolus and terminates at the tuber-

osity of the navicular. If the incision has been made properly, the saphenous vein and nerve will lie anterior to the incision. The posterior artery and venae comitantes and the posterior tibial nerve are located beneath the retinaculum between the tendons of the tibialis posterior and flexor digitorum anteriorly and the flexor hallucis posteriorly. In exposing the medial side of the calcaneus, the dissection may be carrried down superficial to the retinaculum. The retinaculum must be incised to expose the tendons or neurovascular structures for exploration. Several branches of the medial calcaneal nerve course through this area. They should be searched for but unfortunately are rarely observed. These cut nerves will often produce a painful scar (Fig. 18-6, *C*).

Lateral approach to the calcaneus (Banks and Laufman, 1953)

The lateral surface of the calcaneus is readily exposed through a curvilinear inci-

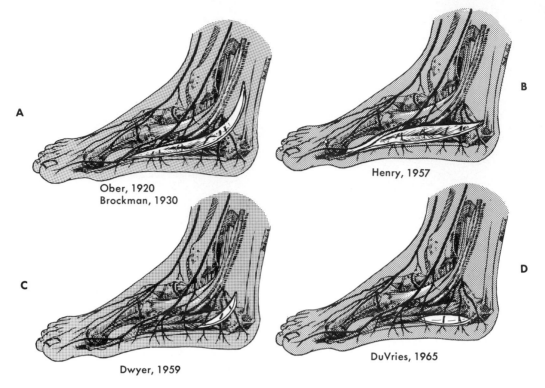

A
Ober, 1920
Brockman, 1930

B
Henry, 1957

C
Dwyer, 1959

D
DuVries, 1965

Fig. 18-6. Medial approaches to the plantar structures.

sion. This approach may be used for wedge osteotomies of the calcaneus (Dwyer, 1959), for osteomyelitis, or for excision of benign tumors.

The skin incision is 8 to 10 cm in length and parallels the underlying peroneal tendons. It begins at a point approximately 1 cm behind the lateral malleolus, curves with an upward concavity (just distal to the tip of the lateral malleolus), and terminates proximal to the base of the fifth metatarsal. Since the incision follows the course of the sural nerve, which lies in the subcutaneus tissue, the nerve should be sought, exposed, and protected. Occasionally the sural nerve divides into two trunks just past the tip of the lateral malleolus and should be looked for in this approach. The thick subcutaneous tissue may be undercut and reflected to expose the underlying bone (Fig. 18-5, *B*).

Posterior approaches to the calcaneus

Circumferential heel incision (Banks and Laufman, 1953). This approach exposes the entire posterior aspect of the calcaneus. It may be employed in open reduction of an avulsion fracture, for osteotomy, or for partial excision of the calcaneus.

With the patient prone, a transverse incision approximately 15 cm long is made along one of the skin creases, extending equally on both sides of the midpoint of the heel. Skin flaps are undercut to permit wide separation of the wound. The entire posterior and inferior aspects of the calcaneus may be exposed (Fig. 18-3, *B*).

Split heel approach (Gaenslen, 1931; Pridie, 1946). This approach has been employed for the complete or partial extirpation of the calcaneus in cases of osteomyelitis (Gaenslen, 1931) or in a markedly comminuted fracture (Pridie, 1946).

The incision is made in the midline of the heel and begins 2 to 3 cm above the attachment of the tendo Achillis to the calcaneus. It extends to the plantar surface of the heel and ends at the level of the calcaneocuboid articulation. The tendo Achillis is split in line with the skin incision for a distance of 2 to 3 cm, as is the plantar aponeurosis. With an osteotome or saw, the calcaneus is cut longitudinally and the two halves are separated. Curettement of abscesses can be done or excision of the calcaneus may be accomplished by shelling out the fragments of bone. The superficial fibers of the tendo Achillis and periosteum, which pass over the bone to become continuous with the plantar fascia, should be preserved (Fig. 18-3, C).

Exposure of the tendo Achillis

Exposure of the tendo Achillis can be readily accomplished by a straight linear incision placed medially, laterally, or directly posteriorly. A medial approach is generally recommended, however, since cosmetically a scar on the medial side is less apparent. As a rule the direct posterior approach to the tendo Achillis should be avoided to prevent a scar which would be irritated by shoewear.

Exposure of an adventitious Achilles bursa

Normally a bursa is present at the attachment of the tendo Achillis to the calcaneus, which lies between the tendon and the posterosuperior edge of the calcaneus. An adventitious bursa may be present between the skin and the tendon. This superficial bursa is readily approached through a transverse or longitudinal incision. A curved transverse incision located above the edge of the counter of the shoe is perhaps the preferable approach.

Resection of the deep bursa, without an osteotomy of the calcaneus, may be accomplished through a posteromedial or a posterolateral approach.

Posteromedial approach (Fowler and Philip, 1945). A curved transverse incision is made with an upward convexity that is sufficiently high to prevent pressure from the counter of a shoe. The flap is reflected downward. A superficial bursa is readily exposed; if a deeper bursa is to be resected, the upward skin flap may be undermined and retracted upward to expose the tendo Achillis. The tendon is split for a distance of 4 cm and is separated to expose the bursa. A sharp posterior edge of the calcaneus can be rounded, but

a transverse osteotomy cannot be performed with ease through this incision (Fig. 18-3, A).

Posterolateral approach (Zadek, 1939). A longitudinal incision 5 to 6 cm in length is made lateral to and parallel with the tendo Achillis. The bursa is readily isolated and removed. In addition, any sharp edge of the calcaneus can be smoothed off. If an excisional wedge is to be removed from the calcaneus, the wedge can be taken by extending this incision distally (Fig. 18-5, A).

EXPOSURE OF THE PLANTAR STRUCTURES
Medial approaches to the plantar structures

Henry (1957). Since the foot is essentially a half hemisphere that is open medially, structures in the plantar surface are most conveniently approached from the medial side. The skin incision should be located in the overlap area between the medial dorsal cutaneous nerve and the saphenous nerve. The incision begins at the first metatarsophalangeal articulation, proceeds in a smooth curve, passes just below the tuberosity of the navicular, and terminates anterior to the attachment of the tendo Achillis to the calcaneus.

The key to exposure of all the deep structures is the abductor hallucis. By isolating its tendon distally and following the tendon proximally, the surgeon carefully detaches the muscle from its attachments extending from the navicular tuberosity to the inner tuberosity of the calcaneus. The nerve supply to the abductor enters the muscle on its deep side and should be exposed and preserved. The muscle is hinged downward with the plantar flap, thus exposing most of the deep structures in the foot (Fig. 18-6, B).

DuVries (1965). This is a simple and direct approach to expose the tuber portion of the calcaneus and the attachment of the plantar aponeurosis. It may be employed for a fasciotomy of the aponeurosis, removal of a calcaneal spur, or resection of a benign tumor.

An incision approximately 5 cm long begins just short of the heel and is carried forward along the line of the junction of the thick plantar skin and the side of the heel. The skin with its fascia is slightly undermined to permit retraction, and the deep fascia is exposed. The deep fascia is incised, and the abductor hallucis, plantar fascia, and anteroinferior aspect of the calcaneus are exposed (Fig. 18-6, *D*). Occasionally terminal branches of the medial calcaneal nerve become caught in the scar; this makes the scar quite sensitive and most frequently occurs in the anterior portion of the scar.

Combined posteromedial and plantar exposure (Ober, 1920; Brockman, 1930). It is sometimes necessary to expose the posterior aspect of the ankle and subtalar articulation together with structures on the medial and plantar surfaces of the midfoot. An approach with such exposure is appropriate for a posterior and medial release in resistant clubfoot. The incision is a combination of the posteromedial and medial exposures of the plantar structures.

The incision begins 5 to 6 cm proximal to the medial malleolus and midway between the border of the tibia and the tendo Achillis.

It is carried distally, curves around the medial malleolus and along the medial side of the foot, and terminates in the region of the medial cuneiform. The saphenous vein and saphenous nerve lie anteriorly. The posterior flap is reflected to expose the tendo Achillis; the anterior flap is reflected to expose the posterior tibial tendon beneath the deep fascia. From this stage on, the extent of the deep dissection depends upon the surgical procedure to be performed. Whatever the procedure, the posterior tibial nerves and vessels must be carefully exposed and retracted if the surgeon wishes to expose the posteromedial aspect of the ankle and subtalar joints. To expose the deep plantar structures, the abductor hallucis must be dissected free of its attachments to the fascia, the navicular, and the calcaneus (Fig. 18-6, *A*).

EXPOSURE OF THE STRUCTURES OF THE FOREFOOT

Many incisions are available for the exposure of specific structures on the dorsum of the foot. Since most of these are essentially

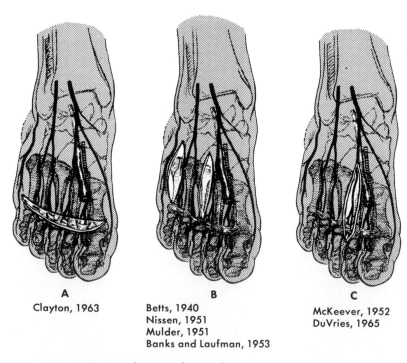

A
Clayton, 1963

B
Betts, 1940
Nissen, 1951
Mulder, 1951
Banks and Laufman, 1953

C
McKeever, 1952
DuVries, 1965

Fig. 18-7. Dorsal approaches to the structures of the forefoot.

subcutaneous, only cutaneous nerves, tendons, and certain vessels need be considered. Surgeons generally agree that surgical exposure of the extensor tendons and the metatarsals can be adequately obtained through longitudinal incisions overlying and roughly paralleling the appropriate structures (Fig. 18-7, *B*).

The choice of a surgical approach when dealing with abnormalities in the area of the metatarsophalangeal articulations is not unanimously agreed upon among surgeons. Some express grave misgivings concerning the placement of a skin incision on the weight-bearing surface of the foot; others recommend such approaches with impunity, stating that surgical exposure is the important criterion. Neither group has presented unequivocal evidence to cause the widespread adoption of a standard approach. Therefore the individual surgeon must base his choice upon his own experience and upon reports in the literature.

The most common indications for the use of surgical procedures in this area of the foot are such disorders of the forefoot as dislocation of the metatarsophalangeal articulations (hammertoes), metatarsalgias, and perineural fibromas.

Approaches to the metatarsal heads for resection

Resection of the metatarsal heads is a procedure that has proved to be of value in cases of marked deformities of the forefoot caused by the ravages of rheumatoid arthritis. These deformities consist of depression of the metatarsal heads, dorsal luxations at the metatarsophalangeal articulations, and hammertoes. The indication for surgical correction is incapacitating pain on weight bearing. When multiple metatarsal heads are to be resected, I (R.A.M.) prefer the following incisions: dorsal centered over the first metatarsophalangeal joint, dorsal web space between the second and third metatarsals, and dorsal web space between the fourth and fifth metatarsals. The other incisions are presented for completeness of the discussion.

Transverse plantar approach (Hoffmann,

1911). Hoffmann was one of the first surgeons to perform resections of the metatarsal heads. After experimenting with dorsal approaches, he proposed a plantar incision. A single transverse curved plantar incision is made just proximal to the web of the toes. A plantar flap of fascia and skin is reflected proximally, immediately exposing the metatarsal heads.

The same approach has been recommended by Kaplan (1950) for exposure of the plantar digital nerves since they lie between the metatarsal heads. The advantage of this incision is its exposure of digital nerves in several interspaces through a single incision (Fig. 18-8, *A*).

Transverse dorsal approach (Clayton, 1963). After trying many dorsal incisions, Clayton proposed a single transverse dorsal approach to the metatarsal heads. The skin incision is made over the metatarsal heads and curves slightly proximally on the medial side to overlie the first metatarsophalangeal joint. The extensor tendons are exposed and may be

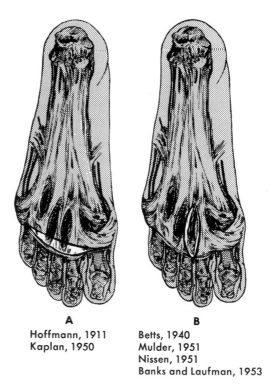

A
Hoffmann, 1911
Kaplan, 1950

B
Betts, 1940
Mulder, 1951
Nissen, 1951
Banks and Laufman, 1953

Fig. 18-8. Plantar incisions for exposure of structures in the area of the metatarsophalangeal articulations.

retracted or, if markedly contracted, cut in the line of the incision. The incision is opened by depressing the toes and the bases of the proximal phalanges; the metatarsal heads are thereby delivered into the wound. The metatarsals are osteotomized at the junction of the shaft to the head, and the metatarsal heads are dissected free. Only subcutaneous tissue and skin are sutured. If the tendon of the extensor hallucis has been cut, it is resutured (Fig. 18-7, *A*).

Approaches to the digital nerves for removal of perineural fibromas

Longitudinal plantar approach (Betts, 1940). This incision was originally proposed as a direct approach to the digital nerves for the removal of perineural fibromas. It offers an excellent view of the digital nerve and preserves the transverse metatarsal ligament. The disadvantages of the incision are (1) it places the scar on the weight-bearing surface and (2) it provides an exposure that is limited to a single metatarsal interspace. This incision is recommended by Mulder (1951), Nissen (1951), and Banks and Laufman (1953).

A straight longitudinal incision is made on the plantar surface of the foot extending from the web between the toes proximally for 3 cm. It is placed midway between the metatarsal heads (Fig. 18-8, *B*).

Transverse plantar approach (Kaplan, 1950). To avoid placing the scar over the metatarsal pads and permit exposure of more than a single digital nerve without section of the transverse metatarsal ligament, a transverse incision was proposed for the removal of perineural fibromas. This approach is similar to the one suggested by Hoffmann (1911) for excision of the metatarsal heads.

The incision is placed transversely, slightly distal to the interdigital folds, and may extend from the medial side of the first toe to the lateral side of the fifth toe. The subcutaneous plantar fat is cut in the line of the skin incision to expose the digital extensions of the plantar fascia. The skin with superficial fascia is retracted, exposing the flexor tendon sheaths that lie superficial to the tendons of the lumbrical muscles and transverse metatarsal ligament (Fig. 18-8, *A*).

Longitudinal dorsal approach (McKeever, 1952; DuVries, 1965). Because of aversion to plantar incisions, many surgeons employ a dorsal approach. Although this avoids placing a scar on the weight-bearing surface, the exposure of the nerve requires deeper dissection and cutting of the transverse metatarsal ligament. Cutting the transverse metatarsal ligament has not been shown to cause any significant postsurgical problems, however.

A skin incision is made between the proper metatarsals, extending proximally from the web for 3 cm. With a hemostat, blunt dissection is achieved between the metatarsal heads. To separate the metatarsal heads adequately in order to expose the digital nerve, the transverse metatarsal ligament must be incised. Firm pressure under the metatarsals will present the nerve. To permit sufficient proximal sectioning of the nerve, it may have to be grasped with a hemostat and delivered into the wound (Fig. 18-7, *C*).

For exposure of a metatarsophalangeal joint, a skin incision is made between the proper metatarsals starting in the web space and continuing obliquely until centered over the metatarsal head and shaft to be exposed. A direct longitudinal incision over the dorsal aspect of a metatarsophalangeal joint should be avoided because of possible contracture of the scar which would cause the toe to be held dorsally so it would not touch the ground.

REFERENCES

Banks, S. W., and Laufman, H.: An atlas of surgical exposures of the extremities, Philadelphia, 1953, W. B. Saunders Co.

Betts, L. O.: Morton's metatarsalgia: neuritis of the fourth digital nerve, Med. J. Aust. 1:514, 1940.

Boyd, H. B.: Surgical approaches. In Crenshaw, A. H., editor: Campbell's operative orthopaedics, ed 5, vol. 1, St. Louis, 1971, The C. V. Mosby Co.

Brockman, E. P.: Congenital club-foot (talipes equinovarus), Bristol, 1930, J. Wright & Sons, Ltd.

Broomhead, R.: Discussion on fractures in the region of the ankle-joint, Proc. R. Soc. Med. 25:1082, 1932.

Clayton, M. L.: Surgery of the lower extremity in rheumatoid arthritis, J. Bone Joint Surg. 45A:1517, 1963.

Colonna, P. C., and Ralston, E. L.: Operative approaches to the ankle joint, Am. J. Surg. 82:44, 1951.

DuVries, H. L. Surgery of the foot, ed. 2, St. Louis, 1965, The C. V. Mosby Co.

Dwyer, F. C.: Osteotomy of the calcaneum for pes cavus, J. Bone Joint Surg. **41B**:80, 1959.

Fowler, A., and Philip, J. F.: Abnormality of the calcaneus as a cause of painful heel: its diagnosis and operative treatment, Br. J. Surg. **32**:494, 1945.

Gaenslen, F. J.: Split-heel approach in osteomyelitis of os calcis, J. Bone Joint Surg. **13**:759, 1931.

Gatellier, J., and Chastang: La voie d'accès juxtarétro-péronière dans le traitement sanglant des fractures malléolaires avec fragment marginal postérieur, J. Chir. **24**:513, 1924.

Grice, D. S.: An extra-articular arthrodesis of the subastragalar joint for correction of paralytic flatfeet in children, J. Bone Joint Surg. **34A**:927, 1952.

Henry, A. K.: Extensile exposure, ed. 2, Baltimore, 1957, The Williams & Wilkins Co.

Hoffmann, P.: An operation for severe grades of contracted or clawed toes, Am. J. Orthop. Surg. **9**:441, 1911.

Jergesen, F.: Open reduction of fractures and dislocations of the ankle, Am. J. Surg. **98**:136, 150, 1959.

Kaplan, E. B.: Surgical approach to the plantar digital nerves, Bull. Hosp. Joint Dis. **11**:96, 1950.

Kocher, T.: Textbook of operative surgery, ed. 3 (translated by H. J. Stiles and C. B. Paul), London, 1911, A. & C. Black.

McKeever, D. C.: Surgical approach for neuroma of plantar digital nerve (Morton's metatarsalgia), J. Bone Joint Surg. **34A**:490, 1952.

McLaughlin, H. L., and Ryder, C. T.: Open reduction and internal fixation for fractures of the tibia and ankle, Surg. Clin. North Am. **29**:1523, 1949.

Mulder, J. D.: The causative mechanism in Morton's metatarsalgia, J. Bone Joint Surg. **33B**:94, 1951.

Nicola, T.: Atlas of surgical approaches to bones and joints, New York, 1945, The Macmillan Co.

Nissen, K. I.: The etiology of Morton's metatarsalgia, J. Bone Joint Surg. **33B**:293, 1951.

Ober, F. R.: An operation for the relief of congenital equino-varus deformity, J. Orthop. Surg. **2**:558, 1920.

Ollier, L.: Traité des résections et des opérations conservatrices qu'on peut practiquer sur le système osseux, vol. 3, Paris, 1891, G. Masson.

Patrick, J.: A direct approach to trimalleolar fractures, J. Bone Joint Surg. **47B**:236, 1965.

Picot, G.: L'intervention sanglante dans les fractures malléolaires, J. Chir. **21**:529, 1923.

Pridie, K. H.: A new method of treatment for severe fractures of the os calcis: a preliminary report, Surg. Gynecol. Obstet. **82**:671, 1946.

Scaglietti, O.: Tecnica e risultati dell'artrodesi della tibiotarsica, Chir. Organi Mov. **26**:244, 254, 1940.

Westin, G. W., and Hall, C. B.: Subtalar extra-articular arthrodesis: a preliminary report of a method of stabilizing feet in children, J. Bone Joint Surg. **39A**:501, 1957.

Zadek, I.: An operation for the cure of achillobursitis, Am. J. Surg. **43**:542, 1939.

19

MAJOR SURGICAL PROCEDURES FOR DISORDERS OF THE ANKLE, TARSUS, AND MIDTARSUS

Verne T. Inman and Roger A. Mann

THE ANKLE
Open reduction of fractures about the ankle

If closed reduction fails to reposition all articular surfaces of the ankle mortise accurately, open reduction and internal fixation are indicated.

Fractures of internal malleolus. The saphenous nerve crosses the medial malleolus midway between the anterior and posterior borders of the malleolus. The nerve can be palpated by passing one's fingernail across the skin. The nerve is felt as a taut cord between the fingernail and the underlying bone. It should be avoided, since its injury or section may produce annoying symptoms. To avoid the nerve, either a posteromedial or an anteromedial approach can be used. (See Chapter 18.)

In the posterior approach, care should be taken not to open the sheath of the posterior tibial tendon or to lacerate the tendon. The posterior approach will avoid the saphenous nerve but affords a less satisfactory view of the interior of the ankle joint.

The anteromedial approach, if extended distally, is more likely to interrupt the saphenous nerve, but this approach provides a better view of the interior of the ankle joint and enables the surgeon to check the accuracy of the reduction.

The distal fragment of the medial malleolus is usually slightly displaced anteriorly. After the fracture site is exposed, soft tissue imposition should be looked for and any tissue found should be removed. The malleolar fracture can be reduced and fixed with a towel clip while a screw or pin is placed through the distal tip of the malleolus into the shaft of the tibia.

Fractures of lateral malleolus. The sural nerve passes along the posterior border of the lateral malleolus and can be palpated beneath the skin between the examiner's fingernail and the underlying bone. Preliminary palpation will help avoid interruption of this nerve.

The lateral malleolus is exposed through a direct longitudinal incision placed over the malleolus. Fractures of the lateral malleolus are usually spiral in nature and occur at the level of the joint or above the joint in the distal shaft. In the latter case the examiner should be suspicious of a possible tibiofibular diastasis. The fracture can usually be reduced with ease and fixed with an intermedullary pin or screw.

Fractures of posterior lip of tibia (trimalleolar fracture; Cotton's fracture). An isolated fracture of the posterior lip of the tibia occurs infrequently; however, it is a common fracture in conjunction with fractures of the malleoli with posterior dislocation of the ankle joint. More than any other type of fracture, it is one that requires open reduction and an accurate realignment of the fragments. Usually the fracture occurs on the lateral side of the plafond; the talus is rotated and displaced backward and laterally.

The posterior aspect of the ankle joint can be approached through a posterolateral or posteromedial incision. A 10 cm linear incision is made 1.5 cm medial or lateral to the tendo Achillis. The tendon is retracted either laterally or medially. The dissection is carried down through the loose fatty areolar tissue until the posterior aspect of the joint is encountered. The tendon of the flexor hallucis longus is located as it crosses the posterior capsule from the lateral side toward the medial side. The tendon is retracted medially and the posterior aspect of the ankle joint is exposed. By keeping lateral to the tendon of the flexor hallucis longus, the surgeon avoids the posterior tibial vessels and the nerve. The fracture can be readily located, and the upwardly displaced posterior lip of the tibia is corrected with a towel clip. After visual confirmation of the reduction, the surgeon may fix the reduction by the insertion of a stainless steel nail or a screw. Since accurate alignment is mandatory, radiographs should be taken after reduction and before closure.

Fractures of anterior lip of tibia. These require accurate reduction. The anterior aspect of the tibia is best exposed through an anteromedial approach. The incision is made in the space between the anterior tibial tendon and the extensor tendons; the tendons are displaced medially to expose the anterior aspect of the joint.

After reduction is carried out, the frag-ments may be fixed with stainless steel pins or screws.

Arthrodesis of the talocrural (ankle) joint

Many methods to arthrodese the ankle have been reported in the literature. The selection of one particular procedure over others has been influenced by such factors as the type of pathologic process present, the preconceived ideas of individual surgeons, and the kind of fusion that is indicated.

Extra-articular fusions have been done for septic arthritis, particularly for tuberculous destruction of the joint. They have also been used when the surgeon has felt that simultaneous fusion of the ankle and subtalar joints was necessary because of the presence of lesions involving both articulations. Such cases fall into a special category and are discussed separately.

In arthrodeses of the ankle joint alone, the objective is to accomplish good bony apposition between the body of the talus and the mortise; after removal of the articular cartilage from the surfaces of the joint, a loose and sloppy articulation is left. To ensure firm contact between the bony surfaces and to stabilize the joint during the period of time required for union, various procedures have been employed. These include the packing of bone chips into the space between the bones, the use of bone grafts to span the joint, and the performance of osteotomies of one or both of the malleoli to narrow the mortise. Any combination of these methods has been used, with or without additional internal fixation with metal pins, rods, and screws.

Most of the basic operations were introduced by the pioneers in orthopaedic surgery at the beginning of this century. An excellent historical review with an extensive bibliography of earlier operative procedures was published in 1946 by Schwartz. Only minor modifications have been introduced by individual surgeons who felt that their contributions either improved the chances of fusion or decreased the time required to achieve a firm union.

The methods used to arthrodese the ankle joint may be divided into the four categories

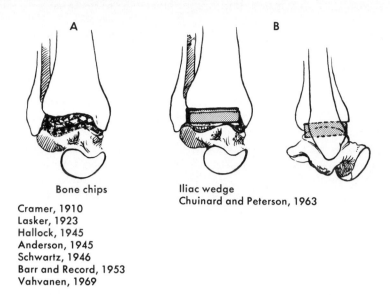

A

B

Bone chips

Cramer, 1910
Lasker, 1923
Hallock, 1945
Anderson, 1945
Schwartz, 1946
Barr and Record, 1953
Vahvanen, 1969

Iliac wedge
Chuinard and Peterson, 1963

Fig. 19-1. Arthrodeses of the talocrural joint using intra-articular bone grafts. **A,** Denuding the articular surfaces of cartilage and packing the interval with bone chips. **B,** Insertion of a single bone graft between the plafond and the talus.

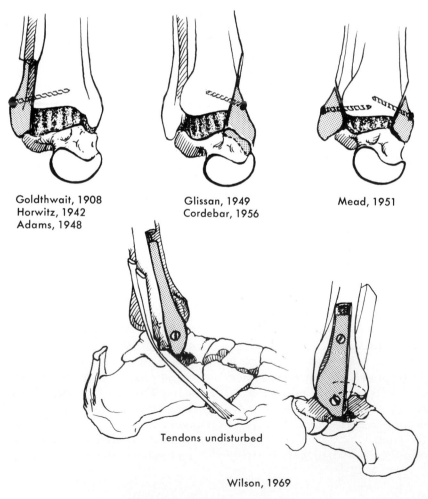

Goldthwait, 1908
Horwitz, 1942
Adams, 1948

Glissan, 1949
Cordebar, 1956

Mead, 1951

Tendons undisturbed

Wilson, 1969

Fig. 19-2. Malleolar osteotomies.

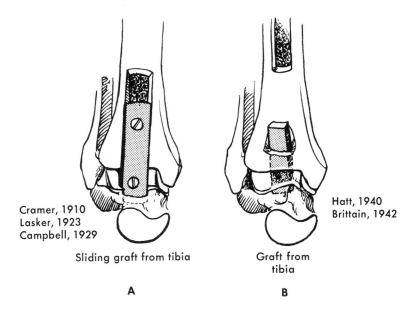

Fig. 19-3. Anterior tibial bone grafts. An anterior bone graft supplements the intra-articular fusion.

listed below. Figs. 19-1 through 19-4 offer a pictorial summary of the various procedures.

1. Intra-articular bone graft
2. Malleolar osteotomy
3. Anterior tibial graft
4. Compression arthrodesis

Intra-articular bone graft. The ankle joint has been exposed through varioius incisions—including a lateral J-shaped incision (Schwartz, 1946), the anterolateral approach (Cramer, 1910; Lasker, 1923; Anderson, 1945; Hallock, 1945; Vahvanen, 1969), and the approach that employs two linear incisions, one along the anterior border of the lateral malleolus and a second along the anterior margin of the medial malleolus (Barr and Record, 1953).

After denuding all cartilage from the articular surfaces to expose bleeding bone, the surgeon fills the joint space with bone chips either "fish-scaled" from the tibial and talar surfaces (Hallock, 1945) or secured from the iliac crest or the anterior surface of the tibia (Fig. 19-1, *A*). Chuinard and Peterson (1963)

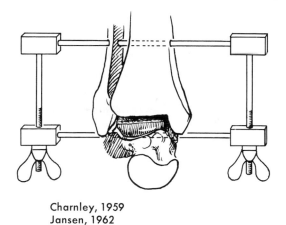

Fig. 19-4. Compression arthrodesis. After removal of articular cartilage from the joint surfaces, the joints are continuously compressed by means of pins, threaded rods, and wing nuts.

inserted a wedge graft taken from the iliac crest between the plafond of the tibia and the talus (Fig. 19-1, *B*). This method of arthrodesis is particularly applicable to young persons, whose epiphyses are still open.

Malleolar osteotomy. The need to achieve

a snug fit between the trochlea of the talus and the mortise after removal of the articular cartilage was recognized early.

Goldthwait (1908) proposed narrowing the mortise by performing an osteotomy of the fibula and displacing the fibula medially. Several modifications of this procedure have appeared (Horwitz, 1942; Adams, 1948). Glissan (1949) and Cordebar (1956) osteotomized the medial malleolus. Mead (1951) osteotomized both malleoli. Wilson (1969) osteotomized only the anterior halves of both malleoli to avoid possible injury to or malfunction of the tendons of the peroneal and posterior tibial muscles (Fig. 19-2).

Various incisions were employed by the several surgeons, depending on the required exposure.

Anterior tibial graft. This procedure has been an old and popular method of arthrodesis (Fig. 19-3). It appears to have been first employed by Cramer (1910), Lasker (1923), and Campbell (1929).

The ankle joint is exposed through an anterior approach. After denuding the articular cartilage from the joint surfaces and correcting the deformity, the surgeon cuts a bone graft from the anterior aspect of the tibia, places it across the joint, and affixes it to the talus and the tibia with screws (Fig. 19-3, A). A modification of this procedure proposed by Hatt (1940) was popularized by Brittain (1942), in which the tibial graft is embedded into the body of the talus through a hole in the plafond (Fig. 19-3, B).

Compression arthrodesis. Whereas Anderson (1945) used an external metal appliance to retain the bones in position and White, in discussing Hallock's (1945) paper, stated that he had been placing pins through the tibia and the calcaneus which were connected by rubber bands to maintain compression, it was Charnley (1959) who popularized compression arthrodesis (Fig. 19-4).

Charnley employed a transverse incision across the anterior aspect of the ankle joint extending 1 cm above the tip of each malleolus. The extensor tendons were divided, the vessels were ligated and cut, and the nerves were severed. The extensor tendons were

resutured during closure. Ratliff (1959), in a review of fifty-five ankles repaired by Charnley's technique, reported a high percentage of fusion. However, minor complications and disabilities also occurred. These residual conditions included extensor tendons adherent to the scar, persistent mild edema of the foot distal to the incision, persistent numbness over the dorsum of the foot, and a decrease in the power of dorsiflexion of the toes.

Jansen (1962) approved the concept of compression arthrodesis but felt that the tranverse incision was unnecessary. He combined compression with the medial and lateral approach of Anderson (1945) and reported twenty-four out of twenty-five solid fusions. Dahmen and Mleyer (1965) published an extensive and critical review of their experience with the various methods of fusion of the talocrural joint.

Recommended procedure. In my experience (R.A.M.) a Charnley-type arthrodesis through the anterior approach utilizing an anterior sliding tibial graft has been most successful in the ankle. To avoid the possibility of a thick scar over the anterior aspect of the ankle, the anterior approach should be a lazy S skin incision. Extreme caution should be exercised in the anterior approach to be sure the superficial branches of the peroneal nerve are identified and retracted.

The position of choice for an ankle arthrodesis is neutral for dorsiflexion and plantar flexion in men and as much as 5° or 10° of plantar flexion in women. When considering varus and valgus, one must place the ankle in 0° to 5° of valgus. When considering the position at the time of surgery, one must keep in mind the overall alignment of the entire lower extremity and not just the relationship of the talus to the distal tibia.

Posterior bone blocks

Posterior bone blocks have been employed as supplementary techniques for the stabilization of the foot. The procedures of Campbell (1923, 1925) and Gill (1933) are illustrated in Fig. 19-5. A case of paralytic dropfoot treated by means of the Gill procedure is illustrated in Fig. 19-6.

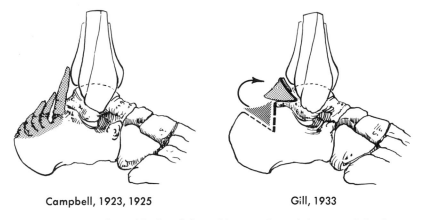

Campbell, 1923, 1925   Gill, 1933

Fig. 19-5. Posterior bone blocks of the ankle joint for stabilization of the foot.

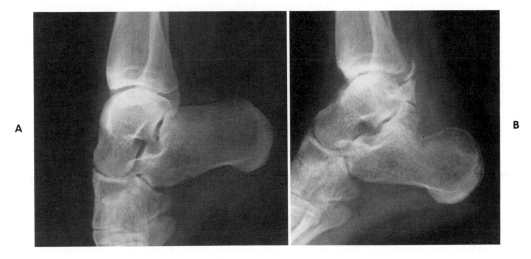

A   B

Fig. 19-6. Treatment of paralytic foot drop in a 25-year-old woman who had had poliomyelitis in childhood. **A,** Preoperative; **B,** postoperative following a Gill procedure.

Indications for these procedures as well as the Inclan (1949) procedure have been recorded in detail by Wheeldon and Clark (1936), Branch (1939), Inclan (1949), and Ingram and Hundley (1951). When used in conjunction with triple arthrodesis and a laterally stable talotibial joint, the posterior bone block limits plantar flexion by contact with the inferior and posterior articular surfaces of the tibia.

Soft tissue procedures

Surgical repair of ankle ligaments. Severe ligamentous injuries of the ankle often masquerade as sprains. For adequate evaluation, radiographs of the ankle in stressed position must be taken; occasionally, arthrograms are necessary as well.

Collateral ligaments. Complete tears of the collateral ligaments necessitate surgical exploration and repair. In acute cases direct surgical repair of the torn ligaments is possible (Ruth, 1961) (Fig. 19-7). In old cases of instability of the ankle, repair of the old tear, particularly of the anterior talofibular ligament (Broström, 1966), or reconstruction of the collateral ligaments is necessary. Broström has pointed out that even after several years it is possible to adequately dissect out and suture the torn end of ankle ligaments. In a few cases in which the ligamentous tissue was inadequate for direct repair, the anterior talofibular ligament was reconstructed using a flap from the lateral talocalcaneal ligament.

Reconstruction of lateral collateral ligament. The lateral collateral ligament of the ankle is composed of three separate structures. With forceful inversion of the ankle, the susceptibility to rupture of each component appears to be as follows (Francillon, 1962): The anterior talofibular ligament is most likely to be torn. With further inversion, disruption

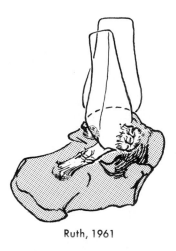

Ruth, 1961

Fig. 19-7. Procedure for reconstruction of the lateral collateral ligament. Resuturing of the ligament is readily accomplished if performed soon after the injury has occurred.

of the calcaneofibular ligament occurs in addition to tear of the anterior talofibular ligament (Ruth, 1961). Isolated tears of the calcaneofibular ligament are infrequent and occur only if the foot is inverted while in a position of full dorsiflexion. Tears of the posterior talofibular ligament seem to occur rarely if at all (Ashhurst and Bromer, 1922; Anderson and LeCocq, 1954).

Various procedures for the reconstruction of the lateral collateral ligament have been employed. Elmslie (1934) attempted to replace the injured ligaments anatomically with a strip of fascia lata (Fig. 19-8). His procedure demonstrated an appreciation of the mechanical relationships that exist between the arrangement of the ligaments and the axes of motion of the ankle and subtalar joints. Some surgeons have questioned the durability of fascia for the repair and have preferred to use tendon. The obvious availability of the peroneal tendons led to their use in these procedures, which differed only according to the personal ingenuity of the surgeon who employed the handy structures. Unfortunately the anatomic arrangements resulting from these procedures placed the newly formed collateral ligaments in such a position as to always compromise the subtalar motion. The Chrisman and Snook (1969) type–reconstruction fairly accurately approximates the normal ligamentous anatomy of the ankle joint.

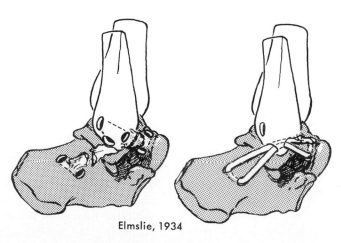

Elmslie, 1934

Fig. 19-8. Reconstructive procedure for old tears of the lateral collateral ligament of the ankle using fascia lata.

Other procedures that have been used for reconstruction of the lateral collateral ligaments in unstable ankle joints are depicted in Fig. 19-9. The surgeons advocating each procedure are referred to. Ligamentous reconstruction on the lateral side of the ankle should be carried out after all conservative methods of treatment have been exhausted. The surgical procedure leaves a significant and frequently symptomatic scar as well as stiffness about the ankle and subtalar joints.

Reconstruction of medial collateral (deltoid) ligament. Isolated tears of this ligament are rare. When the foot has been forcibly everted, the medial malleolus is more likely to be fractured or the ligament is more apt to be avulsed from the tibia. Small fragments of bone are seen on radiographs.

Watson-Jones (1955) warned that in suspected injuries to the medial collateral ligament, one should be alert to the possibility of a diastasis of the distal tibiofibular syndesmosis. Because of the nature of the pathologic findings, direct repair of the ligament in acute cases is indicated, and tightening of the structure for chronic instability of the ankle has been reported.

The technique of Schoolfield (1952) has been adapted for the repair of recurrent sprains of the deltoid ligament. The anterior skin flap is deflected to expose the deltoid ligament, which is detached from the medial malleolus and freed to its insertions. The foot is inverted at this point to permit suturing the deltoid ligament to the periosteal and ligamentous tissues over the medial malleolus

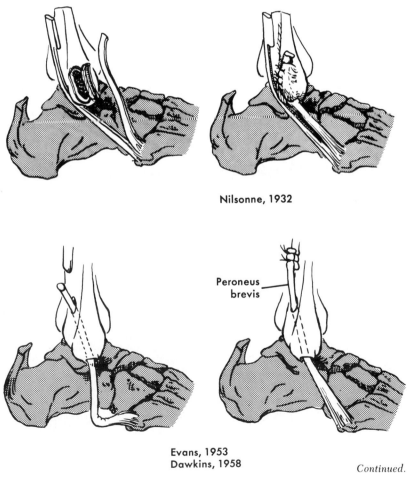

Nilsonne, 1932

Peroneus
brevis

Evans, 1953
Dawkins, 1958

Continued.

Fig. 19-9. Procedures for reconstruction of the lateral collateral ligament.

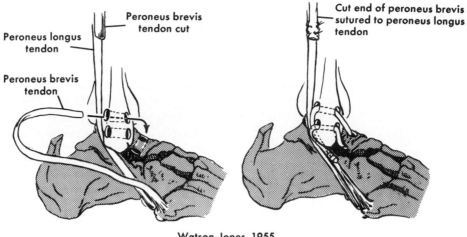

Peroneus longus tendon

Peroneus brevis tendon

Peroneus brevis tendon cut

Cut end of peroneus brevis sutured to peroneus longus tendon

Watson-Jones, 1955
Gillespie and Boucher, 1971

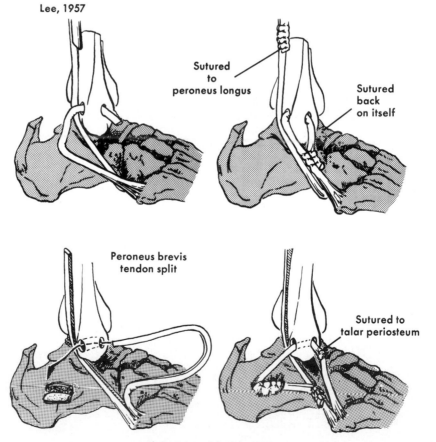

Lee, 1957

Sutured to peroneus longus

Sutured back on itself

Peroneus brevis tendon split

Sutured to talar periosteum

Chrisman and Snook, 1969

Fig. 19-9, cont'd. For legend see p. 537.

just above the natural origin of the deltoid ligament (Fig. 19-10).

For recurrent sprains of the deltoid ligament, DuVries (1965) found that a cruciate incision and cross-shaped scar formation give preferable results. A vertical incision is bisected by a horizontal incision, forming a cross of equal arms. The margins are sutured together to leave a cross-shaped scar which is strong enough to act successfully as a stabilizer of the ankle (Fig. 19-11).

Tendon transfers about hindfoot. Since the talus has no muscular attachments, the stability of this bone within its skeletal compartment is in constant jeopardy. During weight bearing and locomotion, all the muscles be-

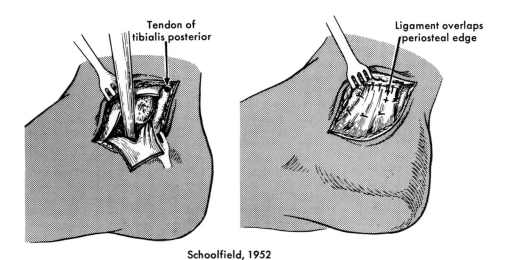

Schoolfield, 1952

Fig. 19-10. Schoolfield's technique for reconstruction of the deltoid ligament. **A,** The ligament is stripped from above downward over the medial malleolus. **B,** Foot held in inversion. The upper margin of the deltoid ligament is sutured to the periosteal edge, which it overlaps.

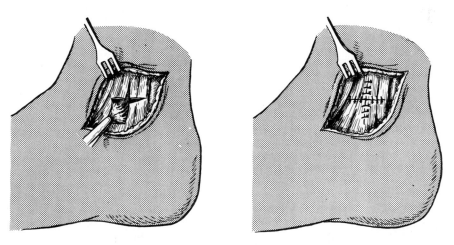

DuVries, 1965

Fig. 19-11. DuVries' technique for reconstruction of the deltoid ligament. **A,** Vertical incision into the ligament bisected at the center by a transverse incision. The resulting four right-angular flaps of the ligament are denuded and freed from the bone. **B,** Four flaps sutured to form a cross-shaped scar which stabilizes the ankle.

tween the leg and the remaining skeletal structures in the foot play varying roles in keeping the talus properly aligned within the ankle mortise above, in maintaining the alignment of the articular surfaces of the calcaneus below, and in preserving functional contact with the navicular in front. Synovitis of tendon sheaths, dislocations and ruptures of tendons, and paralysis or spasticity of muscles may so alter the forces that stability is impaired and deformity results. In attempts to rebalance these forces, many tendon transfers have been carried out. It is impossible to enumerate them all; however, when considering the performance of a tendon transference, the surgeon should bear in mind the following questions:

1. What is the etiology of the functional loss? Is the condition static or progressive? In the child, what effect will growth have upon the function of the transfer?

2. Is the muscle of the tendon to be transferred sufficiently strong, and is its fiber length such that adequate excursion is assured? Will the tendon be long enough to reach the area into which it is to be implanted?

3. Is the phasic action of the donor muscle the same as that of the diseased one which it will replace? Close and Todd (1959) indicated that a complete change in phasic action of muscles in the lower extremity is not likely to occur.

4. What will be the consequences of the loss of the normal function of the donor tendon?

5. Should arthrodesing procedures be performed along with the tendon transfer?

Certain principles are to be followed in tendon transfers. As has been indicated, a muscle having approximately the same phasic action should be selected for transfer. The line of pull of the muscle and its tendon should be as straight as possible from its origin to the new insertion. If at all possible, the tendon should be firmly fixed to bone through a drill hole or an osteoperiosteal tunnel.

The length-tension relationship in striated muscle is such that maximal tension can be developed only if the muscle is at its rest length. If the muscle is activated when it is shorter or longer than its rest length, it will generate less force. Rest length can be determined by gently pulling the tendon and estimating the increase in passive resistance to further stretching. The rest length is the point at which passive resistance can first be determined by the surgeon. Thus the tendon should be implanted in bone with only minimal tension and with the skeletal part in the position of maximal function.

Because of the multiplicity of factors that must be considered, each case presents a unique problem which the surgeon must consider carefully before he attempts a solution by means of a tendon transfer.

Synovectomies. Synovectomies have had a long and variegated history. The reader interested in an excellent historical review may consult the article by Geens (1969).

London (1955) rekindled enthusiasm for synovectomy of the knee in rheumatoid arthritis, and the literature since then has been copious. With the increasing popularity of synovectomy of the knee, the procedure has been applied to almost every joint. This operation is useful for relieving pain in the active stages of the disease before joint destruction has occurred. Heywood (1967), Whitefield (1967), Vahvanen (1968), Jakubowski (1970), and Murray (1972) reported on the use of this procedure on the ankle joint.

The most satisfactory approach is the anterolateral, which permits excision of most of the synovial membrane lining at the front and sides of the joint. As much of the synovial membrane in the posterior part of the joint as possible is removed with a pituitary rongeur.

Tendon dislocations and subluxations in ankle region. There are several tendons in the region of the ankle that are subject to partial or complete dislocation. These dislocations usually result from twisting injuries to the ankle, but they have been reported to occur spontaneously. The peroneals are by far the most frequently injured tendons.

Mounier-Kuhn and Marsan (1968) published a careful review of forty-four cases of tendon dislocation in the ankle. They divided

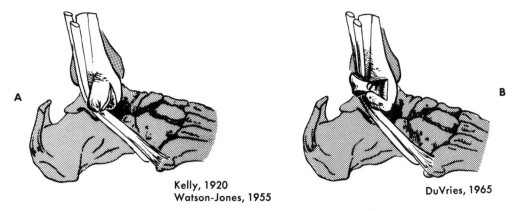

Kelly, 1920
Watson-Jones, 1955

DuVries, 1965

Fig. 19-12. Method of deepening the sulcus for prevention of recurrent dislocations of peroneal tendons.

the cases into five groups according to etiology, pathology, and treatment. In readily reducible acute dislocations that are stable after reduction, conservative treatment consisting of reduction and immobilization of the foot in a cast for 6 to 8 weeks may be used. If the reduction is unstable—as in an osteoperiosteal avulsion (Murr, 1961) or a complete tear of the tendon sheath—surgical repair will be indicated.

Several procedures have been employed. Kelly (1920) and Watson-Jones (1955) displaced an osteoperiosteal graft from the malleolus posteriorly (Fig. 19-12, A). DuVries (1965) cut a wedge-shaped bone graft from the malleolus, displaced it posteriorly, and fixed it with a screw. At the same time the redundant sheath of the peroneal tendons was excised and the tendon sheath repaired (Fig. 19-12, B). These procedures deepened the sulcus and prevented recurrences of the dislocation.

Mounier-Kuhn and Marsan (1968) and Daimant-Berger (1971) plicated and resutured the tendon sheath. Weigert (1969) tightened the sheath by suturing its border to the fibula through drill holes in the malleolus. Folschveiller (1967) and Bogutskaia (1970) reinforced the sheath with a flap of periosteum which was reflected from the fibula and sutured over the repaired tendon sheath. In chronic dislocations and habitually dislocating tendons, osteotomies of the malleolus are required.

The posterior tibial tendon may be dislocated from its sulcus behind the medial malleolus, although such an occurrence appears to be quite rare. Muralt (1956) was the first to describe a case. Scheuba (1969), in reporting two cases, stated the opinion that a habitually dislocating posterior tibial tendon may be more common than is indicated from the literature. He pointed out that when individuals complain of instability and pain in the area of the medial malleolus the possibility of dislocation of the posterior tibial tendon should be kept in mind.

Because of the lack of reported cases, no standard operative procedure has emerged. Based on the experience gained from peroneal dislocations, however, an osteoperiosteal flap from the medial malleolus similar to that in the procedure used by Kelly and Watson-Jones on the lateral malleolus seems indicated.

THE TARSUS
Posterior tarsus

Subtalar and triple arthrodeses. During the first two decades of the twentieth century, the problem of treatment of the deformed or flail foot ocurring as a sequela to poliomyelitis occupied the attention of the orthopaedist. The necessity of stabilizing the articulations of the posterior tarsus was apparent.

The surgical solution to this problem was attempted with two ideas in mind: one was to achieve greater stability by obliterating or limiting ankle and subtalar motion; the other was to displace the foot posteriorly so the body weight would pass more nearly through the midfoot. A variety of surgical procedures were proposed and carried out by different surgeons, ranging from talectomy to pantalar arthrodesis. The majority of the operations were intended to correct pes cavus and to stabilize the subtalar and transverse tarsal articulations.* Numerous modifications, with adjuvant procedures such as tendon transfers, have been used. Some of these procedures have withstood the test of time; others have been abandoned.

Subtalar and triple arthrodeses are now done less frequently since the deformities resulting from poliomyelitis no longer constitute a major part of the practice of orthopaedics. Excellent reviews and discussions concerning surgical arthrodeses, particularly in poliomyelitis, have been presented.†

Although the need for a variety of procedures to deal with the multiplicity of disabilities resulting from poliomyelities is presently not so great, indications for subtalar and triple arthrodeses in specific cases still remain. From the numerous methods employed in the past, two have proved useful and have become accepted as standard procedures.

The first is the Hoke arthrodesis, with numerous modifications (Fig. 19-13). It is an intra-articular arthrodesis and is useful for painful arthritic processes involving the subtalar and transverse tarsal articulations.

The second is the extra-articular arthrodesis of Grice (Fig. 19-14), which is useful in blocking subtalar motion in patients who have no gross skeletal deformities but have instability of the hindfoot. The Grice arthrodesis is particularly applicable in children, since there is little interference with future growth of the foot.

In the Grice extra-articular arthrodesis, the operative technique is relatively simple. The region of the sinus tarsi is exposed through a

---

*Jones, 1908; Davis, 1913; Hoke, 1921; Ryerson, 1923; Dunn, 1928.
†Hart, 1937; Crego and McCarroll, 1938; Hallgrímsson, 1943; Schwartz, 1946.

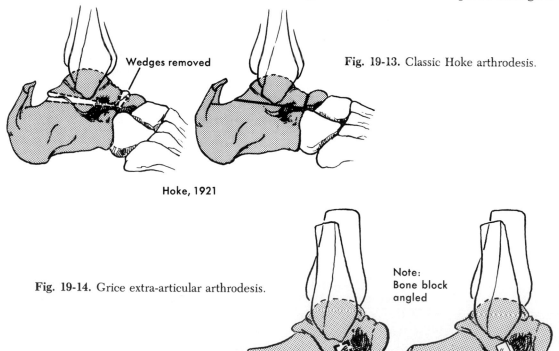

Wedges removed

Hoke, 1921

Fig. 19-13. Classic Hoke arthrodesis.

Fig. 19-14. Grice extra-articular arthrodesis.

Note:
Bone block
angled

Grice, 1952

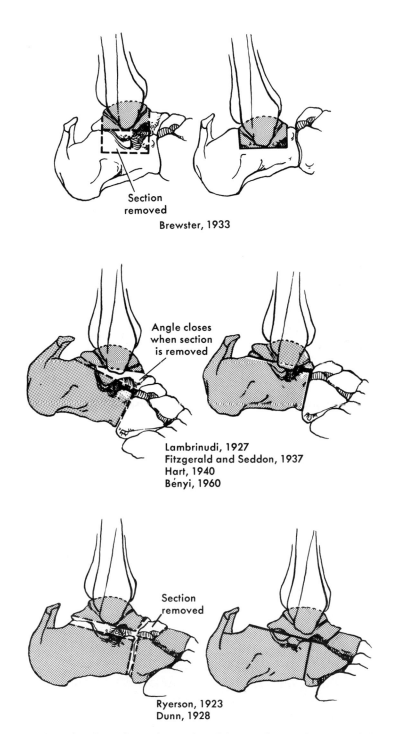

Fig. 19-15. Arthrodeses formerly employed for paralytic deformities of the foot.

short curvilinear incision extending from the peroneal tendons to the extensor tendons. The ligamentous structures and adipose tissue are removed from the sinus tarsi. The origin of the extensor digitorum brevis is dissected from the calcaneus and reflected distally, allowing complete visualization of the interval between the talus and the calcaneus. With an osteotome, slots are cut in the inferior surface of the talus and the superior surface of the calcaneus. The surgeon should recall the direction of the axis of the subtalar joint; the graft, to provide adequate stabilization, must lie in a plane that is perpendicular to this axis (Fig. 19-14). Thus the graft should run distally and anteriorly; otherwise, it will not block motion of the subtalar joint and may become displaced. The graft may be taken from the anterosuperior surface of the tibia or from the iliac crest.

There are several other surgical methods of arthrodesing the articulations of the hindfoot. These procedures were formerly employed for paralytic deformities and are depicted in Fig. 19-15. The surgeons advocating each procedure are indicated. The *beak* triple arthrodesis as advocated by Siffert et al. (1966) is most useful for correction of a severe cavus deformity (Fig. 19-16).

Combined talonavicular, talocrural, and pantalar arthrodesis. Orthopaedic surgeons disagree as to the indications for an arthrodesis of the joints of the posterior tarsus. Furthermore, once the decision has been made to perform such an extensive fusion, there is further disagreement as to the best procedure to follow.

Lorthioir (1911), who originally reported the results of such an operation, extirpated the entire talus and replaced it as a free graft in order to achieve a pantalar arthrodesis. The same procedure (Fig. 19-17) was reported by Crainz (1924) and by Hunt and Thompson (1954); however, most orthopaedic surgeons appear to have been fearful of the possibility of necrosis of the talus when it is employed as a free graft and have used other methods (Marek and Schein, 1945). Whereas Lorthioir (1911), Steindler (1923), Crainz (1924), Hamsa (1936), Hunt and Thompson (1954)

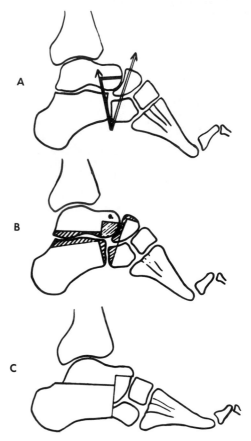

Fig. 19-16. **A,** In the beak triple arthrodesis a large wedge is planned as in the routine triple arthrodesis. Only the inferior cortex of the talus is osteotomized, however, and the surgeon must be careful not to disturb the dorsal talar soft tissues. **B,** Hatching indicates the bone removed in the procedure. **C,** Final position after the forefoot has been displaced downward and the navicular has been locked under the talar beak with flattening of the foot. (From Siffert, R. S., et al.: Clin. Orthop. **45:**101, 1966.)

and Waugh et al. (1965) did their fusions in a single stage, Liebolt (1939) and Patterson et al. (1950) believed fewer complications resulted when the fusion was performed in two stages, with either the subtalar or the talocrural joint being fused first.

Various approaches have been recommended, depending on the surgical procedure to be used. If a single stage arthrodesis is to be performed, the most popular surgical incisions appear to be the anterolateral or the

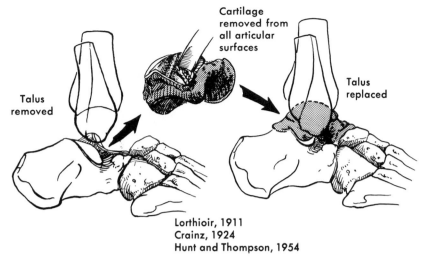

Lorthioir, 1911
Crainz, 1924
Hunt and Thompson, 1954

Fig. 19-17. Pantalar arthrodesis accomplished by removing the entire talus, denuding it of all its articular cartilage, and reinserting it as a graft.

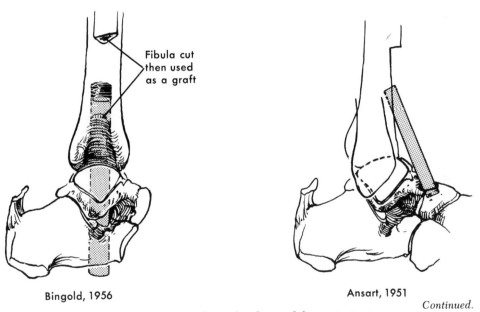

Fibula cut then used as a graft

Bingold, 1956

Ansart, 1951

Continued.

Fig. 19-18. Extra-articular arthrodeses of the posterior tarsus.

Kocher incisions. When an anterior bone graft and/or a posterior bone graft are being considered, the preferred combination seems to be the anterolateral and posterolateral incisions.

The methods employed to achieve bony stabilization of both the talocrural and the subtalar articulations may be divided into two general categories: (1) those that are essentially intra-articular, in which the cartilage is denuded from all articular surfaces of the respective joints, and (2) those that are extra-articular, depending on various types of bone grafts to span the joints. The procedures employed are summarized in Fig. 19-18. Names of the surgeons are indicated under each drawing.

Talectomy (astragalectomy). Talectomy is

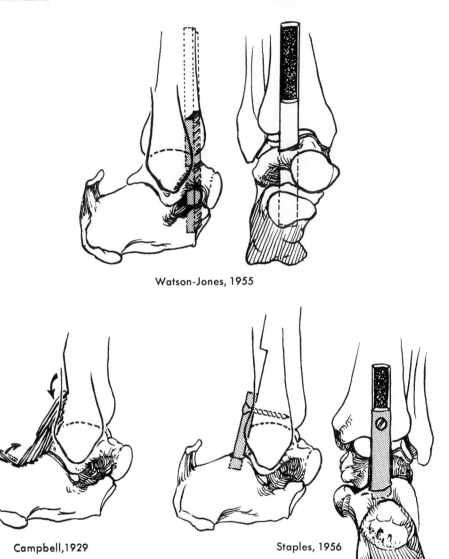

Watson-Jones, 1955

Campbell, 1929   Staples, 1956

Fig. 19-18, cont'd. For legend see p. 545.

a surgical procedure that has been performed for many years. The first talectomy was done in 1608, probably by Fabricius Hildanus, for a compound fracture. After that time the procedure was mainly used for fracture or disease.

In 1901 Whitman published a report of thirteen cases of paralytic talipes of the calcaneus type that he had managed by talectomy. For twenty years the procedure gained popularity in treatment of calcaneus and calcaneal valgus feet. It was also found useful in flail feet, especially when secondary to poliomyelitis

and not associated with varus or equinus deformities. The reason for the apparent success of talectomy was that it provided enough laxity of the tissues in both the equinus and the varus deformities to permit correction without tension. Furthermore, the false joint between the mortise and the calcaneus was sufficiently stable when the foot was plantigrade to permit weight bearing.

Following a peak of popularity during the late 1920s, the enthusiasm for this procedure began to wane. Dunn (1930) stated that "the operation of astragalectomy should not now be taught or practised for the treatment of any type of paralytic deformity of the foot." Commendatory reports continued to appear in the orthopaedic literature, however. Thompson (1939), in an excellent review, surveyed 2,066 records and reported on a sample of 100 patients who had undergone talectomy. His conclusions were that the foot can be corrected and stabilized by removal of the talus, that in children the deformity is apt to recur with growth, and that disabling pain is likely to occur in patients over 15 years of age. Tompkins et al. (1956) stated that "astragalectomy does not deserve either wholesale condemnation or unqualified praise."

With proper application and indications, talectomy remains an excellent procedure. Besides having been used for the correction of paralytic deformity, it has also been employed for diverse pathologic conditions such as osteoblastoma or osteoid osteoma, osteogenic sarcoma, giant cell tumor, Ewing's sarcoma, tuberculosis, fracture and posttraumatic arthritis, and occasionally osteomyelitis. Excision of the talus for traumatic fracture or fracture-dislocation has been done, and the procedure has been utilized for spina bifida and arthrogryposis multiplex congenita (Menelaus, 1971), for the correction of untreated clubfoot in adults, and for rheumatoid arthritis (Murray, 1972).

With the increasing interest in prosthetic replacement of skeletal parts, talectomy for aseptic necrosis following fractures of the talus has been performed. Sohier (1952, 1952-1953), Boron and Viarnaud (1958), and Queinnec and Queinnec (1971) replaced the excised talus with a plastic replica and reported favorable results.

The criteria for a good result with talectomy are (1) even weight distribution on the plantar surface in both stance and gait, (2) good lateral stability, (3) an ankle axis that is forward and at a right angle to the long axis of the foot, (4) limited ankle motion, especially in dorsiflexion, (5) no pain, (6) no necessity for external support, and (7) a good appearance of the foot.

A talectomy may be performed by one of several methods. Whitman (1901) approached the talus through a curved posterolateral incision extending from the attachment of the tendo Achillis, passing below the lateral malleolus, and terminating over the head of the talus. The two peroneal tendons were freed and were either retracted distally or divided. The lateral collateral ligaments of the ankle were cut and the foot was inverted, exposing the talus, which was extracted with comparative ease after the inferior talocalcaneal (interosseous) ligament was severed.

More recently, as talectomy has been employed in avascular necrosis and rheumatoid arthritis, the anterolateral approach has been widely used. In such an approach the talus is readily extirpated with minimal disruption of the supporting soft tissue structures. After the dorsal capsule has been detached and the inferior talocalcaneal ligament in the sinus tarsi cut, the talus is scooped out totally with a curved gouge. To achieve a better fit between the mortise and the superior surface of the calcaneus in cases in which no prosthetic replacement is being considered, it may be necessary to remove a portion of the malleoli and reshape the posterior facet of the calcaneus so the tibial plafond contacts the calcaneus below and the navicular in front.

Although many surgeons prefer arthrodeses and/or tendon transfers for stabilization of a paralytic foot, these procedures are not universally accepted because they often give unpredictable results. The method of talectomy described by Whitman was once judged the best procedure for the stabilization of a paralytic foot by the American Orthopaedic Surgery Committee.

External rotation of the foot not compensated for by internal rotation of the leg in gait can be corrected by osteotomy of the tibia as a secondary procedure, but it is rarely necessary. An important point in the surgical technique is to avoid aligning the foot with the patella, for doing so may lead to an unstable foot with a varus deformity.

The calcaneus

Open reduction and bone grafting for calcaneal fractures. It is well known that the prognosis for fractures involving the articular surfaces of the calcaneus is unfavorable. Accurate realignment of the displaced fragments is mandatory and often can be achieved only under direct vision by an open reduction.

Palmer (1948) stated that in approximately 50% of cases a major longitudinal fracture line through the calcaneus occurs. It extends from the medial side upward and laterally, splitting the calcaneus into two major fragments. The fracture passes through the posterior facet of the calcaneus. The lateral fragment is usually found displaced, and a "ledge" or "step" is produced in the articular surface of the posterior facet. Such fractures are amenable to open reduction and bone grafting. To select the proper cases for such a procedure requires the closest cooperation between the surgeon and the radiologist.

Widén (1954), Vestad (1968), and Hazlette (1969) reported favorable results with open reduction and bone grafting for suitable cases.

The surgical procedure is relatively simple. The calcaneus is approached through a curvilinear incision approximately 15 cm long extending from the back of the calcaneus, passing just below the lateral malleolus, and terminating at the calcaneocuboid articulation. The sheath of the peroneal tendons is incised and the tendons are displaced forward. The talocalcaneal ligament is divided, and the posterior facet of the talocalcaneal (subtalar) joint is exposed. The heel is carefully inverted to reveal the articular surface of the calcaneus; this allows inspection and assessment of the extent of the injury. With a traction pin through the tuber of the calcaneus and with judicious use of an elevator, the joint surfaces may be realigned. However, the reduction is usually very unstable and a large defect, formed by compression of the cancellous bone, is present. A bone graft from the iliac crest is shaped and driven into the defect and acts as a key to hold the reduction. Hazlette (1969) found it necessary in some cases to use screws to supplement the graft and secure reduction of the major fragments. The degree of stability of the reduction should indicate to the surgeon whether or not the transfixing pin should be incorporated into the cast to ensure that the reduction is maintained during the early stages of healing.

Osteotomies of calcaneus. In the so-called normal or average foot the superincumbent body weight is transmitted through a vertical plane to the talus and thence to the tuberosity of the calcaneus. The axes of the subtalar and ankle joints, when projected onto a transverse plane, intersect in the center of the trochlea (Isman and Inman, 1969). The body of the calcaneus has a medial curve, which brings the tuberosity under the weight-bearing line of the leg. With such an arrangement a metastable state is created which requires minimal muscular effort to maintain. The variations in the position of the axis of the subtalar joint and the variability of the anatomic structure of the calcaneus may cause the weight-bearing line of the leg to fall outside the reaction point on the heel. A moment is thus created that, if not resisted by muscular effort, will cause the foot either to pronate or to supinate.

This situation has been recognized for many years and has led to the development and use of shoe modifications and different types of appliances. Surgical procedures designed to bring the weight-bearing line of the leg within the reaction point on the heel and thus improve alignment have also been devised and are of interest historically. Trendelenburg (1889), in cases of flatfoot, moved the weight-bearing line of the leg laterally by carrying out a supramalleolar varus osteotomy of the tivia and fibula. Gleich (1893) osteotomized the calcaneus, moving its posterior segment downward and medialward to retain the motions of the joints and preserve the elasticity of the foot (Fig. 19-19). Operations which fused the midtarsal region of the foot, popular at that time, sacrificed these elements.

Since the pioneering efforts of certain surgeons, osteotomy of the calcaneus has been used for a variety of deformities of the foot, including cosmetic improvement in cases of flatfoot, treatment of congenital flaccid flatfoot, and correction of deformities resulting from spastic or paralytic states. Osteotomy has been employed in pes cavus and pes planus and has consisted of both closing and opening

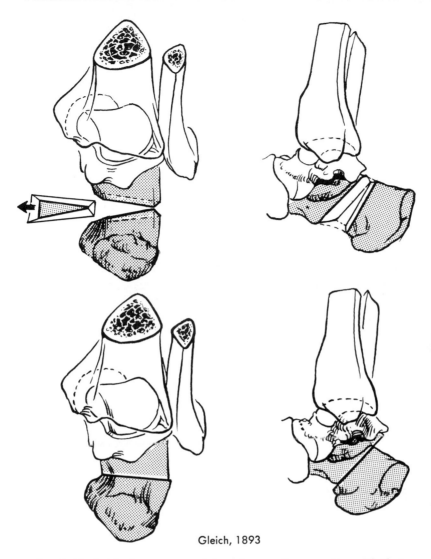

Gleich, 1893

Fig. 19-19. Original osteotomy of the calcaneus for correction of flatfoot.

wedges, with and without lateral or medial displacement of the posterior portion of the calcaneus. The purpose of all the osteotomies is to improve the alignment of the weight-bearing structures of the hindfoot; nevertheless, one should be aware that these procedures may also alter the function of the effective lever arms of the muscles acting on the calcaneus. Unfortunately, the effects have not been adequately studied; but in the reported cases supplementary tendon lengthening and transplants have often been necessary.

The calcaneus may be easily approached from either the medial or the lateral side. Gleich (1893) used a "stirrup" incision passing under the heel to expose the inferior aspect of the calcaneus. Few surgeons have employed this, however, since it places a scar on the weight-bearing surface. An opening wedge tends to increase the normal posterior projection of the heel slightly and may make skin closure more difficult. In employing an opening wedge, many surgeons have believed the defect must be filled with some type of bone graft. Closing wedges that retain a precise contact of the surfaces are technically a little more difficult to achieve. Furthermore, a closing wedge tends to shorten the heel slightly.

The various types of osteotomies of the calcaneus may be roughly divided into three categories: (1) those that are used to treat valgus deformities (Figs. 19-19 to 19-21), (2) those that are employed to improve cavus feet (Fig. 19-22), and (3) those that are used for specific pathologic conditions.

Surgical treatment of Haglund's disease. Undue prominence of the posterosuperior portion of the calcaneus may lead to painful symptoms in the area of the attachment of the tendo Achillis. The majority of these painful heels are seen in adolescent patients, and the condition may be bilateral.

To relieve the symptoms, reduction of the prominent posterior projection of the calcaneus is indicated. This has been accomplished by direct extirpation of the offending bony projection or by the performance of a rotational osteotomy of the calcaneus. The former procedure must be done with considerable care. Nissen (1957) warned that removal of too small a piece of bone might not cure the condition and the removal of too large a piece might weaken the attachment of the tendo Achillis and lead to subsequent rupture. Heller (1971) has reported such a case.

To remove the posterosuperior projection of the calcaneus surgically, Fowler and Philip (1945) employed a transverse curvilinear skin incision and split the tendo Achillis; however, most surgeons prefer a para–tendo Achillis approach. DuVries has successfully employed this method in many cases. He utilizes a lat-

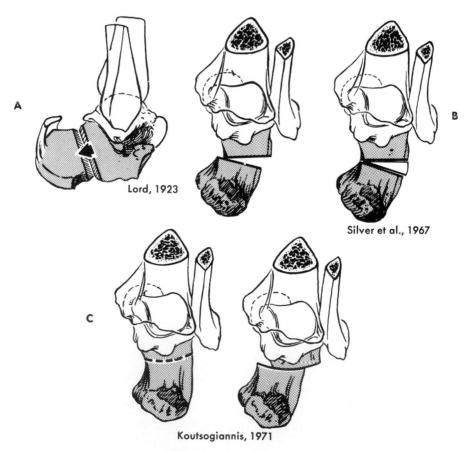

Fig. 19-20. Displacement osteotomies for the treatment of flatfoot.

eral approach and removes a wedge of bone, being careful to avoid any injury to the attachment of the tendo Achillis (Fig. 19-23). Preoperative and postoperative radiographs of a correctly performed osteotomy are shown in Fig. 19-24.

Keck and Kelly (1965) preferred a wedge osteotomy of the calcaneus. In this procedure the posterior portion of the calcaneus is rotated, and the prominence of its posterosuperior margin impinging on the tendo Achillis is reduced (Fig. 19-25).

Surgical treatment of calcaneal spurs. Several operative procedures have been devised for treating calcaneal spurs. All of them

consist of osteotomies of parts of the calcaneus.

Griffith (1910) and Chang and Miltner (1934) exposed the plantar surface of the calcaneus through a circular flap. A U-shaped incision was made completely around the heel, and the skin flap was reflected to expose the plantar surface of the heel at the origin of the plantar fascia (Fig. 19-26). The fascia was severed at its origin, and amputation of the spur was carried out.

Blokhin and Vinogradova (1937) reported thirty-three cases in which they used a modified Chang and Miltner technique successfully in the seventeen patients whom they

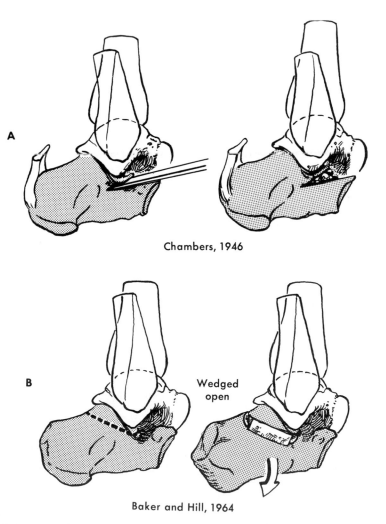

Chambers, 1946

Baker and Hill, 1964

Fig. 19-21. Procedures to restrict pronatory motion without resorting to arthrodesis.

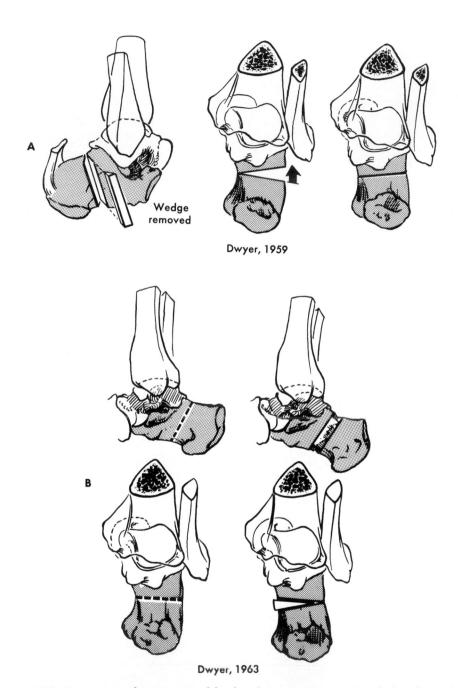

A

Wedge
removed

Dwyer, 1959

B

Dwyer, 1963

Fig. 19-22. Osteotomies for an inverted heel and pes cavus. **A,** Original procedure: closing osteotomy on the lateral side. **B,** Opening wedge with a graft on the medial side. The procedure was proposed by Dwyer to replace a closing osteotomy, which shortened the heel.

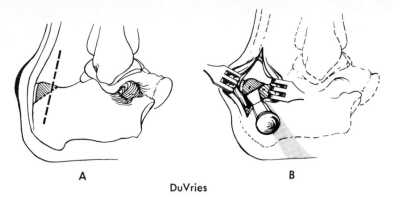

A   B

DuVries

Fig. 19-23. Removal of the posterosuperior prominence of the calcaneus through a lateral incision. **A,** Skin incision; **B,** osteotomizing the prominence.

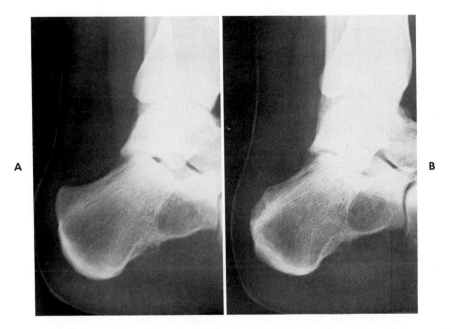

A   B

Fig. 19-24. Correctly performed osteotomy for a prominent posterosuperior tuberosity of the calcaneus in a 16-year-old girl with Haglund's disease. **A,** Preoperative; **B,** one year postoperative.

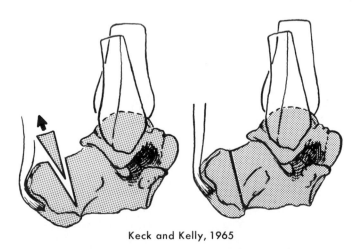

Keck and Kelly, 1965

Fig. 19-25. Osteotomy to decrease the prominence of the calcaneus.

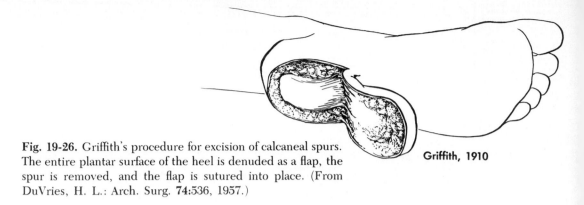

Fig. 19-26. Griffith's procedure for excision of calcaneal spurs. The entire plantar surface of the heel is denuded as a flap, the spur is removed, and the flap is sutured into place. (From DuVries, H. L.: Arch. Surg. **74:**536, 1957.)

Griffith, 1910

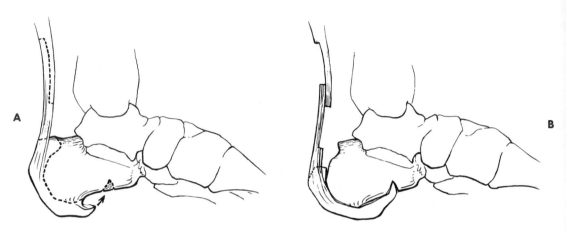

A

B

Fig. 19-27. Steindler and Smith's rotation osteotomy for calcaneal spurs. **A,** The tendo Achillis is lengthened and an osteotomy performed in the posterior portion of the calcaneus. **B,** The posterior portion is rotated. The spur fits into a previously prepared notch in the plantar surface of the body of the calcaneus. (From DuVries, H. L.: Arch. Surg. **74:**536, 1957.)

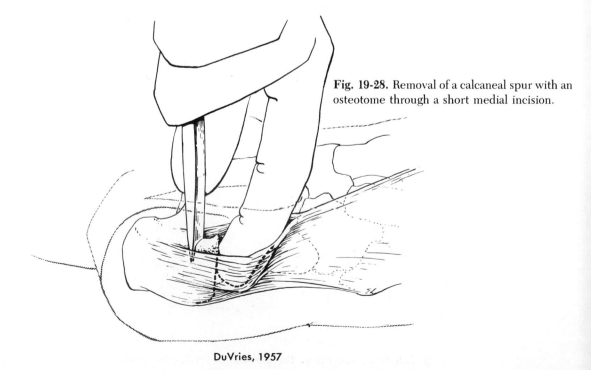

Fig. 19-28. Removal of a calcaneal spur with an osteotome through a short medial incision.

DuVries, 1957

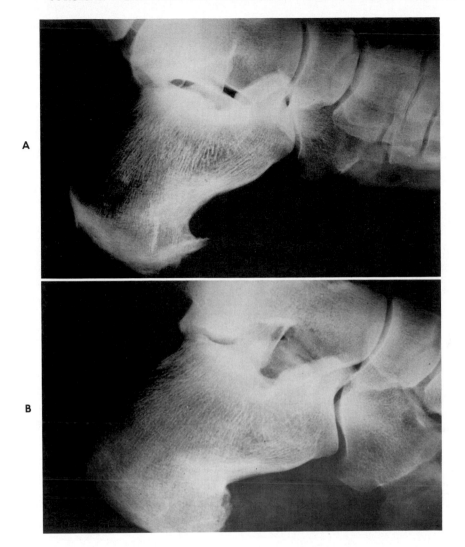

Fig. 19-29. Painful calcaneal spur. **A,** Preoperative. **B,** Three years postoperative; symptom free.

followed for one to four years postoperatively.

Steindler and Smith (1938) reported the use of a rotational osteotomy of the entire tuberosity of the calcaneus which required lengthening of the tendo Achillis. Such an extensive surgical procedure, in most cases, seems unwarranted (Fig. 19-27).

DuVries (1957) recommended a simple medial approach to the plantar surface of the calcaneus, with sectioning of the plantar aponeurosis at its calcaneal attachment and excision of the spur by a small osteotome (Fig. 19-28). Radiographs of a painful spur may demonstrate successful treatment (Fig. 19-29), but unfortunately the surgical treatment of calcaneal spurs gives only 50% to 60% satisfactory results.

THE MIDTARSUS

The surgical correction of some deformities of the foot has been achieved by means of wedge osteotomies or fusions in the area of the midtarsus. Such procedures have been employed in cases of marked pes cavus or pes planus, with or without accompanying adduction or abduction of the forefoot, as well as in cases in which operative procedures on the hindfoot are not indicated because of the absence of an appreciable varus or valgus of the heel.

Pes cavus

Cole (1940) employed a transverse midtarsal osteotomy to treat pes cavus in patients for whom all types of conservative treatment (e.g., soft tissue releases, manipulations, tendon transfers, casts, and external appliances) had failed. The procedure consisted of the removal of a wedge of bone from the navicular, the cuneiforms, and the cuboid (Fig. 19-30, A); closing of the wedge led to the correction of the deformity. When adduction of the forefoot accompanied the cavus deformity, as in persistent or untreated clubfoot, the direction of the wedge of bone could be changed to correct this added deformity (Fig. 19-30, B).

Pes planus

The term peroneal spastic flatfoot has been loosely applied to the type of flatfoot in which passive correction of the deformity is resisted by contracture and reflex spasm of the peroneal muscles (i.e., a rigid flatfoot). Such resistance is indicative of an irritative lesion in the hindfoot or midfoot. These lesions are frequently found in arthritic processes involving the subtalar and transverse articulations and in various types of tarsal coalition. Since the proper remedial procedure must be based on the precise pathologic condition, a careful physical and radiographic examination of the foot is mandatory.

If the condition is caused by the presence of a calcaneonavicular bar, DuVries has found that excision of the bar through a lateral approach to the sinus tarsi will often relieve the disorder, especially in adolescents (Fig. 19-31). If arthritic changes in the subtalar or transverse tarsal articulations are the etiologic factor, subtalar or triple arthrodesis may be the indicated treatment.

The only kind of flexible flatfoot that requires treatment is symptomatic flatfoot. The cosmetic appearance of the foot is not an indication for surgical procedures. Conservative measures (appliances, e.g., heel wedges, higher heels, shoe inserts) may be employed to improve the appearance of the foot and reduce the concomitant deformation of the shoe.

In most cases of flexible flatfoot, an accompanying valgus position of the hindfoot is present. Since inversion of the heel by various means both improves the appearance of the foot and relieves symptoms, the majority of surgical procedures have been done on the hindfoot (e.g., osteotomies of the calcaneus and subtalar fusions). In some individuals, however, pes planus appears to manifest itself as a vertical collapse of the longitudinal arch

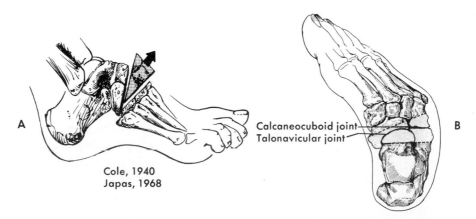

Fig. 19-30. Midtarsal osteotomies. **A,** For correction of pes cavus. **B,** For correction of pes cavus with adduction of the forefoot. (From Crenshaw, A. H., editor: Campbell's operative orthopaedics, ed. 5, vol. 2, St. Louis, 1971, The C. V. Mosby Co.)

without a valgus heel; and in these individuals stabilization procedures of the midfoot are indicated.

Hoke (1921, 1931) and Miller (1927) found that the instability of the medial side of the longitudinal arch appeared to be caused by the malfunctioning of a series of individual articulations between the first metatarsal, the first cuneiform, the navicular, and the head of the talus. Both men believed that stability of the longitudinal arch could be restored without undue loss of mobility by arthrodesing some of these articulations. Hoke arthrodesed the naviculocuneiform articulations, using an

inlay tibial graft after removing the articular cartilage (Fig. 19-32, *A*). Miller resected the articular cartilage between the navicular and the first cuneiform and, in more severe cases, also between the first cuneiform and the base of the first metatarsal. In such a procedure any abduction of the forefoot could be corrected by removing various sizes of wedges of bone (Fig. 19-32, *B*).

L'Episcopo and Sabatelle (1939) reported their observations of sixteen patients with flatfoot after operation by Hoke's procedure; 68% obtained good results and 32% fair results. Butte (1937) reported on seventy-six feet

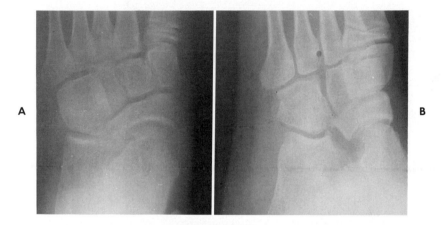

Fig. 19-31. Excision of a calcaneonavicular bar. **A,** Preoperative; **B,** postoperative.

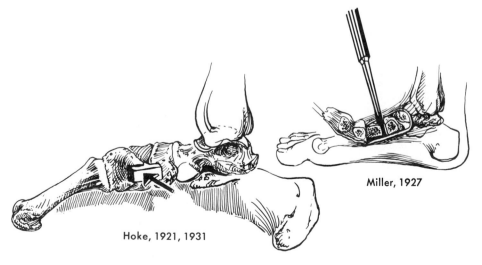

Miller, 1927

Hoke, 1921, 1931

Fig. 19-32. Stabilization procedures. **A,** Bone graft of the naviculocuneiform joints. **B,** Arthrodesis of the talonavicular joint and the cuneiform and first metatarsal without a graft.

Fig. 19-33. Arthrodesis of the talonavicular and calcaneocuboid articulations for treatment of flat-foot with no osseous anomalies.

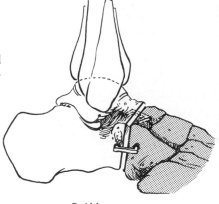

DuVries

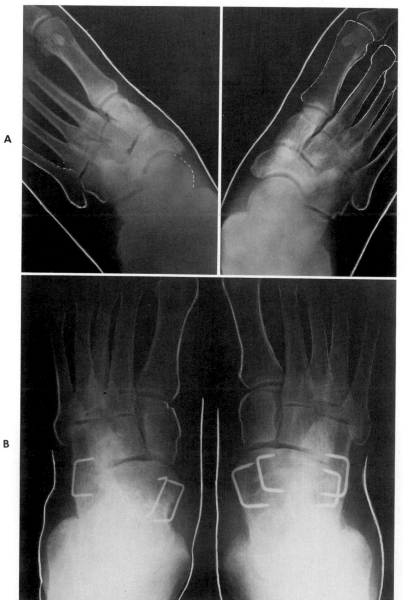

A

B

Fig. 19-34. For legend see opposite page.

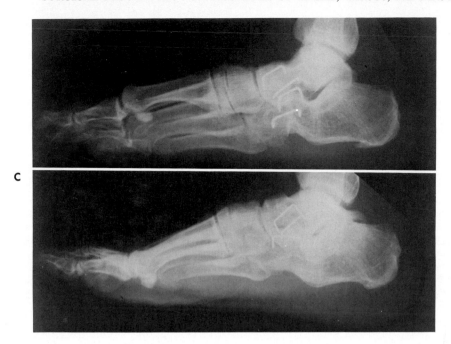

Fig. 19-34. Treatment of bilateral painful flatfoot by double arthrodesis in a 41-year-old man. Note the extreme pronation of both feet. **A,** November, 1963. **B,** February, 1972. **C,** February, 1972; completely asymptomatic.

operated on by Hoke's procedure; results were satisfactory in about 50%. Jack (1953) performed Hoke's operation for flatfoot in forty-six cases and obtained satisfactory results in 82%.

For the treatment of symptomatic flexible flatfoot with no osseous anomalies, DuVries has used an arthrodesis of the talonavicular and calcaneocuboid articulations (Fig. 19-33). He reported good results in more than forty cases (Fig. 19-34). His technique consists of two curvilinear incisions, one to expose the talonavicular joint and the other the calcaneocuboid joint. Cartilage is removed from all articular surfaces and the bones are trimmed so they can be coapted. They are fixed with small staples.

Special mention should be made concerning the possible role played by an accessory navicular in painful flatfoot. Kidner (1929, 1933) presented evidence that the presence of an accessory navicular or an abnormal prolongation of the tuberosity of the navicular resulted in a medial displacement of the attachment of the tendon of the tibialis poste-

rior. Such an anatomic arrangement caused the tibialis posterior to act more as an adductor of the forefoot than as a supinator and elevator of the longitudinal arch. The so-called Kidner procedure consists of careful excision of the accessory navicular and a portion of the medial side of the tarsal navicular, if it is enlarged, as well as transposition of the tendon to lie more laterally and beneath the navicular. Unfortunately, no large series or long-term follow-up of individuals who have undergone the Kidner procedure has been found in the literature. We have had most satisfactory results using the Kidner procedure for a symptomatic accessory navicular in both adults and children.

REFERENCES

Adams, J. C.: Arthrodesis of the ankle joint: experiences with the transfibular approach, J. Bone Joint Surg. **30B:**506, 1948.

Anderson, K. J., and LeCocq, J. F.: Operative treatment of injury to the fibular collateral ligament of the ankle, J. Bone Joint Surg. **36A:**825, 1954.

Anderson, R.: Concentric arthrodesis of the ankle joint: a

transmalleolar approach, J. Bone Joint Surg. **27**:37, 1945.

Ansart, M. B.: Pan-arthrodesis for paralytic flail foot, J. Bone Joint Surg. **33B**:503, 1951.

Ashhurst, A. P. C., and Bromer, R. S.: Classification and mechanism of fractures of the leg bones involving the ankle: based on a study of three hundred cases from the Episcopal Hospital, Arch. Surg. **4**:51, 1922.

Baker, L. D., and Hill, L. M.: Foot alignment in the cerebral palsy patient, J. Bone Joint Surg. **46A**:1, 1964.

Barr, J. S., and Record, E. E.: Arthrodesis of the ankle joint, N. Engl. J. Med. **248**:53, 1953.

Bényi, P.: A modified Lambrinudi operation for drop foot, J. Bone Joint Surg. **42B**:333, 1960.

Bingold, A. C.: Ankle and subtalar fusion by a transarticular graft, J. Bone Joint Surg. **38B**:862, 1956.

Blokhin, V. N., and Vinogradova, T. P.: Shpory pyatochnykh kostey [Calcaneal spurs], Ortop. Travmatol. Protez. **11**:96, 1937.

Bogutskaia, E. V.: Privychnyy vyvikh sukhzuliy malobyertsovykh myshts u sporsmyenov [Habitual dislocation of fibular muscles of athletes], Khirurgiia **46**:83, 1970.

Boron, R., and Viarnaud. E.: Une observation de prothèse astragalienne en acrylique, Mem. Acad. Chir. **84**:549, 1958.

Branch, H. E.: Drop-foot: end results of a series of boneblock operations, J. Bone Joint Surg. **21**:141, 1939.

Brewster, A. H.: Countersinking the astragalus in paralytic feet, N. Engl. J. Med. **209**:71, 1933.

Brittain, H. A.: Architectural principles in arthrodesis, Baltimore, 1942, The Williams & Wilkins Co.

Broström, L.: Sprained ankles. VI. Surgical treatment of "chronic" ligament ruptures, Acta Chir. Scand. **132**:551, 1966.

Butte, F. L.: Navicular-cuneiform arthrodesis for flatfoot: an end-result study, J. Bone Joint Surg. **19**:496, 1937.

Campbell, W. C.: An operation for the correction of "drop-foot," J. Bone Joint Surg. **5**:815, 1923.

Campbell, W. C.: End-results of operation for correction of drop-foot, J.A.M.A. **85**:1927, 1925.

Campbell, W. C.: An operation for the induction of osseous fusion in the ankle joint, Am. J. Surg. **6**:588, 1929.

Chambers, E. F. S.: An operation for the correction of flexible flat feet of adolescents, West. J. Surg. Obstet. Gynecol. **54**:77, 1946.

Chang, C. C., and Miltner, L. J.: Periostitis of the os calcis, J. Bone Joint Surg. **16**:355, 1934.

Charnley, J.: Compression arthrodesis of the ankle and the shoulder, J. Bone Joint Surg. **33B**:180, 1959.

Chrisman, O. D., and Snook, G. A.: Reconstruction of lateral ligament tears of the ankle: an experimental study and clinical evaluation of seven patients treated by a new modification of the Elmslie procedure, J. Bone Joint Surg. **51A**:904, 1969.

Chuinard, E. G., and Peterson, R. E.: Distraction-compression bone-graft arthrodesis of the ankle: a

method especially applicable in children, J. Bone Joint Surg. **45A**:481, 1963

Close, J. R., and Todd, F. N.: The phasic activity of the muscles of the lower extremity and the effect of tendon transfer, J. Bone Joint Surg. **41A**:189, 1959.

Cole, W. H.: The treatment of claw-foot, J. Bone Joint Surg. **22**:895, 1940.

Cordebar, J.: Reconstitution de la mortaise tibiotarsienne, Presse Med. **64**:774, 1956.

Crainz, S.: L'artrodesi del piede per mezzo dell'astragalectomia sequita de reimpianto parziale o totale dell'astragalo, Policlinico (Chir.) **31**:1, 1924.

Cramer, K.: Beitrag zur Arthrodese des Talo-cruralgelenkes, Zentralbl. Chir. Mechan. Orthop. **4**:113, 1910.

Crego, C. H., Jr., and McCarroll, H. R.: Recurrent deformities in stabilized paralytic feet: a report of 1100 consecutive stabilizations in poliomyelitis, J. Bone Joint Surg. **20**:609, 1938.

Dahmen, G., and Meyer, H.: Ueber die verschiedenen Methoden zur Arthrodese des oberen Springgelenkes, Arch. Orthop. Unfallchir. **58**:265, 1965.

Davis, G. G.: The treatment of hollow foot (pes cavus), Am. J. Orthop. Surg. **11**:231, 1913.

Dawkins, A.: The unstable subtalar joint. Proceedings and reports of councils and associations, J. Bone Joint Surg. **40B**:357, 1958.

Diamant-Berger, L.: La luxation des tendons péroniers latéraux, Presse Med. **79**:17, 1971.

Dunn, N.: Suggestions based on ten years' experience of arthrodesis of the tarsus in the treatment of deformities of the foot. In The Robert Jones birthday volume: a collection of surgical essays, London, 1928, Oxford University Press.

Dunn, N: Reconstructive surgery in paralytic deformities of the leg, J. Bone Joint Surg. **12**:299, 1930.

DuVries, H. L.: Heel spur (calcaneal spur), Arch. Surg. **74**:536, 1957.

DuVries, H. L.: Surgery of the foot, ed. 2, St. Louis, 1965, The C. V. Mosby Co.

Dwyer, F. C.: Osteotomy of the calcaneum for pes cavus, J. Bone Joint Surg. **41B**:80, 1959.

Dwyer, F. C.: The treatment of relapsed club foot by the insertion of a wedge into the calcaneum, J. Bone Joint Surg. **45B**:67, 1963.

Elmslie, R.C.: Recurrent subluxation of the ankle-joint, Ann. Surg. **100**:364, 1934.

Evans, D. L.: Recurrent instability of the ankle: a method of surgical treatment, Proc. R. Soc. Med. **46**:343, 1953.

Fitzgerald, F. P., and Seddon, H. J.: Lambrinudi's operation for drop-foot, Br. J. Surg. **25**:283, 1937.

Folschveiller, J.: Abriss des Retinaculum Musculi fibularium proximale und seine Folgen, Hefte Unfallheilkd. **92**:98, 1967.

Fowler, A., and Philip, J. F.: Abnormality of the calcaneus as a cause of painful heel: its diagnosis and operative treatment, Br. J. Surg. **32**:494, 1945.

Francillon, M. R.: Distorsio pedis with an isolated lesion of the ligamentum calcaneo-fibulare, Acta Orthop. Scand. **32**:469, 1962.

Geens, S.: Synovectomy and débridement of the knee in rheumatoid arthritis. Part I. Historical review, J. Bone Joint Surg. **51A**:617, 1969.

Gill, A. B.: An operation to make a posterior bone block at the ankle to limit foot-drop, J. Bone Joint Surg. **15**:166, 1933.

Gillespie, H. S., and Boucher, P.: Watson-Jones repair of lateral instability of the ankle, J. Bone Joint Surg. **53A**:920, 1971.

Gleich, A.: Beitrag zur operativen Plattfussbehandlung, Arch. Klin. Chir. **46**:358, 1893.

Glissan, D. J.: The indications for inducing fusion at the ankle joint by operation, with description of two successful techniques, Aust. N. Z. J. Surg. **19**:64, 1949.

Goldthwait, J. E.: An operation for the stiffening of the ankle joint in infantile paralysis, Am. J. Orthop. Surg. **5**:271, 1908.

Grice, D. S.: An extra-articular arthrodesis of the subastragalar joint for correction of paralytic flat feet in children, J. Bone Joint Surg. **34A**:927, 1952.

Griffith, J. D.: Osteophytes of the os calcis, Am. J. Orthop. Surg. **8**:501, 1910.

Hallgrímsson, S.: Studies on reconstructive and stabilizing operations on the skeleton of the foot. With special reference to subastragalar arthrodesis in the treatment of foot deformities following infantile paralysis, Acta Chir. Scand. (supp. 78) **88**:1, 1943.

Hallock, H.: Arthrodesis of the ankle joint for old painful fractures, J. Bone Joint Surg. **27**:49, 1945.

Hamsa, W. R.: Panastragaloid arthrodesis: a study of end results in eighty-five cases, J. Bone Joint Surg. **28**:732, 1936.

Hart, V. L.: Arthrodesis of the foot in infantile paralysis, Surg. Gynecol. Obstet. **64**:794, 1937.

Hart, V. L.: Lambrinudi operation for drop-foot, J. Bone Joint Surg. **22**:937, 1940.

Hatt, R. N.: The central bone graft in joint arthrodesis, J. Bone Joint Surg. **22**:393, 1940.

Hazlette, J. W.: Open reduction of fractures of the calcaneum, Can. J. Surg. **12**:310, 1969.

Heller, W.: Achillessehnenausriss nach Operation einer Haglund-Ferse, Z. Orthop. **109**:534, 1971.

Heywood, A. W. B.: Rheumatoid arthritis—the orthopaedic contribution. III. The trunk and lower limb, S. Afr. Med. J. **41**:267, 1967.

Hoke, M.: An operation for stabilizing paralytic feet, Am. J. Orthop. Surg. **3**:494, 1921.

Hoke, M.: An operation for the correction of extremely relaxed flat feet, J. Bone Joint Surg. **13**:773, 1931.

Horwitz, T.: The use of the transfibular approach in arthrodesis of the ankle, Am. J. Surg. **55**:550, 1942.

Hunt, W. S., Jr., and Thompson, H. A.: Pantalar arthrodesis: a one-stage operation. J. Bone Joint Surg. **36A**:349, 1954.

Inclan, A.: End results in physiological blocking of flail joints, J. Bone Joint Surg. **31A**:748, 1949.

Ingram, A. J., and Hundley, J. M.: Posterior bone block of the ankle for paralytic equinus: an end-result study, J. Bone Joint Surg. **33A**:679, 1951.

Isman, R. E., and Inman, V. T.: Anthropometric studies of the human foot and ankle, Bull. Prosthet. Res. **10-11**:97, 1969.

Jack, E. A.: Naviculo-cuneiform fusion in the treatment of flat foot, J. Bone Joint Surg. **35B**:75, 1953.

Jakubowski, S.: Synowektomia stawv skokowogelenio-wego goś ću przewleklym postepujacym (Ankle joint synovectomy in rheumatoid arthritis), Chir. Narzadow Ruchu Ortop. Pol. **35**:683, 1970.

Jansen, K.: Arthrodesis of the ankle joint, Acta Orthop. Scand. **32**:476, 1962.

Japas, L. M.: Surgical treatment of pes cavus by tarsal V-osteotomy: preliminary report, J. Bone Joint Surg. **50A**:927, 1968.

Jones, R.: An operation for paralytic calcaneocavus, Am. J. Orthop. Surg. **5**:371, 1908.

Keck, S. W., and Kelly, P. J.: Bursitis of the posterior part of the heel: evaluation of surgical treatment of eighteen patients, J. Bone Joint Surg. **47A**:267, 1965.

Kelly, R. E.: An operation for the chronic dislocation of the peroneal tendons, Br. J. Surg. **7**:502, 1920.

Kidner, F. C.: The prehallux (accessory scaphoid) in its relation to flat-foot, J. Bone Joint Surg. **11**:831, 1929.

Kidner, F. C.: The prehallux in relation to flat-foot, J.A.M.A. **101**:1539, 1933.

Koutsogiannis, E.: Treatment of mobile flat foot by displacement osteotomy of the calcaneus, J. Bone Joint Surg. **53B**:96, 1971.

Lambrinudi, C.: New operation on drop-foot, Br. J. Surg. **15**:193, 1927.

Lasker, W.: Spätresultate der Arthrodesenoperation nach Cramer, zugleich ein Beitrag zur Frage der Knochentransplantation, Beitr. Klin. Chir. **128**:499, 1923.

Lee, H. G.: Surgical repair in recurrent dislocation of the ankle joint, J. Bone Joint Surg. **39A**:828, 1957.

L'Episcopo, J. B., and Sabatelle, P. E.: The Hoke operation for flat feet, J. Bone Joint Surg. **21**:92, 1939.

Liebolt, F. L.: Pantalar arthrodesis in poliomyelitis, Surgery **6**:31, 1939.

London, P. S.: Synovectomy of the knee in rheumatoid arthritis: an essay in surgical salvage, J. Bone Joint Surg. **37B**:392, 1955.

Lord, J. P.: Correction of extreme flatfoot: value of osteotomy of os calcis and inward displacement of posterior fragment (Gleich operation), J.A.M.A. **81**:1502, 1923.

Lorthioir, J.: Huit cas d'arthrodèse du pied avec extirpation temporaire de l'astragale, J. Chir. Ann. Soc. Belge Chir. **11**:184, 1911.

Marek, F. M., and Schein, A. J.: Aseptic necrosis of the astragalus following arthrodesing procedures of the tarsus, J. Bone Joint Surg. **27**:587, 1945.

Mead, N. C.: Arthrodesis of the ankle joint: a simple efficient method, Q. Bull. Northwestern Univ. Med. Sch. **25**:248, 1951.

Menelaus, M. B.: Talectomy for equinovarus deformity in arthrogryposis and spina bifida, J. Bone Joint Surg. **53B**:468, 1971.

Miller, O. L.: A plastic flat foot operation, J. Bone Joint Surg. 9:84, 1927.

Mounier-Kuhn, A., and Marsan, C.: Le syndrome des tendons péroniers, Ann. Chir. 22:641, 1968.

Muralt, R. H.: Luxation der Peronäalsehnen, Z. Orthop. 87:263-274, 1956.

Murr, S.: Dislocation of the peroneal tendons with marginal fracture of the lateral malleolus, J. Bone Joint Surg. 43B:563, 1961.

Murray, W. R.: Personal communication, 1972.

Nilsonne, H.: Making a new ligament in ankle sprain, J. Bone Joint Surg. 14:380, 1932.

Nissen, K. I.: Remodelling of the posterior tuberosity of the calcaneum. In Rob, C., and Smith, R., editors: Operative surgery, vol. 5, London, 1957, Butterworth & Co., Ltd.

Palmer, I.: The mechanism and treatment of fractures of the calcaneus, J. Bone Joint Surg. 30A:2, 1948.

Patterson, R. L., Jr., Parrish, F. F., and Hathaway, E. N.: Stabilizing operations on the foot: a study of the indications, techniques used, and end results, J. Bone Joint Surg. 32A:1, 1950.

Queinnec, A., and Queinnec, J.: Résultats éloignés de deux cas de prothèse de l'astragale par des pièces en "plastique," Chirurgie 97:193, 1971.

Ratliff, A. H. C.: Compression arthrodesis of the ankle, J. Bone Joint Surg. 41B:524, 1959.

Ruth, C. J.: The surgical treatment of injuries of the fibular collateral ligaments of the ankle, J. Bone Joint Surg. 43A:229, 1961.

Ryerson, E. W.: Arthrodesing operations on the feet, J. Bone Joint Surg. 5:453, 1923.

Scheuba, G.: Die Luxation der Tibialis posterior-Sehne, Monatsschr. Unfallheilkd. 72:540, 1969.

Schoolfield, B. L.: Operative treatment of flatfoot, Surg. Gynecol. Obstet. 94:136, 1952.

Schwartz, R. P.: Arthrodesis of subtalus and midtarsal joints of the foot: historical review, pre-operative determinations and operative procedure, Surgery 20:619, 1946.

Siffert, R. S., Forster, R. I., and Nachamie, B.: "Beak" triple arthrodeses for correction of severe cavus deformity, Clin. Orthop. 45:101, 1966.

Silver, C. M., Simon, S. D., Spindell, E., Litchman, H. M., and Scala, M.: Calcaneal osteotomy for valgus and varus deformities of the foot in cerebral palsy: a preliminary report on twenty-seven operations, J. Bone Joint Surg. 49A:232, 1967.

Sohier, H. M. L.: Astragale en acrylic employée comme prothèse après astragalectomie pour fracture, Mem. Acad. Chir. 78:666, 1952.

Sohier, H. M. L.: Astragales en matière plastique, Bull. Mem. Ec. Prep. Med. Pharm. Dakar 1:132, 1952-1953.

Staples, S.: Posterior arthrodesis of the ankle and subtalar joints, J. Bone Joint Surg. 38A:50, 1956.

Steindler, A.: The treatment of flail ankle: panastragaloid arthrodesis, J. Bone Joint Surg. 5:284, 1923.

Steindler, A., and Smith, A. R: Spurs of the os calcis, Surg. Gynecol. Obstet. 66:663, 1938.

Thompson, T. C.: Astragalectomy and the treatment of calcaneovalgus, J. Bone Joint Surg. 21:627, 1939.

Tompkins, S. F., Miller, R. J., and O'Donoghue, D. H.: An evaluation of astragalectomy, South. Med. J. 49:1128, 1956.

Trendelenburg, F.: Ueber Plattfussoperationen, Arch. Klin. Chir. 39:751, 1889.

Vahvanen, V.: Synovectomy of the talocrural joint in rheumatoid arthritis, Ann. Chir. Gynaecol. Fenn. 57:576, 1968.

Vahvanen, V.: Arthrodesis of the TC or pantalar joints in rheumatoid arthritis, Acta Orthop. Scand. 40:642, 1969.

Vestad, E.: Fractures of the calcaneum: open reduction and bone grafting, Acta Chir. Scand. 34:617, 1968.

Watson-Jones, R.: Fractures and joint injuries, ed. 4, Baltimore, 1955, The William & Wilkins Co.

Waugh, T. R., Wagner, J., and Stinchfield, F. E.: An evaluation of pantalar arthrodesis: a followup study of one hundred and sixteen operations, J. Bone Joint Surg. 47A:1315, 1965.

Weigert, M.: Ein einfaches Verfahren zur operativen Behandlung der habituellen Peronaealsehnenluxation, Z. Orthop. 105:273, 1968.

Wheeldon, T. F., and Clark, M. M.: The Gill bone block operation for foot drop, J.A.M.A. 106:447, 1936.

Whitefield, G. A.: Surgical management of rheumatoid arthritis, Scott. Med. J. 12:107, 1967.

Whitman, R.: The operative treatment of paralytic talipes of the calcaneus type, Am. J. Med. Sci. 122:593, 1901.

Widén, A.: Fractures of the calcaneus: a clinical study with special reference to the technique and results of open-reduction, Acta Chir. Scand., supp. 188, 1954.

Wilson, H. J.: Arthrodesis of the ankle: a technique using bilateral hemimalleolar onlay grafts with screw fixation, J. Bone Joint Surg. 51A:775, 1969.

20

MAJOR SURGICAL PROCEDURES FOR DISORDERS OF THE FOREFOOT

Roger A. Mann and Henri L. DuVries

FIRST METATARSOPHALANGEAL JOINT

General principles in the treatment of hallux valgus

The objective in the treatment of a hallux valgus deformity is to correct the deformity and at the same time produce no residual disability. Based on the number and variety of surgical procedures which have been described to correct a hallux valgus, obviously this goal has not been achieved.

As pointed out in the discussion of the pathologic anatomy of hallux valgus (p. 254), the basic pathology is a contracture of the capsular structures on the lateral side of the metatarsophalangeal joint, attentuation of the capsular structures on the medial side of the metatarsophalangeal joint, attentuation of the capsular structures on the medial side of the metatarsophalangeal joint, axial rotation of the great toe, and a medial prominence of the first metatarsal head. In the majority of cases, we believe the metatarsus primus varus is a secondary phenomenon and not the underlying pathologic process of hallux valgus. This is not to say that metatarsus primus varus does not exist; rather it is usually responsible for the juvenile hallux valgus as opposed to the common type which develops in later years.

There may also be a deformity of the first metatarsocuneiform joint with medial deviation of the joint; and this too may present in the juvenile and adult types of hallux valgus. When these particular deformities are present, they must be corrected at the time of surgery or the deformity will recur.

It is true that no procedure alone is adequate to correct all types of bunion deformities since there is a variety of types of hallux valgus as well as variations in severity.

Generally the surgical procedure should correct the deformity at the metatarsophalangeal joint without significantly altering the normal weight-bearing pattern of the forefoot. Unfortunately any procedure which shortens the first metatarsal significantly will result in increased weight bearing by the second and third metatarsal shafts; and this often leads to metatarsalgia. Therefore we believe that the McBride type of repair offers the most logical repair of the pathologic anatomy of hallux valgus. The procedure releases the contracture on the lateral side of the metatarsophalangeal joint, plicates the capsule on the medial side of the metatarsophalangeal joint, removes the medial prominence of the metatarsal head, and corrects the axial rotation of the hallux.

Silver (1923) was one of the first authors to call attention to an imbalance of the intrinsic muscles in the etiology of hallux valgus. He considered these muscles to be basic in producing the deformity. McBride (1928, 1935, 1954) supported Silver regarding the influence of the intrinsic muscles on the deformity—particularly that of the adductor hallucis, whose conjoint tendon inserts into the base of the proximal phalanx of the great toe (Fig. 8-12, A). He further called attention to the usual displacement of the fibular sesamoid into the space between the first and second metatarsal heads.

Lapidus (1934) believed that the varus of the first metatarsal shaft was an extremely important factor in hallux valgus. He advised arthrodesis of the first metatarsocuneiform joint and the tibial side of the base of the second metatarsal. He also excised the tibial condyle of the first metatarsal head (Fig. 20-1).

The procedure is of definite value in cases of juvenile hallux valgus and also in adult patients in whom the first metatarsal is in extreme varus.

Surgical procedures for hallux valgus

Since the causative factors and the pathologic changes in hallux valgus vary from case to case, apparently no single procedure can be successful in all cases. Reports of operative procedures for correction of the problem (Fig. 20-2) are numerous (Galland and Jordan, 1938). The surgeon must study each case of hallux valgus and decide on a procedure or combination of procedures which suits that particular case. After he has decided what type of procedure is indicated for the patient, he must ask himself what can be done for the patient if the selected procedure fails to provide the optimal results. By carefully pondering this question prior to the surgery, he will prevent many unsalvageable failures.

Recommended procedures for reduction of hallux valgus. For the purpose of surgical correction, hallux valgus is generally classified by type as follows:

1. The common adult type, without congenital or hereditary abnormalities or abnormalities from disease, comprising about 80% of the cases; the majority of

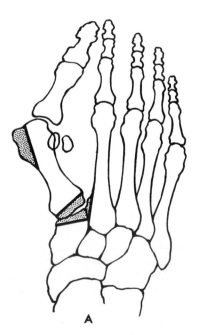
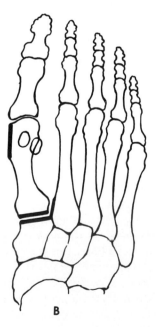

Fig. 20-1. Lapidus operation for correction of hallux valgus. **A,** Bone excised; **B,** deformity corrected.

these persons tend to have a rather broad forefoot and mild pronation of the hindfoot

2. The juvenile type (seen occasionally) with congenital predisposing factors such as a round first metatarsal head, metatarsus primus varus, pronation of the hindfoot, congenital laxity of the ligaments, or a neuromuscular disorder (Fig. 20-3)

3. An infrequently seen type in which the first metatarsal is markedly longer than the second (Figs. 8-11 and 20-14, *A*)

4. A type sometimes accompanied by severe splayfoot

5. A type occurring in the rheumatoid foot

The following procedures have proved effective for the types listed.

Type 1. DuVries' modified McBride technique is indicated for the common adult type of hallux valgus. In a series of 2,700 cases of hallux valgus over a forty-year span, reduction by means of a modified McBride procedure proved good to excellent in 90% of the cases, fair in 8%, and poor in 2%.

1. After hemostasis has been achieved by means of a pneumatic cuff about the calf or thigh, make an incision in the first interspace (Fig. 20-4, *A*) starting in the web space and

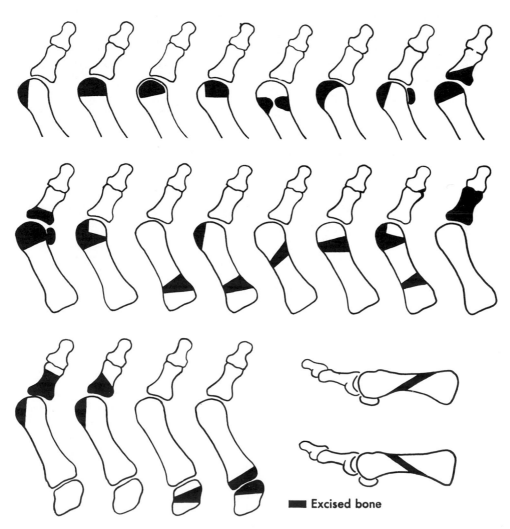

■ Excised bone

Fig. 20-2. Some methods of excising bone for hallux valgus.

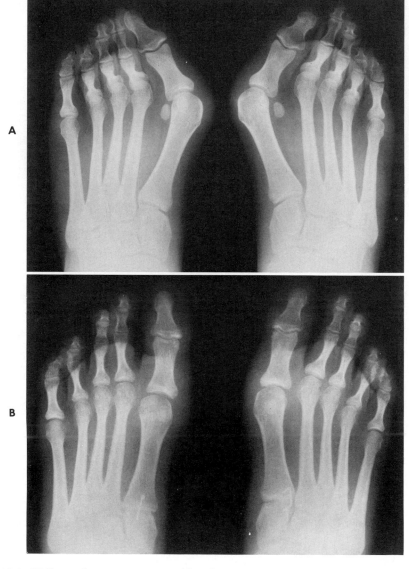

Fig. 20-3. Hallux valgus in a 16-year-old girl. **A.** Preoperative. **B,** One year postoperative following a modified McBride procedure with stabilization of the base of the first metatarso-cuneiform joints. Note the staple, which aids in arthrodesis.

Fig. 20-4. A, Location of the initial incision in the first web space. **B,** Releasing of the adductor hallucis from the base of the proximal phalanx and excision of the lateral sesamoid. Note the cuff of capsule left on the lateral aspect of the metatarsal head, which is used later in the repair. *MS,* Medial sesamoid; *LS,* lateral sesamoid: *FHL,* flexor hallucis longus; *ADD,* adductor hallucis. **C,** Medial incision; may be slightly curved dorsally or straight. Capsular incision; seen in cross section. **D,** Excision of the exostosis, starting the cut in the sagittal groove and proceeding proximally. **E,** Prior to plication of the medial capsule, derotate the hallux to bring the edge of the medial sesamoid into view in the medial incision. The toenails should all be in the same plane. **F,** Plication of the medial capsule with 1-0 chromic. Start the plication in the tendon of the abductor hallucis. **G,** After plication of the medial capsule, place three sutures of 2-0 chromic in the first web space—incorporating the cuff of capsule on the first metatarsal head, the adductor hallucis tendon, and the medial capsule of the second metatarsophalangeal joint. Squeeze the metatarsal heads together and tie the sutures.

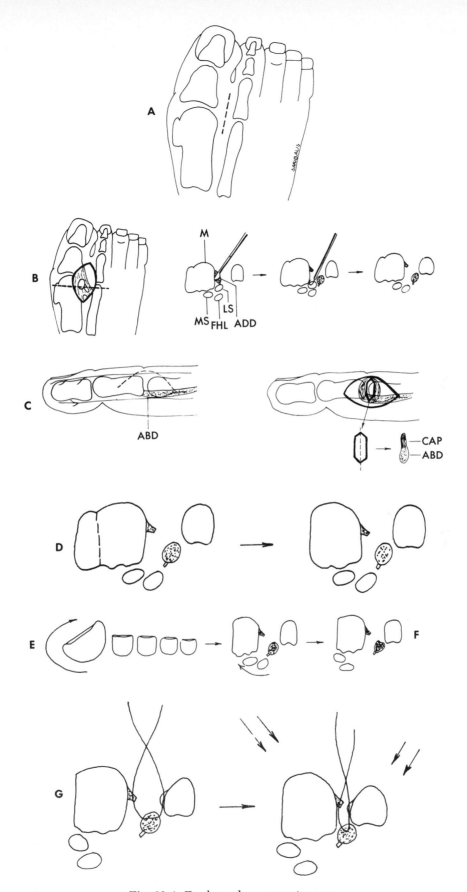

Fig. 20-4. For legend see opposite page.

proceeding proximally about 2.5 cm. Do not go too far proximal with this incision, for fear of cutting the superficial portion of the deep peroneal nerve in the first web space. Continue the dissection down in the midline to avoid disrupting the superficial branch of the deep peroneal nerve on both sides of the web space. Deepen the incision down through the subcutaneous tissue until a small but easily recognizable adventitious bursa is noted. This marks the area of the insertion of the adductor hallucis tendon into the lateral head of the flexor digitorum brevis and proximal phalanx. At this point, place a Weitlander retractor in the web space and spread so the structures in the base of the wound can be accurately identified.

2. By sharp dissection, carefully identify the adductor tendon as it passes from lateral to medial to insert into the flexor digitorum brevis tendon and then into the base of the proximal phalanx (Fig. 20-4, *B*). With a no. 15 blade, make an incision along the lateral aspect of the first metatarsal head in the interval between the capsule and the lateral sesamoid. A cuff of capsule has been created above this incision along the lateral aspect of the first metatarsal head and will be utilized later in the procedure. Once the interval between the capsule and the sesamoid has been identified, the knife is readily passed between the sesamoid and the metatarsal head distally to the base of the proximal phalanx. Upon reaching the base of the proximal phalanx, pass the knife laterally thereby detaching the adductor tendon as well as a portion of the flexor digitorum brevis tendon from the base of the proximal phalanx.

3. By sharp dissection, remove the lateral sesamoid. Removal of the sesamoid is facilitated by being sure the metatarsal heads are widely spread by the Weitlander. The intersesamoid ligament should be cut initially when excising a sesamoid because the sesamoid can thereby be pulled into the interspace and readily dissected out of the lateral conjoint tendon. Once this has been achieved, carefully inspect the base of the wound to be sure the flexor hallucis longus tendon is still intact. The neurovascular bun-

dle of the first web space will be noted in the plantar aspect of the wound and should not have been disturbed by removal of the sesamoid.

4. Cut the lateral capsule of the metatarsophalangeal joint by making a vertical incision just proximal to the base of the proximal phalanx of the great toe. Once this has been achieved, the great toe can be readily brought into correct alignment. Then remove the Weitlander and place a finger between the first and second metatarsal heads. As the great toe is brought into proper alignment, note the way the interspace between the first and second metatarsal heads is closed down and actually pinches one's finger. This, I believe, demonstrates that the widening between the first and second metatarsals is a secondary rather than a primary change in the production of a hallux valgus deformity.

5. Make a second incision about 3 cm long over the medial aspect of the metatarsophalangeal joint (Fig. 20-4, *C*). This incision may be slightly curved dorsally or in the midline. Carry it down to the capsule of the first metatarsophalangeal joint and then dissect a dorsal and a plantar flap along the plane of the capsule. The dorsal flap should be dissected until the medial dorsal cutaneous nerve of the great toe is identified and can be safely retracted. The plantar flap is dissected plantarward until the abductor hallucis tendon and the medial plantar nerve to the great toe are identified.

6. With an assistant retracting the dorsal and plantar flaps, make two vertical incisions with a no. 11 blade in the medial capsule: the initial incision 2 mm proximal to the base of the proximal phalanx, and a second parallel incision anywhere from 3 to 6 mm proximal to the initial incision. The width of the capsular section is dependent on the degree of deformity of the first metatarsophalangeal joint. This part of the procedure must be learned by trial and error; and needless to say, it is advisable to take off too little capsule and then have to take out another section rather than take off too much primarily. Bring the capsular incision down to the dorsal border of the abductor hallucis tendon, at which time the incision is

made V shaped through the abductor hallucis tendon so the apex of the incision rests against the medial sesamoid. Dorsally the incision is likewise V shaped to end at the dorsomedial aspect of the metatarsophalangeal joint. This capsule is then discarded.

7. Free the capsule from the medial prominence by sharp dissection. This is most easily done by starting at the plantar medial aspect where there is an anatomic space and carrying the dissection dorsally. The capsule is the thickest in the plantar half and becomes quite thin at times in the dorsal half.

8. Now excise the medial prominence using an osteotome (Fig. 20-4, *D*). The excision begins approximately 1 mm medial to the end of the articular cartilage of the metatarsal head, where the anatomic sagittal groove is located. Direct the osteotome proximally in the vertical plane so the cut will end just proximal to the prominence. Once the prominence has been removed, rongeur the edges so there will be no bony prominences over the dorsal aspect and so the cut will be vertical on the plantar aspect.

9. The assistant now holds the great toe in the corrected position so the medial capsular structures can be adequately repaired. Proper alignment consists of correcting the malrotation of the great toe along its longitudinal axis so the toenails are all aligned and the toe is brought out of its valgus position (Fig. 20-4, *E* and *F*). Four sutures of 2-0 chromic are used to repair the medial capsule. The first suture must be placed in the tendon of the abductor hallucis, and the second just dorsal to the first. Then place the other two sutures above these, being sure to use the best capsular material available for the repair. Once this has been accomplished and the assistant releases the great toe, both the rotational deformity and the valgus deformity should be corrected. If not, consideration must then be given to removing the sutures that have just been placed, correcting the alignment of the great toe, and resuturing it.

10. Attention is now redirected to the incision in the first web space. Place a Weitlander in the top of the incision to gently spread the metatarsal heads apart. Then place three sutures of 2-0 chromic between the first and second metatarsal heads, incorporating the adductor tendon (Fig. 20-4, *G*). These pass from the remaining cuff of capsule along the lateral aspect of the first metatarsal head through the adductor tendon and into the medial capsule of the second metatarsophalangeal joint just distal to the interosseous tendon. After the three sutures have been placed, remove the Weitlander retractor and with the assistant squeezing the metatarsal heads together, being careful not to put any pressure on the great toe, tie the three sutures. Once this has been accomplished, the space between the first and second metatarsal heads has been eliminated and the great toe should be well aligned. If the toe is not well aligned, reevaluate carefully in order to obtain adequate alignment.

11. The skin is now sutured with interrupted 5-0 cotton. Care must be taken to be sure the skin edges are everted. Apply a sterile compression dressing over at least 1.5 cm of gauze fluffs.

12. After the compression dressing is in place, release the tourniquet. If bleeding appears within the first 5 minutes after the surgery, the compression dressings should be made tighter.

The postoperative regimen is almost as important as the original surgery. The compression dressing remains in place for approximately 18 hours, at which time it is released and the patient remains at bed rest with the foot elevated; 48 hours after the surgery, the foot is redressed in a snug compression dressing with 2-inch kling and ½-inch adhesive tape. The dressing is applied initially circumferentially around the metatarsal heads to support the suture line between the first and second metatarsals (Fig. 20-5). It is then brought around the great toe to finely adjust the position of the great toe. If slight overcorrection has been obtained at surgery, the great toe should be gently splinted to the second toe to ensure that a varus deformity will not result. If, however, slight valgus of great toe still remains, the dressing should be applied in such a way as to help support the suture line along the medial side of the toe and

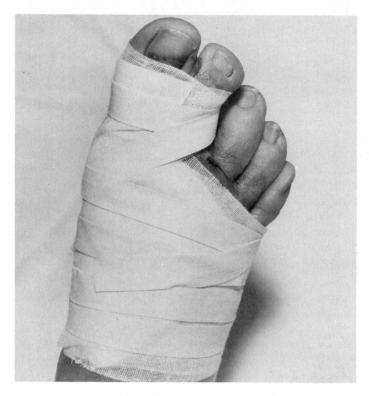

Fig. 20-5. Postoperative dressings for hallux valgus. The second toe serves as a splint. Sometimes the third digit is also included in the splint.

achieve as much correction as possible.

The dressing is changed every week for the first 4 weeks and then every 10 days for the second 4-week period. The patient is ambulatory in a commercially available postsurgical wooden shoe. It is important that the patient not cover the foot with a tight stocking because this will place undue stress along the medial suture line and can result in a possible recurrence of the deformity. After 8 weeks of immobilization, the patient is started on range-of-motion exercises and placed in a round-toed shoe or sandal. Any form of tight shoe should be avoided for a period of 4 to 6 months from the time of surgery. The patient will continue to experience a certain amount of stiffness and swelling after removal of the dressings (for 3 to 6 months). It is extremely important to encourage patients to work their toes after the dressing has been removed to regain mobility; they should also elevate the foot when sitting to keep swelling at a minimum.

Results of the foregoing technique are illustrated in Figs. 20-6 and 20-7.

There are several questions frequently asked regarding this surgical procedure:

1. When should the fibular sesamoid be removed? The fibular sesamoid should be excised if on a weight-bearing radiograph more than one third of the sesamoid is subluxed into the webspace. If the sesamoid is not excised, the surgeon must be absolutely sure to adequately remove the adductor tendon from the lateral aspect of the sesamoid as well as remove it from the base of the proximal phalanx. This is important because, as pointed out earlier (p. 254), the adductor tendon and its surrounding capsular structures are contracted and holding the toe in a valgus position.

2. When should the extensor hallucis longus tendon be lengthened? It is often thought that the extensor hallucis longus tendon should be frequently lengthened during repair of a bunion deformity; in reality, this

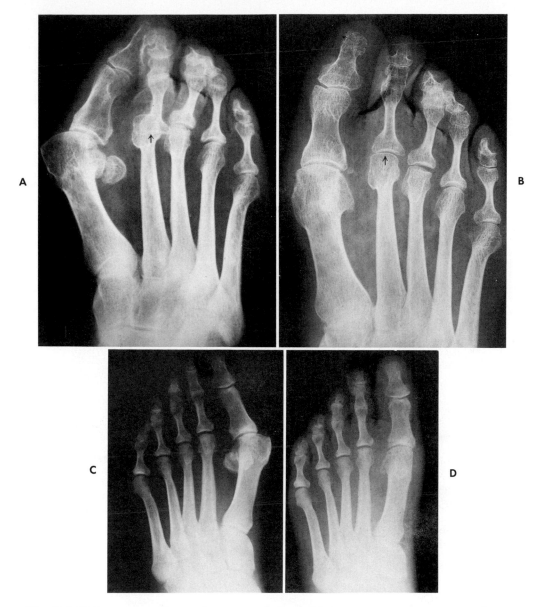

Fig. 20-6. Hallux valgus and second metatarsophalangeal dislocation. **A,** Preoperative. **B,** Three years following a modified McBride procedure. Note that the second metatarsophalangeal dislocation is reduced without bone excision. (See static second metatarsophalangeal dislocation in Fig. 8-42.) **C,** Preoperative view of another hallux valgus. **D,** Two years postoperative following a modified McBride procedure.

should rarely be done. One must, when evaluating the tension of the extensor hallucis longus tendon, be sure that the ankle is held at a right angle. Normally at the operating table the foot is in marked plantar flexion, thereby creating tension on the extensor hallucis longus tendon that normally is not present.

When the ankle is brought up into neutral position, the extensor hallucis longus tendon is rarely if ever too tight.

3. Should the hallux be overcorrected in a McBride procedure? At surgery, one should strive to precisely correct the alignment of the first metatarsophalangeal joint and not over-

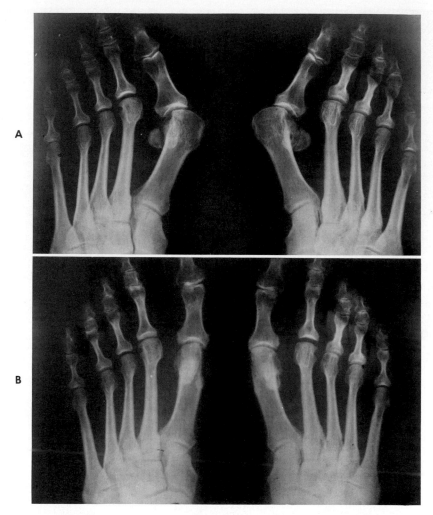

Fig. 20-7. Severe hallux valgus. **A,** Preoperative; **B,** twelve years postoperative following a modified McBride procedure.

correct the great toe. If, however, the great toe is slightly overcorrected the postoperative dressings will usually adequately compensate and produce satisfactory alignment. With improper postoperative dressing a hallux varus may result.

4. When do you perform an osteotomy of the first metatarsal in an adult patient with hallux valgus deformity? A metatarsal osteotomy is usually not necessary in the correction of an adult type—hallux valgus. As stated previously (p. 251), we believe that the metatarsus primus varus present is a secondary change to the deviation of the proximal pha-

lanx so that once the proximal phalanx has been brought back into proper alignment the metatarsus primus varus is no longer present. In a few adults there is medial deviation of the metatarsal shaft on an anatomic basis; and in these persons an osteotomy at the base of the metatarsal would be indicated. Occasionally there is marked obliquity of the first metatarsocunieform joint which should be corrected by an arthrodesis of the first metatarsocuneiform joint.

Complications following repair of a hallux valgus deformity are rare. If a pyogenic infection occurs, it is imperative that specific antibiotic therapy with a bactericidal drug be instituted on a parenteral basis until the acute infection subsides, following which oral antibiotics can be used. Occasionally the skin edges appear inflamed postoperatively but the other signs and symptoms of a postoperative infection are absent. This is often secondary to spores of a tinea infection. Local treatment, i.e., painting a fungicide on the skin margins, will then usually induce uneventful healing.

The common postoperative deformities of this procedure which have been seen by us are (1) recurrent hallux valgus, (2) postoperative hallux varus, and (3) dorsal contracture of the hallux often accompanied by a hammered interphalangeal joint of the great toe.

A *recurrent hallux valgus* is usually due to the fact that the fibular sesamoid was not excised at the time of the original procedure. If all the contracture on the fibular side of the metatarsophalangeal joint is not released at the time of surgical correction, then recurrent deformity is a distinct possiblity. At times the capsular repair on the medial side of the metatarsophalangeal joint has not been adequate; hence a recurrence of the deformity. If the patient has a severely pronated foot which is not or cannot be adequately accommodated postoperatively, a recurrence can result. The treatment of the recurrent deformity if warranted would be to repeat the original procedure so any deficiencies that might still be present would be corrected.

The treatment of a *postoperative hallux varus* has already been presented in detail (p. 261).

The *dorsal contracture of the hallux* along with *hammering of the interphalangeal joint* is usually caused by the functional loss of the flexor hallucis brevis as a result of the surgical procedure. This occasionally develops when the fibular sesamoid has been removed and the tibial sesamoid slips medially to the metatarsal head. The resulting extension of the metatarsophalangeal joint and flexion of the interphalangeal joint can be most difficult to treat. Initially one must be sure that the interphalangeal joint of the great toe and the metatarsophalangeal joint are kept mobile by having the patient manually exercise the joints. The condition can then be surgically corrected by freeing the tibial sesamoid from the medial side of the metatarsal head and replacing it underneath the metatarsal so it can resume its normal function as an intrinsic muscle.

Another complication occasionally seen after any type of foot procedure is the entrapment of a cutaneous nerve, which can produce either dysesthesia or anesthesia at the site of the involved nerve. Needless to say, prevention is the best treatment; but once the condition exists, I find it most helpful to have the patient try to desensitize the involved area by massaging, rubbing, and tapping over the sensitive area. This will often, over a period of several months, produce a satisfactory response. Occasionally it is necessary to reoperate and further resect the involved nerve to an area of soft fatty tissue so the condition will no longer be symptomatic.

Type 2. The adolescent type of hallux valgus is seen in patients who are between the ages of 10 and 20 years. As mentioned before, the deformity has often been caused by predisposing factors—such as a round first metatarsal head, metatarsus primus varus, pronation of the hindfoot, congenital laxity of the ligaments, or a neuromuscular disorder. The usual adolescent type of hallux valgus is associated with a round metatarsal head, metatarsus primus varus, and mild pronation of the foot. In patients with congenital laxity of the ligaments and/or a neuromuscular disorder, correction of the hallux valgus deformity is associated with a greater than 50% recurrence rate. For this reason, unless the underlying predisposing factors are corrected, repair of the deformity will not be fruitful.

In the usual type of adolescent hallux valgus, if a metatarsus primus varus is present it should be corrected by a dome-shaped osteotomy concave proximally at the base of the metatarsal. If, however, the deformity of the first metatarsal is due to marked obliquity of the first metatarsocuneiform joint, then an arthrodesis of the joint correcting the obliquity should be done.

The procedure for correcting the metatarsophalangeal joint in an adolescent type of hallux valgus is the same as in an adult except that the fibular sesamoid is usually not excised unless more than 50% of it is subluxated into the web space on a weight-bearing radiograph (Fig. 20-8).

From a technical standpoint, the metatarsophalangeal joint is surgically approached in the usual manner, following which the osteotomy or arthrodesis site is prepared. If only an osteotomy is used, then after the osteotomy has been properly realigned, insert the sutures in the web space between the first and second metatarsals. Be sure to incorporate the adductor tendon; by so doing, one will maintain the osteotomy in proper alignment. If there is any question, a threaded Steinmann pin can be inserted from the medial side of the first metatarsal into the second metatarsal to maintain the alignment of the two metatarsal shafts.

To bring the great toe into proper alignment, plicate the capsular structure on the medial side of the metatarsophalangeal joint. If the procedure is not carried out in this

sequence, overcorrection of the metatarsophalangeal joint can occur. If an arthrodesis of the metatarsocuneiform joint is performed, the staple is placed from dorsal to plantar after the joint surfaces have been denuded. By so doing, one again maintains the metatarsal shaft in proper alignment with the sutures in the web space between the first and second metatarsal heads (Fig. 20-4, G).

If the epiphysis at the base of the first metatarsal is still open, the osteotomy should be done about 1 cm distal to the epiphyseal plate; and if an arthodesis is performed, the staple must be distal to the epiphysis. After the arthrodesis site has fused in a patient with an open epiphyseal plate, the staple must be removed to prevent retardation of the growth of the epiphysis.

Postoperatively the foot is dressed as for an adult hallux valgus deformity. The dressing should be tight around the metatarsal heads to maintain the narrowed space between the metatarsals, and the position of the great toe is likewise carefully adjusted. Patients are kept non–weight bearing on crutches for 4 weeks,

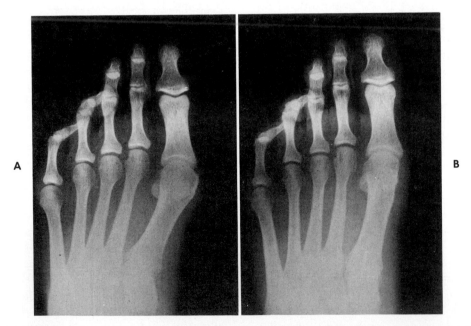

Fig. 20-8. Moderate hallux valgus and metatarsus primus varus of the left foot in an 18-year-old girl. **A,** Preoperative. **B,** Two years postoperative. It was not necessary to excise the fibular sesamoid or do an osteotomy. The three middle metatarsals have assumed normal alignment.

after which they are allowed to walk in a wooden shoe until the arthrodesis site or osteotomy site is healed (usually 8 to 10 weeks). The great toe is held in correct alignment with kling and tape for 8 weeks.

Type 3. For the abnormally long first metatarsal with hallux valgus, the Hawkins et al. (1945) step-cut osteotomy (Fig. 20-9) offers the most rational approach.

Type 4. Hallux valgus with marked splayfoot should be treated as is the adolescent type (Fig. 20-10).

If a component of the splayfoot is marked lateral deviation of the fifth metatarsal shaft and head, consideration should be given to doing an osteotomy of the fifth metatarsal shaft at the time the hallux valgus is repaired. By so doing, one somewhat narrows the forefoot. The other approach to a splayfoot is by using a plantar sling as described by Joplin (1950).

Joplin fashioned a transverse plantar sling of the extensor digitorum longus tendon from the fifth toe (Fig. 20-11), which he brought under the metatarsal arch and passed through a drill hole in the first metatarsal head with the

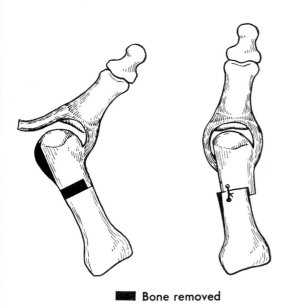

Bone removed

Fig. 20-9. Hawkins et al. (1945) step-cut osteotomy of the first metatarsal shaft for hallux valgus.

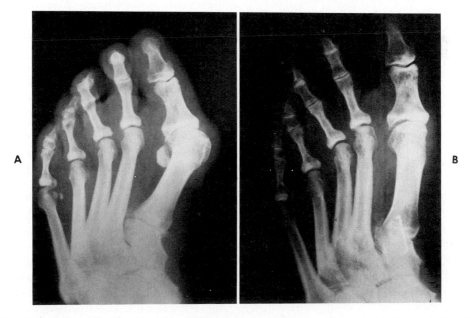

Fig. 20-10. Marked left hallux valgus and splayfoot in a 58-year-old woman. **A,** Preoperative. **B,** Two years postoperative following a modified McBride and arthrodesis of the metatarsocuneiform joint.

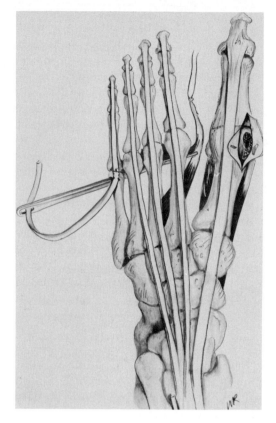

Fig. 20-11. Joplin plantar sling technique for hallux valgus. The extensor tendon of the fifth digit is threaded under the metatarsal heads. Then, together with the tendon of the adductor hallucis, it is threaded through a drill hole in the first metatarsal head and sutured to the capsule on the tibial side. (Courtesy American Academy of Orthopaedic Surgeons, Inc.)

freed adductor hallucis tendon. He then sutured it to the capsule on the tibial side of the first metatarsophalangeal joint. The procedure combines some of the features of an operation that laces a strip of fascia lata around the metatarsal heads to bind them for splayfoot, as reported by Krida (1939). McBride (1928) also employed fascia lata lacing as part of his technique.

These procedures have value in severe splayfoot. Blosser (1964) performed a modified Krida procedure in forty cases of hallux valgus, with good results. It would appear that a strip of fascia lata would bind and hold the distal part of the metatarsals together more securely than would the long extensor, which is a very thin tendon.

Type 5. The treatment of hallux valgus in the rheumatoid foot was discussed by Clayton (1960), who outlined an operative procedure which he had used with success. Marmor (1964) used the Clayton procedure with slight modification and found it to be efficacious.

Clayton's basic technique is a metatarsophalangeal joint resection as outlined by Hoffman (1912). The degree of deformity determines the extent of excision: in severe cases all the metatarsal heads and bases of the proximal phalanges are excised whereas in lesser deformities modification of bone excision is practiced.

DuVries and Dickson modified the Clayton procedure for repair of a rheumatoid foot by doing an arthrodesis of the first metatarsophalangeal joint. This modification was made to prevent the recurrence of the valgus deformity of the great toe and sometimes of the lesser toes that follow the Clayton procedure. Besides preventing any recurrence of the valgus deformity of the great toe, the arthrodesis, we believe, gives the foot greater stability. High-speed motion picture studies of a rheumatoid foot treated in this manner demonstrate how with an arthrodesed first metatarsophalangeal joint toe-off occurs somewhat earlier, thereby helping to decrease weight bearing on the lesser metatarsals and prevent further callus formation.

The pathologic anatomy of the rheumatoid foot is the result of the loss of stability of the metatarsophalangeal joints due to the destructive nature of the synovial proliferation seen in rheumatoid arthritis. With the loss of stability of the joint capsules, the metatarsophalangeal joints are forced into progressive dorsiflexion during normal walking until they eventually are subluxated onto the heads of the metatarsals. As this occurs, the fat pad is dragged distally over the metatarsal heads into an ineffective weight-bearing position. With the metatarsal heads held in a fixed position in the plantar aspect of the foot, there is progressive callus formation beneath the metatarsal heads. These calluses become very thick and painful and eventually ulcerate unless adequately treated.

The surgical procedure essentially reverses this process by excising the base of the proximal phalanx, which releases the insertion of the intrinsic muscles and plantar aponeurosis. Then the displaced structures can be stripped off the dorsal aspect of the metatarsal head and neck and brought back onto the plantar aspect of the foot. Once this has been achieved, the fat pad can be pulled back under the metatarsal heads into a normal weight-bearing position.

We strongly agree with Clayton's basic idea that one need excise only as much metatarsal head as is necessary in each particular case. At times, in patients with mild rheumatoid arthritis, only a synovectomy of the joints will be necessary whereas at the other extreme, in patients with severe dislocations of the metatarsophalangeal joints, all the lesser metatarsophalangeal joints will have to be resected. In doing the operation, the surgeon must be sure that the metatarsal heads form a smooth curve so a single metatarsal is not too prominent lest a callus form beneath it.

Since the operation for a rheumatoid foot is so extensive, we believe only one foot should be done at a time. In our experience with over 200 rheumatoid feet, no patient has failed to return to have the second foot operated upon.

Surgical technique for DuVries-Dickson procedure

1. The first incision is over the first metatarsophalangeal joint. Incise longitudinally on the dorsal aspect of the foot just medial to the extensor hallucis longus tendon, deepening directly to the metatarsophalangeal joint.

2. Insert a Weitlander into the wound to gain adequate exposure. By sharp dissection, remove the joint capsule as well as any proliferative synovial tissue.

3. Detach the adductor hallucis tendon from its insertion in the base of the proximal phalanx.

4. If the medial prominence on the metatarsal head is significantly enlarged, remove it.

5. Cut the distal portion of the metatarsal head and base of the proximal phalanx with an osteotome. Prepare to arthrodese the metatarsophalangeal joint.

6. At this point, approach the lesser metatarsophalangeal joints before placing the pins to arthrodese the first metatarsophalangeal joint.

7. Make a longitudinal incision in the second and fourth dorsal web spaces. Through this incision the metatarsophalangeal joint to the medial and lateral sides can be readily approached.

8. By blunt dissection, expose the base of the proximal phalanx and excise with a bone cutter. This is done for all the lesser toes.

9. Then, by sharp and blunt dissection, strip the plantar structures that are adherent around the metatarsal head so they can again be placed on the plantar aspect of the foot. Once this has been achieved for all the metatarsal heads, the fat pad can be returned to its proper place under the metatarsal heads.

10. If because of soft tissue contracture the fat pad cannot be adequately replaced under the metatarsal heads, remove a sufficient amount of metatarsal head to permit adequate replacement of the fat pad on the plantar weight-bearing aspect of the foot. This will require resection of from half to all of the metatarsal head depending on the degree of contracture of the forefoot. The metatarsal necks must form a smooth arc, and no one metatarsal may be more prominent than the others lest a callosity form beneath it.

11. Attention is now redirected to the first metatarsophalangeal joint, where the raw bone surfaces are brought into position. Check the overall length of the great toe relative to the remainder of the forefoot. If extensive resections have been done on the other metatarsophalangeal joints, the great toe should be shortened somewhat so it will not protude too far beyond the lesser toes. Sometimes the first metatarsophalangeal joint will have to be shortened approximately 1 cm to achieve balance among the toes. Then 0.5 cm is taken from the proximal phalanx and 0.5 cm from the first metatarsal head.

12. Stabilize the arthrodesis site with either staples or (as I prefer) heavy threaded Steinmann pins driven retrograde through the tip of the toe and back across the site to be arthrodesed. The arthrodesis should be so performed that the toe is in 10° of dorsiflexion and 5° of valgus.

13. Close the skin with interrupted 5-0

cotton and apply a sterile compression dressing. The dressing is left in place for approximately 18 hours and then released.

14. Approximately 36 hours after surgery, redress the foot using 2-inch kling. The lesser toes must be splinted with the gauze toward the great toe and plantarward to maintain adequate alignment of the lesser toes because they scar down following the operation.

15. Using the Steinmann pin method of fixation, I allow the patient to walk on the third postoperative day; however, if a staple is used, weight bearing should be restricted for approximately 1 month.

Figs. 20-12 and 20-13 show typical results of rheumatoid foot surgery.

Other procedures for hallux valgus

Simple and modified condylectomies. Be-

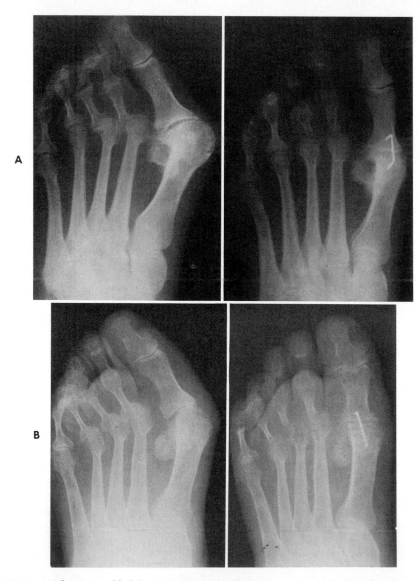

Fig. 20-12. A, Rheumatoid left foot of a 52-year-old woman preoperatively and postoperatively. Note the hypertrophic changes around the first metatarsal head, which has been remodeled. **B,** Preoperative and postoperative views of the left foot of a 56-year-old woman who had severe rheumatoid arthritis of the feet. The staple was removed one year postoperatively when she returned for correction of the right foot.

cause it is seldom disabling, simple condylectomy or exostosectomy of the tibial side of the first metatarsal head is one of the most common procedures advocated for hallux valgus. It produces disability only if performed in cases of severe dislocation of the great toe, if too much of the tibial side of the head of the first metatarsal has been removed, or if the abductor hallucis tendon has been interrupted and improperly repaired.

Levine (1938) and McElvenny and Thompson (1940) removed the tibial condylar lip of the base of the first proximal phalanx; however, that is of value only when the protuber-ance is caused entirely by an unusually wide first metatarsal head. It is of little or no value when there is extreme hallux valgus, and it may even worsen the deformity.

We believe the simple and modified condylectomies are rarely indicated except in older patients who are not good surgical candidates for a routine type of bunion procedure. In these patients, condylectomy may prevent an ulcer from forming over the dorsomedial aspect of the first metatarsal and thus create a more severe problem which could result in loss of the limb. If a younger person has a mild dorsomedial or medial

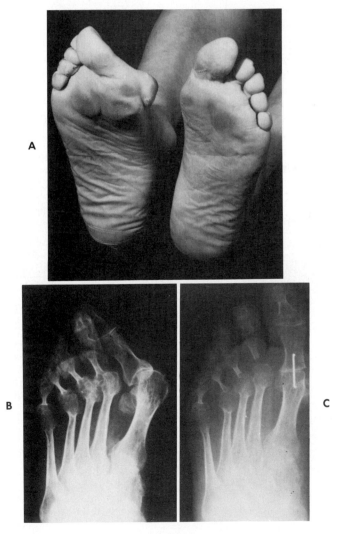

Fig. 20-13. Rheumatoid foot. **A,** Preoperative right foot and one-year postoperative left foot. **B,** Preoperative left foot. **C,** Postoperative left foot.

prominence on the tibial side of the first metatarsal head without significant deformity of the metatarsophalangeal joint, the problem is best treated with a broad-toed shoe.

Silver's (1923) technique for reduction of hallux valgus. A semilunar incision, its vertex placed dorsally, is made over the medial surface of the great toe joint. A Y-shaped incision is then made in the capsule to form three flaps: one distal, one dorsal, and one plantar. The flaps are dissected so the head of the metatarsal is exposed. While the great toe is plantar flexed, a tenotome is inserted just above the plantar capsule of the joint and a longitudinal incision is made on the fibular side of the capsule. With the toe dorsiflexed, a longitudinal incision is made in the dorsal margin of the capsule on the fibular side. The toe is strongly adducted. A vertical incision is made on the fibular capsule between the two longitudinal incisions. This capsulotomy releases the tension on the fibular side of the joint. The toe is overcorrected and the distal flap on the medial side is sutured to the periosteum just behind the head of the first metatarsal. The dorsal and plantar flaps are sutured over the distal flap.

Condylectomy combined with step-down osteotomy. Hawkins et al.(1945) and Mitchell (1958), in addition to removing the tibial condylar side of the first metatarsal head, performed a step-down osteotomy on the first metatarsal shaft (Fig. 20-9). They reported excellent results in a large series of cases.

This procedure has much to recommend it in the uncommon cases of hallux valgus accompanied by a first metatarsal that is longer than the lesser metatarsals (Fig. 20-14, *A*). When the first metatarsal is shorter than the second, however, the resultant additional shortening places an excessive amount of weight bearing on the head of the second metatarsal and often a new problem is produced (Fig. 20-14, *B*).

Wilson (1963) reported the use of an oblique osteotomy of the distal third of the first metatarsal combined with trimming of the exostosis. The distal fragment was displaced laterally, the metatarsal shortened, and the position stabilized by placing the great toe in a position of overcorrection. Wilson believed this operation was particu-

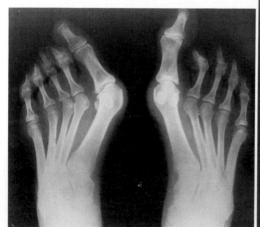
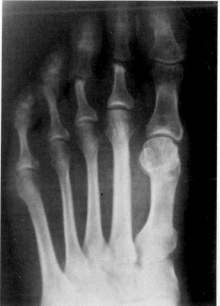

Fig. 20-14. A, Hallux valgus with an abnormally long first metatarsal. A Hawkins et al. (1945) step-cut osteotomy is the procedure of choice in this case. **B,** Result of a step-down osteotomy for hallux valgus. The first metatarsal of this 24-year-old woman was shorter than the second before the operation. A painful plantar keratosis ensued caused by excessive weight bearing on the second metatarsal. A Giannestras step-down osteotomy was done on the second metatarsal.

larly useful for active adolescents since it did not interfere with the efficiency of the foot. Holstein and Lewis (1976) have reported uniformly good results with ninety-eight Wilson-type procedures on sixty-four patients. They used the procedure on both young and middle-aged patients. The overall cosmetic result was good, as was the mobility of the metatarsophalangeal joint. There were a significant number of patients with postoperative metatarsalgia (27% of the series) probably due to the shortening of the first metatarsal.

Akin (1925) described an osteotomy of the base of the proximal phalanx along with excision of the medial prominence and adjacent lip of the proximal phalanx for correction of hallux valgus. The osteotomy of the proximal phalanx has been used alone to correct hallux valgus interphalangeus or in combination with other procedures on the first metatarsal to correct hallux valgus (Giannestras, 1972). The procedure is also useful in reverse, namely a lateral closing wedge osteotomy in cases of mild hallux varus.

Amputation of base of proximal phalanx. Keller (1904) described his operation for amputating the proximal half of the first prox-imal phalanx for hallux valgus correction; later (1912) he reported refinements. His procedure has acquired support, notably by Brandes (1929), Galland and Jordan (1938), Schein (1940), and Cleveland and Winant (1950). It is probably the most widely used procedure in the United States.

Keller's technique. An elliptical incision, having its base dorsally, is made over the great toe joint. A U-shaped incision with its base about 1 cm distal to the base of the proximal phalanx is made in the tibial capsule of the great toe joint. The flap is dissected distally to expose the medial surface of the head of the first metatarsal and the base of the proximal phalanx. The tibial condyle of the first metatarsal is amputated. The attachments to the base of the proximal phalanx are freed. Approximately 1.5 cm or the proximal third of the base of the proximal phalanx is amputated and smoothed with a rasp. The toe is brought into alignment, and the U-shaped flap is sutured to the periosteum just behind the tibial side of the head of the first metatarsal. This is done under mild tenson, with the toe in a slightly overcorrected position. The skin is then sutured (Fig. 20-15).

The Keller method is perhaps the most

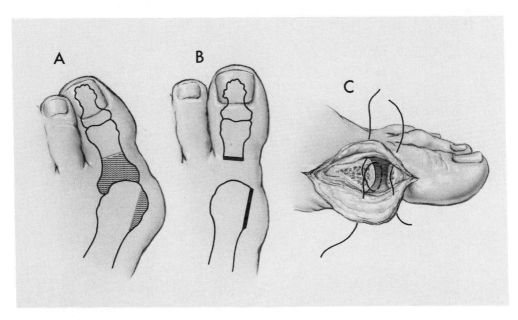

Fig. 20-15. Keller operation for correction of hallux valgus.

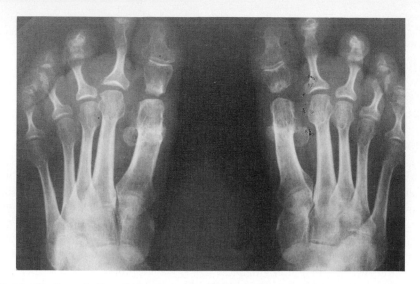

Fig. 20-16. The flexor hallucis brevis insertion had been destroyed during the Keller procedure in the preceding figure. The sesamoids are recessed to the middle of the first metatarsal shaft.

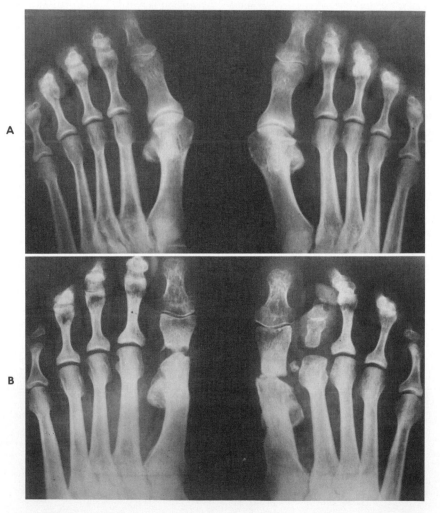

Fig. 20-17. Mild hallux valgus. **A,** Preoperative. **B,** Postoperative following a Keller procedure. The patient was in constant pain because the proximal surface of what remained of the proximal phalanx had been roughened. Amputation of the base of the right second proximal phalanx made that ray unstable also.

common procedure practiced for the surgical treatment of hallux valgus, mainly because the procedure is simple and usually gives a satisfactory cosmetic result. However, the great toe is always shortened, its function in walking is diminished, and in some cases it becomes a useless appendage. Those effects occur because the intrinsic muscles and the plantar aponeurosis insert into the base of the proximal phalanx and in the Keller procedure this part of the bone is excised, thereby destroying the function of these muscles.

Henry and Waugh (1975) have demonstrated that the great toe is unlikely to bear weight when more than one third of the proximal phalanx has been removed. Because of this loss of weight bearing by the first metatarsophalangeal joint, metatarsalgia is an inherent problem following the Keller procedure.

The sesamoids usually recede proximally (Figs. 20-16 and 20-17) because the flexor hallucis brevis insertion has been destroyed and the weight-bearing function of the sesamoids has been lost. Hallux extensus may also follow the Keller procedure as a result of the severance of the flexor hallucis brevis.

Pain in the first metatarsocuneiform joint occurs occasionally after the Keller procedure because removal of the base of the proximal phalanx reduces the stability of the first metatarsal head, thereby putting extra stress at the base of this ray (Fig. 20-18).

Over 150 cases have come into my hands (H.L.D.) because of disability after a Keller procedure. In my experience, a larger group seeks help for postoperative disability resulting from this procedure than from any other operation employed in the alleviation of hallux valgus. Unfortunately, once the base of the proximal phalanx has been destroyed, little can be done to restore normal function. It is difficult to visualize a static deformity of the first metatarsophalangeal joint in which this procedure is indicated.

A person who has undergone a Keller

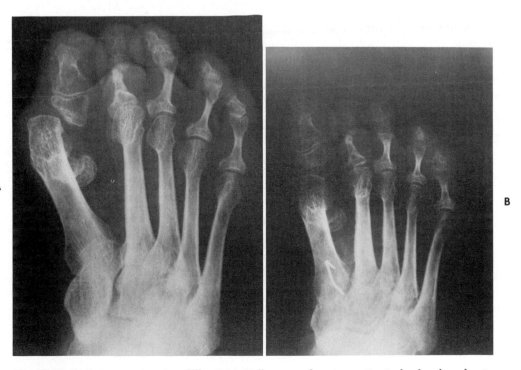

Fig. 20-18. A, Postoperative view following a Keller procedure in a patient who developed pain in the first metatarsocuneiform joint. **B,** Eighteen months after stabilization of the first metatarsocuneiform joint; symptoms disappeared.

procedure and develops metatarsalgia secondary to lack of adequate stability and weight bearing by the first metatarsophalangeal joint can often be made asymptomatic by an arthrodesis of the remaining proximal phalanx and first metatarsal. If at least 50% of the proximal phalanx or more is present, a most successful arthrodesis can be done without adding any bone graft. In these cases the toes should be arthrodesed in only 5° to 10° of dorsiflexion to increase the weight bearing of the great toe. If the great toe is arthrodesed in more dorsiflexion, it will not carry enough weight to relieve the metatarsalgia under the second and third metatarsal heads.

We believe that the only time a Keller procedure is indicated is in an older patient with a severe hallux valgus deformity which has produced an ulcer or is on the verge of ulcerating the skin over the metatarsal head. In such a case the Keller procedure will relieve the tension of the skin over the metatarsal head and, by shortening of the proximal phalanx, the great toe can be brought into better alignment so the patient can resume wearing adequate shoes.

Arthrodesis

Arthrodesis of the first metatarsophalangeal joint is an excellent procedure for treatment of degenerative arthritis of the first metatarsophalangeal joint, for treatment of rheumatoid arthritis, or as a salvage procedure for failed bunion procedures. In an otherwise normal foot the arthrodesed joint should be placed in about 15° of dorsiflexion and 5° of valgus. If, however, the patient has lost stability of the lesser metatarsophalangeal joints such as in rheumatoid arthritis or possibly metatarsal head resections, the arthrodesed joint should be placed in only 5° of dorsiflexion. By decreasing the amount of dorsiflexion at the metatarsophalangeal joint, the procedure causes the person to toe off somewhat sooner and thus has the effect of decreasing the pressure on the other metatarsal heads, thereby helping to alleviate any metatarsalgia that may exist.

The manner in which the arthrodesis is done is not too critical, provided the articular cartilage has been adequately removed and good bony contact is achieved so a successful arthrodesis can take place. We prefer to stabilize the interphalangeal joint by running two heavy threaded Steinmann pins across it and to the tip of the toe; next the arthrodesis site is placed in proper alignment, and the Steinmann pins then run retrograde to the metatarsal head and shaft. By so doing, we are able to have the patient walking 2 days after surgery in a wooden shoe with weight bearing as tolerated. Usually 10 to 12 weeks are needed for the arthrodesis to become solid, at which time the pins are removed. We have had a 95% fusion rate using this particular procedure. The placement of the pins has caused some stiffness of the interphalangeal joint but not enough to create problems in our cases to date (Fig. 20-19).

There are other ways to do an arthrodesis of the first metatarsophalangeal joint:

McKeever (1952) discussed arthrodesis of the first metatarsophalangeal joint in great detail, emphasizing the importance of the position in which the great toe is placed. He prefered to fix the joint with a screw inserted from the plantar aspect of the foot.

Moynihan (1967) recommended arthrodesing the first metatarsophalangeal joint of the great toe by two similar procedures: a peg-and-socket arthrodesis and a procedure in which the cartilage, subchondral bone, and exostosis were excised. In both procedures the arthrodesed joint was fixed with a screw. He performed these operations on 108 patients, with good results in 86% of cases.

Wilson (1967) reported his use of a cone arthrodesis of the first metatarsophalangeal joint. His procedure consisted of making a cone fit between the metatarsal head and the base of the proximal phalanx of the great toe. He stated that by careful positioning of the reamers, it was possible to fuse the joint in as much as 10° or even 15° of dorsiflexion or valgus.

Subcapital amputation

Subcapital amputation as advocated by Heuter (1870-1871) and later modified by Mayo (1908) and Soresi (1931) is mentioned only to point out that the overall results of these procedures are poor, because the

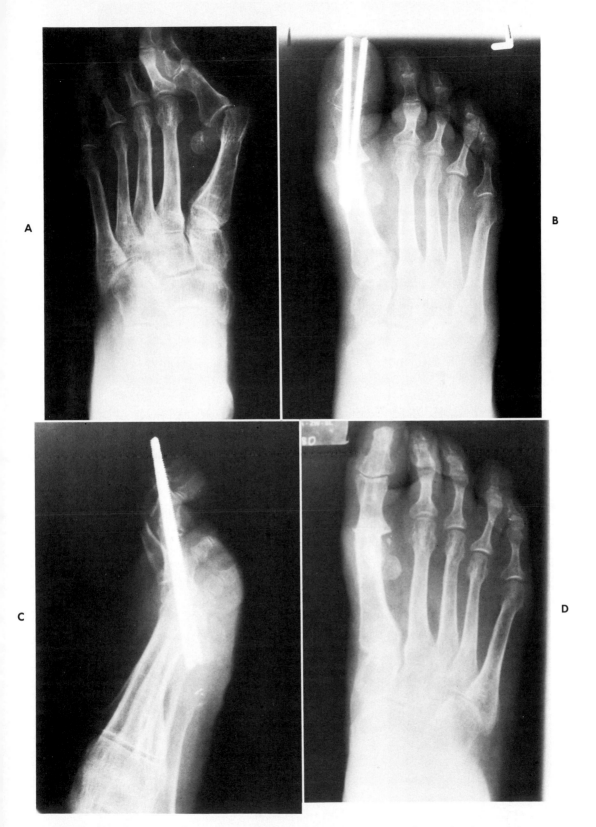

Fig. 20-19. Advanced hallux valgus. **A,** Preoperative. **B,** AP view of an arthrodesis of the metatarsophalangeal joint utilizing heavy threaded Steinmann pins. **C,** Lateral view. Note about 20° of dorsiflexion at the metatarsophalangeal joint. **D,** Postoperative.

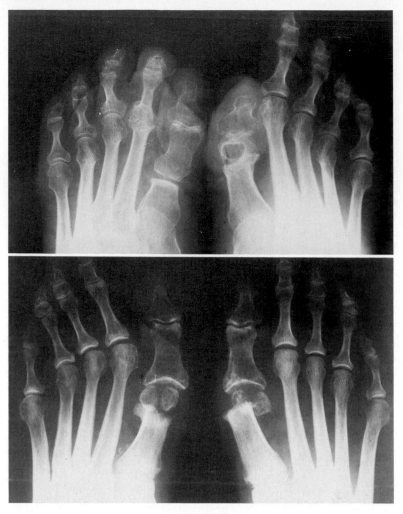

Fig. 20-20. Postoperative views following subcapital amputation of the first metatarsal head for hallux valgus (two patients).

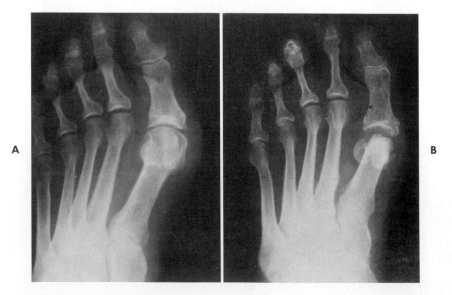

Fig. 20-21. Moderate hallux valgus in a 55-year-old woman. **A,** Preoperative, showing the subcapital amputation that was performed in 1961. **B,** Two years postoperatively. Severe bilateral disability ensued after the subcapital amputation.

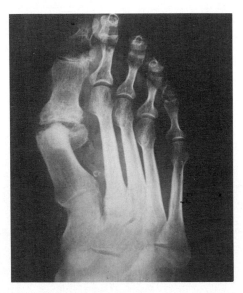

Fig. 20-22. Pointed articulation of the head of the first metatarsal with the base of the proximal phalanx after subcapital amputation. The patient was in constant pain during walking.

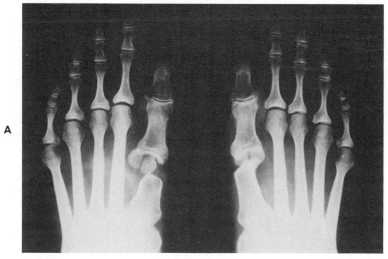

Continued.

Fig. 20-23. Subcapital amputation of the first metatarsal heads for hallux valgus performed elsewhere in 1954. In 1960 this 38-year-old woman sought relief for disability caused by sesamoids wedged between the base of the proximal phalanx and the remains of the first metatarsal of the left foot. A fibular bone graft was performed. **A,** Postoperative view (1954). **B,** Postoperative view (1961). **C,** Postoperative (1964); asymptomatic.

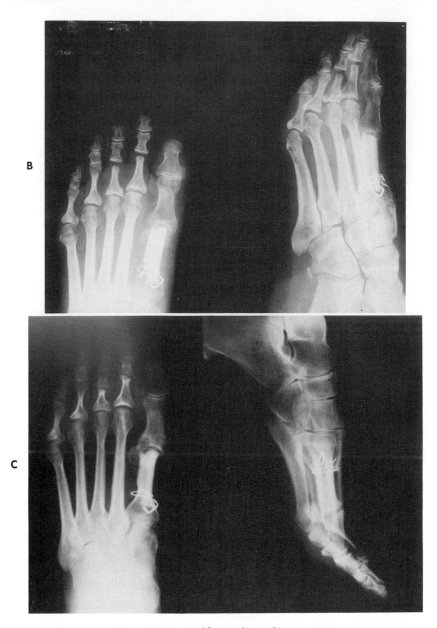

Fig. 20-23, cont'd. For legend see p. 587.

weight-bearing function of the first metatarsal head has been destroyed. Several examples of subcapital amputation are presented to show the marked destruction that has occurred in the weight-bearing function of the foot as a result of such procedures (Figs. 20-20 to 20-24).

DEFORMED TOES
Surgical procedures for the correction of hammertoes

Many complex procedures have been offered for the correction of hammertoes, especially of the middle three toes (Fig. 20-25).

Lorenz (1929), Lapidus (1939), Michele and

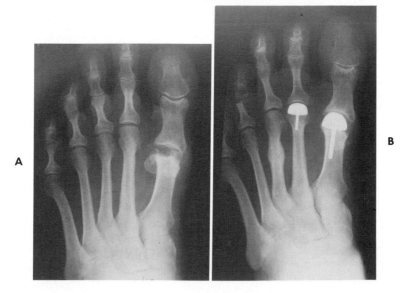

Fig. 20-24. A, Postoperative subcapital amputation for correction of hallux valgus. The foot was symptomatic. **B,** Metallic prostheses inserted for a better articular surface of the metatarsal heads. Note the fatigue fracture of the third metatarsal. (Courtesy Dr. R. H. Seeburger.)

Krueger (1948), and Borg (1950) excised different parts of the phalanges. Tierney (1937) and Young (1938) advised forming a cup and ball of the distal end of the proximal joint. Wagner (1934) and Forrester-Brown (1938) advocated tendon transplantation to correct the hammered great toe. Taylor (1940) and Selig (1941) suggested drawing a Kirschner wire through all the phalanges.

Recommended procedures for reduction of hammered great toe. The procedure outlined here is intended for mild cases in which the deformity is not fixed and can be reduced passively, although it cannot be held in reduction.

1. From the dorsal aspect of the interphalangeal joint, remove a transverse elliptical section (about 0.5 cm in width) of skin, capsule, and tendon of the extensor hallucis longus.

2. Remove 2 or 3 mm of the head of the proximal phalanx and round it with a nasal rasp.

3. Suture the dorsal capsule and the tendon of the extensor hallucis longus in the shortened position and suture the skin.

4. Partly immobilize the toe by adhesive splinting for 2 to 3 weeks. The splinting may be achieved by bandaging the great toe to the three adjacent toes and carrying the bandage over all the metatarsophalangeal joints.

An alternative procedure for a hammertoe deformity of the great toe is an arthrodesis of the interphalangeal joint. When this is done, two threaded pins should be used to fix the joint to prevent motion.

Jones' tendon transfer. In the case of a congenital hammered great toe, the articular surface of the interphalangeal joint is abnormal and soft tissue repair alone will not permanently reduce the deformity. Arthrodesis of the joint as described in Jones' technique without transference of the extensor hallucis longus will usually best correct this condition (Fig. 20-26).

In patients who have developed hyperextension of the metatarsophalangeal joint of the great toe secondary to a combination of weakness of ankle dorsiflexors but with a normally functioning extensor hallucis longus, the Jones technique for transferring the tendon of the extensor hallucis longus and arthrodesing

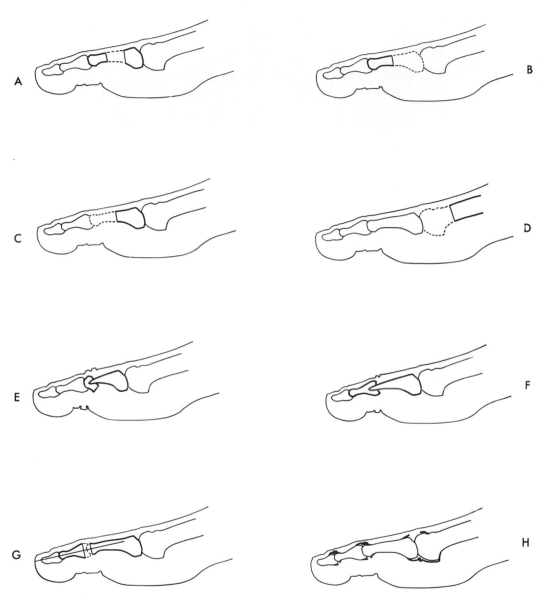

Fig. 20-25. Various operations for correction of hammered middle three toes. **A,** Excision of the middle third of the proximal phalanx. **B,** Excision of the proximal half of the proximal phalanx. **C,** Excision of the distal half of the proximal phalanx. **D,** Excision of the head of the metatarsal. **E,** Shaft of the proximal phalanx cupped into the base of the middle phalanx. **G,** Proximal phalangeal joint denuded of cartilage. A Kirschner wire is passed through the three phalanges. **H,** All contracted capsules sectioned and the elongated capsules shortened.

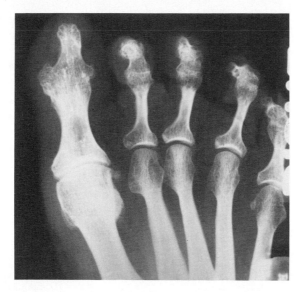

Fig. 20-26. Arthrodesed interphalangeal joint for a hammered great toe.

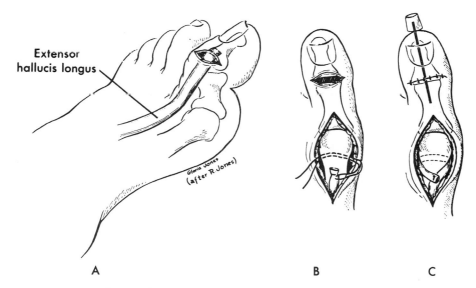

Extensor hallucis longus

A   B   C

Fig. 20-27. Jones reduction for a static clawed great toe. **A,** Incision for cut and release of the tendon. **B,** Phalangeal joint denuded of cartilage and tendon threaded through a drill hole. **C,** Tendon sutured to itself and a pin inserted into the arthrodesed phalangeal joint. The exposed pin is covered with cork.

the interphalangeal joint still offers the best results.

1. Make an elliptical transverse incision centered over the interphalangeal joint of the great toe and carry it down through the extensor tendon to bone (Fig. 20-27, *A* and *B*).

2. Remove all articular cartilage from the head of the proximal phalanx and base of the distal phalanx, shortening the former enough to correct any deformity at the interphalangeal joint. The arthrodesis site is then fixed with two threaded Steinmann pins.

3. Make a second longitudinal incision along the border of the extensor hallucis longus tendon, starting at the level of the metatarsophalangeal joint and extending proximally to the middle of the first metatarsal shaft (Fig. 20-27, A).

4. Dissect out the extensor hallucis longus tendon both proximally and distally and pull it into the proximal wound.

5. Drill a transverse hole through the first metatarsal just proximal to the metatarsal neck.

6. Thread the extensor tendon through the hole and then, pushing the foot into as much

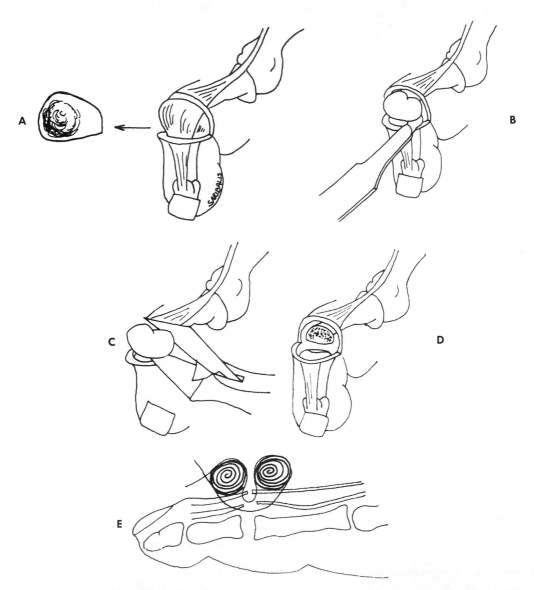

Fig. 20-28. A, Hammertoe deformity. Excise an ellipse of skin including the extensor tendon. **B,** Cut the medial and lateral collateral ligaments. This frees the head of the proximal phalanx. **C,** Excise the head of the proximal phalanx proximal to the condyles. **D,** Toe after excision of the head of the phalanx. **E,** Figure-8 suture of 3-0 silk, incorporating Telfa bolsters to hold the toe in extension.

dorsiflexion as possible, suture the extensor tendon back onto itself using interrupted 0 silk sutures (Fig. 20-27, *C*).

7. Close the wounds in a routine manner and place the patient in a short leg cast for a period of 6 weeks.

8. After 6 weeks of immobilization, the tendon transfer has healed but the interphalangeal joint usually requires about 1 month of healing time. We allow the patient to walk in a wooden shoe the last 4 weeks until the interphalangeal joint has become arthrodesed.

Reduction of hammered middle three toes. The following procedure is recommended for reduction of fixed hammertoes involving the three middle toes.

1. Make an elliptical incision over the dorsal aspect of the proximal interphalangeal joint, excising the callus (Fig. 20-28, *A*). Carry it down through the extensor tendon to include the joint capsule. This ellipse is then discarded.

2. Cut the collateral ligament on the medial and lateral aspects of the proximal interphalangeal joint to allow the head of the proximal phalanx to be delivered into the wound (Fig. 20-28, *B*).

3. Resect the head of the proximal phalanx just proximal to the flare of the condyles. Smooth the edges with a rongeur (Fig. 20-28, *C* and *D*).

4. Insert a horizontal figure-8 suture, utilizing 3-0 silk and incorporating two Telfa bolsters. When the suture is inserted in this manner, there is a moderate degree of leverage holding the great toe in satisfactory alignment (Fig. 20-28, *E*).

5. Dress the toe with a compression dressing, holding it in dorsiflexion.

6. After 1 week, remove the bolster and support the toe with adhesive tape for 6 to 8 weeks until complete healing of the tissues has occurred.

7. This procedure has been very successful in our experience. Complications and failures are quite uncommon. If the patient has an extremely tight flexor digitorum longus tendon, it should be exposed in the plantar aspect of the wound and cut at the time of the procedure to prevent any recurrence of the hammertoe deformity.

The bolster should be left in place only 1 week; if it is left in place longer than this, there is a distinct possibility that necrosis will develop underneath it. The toe should be held in correct alignment with tape for 6 weeks to prevent recurrence of the deformity.

Of academic interest is the case illustrated in Fig. 20-29, in which complete regeneration of the head of a phalanx occurred within five

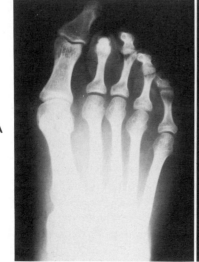
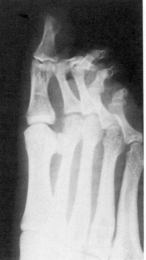

Fig. 20-29. Complete regeneration of the head of the phalanx. This occurred within five years after amputation for hammertoe. **A,** Preoperative (September, 1956).   *Continued.*

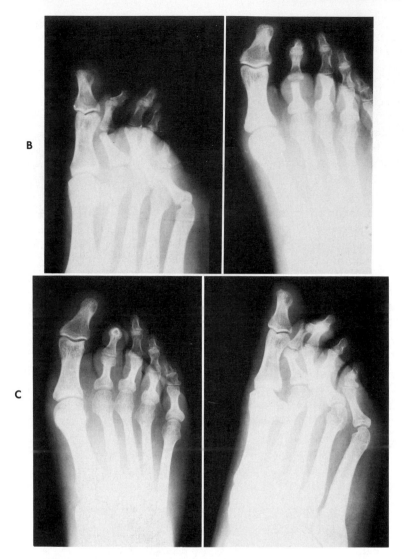

Fig. 20-29, cont'd. B, Postoperative (March, 1957). **C,** Four years postoperative (August, 1961); regenerated head showing.

years after an amputation for hammertoe (DuVries and Shogren, 1962). Franklin (1968) described a similar regeneration phenomenon in a patient on whom he performed three operations for contracted toes. Scheck (1968) reported the presence of degenerative changes in the metatarsophalangeal joints of three patients who had undergone surgical correction of severe hammertoe deformities.

Reduction of hammered fifth toe. A hammertoe deformity involving the fifth toe may be corrected in the same manner as was done

in treating the middle three toes except that a longitudinal incision is made on the dorsal aspect of the toe, starting over the middle phalanx and proceeding near the base of the proximal phalanx.

In patients with a severe cock-up deformity of the small toe, in which the proximal phalanx is sitting at nearly a right angle to the fifth metatarsal shaft, a Ruiz-Mora (1954) procedure is recommended. This is done by making an elliptical incision on the plantar aspect of the fifth toe following the long axis of the small toe but deviating slightly medialward at the base of the toe. The ellipse of skin is then discarded, after which the proximal phalanx of the fifth toe is removed. The elliptical incision in the long axis of the toe is closed at right angles to the long axis so the toe will be drawn out of its cocked position into a more normal plantar position. This procedure has been most successful in correcting the cock-up deformity.

Reduction of flexible or dynamic hammertoe. In patients with a flexible or dynamic hammertoe, there is deformity when the patient stands but practically none when the patient is sitting on the examining table. No contracture is present at the interphalangeal joints of the toe. This is not a clawtoe deformity because the metatarsophalangeal joint is not involved. The deformity seems to be caused by a contracture of the flexor digitorum longus tendons. We correct this deformity by carrying out a flexor tendon transfer. Using a tendon transfer procedure, Parrish (1973) had good to excellent results in twenty of twenty-three patients. The technique is as follows:

1. Under hemostasis by a thigh tourniquet, make a transverse incision 4 to 5 mm long in the proximal flexion crease at the base of the involved toe. Spread the tissue with a clamp until the flexor tendon sheath is identified in the base of the wound (Fig. 20-30, A).

2. Using a no. 11 blade, open the flexor tendon sheath longitudinally. When observing the contents of the flexor tendon sheath, note that the flexor digitorum longus is the central of three tendons. Place a curved

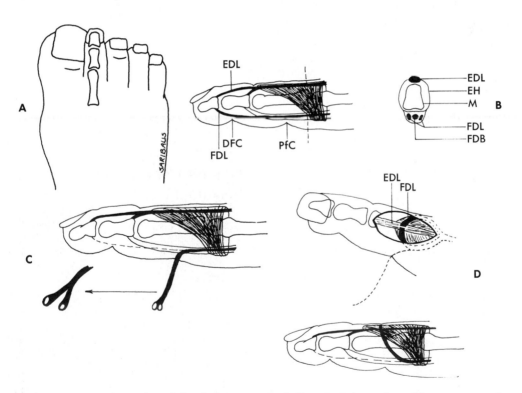

Fig. 20-30. A, Relationship of the phalanges to the hallux. **B,** Relationship of the extensor and flexor tendons to the phalanges. *EDL* Extensor digitorum longus tendon; *FDL,* flexor digitorum longus tendon; *FDB,* flexor digitorum brevis; *EH,* extensor hood; *DFC,* distal flexion crease; *PFC,* proximal flexion crease; *m,* metatarsal head. **C,** The flexor digitorum longus tendon is cut percutaneously from the insertion, pulled out through the proximal flexion crease, and divided into two tails. **D,** The two tails are brought up along the extensor hood and sutured into the top of the extensor tendon with the toe held in plantar flexion.

mosquito clamp under the tendon and bring it out through the wound under tension (Fig. 20-30, *B*).

3. Percutaneously with a no. 11 blade, release the long flexor tendon at its insertion into the base of the distal phalanx (Fig. 20-30, *C*).

4. Observation of the flexor digitorum longus tendon demonstrates that there is a natural cleavage plane. Utilize this plane to create two tails of the tendon.

5. Make a second longitudinal incision in the dorsal aspect of the involved toe centered over the proximal phalanx and deepen this into the extensor tendon.

6. Create a tunnel along the extensor expansion which presents in the plantar wound.

7. Bring a tail of flexor digitorum longus up on the medial aspect and on the lateral aspect of the extensor hood to the dorsal aspect of the proximal phalanx. With the metatarsophalangeal joint held in a plantar-flexed position, suture the extensor tendon tails into the extensor tendon using 4-0 silk (Fig. 20-30, *D*).

8. Close the skin in a routine manner and apply a compression dressing.

9. The patient can walk 24 hours after surgery in a wooden shoe. This procedure has been most satisfactory in our hands. It can be applied to flexible hammertoes as a result of cerebral palsy and stroke as well as to idiopathic flexible hammertoes.

Reduction of mallet toe

The procedure for reduction of mallet toe is essentially the same as for the reduction of hammered toes except that the incision is made over the distal interphalangeal joint and the head of the middle phalanx is excised. When the deformity occurs on the fourth toe, the distal end of the toe occasionally also underlaps the third toe. Then the dorsal elliptical skin incision should be made slightly fibularward to help straighten the toe.

Surgical treatment of clawtoe

Frank and Johnson (1966) described the use of an extensor shift procedure in a series of

twenty-two feet with clawtoe deformities. Results were excellent in nine and satisfactory in eleven; there was no improvement in two. Sandeman (1967) stated that in the correction of clawtoes, structures on both the dorsum and the lateral aspects of the metatarsophalangeal joints must be adequately tenotomized to make full reduction possible.

Recommended technique. In most cases of clawtoe, a Jones tendon transfer of the great toe (Fig. 20-27) and hammertoe reduction of the lesser toes (Fig. 20-28) with sectioning of the long extensor tendons and the contracted dorsal metatarsophalangeal joint capsules to the lesser toes usually produce satisfactory results (Fig. 20-31). Occasionally, when the lesser toes do not flatten into a normal position at the time of surgery, arthrodesis of the proximal interphalangeal joints will correct the deformity. In the few cases in which the hindfoot is deformed to a degree that requires major stabilization, the aforementioned pro-

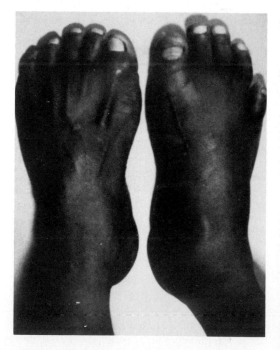

Fig. 20-31. Bilateral congenital clawtoes. Left, Uncorrected. Right, Reduced by a Jones tendon transfer and hammertoe reduction with sectioning of the long extensor tendons and the dorsal metatarsophalangeal joint capsules.

cedure is a valuable adjunct to the restoration of a well-functioning foot.

Surgical treatment of overlapping toes

Overlapping fifth toe. Several procedures have been used to correct overlapping fifth toe.

Lantzounis procedure. Lantzounis (1940) divided the tendon of the extensor digitorum longus of the fifth toe at a point over the shaft of the proximal phalanx and drilled a tunnel behind the head of the fifth metatarsal. Through the tunnel he threaded the proximal end of the severed tendon, and he sutured the tendon onto itself.

Lapidus procedure. In 1942 Lapidus described a radical operation for correcting fifth toe overlap (Fig. 20-32) which consisted of transferring the proximal end of the distal

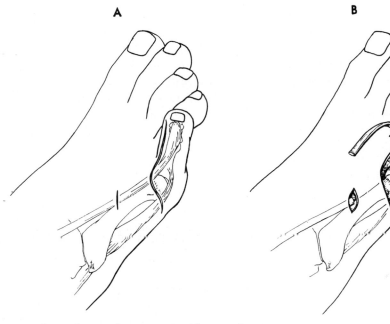

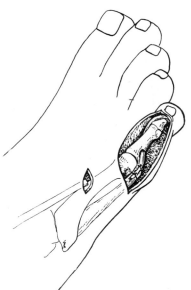

Fig. 20-32. Lapidus technique for correction of an overlapping fifth toe. **A,** Hockey stick–shaped incision over the dorsum of the fifth toe. A second incision is made over the middle of the shaft of the fifth metatarsal. **B,** Sectioning of the extensor digitorum longus tendon to the fifth toe at a second incision. The distal portion is retracted. **C,** Threading of the freed tendon through a drill hole in the proximal phalanx from the tibial to the fibular side. There it is sutured to the abductor digiti minimi tendon.

terminal portion of the extensor digitorum longus tendon of the fifth toe into the tendon of the abductor digiti minimi.

The procedure is performed through two incisions, one extending from the dorsal surface of the middle phalanx of the fifth toe to the lateral side of the fifth metatarsophalangeal joint, and the other placed over the middle third of the fifth metatarsal. Through the second incision the extensor digitorum longus tendon is severed. The distal end of this tendon is extracted through the first incision and is sutured to the lateral side of the fifth metatarsophalangeal joint.

Wilson procedure. Wilson (1953) advocated a procedure consisting of a V-shaped incision over the base of the fifth proximal phalanx. The extensor tendons and the dorsal capsule of the fifth metatarsophalangeal joint were sectioned and the fifth digit was plantar flexed. This pulled the tongue of the incision distally, forming a Y-shaped opening. The skin was sutured in the Y shape (Fig. 20-33).

Recommended technique for correction of fifth toe overlapping when skin is not involved. The dorsal skin is not involved in maintaining the deformity if the fifth toe can be forcibly held in a plantar-flexed position without the skin's becoming very tight; in such a case, the following procedure is recommended:

1. Make an incision about 2 cm long on the tibial side of the fifth metatarsophalangeal joint.

2. Section the tendon and capsule over this joint with a tenotome. At times the sectioning of the capsule needs to be carried to the sides of the joint until the toe maintains itself in a normal position.

3. Close the skin.

4. Place the toe in an overcorrected position with adhesive tape for about 6 weeks.

Recommended technique for correction of fifth toe overlapping when dorsal skin is moderately contracted. DuVries' technique for correction of overlapping of the fifth toe is recommended:

1. Make a longitudinal incision over the fourth metatarsal interspace, beginning in the web between the fourth and fifth toes and extending over the dorsum to about the proximal third of the metatarsal shafts.

2. Carry the incision to a depth sufficient to sever all adhesive fibers holding the toe in deformity.

3. Perform a tenotomy and a capsulotomy of the dorsum of the fifth metatarsophalangeal

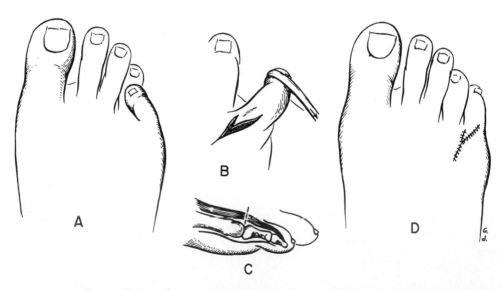

Fig. 20-33. Wilson technique for correction of an overlapping fifth toe. **A,** Preoperative. **B,** Y-shaped incision over the fifth metatarsophalangeal joint. **C,** Sectioning of the dorsal tendon and capsule of the metatarsophalangeal joint. **D,** Correction of the deformity and suturing of the skin.

joint if necessary so the toe can lie in a normal position by its own weight (Fig. 20-34, *A*).

4. Stretch the fibular skin margin distally and the tibial margin proximally by plantar flexing the fifth toe, forming a pucker ("dog ear") at both ends of the incision. The puckered portion is excised (Fig. 20-34, *B*).

5. Suture the skin margins in the new position. Also suture the small transverse incision left by excision of the pucker (Fig. 20-34, *C*).

6. Place the toe in an overcorrected position with adhesive tape for about 8 weeks. When the skin is severely contracted, the

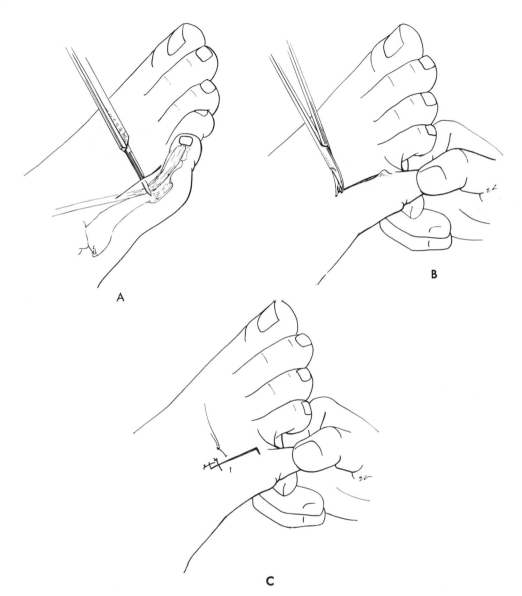

Fig. 20-34. DuVries technique for an overlapping fifth toe with moderate skin contracture. (For severe skin contracture, see Fig. 20-35.) **A,** Longitudinal incision made over the fourth metatarsal interspace. Tenotomy and a capsulotomy over the fifth metatarsophalangeal joint are then performed. **B,** The fifth toe is plantar flexed to force the fibular margin of the incision distally and the tibial margin proximally. This forms a fold at each end of the incision. The folds are then excised. **C,** Incision sutured in the new position.

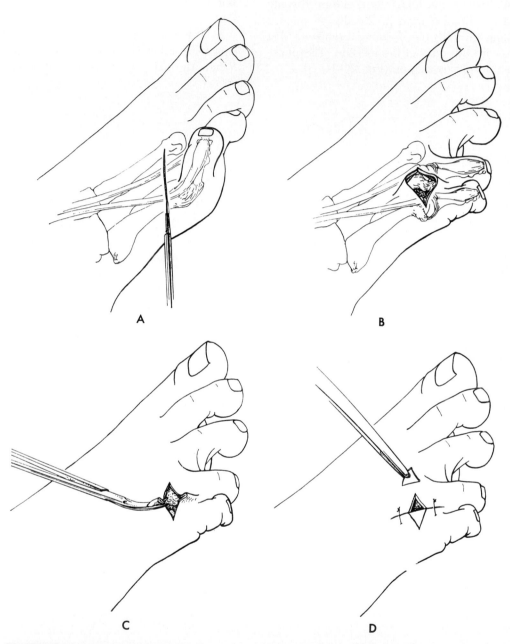

Fig. 20-35. DuVries technique for reduction of a hammered toe with severe skin contracture. (For mild skin contracture, see Fig. 20-34.) **A,** Transverse incision over the dorsum of the fourth and fifth metatarsophalangeal joints just behind the metatarsal necks. **B,** Dorsal tendon and capsule of the fifth metatarsophalangeal joint sectioned. All other subdermal adhesive fibers are severed. The fourth and fifth toes are plantar flexed to form a diamond-shaped incision. The transverse axis is narrowed. The middle of both skin margins is puckered. **C,** Skin puckering excised. The pucker forms a triangular section of skin. **D,** Rotation of the triangular pieces of skin. The skin fits perfectly into the defect and is sutured in that position.

procedure described in Fig. 20-35 is indicated.

Correction of second toe overlapping. In second toe overlapping, the second toe usually overlaps the great toe. Usually this deformity is static and accompanied by hallux valgus. The two conditions must be reduced simultaneously.

Overlapping in the flaccid foot may be reduced when dislocation of the metatarsophalangeal joint is not present. This is accomplished by dorsal tenotomy and capsulotomy of the second metatarsophalangeal joint. The toe is then fixed with adhesive tape in an overcorrected plantar attitude and maintained for 6 to 8 weeks.

REFERENCES

Akin, O. F.: The treatment of hallux valgus—a new operative procedure and its results, Med. Sentinel **33:**678, 1925.

Blosser, J.: Fascia lata lacing for hallux valgus. Personal communication, 1964.

Borg, I.: Operation for hammer-toe, Acta Chir. Scand. **100:**619, 1950.

Brandes, M.: Zur operativen Therapie des Hallux valgus, Zentralbl. Chir. **56:**2434, 1929.

Clayton, M. L.: Surgery of the forefoot in rheumatoid arthritis, Clin. Orthop. **16:**136, 1960.

Cleveland, M., and Winant, E. M.: An end-result study of the Keller operation, J. Bone Joint Surg. **32A:**163, 1950.

DuVries, H. L., and Shogren, C. V.: Spontaneous restoration of the head of a proximal phalanx following amputation: a case report, J. Am. Podiatry Assoc. **52:**126, 1962.

Forrester-Brown, M. F.: Tendon transplantation for clawing of the great toe, J. Bone Joint Surg. **20:**57, 1938.

Fowler, A. W.: The surgery of fixed claw toes, J. Bone Joint Surg. **39B:**585, 1957.

Fowler, A. W.: A method of forefoot reconstruction, J. Bone Joint Surg. **41B:**507, 1959.

Frank, G. R., and Johnson, W. M.: The extensor shift procedure in the correction of clawtoe deformities in children, South. Med. J. **59:**889, 1966.

Franklin, L.: Regeneration of resected phalangeal heads, J. Am. Podiatry Assoc. **58:**511, 1968.

Galland, W. I., and Jordan, H.: Hallux valgus, Surg. Gynecol Obstet. **66:**95, 1938.

Giannestras, N. J.: Modified Akin procedure for the correction of hallux valgus. In Instructional Course Lectures, American Academy of Orthopaedic Surgeons, vol. 21, St. Louis, 1972, The C. V. Mosby Co.

Hawkins, F. B., Mitchell, C. L., and Hedrick, D. W.:

Correction of hallux valgus by metatarsal osteotomy, J. Bone Joint Surg. **27:**387, 1945.

Henry, A. P. J., Waugh, W., and Wood, H.: The use of footprints in assessing the results of operations for hallux valgus, J. Bone Joint Surg. **54B:**478, 1975.

Hoffmann, P.: An operation for severe grades of contracted or clawed toes, Am. J. Orthop. Surg. **9:**441, 1912.

Holstein, A., and Lewis, G. B.: Experience with Wilson's oblique displacement osteotomy for hallux valgus. In Bateman, J. E., editor: Foot science, Philadelphia, 1976, W. B. Saunders, Co.

Hueter, C.: Klinik der Gelenkkrankheiten mit Einschluss der Orthopädie, Leipzig, 1870-1871, F. C. W. Vogel.

Jones, R.: Notes on military orthopedics, London, 1917, Cassel & Co.

Joplin, R. J.: Sling procedure for correction of splay-foot, metartarsus primus varus, and hallux valgus, J. Bone Joint Surg. **32A:**779, 1950.

Keller, W. L.: The surgical treatment of bunions and hallux valgus. N.Y. Med. J., **80:**741, 1904.

Keller, W. L.: Further observations on the surgical treatment of hallux valgus and bunions, N.Y. Med. J. **95:**696, 1912.

Krida, A.: A new operation for metatarsalgia and splay-foot, Surg. Gynecol. Obstet. **69:**106, 1939.

Lantzounis, L. A.: Congenital subluxation of the fifth toe and its correction by periosteocapsuloplasty and tendon transplantation, J. Bone Joint Surg. **22:**147, 1940.

Lapidus, P. W.: Operative correction of metatarsus varus primus in hallux valgus, Surg. Gynecol. Obstet. **58:**183, 1934.

Lapidus, P. W.: Operation for correction of hammer-toe, J. Bone Joint Surg. **21:**977, 1939.

Lapidus, P. W.: Transplantation of the extensor tendon for correction of the overlapping fifth toe, J. Bone Joint Surg. **24:**555, 1942.

Levine, M. A.: An operative technique for hallux valgus, J. Bone Joint Surg. **20:**923, 1938.

Lorenz, H.: Zur operativen Therapie des Hallux valgus, der Hammerzehe und unerträglicher Clavi, Wien. Med. Wochenschr. **79:**713, 1929.

Marmor, L.: Surgery of the rheumatoid foot, Surg. Gynecol. Obstet. **119:**1009, 1964.

Mayo, C. H.: The surgical treatment of bunion, Ann. Surg. **48:**300, 1908.

McBride, E. D.: A conservative operation for bunions, J. Bone Joint Surg. **10:**735, 1928.

McBride, E. D.: The conservative operation for "bunions": end results and refinements of technic, J. A.M.A. **105:**1164, 1935.

McBride, E. D.: Hallux valgus, bunion deformity: its treatment in mild, moderate and severe stages, J. Int. Coll. Surg. **21:**99, 1954.

McElvenny, R. T., and Thompson, F. R.: A clinical study of one hundred patients subjected to simple exostosectomy for the relief of bunion pain, J. Bone Joint Surg. **22:**942, 1940.

Michele, A. A., and Krueger, F. J.: Operative correction for hammertoe, Milit. Surg. **103:**52, 1948.

Mitchell, C. L., Fleming, J. L.. Allen, R., Glenney, C., and Sanford, G. A.: Osteotomy-bunionectomy for hallux valgus, J. Bone Joint Surg. **40A:**41, 1958.

Moynihan, F. J.: Arthrodesis of the metatarsophalangeal joint of the great toe, J. Bone Joint Surg. **49B:**544, 1967.

Parrish, T. F.: Dynamic correction of claw toes, Orthop. Clin. North Am. **4:**97, 1973.

Ruiz-Mora, J.: Plastic correction of over-riding 5th toe, Orthopaedic Letters Club, vol. 6, 1954.

Sandeman, J. C.: The role of soft tissue correction of claw toes, J. Clin. Pract. **21:**489, 1967.

Scheck, M.: Degenerative changes in the metatarsophalangeal joints after surgical correction of severe hammer-toe deformities: a complication associated with avascular necrosis in three cases, J. Bone Joint Surg. **50A:**727, 1968.

Schein, A. J.: Keller operation—partial phalangectomy in hallux valgus and hallux rigidus: report of operations in 32 cases, Surgery **7:**342, 1940.

Selig, S.: Hammer-toe: a new procedure for its correction, Surg. Gynecol. Obstet. **72:**101, 1941.

Silver, D. : The operative treatment of hallux valgus, J. Bone Joint Surg. **5:**225, 1923.

Soresi, A. L.: The radical cure of hallux valgus (bunion): Subarticular resection of the head of the metatarsal bone, Surg. Gynecol. Obstet. **52:**776, 1931.

Taylor, R. G.: An operative procedure for the treatment of hammer-toe and claw-toe, J. Bone Joint Surg. **22:**608, 1940.

Tierney, A. : Hammer-toe: the cup and ball procedure. In Pauchet, V., editor: La pratique chirurgicale illustrée, ed. 2, Paris, 1937, Gaston Doin & Cie.

Wagner, L. C.: The operative correction of extreme flexion contraction of the great toe, J. Bone Joint Surg. **16:**914, 1934.

Wilson, J. N.: V-Y correction for varus deformity of the fifth toe, Br. J. Surg. **41:**133, 1953.

Wilson, J. N.: Oblique displacement osteotomy for hallux valgus, J. Bone Joint Surg. **45B:**552, 1963.

Wilson, J. N.: Cone arthrodesis of the first metatarsophalangeal joint, J. Bone Joint Surg. **49B:**98, 1967.

Young, C. S.: An operation for the correction of hammer-toe and claw-toe, J. Bone Joint Surg. **20:**715, 1938.

Index